FIFTH EDITION

FETAL HEART MONITORING

PRINCIPLES AND PRACTICES

Editors

Audrey Lyndon, PhD, RNC, FAAN
Linda Usher Ali, MS, CNS, RNC

Contributors

Linda Usher Ali, MS, CNS, RNC
Joanne D. Barnes, MS, RNC
Rebecca L. Cypher, MSN, PNNP
Dodi Gauthier, M.Ed, BSN, RNC-OB, C-EFM
Molly M. Killion, MS, RN, CNS
Audrey Lyndon, PhD, RNC, FAAN
Patricia Robin McCartney, PhD, RNC, FAAN
Barbara T. O'Brien, MS, RN
Nancy O'Brien-Abel, MN, RNC-OB
Kathleen Rice Simpson, PhD, RNC, CNS-BC, FAAN
Catharine M. Treanor, MS, RNC-OB, C-EFM
Kirsten Wisner, MS, RNC-OB, CNS, C-EFM
Marya G. Zlatnik, MD, MMS

AWHONN Fetal Heart Monitoring PROGRAM

AWHONN
PROMOTING THE HEALTH OF WOMEN AND NEWBORNS

Kendall Hunt
publishing company

Any procedure or practice described in this book should be applied by the health care provider only under appropriate supervision in accordance with professional guidelines, and in light of the specific circumstances of each practice situation. The information contained in this book does not define a standard of care, nor is it intended to dictate an exclusive course of management. It presents general methods and techniques of practice that are currently viewed widely as acceptable, based on current research and used by recognized authorities. Proper care of individual patients may depend on many individual factors as well as professional judgment. The information presented here is not designed to define standards of practice for employment, licensure, discipline, legal or other purposes. Variations and innovations that are consistent with law and that demonstrably improve the quality of patient care should be encouraged. Care has been taken to confirm the accuracy of information presented and to describe generally accepted practices. However, the authors, editors, and publisher expressly disclaim any responsibility for errors or omissions or for any consequences resulting from the application of the information in this book and make no warranty, express or implied, with respect to the contents of the book.

The author and publisher have endeavored to ensure that drug selection and dosage set forth in this text are in accordance with current recommendations and practice at the time of publication. However, in view of ongoing changes in government regulations, and the constant flow of information relating to drug therapy and drug reactions, the reader is urged to check the package insert for each drug for any changes in indications and dosage and for added warnings and precautions. This is particularly important when the recommended agent is a new or infrequently used drug. It is the responsibility of the health care provider to ascertain the most current FDA status and guidance on drugs and devices planned for use in their clinical practice.

ISBN 978-1-4652-6970-6

Printed in the United States of America

Contents

SECTION FOUR
Application of Fetal Heart Monitoring Data

Preface

When developed in 1992, the Association of Women's Health, Obstetric and Neonatal Nurses (AWHONN) Fetal Heart Monitoring Principles and Practices (FHMPP) Workshop consisted of a single 2-day event designed to validate registered nurses' knowledge and skills in the use of fetal heart monitoring technologies. In the intervening years, the course evolved into the AWHONN Fetal Heart Monitoring Program (FHMP) and includes courses and supporting materials addressing the needs of the novice clinician as well as those of the expert-level clinician. Today the AWHONN FHMP is a dynamic, comprehensive series of fetal heart monitoring courses and resources designed for use by a multidisciplinary clinical audience including professional nurses, midwives, and physicians. While the purpose of this book is primarily to support the AWHONN FHMP courses, perinatal health care providers also find it a useful stand-alone practice resource.

This edition of *Fetal Heart Monitoring Principles and Practices* continues the use of the 2008 National Institutes of Child Health and Development (NICHD) definitions for terms to describe fetal heart rate and uterine activity findings. Use of standardized terminology among health care providers to communicate fetal heart monitoring information is important to the promotion of patient safety and is consistent with Joint Commission recommendations (*Sentinel Event Alert* #30). AWHONN, the American College of Nurse Midwives (ACNM), and the American College of Obstetricians and Gynecologists (ACOG) all support adoption of a common language for fetal heart monitoring as one step toward improving communication between providers during labor and birth.

The 2008 NICHD guidelines for interpretation of EFM tracings also have implications for the interpretation and communication of fetal heart rate (FHR) data obtained by intermittent auscultation (IA). In order to maintain a consistent language for discussion of FHR findings, two categories for interpretation of IA that are consistent with the three-tiered electronic fetal monitoring (EFM) system are retained from the previous edition of this text. This format for interpretation of auscultation findings is also supported by ACNM. Thus the terms category I (normal) and category II (indeterminate) are used for interpretation of auscultation findings, and category I (normal), category II (indeterminate), and category III (abnormal) are used for interpretation of electronic fetal monitoring findings in this text. While providers may have some concerns about the breadth of EFM tracings that fall into category II (indeterminate) classification, no consensus has been developed on any further breakdown of classification of category II tracings. All providers are encouraged to continue the important focus on using a common language for communicating FHR findings and responding to the clinical situation at hand with timely assessment, collegial communication, shared decision making, and appropriate action.

The core principles of the FHMP continue in this edition. These principles include an emphasis on a physiologic framework for decision making, an evidence-based approach to the care of laboring women and their families, and a commitment to supporting the full range of FHR assessment technology, including auscultation. AWHONN participated in the 2008 NICHD Workshop on definitions, interpretation, and research guidelines for EFM. The three-tiered classification system for EFM patterns fits well with the AWHONN dynamic physiologic response model for interpreting FHR characteristics, and the 2008 classification system is integrated into this text.

One of the challenges in presenting the literature on FHM is that many of the important studies are now "classics" from an earlier time. We have incorporated new EFM studies where available, but we continue to rely on many of the older original research articles that established the field; thus, the book contains many older citations to original research. The terms "reassuring" and "nonreassuring" are used in a limited way in the text to discuss interpretation of some types of testing (e.g., biophysical profile results), and are also used in quotation marks when discussing research findings that were originally reported using these terms.

Major changes for the fifth edition include transition to an ebook format with interactive materials, significant expansion of the assessment chapter, and reorganization of the communication chapter into two chapters, one devoted to communication and another devoted solely to documentation.

In this text "clinician" refers to professional nurses, midwives, and physicians practicing in accordance with their education and training and within the parameters of their institutional, state, provincial, regional, or other regulatory scope of practice and professional guidelines. The term "midwife" refers to certified nurse midwives and certified midwives in the United States and registered midwives in Canada.

Reviewers

AWHONN gratefully acknowledges the work of the individuals who have contributed their time and expertise to creating and reviewing the material for this book.

Reviewers

Patricia Bielecki, MSN, CNS, RNC
Mary Katherine Carson, MSN, RNC-OB, C-EFM
Carol J. Craig, MSN, BSN, RNC-OB
Deborah Anne Cruz, MSN, BSN, CRNP, RNC
Lawrence D. Devoe, MD
Susan Drummond, MSN, RN, C-EFM
Ann C. Holden, MSc (T), BScN, RN, PNC
Helain Landy, MD
Karen P. Langston, MSN, RNC-OB, C-EFM
Kathleen J. Murray, MN, RN
Barbara T. O'Brien, MS, RN
Katherine O'Connell, MN, RN
Cheryl K. Roth, PhD, WHNP-BC, RNC-OB, RNFA
Christina L. Rust, DNP, MSN, RNC-OB, C-EFM
Frann Teplick, MSN, RN-BC, CNS
Karin P. Van Doren, MSN, RNC-OB, CNS, WHNP-BC
Julie Zimmerman, MSN, RNC-OB, C-EFM

SECTION ONE

Theoretical Basis for Fetal Heart Monitoring

CHAPTER 1

Intrapartum Fetal Monitoring: A Historical Perspective

Patricia Robin McCartney

INTRODUCTION

Fetal heart rate (FHR) assessment is performed in nearly all births, and electronic fetal monitoring is a common obstetric procedure in the United States and Canada today. This introduction to fetal heart monitoring (FHM) education includes an overview of the history of FHR assessment, evidence about FHM practice, development of professional guidelines, standardization of terminology, evolution of FHM education, and use of a collaborative fetal monitoring process as a framework for applying FHM education to practice. These components provide a historical context and understanding of the state of the science as a basis for the AWHONN Fetal Heart Monitoring Program.

HISTORY OF FETAL HEART RATE SURVEILLANCE

Assessment of the FHR is an indirect measure of fetal oxygenation in antepartum and intrapartum care. This overview highlights the development of techniques to assess the fetus by assessing FHR and uterine activity (UA) along with adjunct assessment techniques such as ultrasonography, fetal scalp blood sampling, fetal scalp stimulation, acoustic stimulation, pulse oximetry, and computer analysis. This review is based on material from several more comprehensive sources, including Goodlin (1979), Schmidt and McCartney (2000), Wulf (1985), Association of Women's Health, Obstetric and Neonatal Nurses (AWHONN; 2005), and Bloom et al. (2006). Key events are summarized in Table 1-1.

Clinicians and researchers seeking ways to prevent fetal death (mortality) and neurologic damage (morbidity) shaped the evolution of FHM techniques. Clinical assessment of FHR and UA began with unassisted auscultation (examiner's ear on the maternal abdomen) and palpation (examiner's hands on the abdomen) and expanded with the addition of mechanical devices, electronic technology, and health information technology. Contemporary practice is the result of more than a century of development by practitioners dedicated to promoting optimal birth outcomes by identifying and implementing best practices for fetal heart assessment, interpretation, and intervention.

Fetal Heart Rate

Clinical assessment of the FHR began almost 200 years ago, when the Swiss surgeon Mayor in 1818 and the French physician and nobleman Kergaradec (Jean-Alexandre Le Jumeau, Vicomte de Kergaradec) in 1821 reported the presence of fetal heart sounds obtained by auscultation.

TABLE 1-1 A Chronology of Major Fetal Heart Monitoring Developments

Date	Development
1818	Mayor listens to FHR with ear on woman's abdomen.
1821	Kergaradec obtains FHR by stethoscope and relates FHR to fetal life and well-being.
1893	Von Winckel publishes text with auscultation criteria for diagnosing fetal distress.
1906	Cremer uses abdominal and intravaginal leads for fetal ECG.
1917	Hillis describes the head fetoscope.
1958	Hon reports preliminary EFM research.
1961	Saling measures fetal scalp pH.
1964	Callagan adapts Doppler ultrasonography to detect FHR.
1968	Hammacher and Hewlett-Packard market commercial EFM.
1971	International panel approves EFM pattern terminology.
1972	Hon develops the spiral fetal scalp electrode.
1976	Haverkamp reports randomized trial comparing EFM and auscultation.
1977	Read uses acoustical stimulation to assess fetal well-being.
1978	Dawes-Redman criteria created for computer analysis of FHR.
1982	Clark uses scalp stimulation to assess fetal well-being.
1985	Manning reports findings on the biophysical profile.
1986	Paine publishes the auscultation acceleration test.
1992	AWHONN introduces a standardized FHR monitoring education program.
1997	NICHD panel recommends standardized EFM definitions.
1999	Thacker and Stroup report meta-analysis of EFM clinical trials.
2000	FDA conditionally approves the fetal pulse oximeter.
2005	FDA premarket approval of fetal heart ST analysis (STAN).
2006	AWHONN and ACOG incorporate 1997 NICHD standardized EFM definitions in educational resources.
2008	NICHD panel recommends standardized categories for interpretation of EFM patterns. AWHONN incorporates interpretation categories into educational resources.
2009	Health Information Technology for Economic and Clinical Health (HITECH) Act drives use of certified clinical information systems for medical record. ACOG incorporates 2008 NICHD terminologies into practice bulletin, noting definitions are developed for visual interpretation but should be adaptable to computerized systems of interpretation.
2010	ACOG incorporates 2008 NICHD interpretation categories into a framework for evaluation and management of intrapartum EFM patterns.

AWHONN, Association of Women's Health, Obstetric and Neonatal Nurses; ECG, electrocardiogram; EFM, electronic fetal monitoring; FDA, U.S. Food and Drug Administration; FHM, fetal heart monitoring; FHMPP, Fetal Heart Monitoring Principles and Practices; FHR, fetal heart rate; NICHD, National Institute of Child Health and Human Development.

Mayor used the ear-to-abdomen method, but Kergaradec used a wooden stethoscope and is credited as the first practitioner to recommend assessing fetal heart sounds for diagnostic purposes. In 1833, Evory Kennedy in Dublin wrote a comprehensive monograph, *Observations on Obstetric Auscultation*, intended to convince doubting colleagues to use Kergaradec's auscultation technique. Kennedy's textbook described the slowness of FHR return when a contraction "is passing on" and the effects of fetal head and funic compression on the FHR.

During the mid-1800s, a number of investigations using auscultation were reported, including identifying the normal FHR range and correlating FHR with other clinical findings, such as maternal fever, gestational age, fetal weight, fetal sex, and fetal movement. Clinicians debated the methods of auscultation (stethoscope vs. ear-to-abdomen), the ideal positioning of the mother (standing vs. supine), and the necessity of exposing the pregnant woman's abdomen during the procedure. Clinicians also investigated physiologic causes for changes in FHR. In Germany in 1858, Schwartz wrote in a text that FHR should be counted during labor, both between and during contractions, as a method of assessing fetal well-being. Schwartz related fetal bradycardia to both fetal head compression and decreased placental function caused by the reduction in blood flow during uterine contractions. He was the first to investigate fetal breathing activity. In 1885, Schatz described umbilical cord compression; in 1903, Seitz claimed that FHR decelerations were indicators of fetal oxygenation and described head compression.

In 1849 in the United States, Kilian proposed that finding a FHR of less than 100 beats per minute (bpm) or greater than 180 bpm could identify "fetal distress" that required forceps intervention. Von Winckel in Germany in 1893 formulated specific criteria to identify "fetal distress" as determined by auscultation: tachycardia greater than 160 bpm, bradycardia less than 120 bpm, or irregularity of FHR. Von Winckel's criteria and auscultation guidelines were followed for the next 75 years (Wulf, 1985).

In the early 1900s, the fetoscope replaced auscultation with the ear or binaural or monaural stethoscope. The head fetoscope was first described in the literature by Hillis (1917) as a metal band over the head attached to a common binaural stethoscope. The original purpose for the device was to enable the obstetrician to listen to second-stage fetal heart tones without using any hands, thus remaining "surgically prepared" for the birth. However, additional benefits were improved assessment from bone conduction and the ability to press the bell of the stethoscope firmly against the abdomen. This device came to be known as the DeLee-Hillis fetoscope to acknowledge both obstetrician inventors.

The use of technology to assess FHR began with indirect measurement using abdominal devices and direct measurement using fetal devices. Pestalozza in 1891 and Hofbauer and Weiss in 1908 reported use of phonocardiography, a mechanical process using a microphone-like apparatus that amplified and continuously recorded FHR through the maternal abdominal wall. Many years later, Hammacher in 1962 improved the clarity of the phonocardiographic signal and connected the FHR with the recording of uterine contractions. One hundred years ago, the cardiologist Cremer applied abdominal and vaginal electrodes to obtain a fetal electrocardiogram (ECG) on the fetus of a woman who was not in labor.

In the 1950s, Hon in the United States, Caldeyro-Barcia in Uruguay, and Hammacher in Germany began to report success with electronic monitors that could continuously record indirect abdominal phonocardiography and electrocardiography. In one of the earliest reports, Hon (1958) described using silver electrodes inside light plastic shells on the mother's abdomen and thigh. Hon compared FHR and patterns of FHR changes with labor variables and neonatal outcomes. Because of poor signal quality of the early abdominal fetal ECG, clinicians experimented with multiple devices to record FHR directly from the fetus. Hon developed a disposable fetal scalp electrode in 1972 that successfully obtained a direct fetal ECG; this remains the basis for the devices used today. In 1964, Callagan adapted Doppler ultrasound technology to indirectly assess fetal heart motion through the maternal abdomen. This external measurement technique became widespread in both antepartum and intrapartum settings, with progressive engineering improvement in the signal quality and accuracy.

Uterine Activity

Clinical assessment of UA with technological devices actually began a little earlier than FHR technology. In 1872, Schatz reported measuring UA by placing balloons within the uterus to record intrauterine pressures on a graph called a "pain tracing." Two decades later, Schaeffer measured UA externally by placing a hood with a tube connected to a spirometer over the pregnant woman's abdomen. These early investigators examined normal UA and uterine response to drugs such as epinephrine, ether, and morphine. By 1947, an external device, the tocodynamometer, was designed to detect and eventually to continuously record tension changes in the abdomen resulting from uterine contractions. This device provided a visual wave displaying the frequency, duration, and relative strength of uterine contractions.

The first internal assessment of UA was reported by Williams and Stallworthy in 1952; they inserted a polyethylene catheter through the cervix of a woman in labor but concluded, "No instrument was as discerning as the experienced hand in assessing the quality of uterine contractions." Also in 1952, Caldeyro-Barcia reported inserting catheters into the uterus through an amniocentesis needle in the abdominal wall. Caldeyro-Barcia coined the term "Montevideo units" (see Glossary) as a quantifiable measure of intrauterine pressure. Later, a commercial fluid-filled intrauterine pressure catheter (IUPC) was developed to be inserted into the uterus through the cervix and attached to an external strain gauge transducer to record pressure changes. Current IUPCs have either a microchip transducer–tipped catheter to detect pressure changes, or an air sensor–tipped catheter.

Electronic Fetal Monitoring

The simultaneous measurement of FHR and uterine contractions came to be called either cardiotocography (CTG) or electronic fetal monitoring (EFM). Hammacher and Hewlett-Packard developed the first commercially available electronic FHR monitor in 1968, initially using external microphone phonocardiography and later adding external ultrasound and internal fetal ECG devices (Freeman, Garite, Nageotte, & Miller, 2012). Today, the term "phonocardiography" refers to the reflected sound wave from ultrasound technology. The computerized sampling of the raw ultrasound signal, the mathematical calculation of rate, and the visual representation all progressively improved. As ultrasound FHR signal sampling and calculation were improved through engineering (autocorrelation techniques), the devices came to be called "second-generation monitors" (see Chapter 4). Wireless transmission of the ultrasound signal later enabled ambulatory telemetry. Today, it is assumed that all ultrasound FHR signal processing uses autocorrelation, and FHR interpretation is based on this assumption (Macones, Hankins, Spong, Hauth, & Moore, 2008).

An important result of electronic technology was the conversion of an auditory signal into a visual waveform and the creation of a continuous visual pattern of FHR, recorded on paper. Thus, FHR assessment changed from unassisted auscultation using auditory skills to visual assessment of data generated by an electronic fetal monitor. The development of EFM dramatically altered obstetric practice. In many settings, EFM became the primary technique for FHR monitoring and intermittent auscultation became a screening or secondary technique. In some settings, auscultation remained the primary technique for FHM.

Technology and Intrapartal Nursing Practice

With the introduction of technological advances, nurses had to make EFM fit into their clinical practice. Nurses who experienced the introduction of EFM in their clinical settings were challenged to reconcile the conflict between using technology for greater biomedical objectivity and personalized, nontechnologically assessed childbirth (Sandelowski, 2000). The profession of perinatal nursing has had to focus to ensure that constant attention to the glamour of new technology does not overshadow the fundamental practices of labor support. With research showing no benefit of EFM when compared with IA for low-risk mothers, nurses should consider the mother's informed consent and choice regarding monitoring method (Wood, 2003).

Adjunct Surveillance Methods

EFM was originally intended as a screening methodology to identify or predict fetal compromise early enough to accomplish intervention that would prevent adverse neurologic outcome or death related to oxygen deprivation. The accuracy of any screening test is measured by sensitivity and specificity (Table 1-2). A normal/category I EFM tracing (see Box 1-1) correctly identifies an oxygenated fetus with a high level of sensitivity and is unlikely to have false-negative interpretations (i.e., incorrectly identify a compromised fetus as adequately oxygenated). When a tracing is normal/category I, clinicians usually agree with the interpretation that the fetus is adequately oxygenated. However, a category II EFM tracing is indeterminate, has a low level of specificity, and may have false-positive interpretations

TABLE 1-2 Research Term Definitions Related to Fetal Heart Monitoring

TERM	DEFINITION	FHR EXAMPLE
Sensitivity	Correct identification of the compromised fetus as compromised and not as oxygenated. Reported as a percent. False-negative results are incorrect identification of a compromised fetus as an oxygenated fetus.	A normal/category I FHR tracing has high sensitivity and is unlikely to incorrectly identify a compromised fetus as one that is oxygenated. When a tracing is normal, this indicates the fetus is adequately oxygenated.
Specificity	Correct identification of the oxygenated fetus as oxygenated and not as compromised. Reported as a percent. False-positive results are incorrect identification of an oxygenated fetus as a compromised fetus.	A category II tracing is indeterminate, has poor specificity, and may incorrectly identify an oxygenated fetus as compromised. When an indeterminate tracing indicates a compromised fetus, the fetus may actually be adequately oxygenated.
Reliability	The measurement technique is accurate or consistent. There is agreement when two observers measure (interrater reliability) or when one observer makes two separate measurements (intrarater reliability). Reported as a kappa coefficient.	Two clinicians agree on the interpretation of an FHR tracing; or one clinician agrees with his or her own previous interpretation.
Validity (predictive or concurrent)	The measurement of a particular characteristic is statistically associated with the outcome of interest.	An FHR tracing interpretation is related to a newborn outcome (e.g., metabolic acidosis, healthy newborn, poor Apgar score, adverse neurologic outcome, or death).
Efficacy	The intervention to prevent or treat a particular outcome has true effects on the outcome.	The FHR tracing interpretation and management have an effect on newborn outcome.

FHR, fetal heart rate.

BOX 1-1 2008 Three-Tier Fetal Heart Rate Interpretation System

CATEGORY I

Category I fetal heart rate (FHR) tracings include **all** of the following:

- Baseline rate: 110–160 beats per minute (bpm)
- Baseline FHR variability: moderate
- Late or variable decelerations: absent
- Early decelerations: present or absent
- Accelerations: present or absent

CATEGORY II

Category II FHR tracings include all FHR tracings not categorized as Category I or Category III. Category II tracings may represent an appreciable fraction of those encountered in clinical care. Examples of Category II FHR tracings include any of the following:

Baseline Rate

- Bradycardia not accompanied by absent baseline variability
- Tachycardia

Baseline FHR Variability

- Minimal baseline variability
- Absent baseline variability not accompanied by recurrent decelerations
- Marked baseline variability

Accelerations

- Absence of induced accelerations after fetal stimulation

Periodic or Episodic Decelerations

- Recurrent variable decelerations accompanied by minimal or moderate baseline variability
- Prolonged deceleration $\geq$2 minutes but $<$10 minutes
- Recurrent late decelerations with moderate baseline variability
- Variable decelerations with other characteristics, such as slow return to baseline, "overshoots," or "shoulders"

CATEGORY III

Category III FHR tracings include either

- Absent baseline FHR variability **and** any of the following:
  - Recurrent late decelerations
  - Recurrent variable decelerations
  - Bradycardia
- Sinusoidal pattern

Note From: "The 2008 National Institute of Child Health Human Development Workshop Report on Electronic Fetal Monitoring: Update on Definitions, Interpretations, and Research Guidelines," by G. A. Macones, G. D. Hankins, C. Y. Spong, J. D. Hauth, & T. Moore, 2008, *Journal of Obstetric, Gynecologic and Neonatal Nursing, 37*, 510–515; *Obstetrics & Gynecology, 112*, p. 665. Copyright 2008 by the American College of Obstetricians and Gynecologists. Reprinted with permission.

(i.e., incorrectly identify an oxygenated fetus as compromised). Category II tracings are not predictive of abnormal acid-base status, but also cannot be classified as category I or category III/abnormal (Macones et al., 2008). Therefore, clinicians may differ in opinion about interpretation and need more information to assess oxygenation and avoid unnecessary intervention. Adjunct surveillance methods were developed to provide additional information, and may be especially helpful with the interpretation and management of category II tracings. Category III EFM patterns are defined as abnormal (Macones et al., 2008). The positive predictive value of an abnormal FHR tracing is also quite low. However, in the case of abnormal tracings there is general consensus among experts that the risk of fetal acidemia is high enough to warrant intervention despite the low positive predictive value of the tracing.

Adjunct methods were developed to complement the assessment of the FHR, not only during labor but also in the late antepartum period. These innovations enhanced FHM techniques, provided additional information about fetal oxygenation status, or improved FHM information management. Fetal assessment in late pregnancy introduced a new field of care: antepartum fetal surveillance. This expansion of fetal evaluation led to the development of specialized antepartum testing centers and a new obstetric subspecialty practice, Perinatal Medicine, also known as Maternal-Fetal Medicine.

In the 1960s, clinicians observed that late decelerations during labor were associated with an increased risk of metabolic acidosis. In the 1970s, physicians began using low-dose oxytocin in antepartum testing, and the term "oxytocin challenge test" (OCT) was introduced (Freeman, 1975). Clinicians observed that the FHR response to mild induced contractions could predict the FHR response to the stress of labor. The technique was broadened to become the "contraction stress test" using either oxytocin or stimulation of the breast or nipple (breast stimulation test). Use of the CST has been criticized because of its high false-positive rates.

Schifrin and colleagues adopted the observations by Hammacher and Kubli to create the nonstress test (NST) as a noninvasive predictor of fetal well-being (Rochard et al., 1976). The NST was based on spontaneous FHR accelerations occurring without inducing contractions. The NST required electronic monitors available only in hospitals or at fetal testing centers; however, manufacturers developed more portable monitors specifically suited for antepartum testing in clinicians' offices and in homes. In 1986, Paine and colleagues reported an auscultated acceleration test (AAT) using a fetoscope to graph FHR and accelerations for a 6-minute period (Paine, Zanardi, Johnson, Rorie, & Barger, 2001). A reactive AAT was at least one increase in FHR of at least two beats per 5-second sampling period above baseline during the 6-minute procedure. The test was shown to be a valid and better predictor than the NST for both favorable and poor outcomes. This "low-tech" AAT has been tested internationally and is recommended for settings without EFM technology (Paine et al., 2001).

Ultrasound was first used in the late 1950s to measure the fetal biparietal diameter. By the 1970s, ultrasound became widely used to identify fetal and placental structure and position. Real-time scanning technology was added, and evaluation of the fetal heart became possible. The biophysical profile was pioneered in the 1970s (Manning, Platt, & Silos, 1980) and became a standard fetal assessment test by the 1980s. Ultrasonography, or Doppler velocimetry (Doppler flow), is now used to measure blood flow in the uterine artery, umbilical arteries, and fetal middle cerebral artery as indicators of vascular status and fetal compensatory responses.

Saling reported a technique to assess the presence or absence of fetal acidosis through scalp blood pH sampling in 1961, long before continuous EFM was widely used in labor. The analysis of fetal capillary blood correlated with subsequent umbilical cord blood samples taken at birth, and together these biochemical assessments of pH were viewed as primary physiologic measures of fetal status. Scalp sampling later fell into disfavor because the technique was invasive and technically challenging, often requiring a prolonged maternal supine position, and resulting pH measures had poor specificity (Clark & Paul, 1985).

Several investigators identified methods to stimulate an FHR acceleration now known to be associated with a nonacidotic fetus. Clark, Gimovsky, and Miller (1982, 1984) reported that an FHR acceleration following the stimulation of the scalp during a fetal blood sampling procedure (puncture) was associated with a nonacidotic fetus. These researchers found that an FHR acceleration following fetal scalp stimulation with pinching and pressure was also associated with a nonacidotic fetus. Prior to Clark's work, Read and Miller (1977) reported that an FHR acceleration in response to abdominal acoustic stimulation correlated with OCT outcomes and fetal well-being. This association was later tested using an artificial larynx for intrapartum acoustic stimulation (or vibroacoustic stimulation) and fetal scalp pH levels for measures of fetal well-being (Smith, Nguyen, Phelan, & Paul, 1986). FHR accelerations were consistently shown to be associated with the absence of acidosis. Both scalp stimulation and acoustic stimulation are now recognized as effective assessments of fetal well-being.

Fetal pulse oximetry, developed and commercially available in Europe in the 1990s, was conditionally approved for use in the United States in 2000 (Bloom et al., 2006). Adult pulse oxygen saturation technology (pulse oximetry) was adapted for fetal use with a single, thin fetal sensor that both emits and receives light. In an effort to reduce unnecessary cesarean births and improve newborn outcomes, fetal oxygen saturation has been used as an adjunct to EFM to assess oxygen status when the EFM tracing is category II (indeterminate) or uninterpretable. The American College of Obstetricians and Gynecologists (ACOG; 2001) and the Society of Obstetricians and Gynaecologists of Canada (SOGC; 2002) did not endorse fetal pulse oximetry as a standard of care because the preliminary research was not convincing. A federally funded multisite post-approval trial found no benefit; neither the rate of cesarean births nor newborn outcomes were improved with the use of fetal pulse oximetry (Bloom et al., 2006). The manufacturer ceased sales of the fetal pulse oximeter just before the study was published because of a lack of demand.

Human visual analysis is subjective and limited by human sensory capacities, so from the start clinicians have investigated and reported how computer technology could aid clinician FHR pattern assessment (McCartney, 2000). One early device had flashing yellow and red lights for detection of "ominous FHR patterns" (Yeh, Jilek, & Hon, 1974). In 1978 Dawes and colleagues developed software and rules (Dawes-Redman criteria), now available in Sonicaid (ArjoHuntleigh, Addison, IL) monitors and widely used for CTG analysis in practice and research. Computer analysis of the FHR uses artificial intelligence (AI) to objectively analyze the auditory signal according to predetermined criteria and alert care providers, interpret patterns, or even suggest management options (McCartney, 2011). Through the years, automated analysis has provided objective, standardized, and reproducible data for research on FHR responses in the antepartum and intrapartum setting. One system for FHR pattern analysis is currently used in practice and has been shown to assist in the assessment of FHR patterns that could be associated with metabolic acidosis (Elliott, Warrick, Graham, & Hamilton, 2010; Gabbe et al., 2012).

Fetal electrocardiogram (ECG) ST segment analysis (STAN), obtained through a fetal electrode, is a technology used to provide adjunctive information to aid in the interpretation of FHR patterns in term fetuses considered at risk for intrapartum hypoxia. Fetal myocardial hypoxemia alters the ST-segment resulting in an "ST event" that is associated with cord blood metabolic acidosis (Devoe, 2011) (see Chapter 4 for discussion of the STAN technique). STAN also introduced a new type of requirement for use; the clinician must pass a certifying exam and be credentialed on clinical usage to ensure that STAN is correctly used. STAN received premarket approval from the U.S. Food and Drug Administration in 2005. A recent meta-analysis concluded more evidence is needed on the efficacy of STAN (Garite, 2013; Schuit et al., 2013). A Phase III multisite trial is now in progress in the United States ("A Randomized Trial of Fetal ECG ST Segment and T Wave Analysis as an Adjunct to Electronic Fetal Heart Rate Monitoring," http://clinicaltrials.gov/ct2/show/NCT01131260).

Obstetric computers, also known as perinatal information systems, became commercially available in the 1990s. These computer systems offer more than simultaneous "central fetal monitoring," displays of EFM tracings. Information systems that interface with fetal monitors can be used to enter, display, transmit, analyze, archive, and retrieve FHR data. Perinatal systems can provide alerts, pattern analysis, decision support, and research data collection. The 2009 Health Information Technology for Economic and Clinical Health (HITECH) Act reinforced the trend of computer-based fetal heart monitoring with incentives for meaningful use of certified clinical information systems that enable digital information exchange and analytic decision support (McCartney, 2009, 2013; McCartney & Barnes, 2012).

EVIDENCE FOR FHR ASSESSMENT

When clinicians first experimented with FHM techniques, they recorded their observations as evidence for practice. This kind of anecdotal reporting gradually evolved into the current expectations for (1) rigorous research methods in both observational and interventional clinical trials and (2) complete descriptions of the methods and results in publications.

The initial purpose of EFM was to identify unfavorable FHR characteristics that indicated a fetus at risk for asphyxia, thus enabling intervention to prevent poor outcomes. Years of research and practice with FHM have produced considerable information about favorable and unfavorable FHR characteristics and implications, as well as elucidating the limitations of EFM technology to predict fetal outcomes. Currently, FHM is used to identify FHR characteristics indicating fetal well-being as well as those suggesting risk. Information about normal FHR characteristics is equally helpful in clinical care.

As the practice of FHM (both auscultation and electronic) developed, researchers began to study the accuracy of interpretation by clinicians (reliability) and the relationship between FHR interpretations and neonatal outcomes (validity) (see Table 1-2). Research about the reliability, validity, and efficacy of both auscultated and electronic FHR assessment has stimulated discussion and debate in the literature. Both methods were originally incorporated into clinical practice without sufficient research evidence confirming the benefits and risks of the respective methodologies.

Early proponents of EFM promoted its benefits compared with auscultation. Two early studies on auscultation skill and outcomes have been widely cited in the literature, despite concerns raised about their methodologies. The first study is only briefly described in a paragraph at the beginning of a paper by Hon (1958). This paragraph is all that was ever presented, and this original source is not a complete report. Hon proposed that periodic auscultatory sampling between contractions was inaccurate; therefore, he engaged 15 obstetricians to "count" eight rates recorded on a magnetic audiotape (ranging from 75 to 204 bpm). The counted values varied within a range of 6 to 68 bpm of the true, recorded FHR. Hon subsequently concluded that human auditory interpretation of FHR had poor reliability and that electronic techniques could prevent human error. The report did not describe the counting method, the nature of the recording, or the obstetricians' experience with auscultation.

The second report was a federally funded, multicenter, prospective observational study on auscultated FHR related to "fetal distress," titled the "Collaborative Study of Cerebral Palsy, Mental Retardation, and Other Neurological Diseases and Blindness" (Benson, Shubeck, Deutschberger, Weiss, & Berendes, 1968). In this study, FHR was auscultated by observers who were specially trained (but whose qualifications were not identified) every 15 minutes during the first stage of labor. The FHR was not obtained during a contraction or for 30 seconds following a contraction, and FHRs obtained during the second stage of labor were not used in the final study analysis. The short report states that four auscultated FHR measures (based on Von Winckel's 1893 criteria) were related to "fetal distress" (p. 259) based on the computer analysis of the data. However, the author could not identify one auscultatory FHR measure that was a reliable indicator of "fetal distress" except for bradycardia, which the authors call "save in extreme degree" (p. 262). The authors acknowledged that the study was limited because "even a generally acceptable definition of fetal distress based upon the fetal heart rate is yet to be achieved" (p. 262) but concluded that auscultated FHR findings had poor validity. These two studies have been commonly cited as support for the rejection of auscultation and increased use of electronic monitoring. A number of subsequent publications have examined individuals' skill in assessing FHR, rhythm, and accelerations; compared auscultatory devices such as Doppler and

Pinard devices (Mahomed, Nyoni, Mulambo, Kasule, & Jacobus, 1994); and compared the cost-effectiveness of auscultation to EFM in labor (Feinstein, Sprague, & Trépanier, 2009; Miller, Pearse, & Paul, 1984) (see Chapter 4).

As the use of EFM increased in the late 1970s, clinicians and consumers considered the invasive nature and high equipment costs associated with EFM and questioned the widespread application of an untested technology (Banta & Thacker, 2001). Skepticism grew when the first EFM clinical trials failed to show any benefit over auscultation in low-risk births. The first reports on randomized clinical trials comparing EFM and auscultation, from Haverkamp, Thompson, McFee, and Cetrulo (1976) and the Dublin Trial (MacDonald, Grant, Sheridan-Pereira, Boylan, and Chalmers, 1985), showed that although the use of EFM reduced neonatal seizures, there was no difference in a number of neonatal outcome measures (including cerebral palsy) and there was an increase in the rate of cesarean and operative births. Supporters of EFM debated the methodology of these studies and their implications. Collectively, the findings from 12 randomized controlled trials (RCTs) published between 1976 and 1994 and subsequent meta-analyses of these RCTs demonstrated no benefit with EFM when compared with auscultation (Thacker & Stroup, 1999; Thacker, Stroup, & Chang, 2006).

Clinicians continue to research relationships between EFM patterns and outcomes. Parer, King, Flanders, Fox, and Kilpatrick (2006) used the standardized 1997 National Institute of Child Health and Human Development (NICHD) EFM definitions in a retrospective review of reported research and did identify relationships between FHR patterns and fetal acidemia and/or newborn vigor. Graham, Petersen, Christo, and Fox (2006) also used the 1997 NICHD definitions in a retrospective review and found no relationships between EFM tracings and perinatal brain injury or death. FHR pattern analysis did show accuracy in identifying some FHR tracing characteristics associated with cord blood metabolic acidosis (Elliott et al., 2010; Gabbe et al., 2012) (see Chapter 5 for further discussion).

Studies on reliability (accuracy of clinicians' assessments) with EFM patterns show that clinicians differ in their interpretations of an EFM pattern (interrater or interobserver reliability) and that the same clinician may give different interpretations of the same EFM pattern when it is reviewed at different times (intrarater or intra-observer reliability). Investigators have examined if standardized definitions improve the reliability of clinician analysis of FHR characteristics, and if computer analysis of FHR characteristics is equally as accurate as clinicians. A study comparing clinician analysis using 1997 NICHD definitions with computer analysis found the standardized definitions did not reduce human interobserver differences in pattern interpretation (Devoe et al., 2000). Blackwell, Grobman, Antoniewicz, Hutchinson, and Bannerman (2011) report only moderate agreement in clinician visual analysis using 2008 NICHD criteria and present a table of previous studies on interpretation reliability with visual and computer analysis. A study comparing expert clinician analysis using the 2008 NICHD definitions with computer analysis found similar performance with the computer analysis (Parer & Hamilton, 2010).

Perinatal health care professionals generally agree that additional research is needed to validate the efficacy of FHM practice. Areas for further research include examining clinician education and FHM assessment, interpretation, and intervention. The research needed about assessment includes investigation of clinicians' skills with each monitoring method, clinician reliability, optimal assessment frequency, and computer analysis. Research needed about interpretation includes describing the relationships between FHR characteristics and neonatal outcomes. The research needed about intervention includes testing relationships among interpretations, interventions, and neonatal outcomes. Researchers may capitalize on the opportunity to collect data using perinatal information systems. More evidence is needed to design clinician education and competence validation that is based on knowledge and skill development, differences between a novice and an expert, and effective instruction and evaluation methods.

Despite research and guidelines recommending auscultation for low-risk women, clinicians began to question why evidence was not being translated into practice (Haggerty, 1999). A Canadian study investigated the barriers and supports that influenced successful or unsuccessful implementation of an evidence-based guideline on intermittent auscultation in low-risk births (Graham, Logan, Davies, & Nimrod, 2004). Using focus groups and interviews, these authors found that implementation was influenced by nursing and medical leadership, unit philosophy, unit policies, medicolegal concerns, equipment availability, and auscultation skill. More evidence on research translation is needed to identify the most successful approaches to accomplish changes in practice.

STANDARDIZATION AND PROFESSIONAL GUIDELINES

The Institute of Medicine (IOM) published a comprehensive report that detailed the nature and scope of circumstances within health care systems and facilities and among health care providers that contribute to morbidity and mortality among hospitalized patients. The IOM recommended measures to reduce the incidence of health care errors and promote patient safety (Kohn, Corrigan, & Donaldson, 2000). The report cited many measures that can significantly improve safety, including the use of standardized medical terminology, standardization of education for clinicians, and use of simulation in multidisciplinary training. The IOM report specifically encourages professional organizations to facilitate patient safety by developing and promoting practice guidelines that address patient safety issues and by standardizing technology and education. The Association of Women's Health, Obstetric and Neonatal Nurses (2000) publicly responded to the IOM by emphasizing its commitment to solutions that ensure maternal–fetal safety, including the Fetal Heart Monitoring Principles and Practices (FHMPP) workshop. The efforts taken to move toward consensus and standardization in FHM are summarized in the next section.

Standardized Language, Controversy, and Consensus

Uniform FHR terminology and interpretation are necessary to facilitate meaningful communication, appropriate documentation, establishment of functional information databases, and sound research. A standardized approach to both auscultation and electronic monitoring requires criteria that are quantifiable, objectively measurable, unambiguous, reproducible, and generally accepted.

Historically, clinicians and researchers have sometimes disagreed about elements of FHR assessment, interpretation, and intervention. For example, physicians began to describe slight variations in baseline FHRs using different terminology as early as the 1950s. FHR pattern definitions used in current practice evolved from the pioneering work of Hon, Hammacher, and Caldeyro-Barcia and colleagues during the 1950s and 1960s. These physicians agreed on descriptions of characteristics but disagreed on terms (baseline rates, changes from the baseline rate [called "accelerations" and "decelerations"], and fluctuations of the baseline rate [called "variability"] as classified by the amplitude of FHR changes and the number of cycles of change per minute) (Freeman et al., 2012). Some international agreement on deceleration patterns was first achieved at the Fifth World Congress of Gynecology and Obstetrics in 1967. An international panel on fetal monitoring convened in 1971 in the United States and again in 1972 in Amsterdam to develop consensus on terminology and measurement (Freeman et al., 2012). The panel agreed on the terminology of baseline "variability" and "early, late, and variable" decelerations. No agreement was reached on a monitor paper scale or speed or on the categorization of variability. Consequently, discrepant terminology and categorizations of variability evolved, for example, oscillations, variability, beat-to-beat variability, and variation.

In 1995, the NICHD convened an international panel of researchers and clinicians that developed standardized, quantitative definitions for EFM to be used for both visual and computer interpretation. These definitions, published simultaneously in nursing and medical specialty journals, were recommended to improve the reliability of pattern interpretation in studies and to better compare findings among studies. In 2005, both AWHONN and ACOG incorporated the NICHD definitions into practice resources (ACOG, 2005b; AWHONN, 2005). In 2008 the NICHD, ACOG, and the Society for Maternal–Fetal Medicine (SMFM) jointly sponsored an interdisciplinary workshop to review and update the 1997 NICHD definitions and to assess the need for a standardized system for interpretation of intrapartum EFM findings in the United States (Macones et al., 2008) (described in Box 1-1 and Chapter 5). Key changes resulting from this meeting include revised terminology for excessive uterine activity (Box 1-2) and the adoption of a three-tiered system for classifying EFM findings (Box 1-1 and Chapter 5). The definitions resulting from the 2008 meeting are incorporated throughout this text.

The automated analysis systems, such as Sonicaid, PeriCalm, and SisPorto (SisPorto; Oporto University, Portugal) apply standard criteria for computer analysis (Ayres-de Campos, Bernardes, Garrido, Marques-de-Sá, & Pereira-Leite, 2000). Commercial systems increasingly incorporate the NICHD standardized definitions, but may allow individual users to configure their own criteria for pattern alerting functions.

In the 1970s, nurses began to work on a standardized language or classification system for nursing practice that could be used in a computerized database to help nurses document their contributions to patient care, including intrapartum care (Eganhouse, McCloskey, & Bulechek, 1996). One example of standardized nursing language is the Nursing Intervention Classification (NIC) system, which includes the relevant intervention "6772: Electronic Fetal Monitoring: Intrapartum Intervention." This intervention is defined and detailed with actions that are supported with this textbook as a reference (Dochterman & Bulechek, 2004). This standard intervention could be used for FHM nursing practice (uniform documentation) and nursing research (relating nursing interventions to newborn outcomes).

Standardized nomenclature is necessary for many aspects of clinical practice, including the following examples used in documentation, reimbursement, and bibliographic databases. Experts have expressed concern about the continued use of imprecise terms such as "fetal distress" and "birth asphyxia." In 1998 and 2005, ACOG

BOX 1-2 Uterine Activity

Uterine contractions are quantified as the number of contractions present in a 10-minute window, averaged over 30 minutes. Contraction frequency alone is a partial assessment of uterine activity. Other factors such as duration, intensity, and relaxation time between contractions are equally important in clinical practice. The following represents terminology to describe uterine activity:

A. Normal: $\leq$ 5 contractions in 10 minutes, averaged over a 30-minute window.
B. Tachysystole: $>$ 5 contractions in 10 minutes, averaged over a 30-minute window.
C. Characteristics of uterine contractions:
- Tachysystole should always be qualified as to the presence or absence of associated FHR decelerations.
- The term "tachysystole" applies to both spontaneous or stimulated labor. The clinical response to tachysystole may differ depending on whether contractions are spontaneous or stimulated.
- The terms "hyperstimulation" and "hypercontractility" are not defined and should be abandoned.

Note From: "The 2008 National Institute of Child Health Human Development Workshop Report on Electronic Fetal Monitoring: Update on Definitions, Interpretations, and Research Guidelines," by G. A. Macones, G. D. Hankins, C. Y. Spong, J. D. Hauth, & T. Moore, 2008, *Journal of Obstetric, Gynecologic and Neonatal Nursing, 37,* 510–515; *Obstetrics & Gynecology, 112,* p. 665.

recommended that the term "fetal distress" be replaced with "nonreassuring fetal status," followed by a description of the assessment findings. This recommendation changed with the publication of the 2008 NICHD definitions when clinicians were advised to apply standardized language to most accurately reflect the EFM findings present in tracings. The term "fetal distress" and all inclusive terms for "fetal distress" except "metabolic acidemia" were removed from the perinatal International Classification of Disease code (ACOG, 1998). In 2008 the NICHD Workshop participants also recommended use of the term "tachysystole" to describe excessive uterine activity and recommended the terms "hyperstimulation" and "hypercontractility" be abandoned due to lack of consistent definitions (Box 1-2) (Macones et al., 2008).

The standard language used to organize and effectively search bibliographic databases (Medical Subject Headings [MeSH]) assigns the standard terms "fetal heart rate," "fetal monitoring," "cardiotocography," and "phonocardiography" for articles on FHR assessment (National Library of Medicine, 2013).

Professional Guidelines

As FHM developed, professional organizations issued a number of guidelines to promote standardization and competence in fetal heart assessment. These resources are periodically revised on the basis of new research findings, technological developments, and practice changes. Some resources focus on a specific assessment technique, whereas others are comprehensive. Some resources are interdisciplinary or international in scope.

Professional guidelines have been useful for establishing consistency in FHR assessment in labor. Several guidelines address the choice of FHM method. No professional association of providers involved in childbirth has ever authored a guideline recommending EFM over intermittent auscultation for low-risk births. Because clinical trials have demonstrated that auscultation is as effective as EFM, guidelines include the option of intermittent auscultation for low-risk births (ACOG, 1995, 2005a, 2009). AWHONN supports the use of fetal auscultation as well as the "judicious application of intrapartum EFM and does not support the use of EFM as a substitute for appropriate professional nursing care" (AWHONN, 2008, p. 1). Furthermore, AWHONN recommends that each facility develop a policy regarding appropriate use of each FHR monitoring method. SOGC states that intermittent auscultation is the recommended method of FHR surveillance for women at low risk during labor (SOGC, 1995, 2002, 2007).

FETAL MONITORING EDUCATION

Implementation of EFM requires skilled personnel at the bedside to interpret patterns throughout labor, and this responsibility became part of nurses' work. Nurses quickly found themselves in need of new knowledge and skills to use this technology. Collectively and diligently, nurses initially addressed their immediate needs for education and later emerged as the leaders in fetal monitoring education. Comprehensive professional education should include the knowledge and skills for FHR assessment by both auscultation and electronic fetal heart monitoring.

Development of FHM Education

When EFM was introduced in the 1960s, most nurses learned basic skills through on-the-job and vendor-sponsored training. Textbooks and journals did not include basic instruction on EFM until the late 1970s. Nurses began to develop and teach EFM education programs throughout the United States. These independent educators were instrumental in early EFM instruction and continue to be primary providers of basic and advanced instruction today. Some educators went on to develop train-the-trainer programs that prepared other nurses with the knowledge and skills necessary to teach basic EFM (Adelsperger, 1990). However, the content, style, and emphasis in these education programs had become quite diverse. Nurses identified the need for resources to (1) identify a standard core of FHM knowledge and skills and (2) establish a mechanism for validating knowledge and skills. Nurses turned to professional organizations such as AWHONN (formally known as the Nurses Association of the American College of Obstetricians and Gynecologists [NAACOG]) to meet these needs.

NAACOG responded with a technical bulletin on EFM, followed by a joint position statement with ACOG and educational guidelines. These resources were followed in the years to come with numerous other position statements, standards, guidelines, and educational resources on EFM and FHM for nurses. AWHONN remains the recognized source for FHM guidelines and education, including the AWHONN Fetal Heart Monitoring Program (www.awhonn.org).

Competence Validation and Certification

Competence validation is the process of evaluating an individual's knowledge and clinical skills. A variety of instruction and performance evaluation tools can be used for competence validation. Certification is recognition awarded by an accredited credentialing body to an individual who meets predetermined criteria, usually limited to testing of knowledge, demonstrated by means of a psychometrically sound exam. The advantages and disadvantages of subspecialty certification in didactic EFM knowledge have been debated (Afriat, Simpson, Chez, & Miller, 1994; McCartney, 1999; Murray, 1999). Currently there are no national requirements for certification, and facilities may vary in their requirements for credentialing and competence validation of staff responsible for fetal heart monitoring and assessment.

Instruction and Evaluation Methods

Competence in fetal monitoring requires both didactic knowledge and psychomotor skills. A core (basic) instructional program includes knowledge and skills needed to achieve minimal competence. An educational program for ongoing competence validation includes additional or more complex knowledge and skills. Programs for novices include the content and structure for basic assessment and intervention. Programs for experienced clinicians should provide opportunities for more advanced problem solving through case studies, discussion, and reflection. Both basic education and experience are necessary to achieve competence in clinical judgment and decision making.

Today, many continuing education resources exist for FHM didactic knowledge and some measure of skill proficiency at the basic and experienced levels. A number of providers (professional organizations, nurse entrepreneurs, commercial companies, and health care institutions) offer activities with a variety of formats (conferences; hands-on skills workshops; case studies; independent or home self-study assessment modules; journals; computer simulation; online, audio, video, and satellite conferencing). Instruction and evaluation methods include examination, case-study analysis, tracing interpretation, computer-based evaluation, role-playing, policy debate, documentation audit, and skill demonstration. Some computerized simulation manikins are used for interdisciplinary team training and evaluation of assessment, interpretation, and response to FHR patterns (MacEachin, Lopez, Powell, & Corbett, 2009).

Research about FHM instruction and evaluation methods is limited. Reports include studies about educational content and methods (Kinnick, 1989, 1990; Murray & Higgins, 1996; Sauer, 1993; Trépanier et al., 1996) and studies on assessment of skill (Chez et al., 1990; Haggerty, 1996; Haggerty & Nuttall, 2000; Morrison et al., 1993). Haggerty found that expert intrapartal nurses identified four clinical parameters to assess the severity of fetal stress: duration of stress, fetal reserve status, reversibility, and specific signs of stress. Later, Haggerty and Nuttall (2000) reported that the most important clinical factors that experienced nurses considered in determining fetal risk were scalp pH, maternal parity, amniotic fluid color, and long-term FHR variability. Findings from a systematic review of 20 publications on FHR training programs showed training did increase knowledge and skills, but evidence on long-term effects and clinical outcomes is lacking (Pehrson, Sorenson, & Amer-Wåhlin, 2011). Further studies are needed to identify the best instruction and evaluation methods.

DEVELOPMENT OF THE AWHONN FETAL HEART MONITORING PROGRAM

FHM is a common obstetric procedure in North America, and clinicians need resources to practice in a safe, standardized, and competent manner. The AWHONN Fetal Heart Monitoring Program is designed to be part of an overall plan for competence validation in specialty practice for the individual or institution.

In 1990, NAACOG initiated the development of a standardized fetal monitoring course to validate the cognitive knowledge and psychomotor skills of the experienced nurse in comprehensive FHM (both auscultation and EFM). The course would emphasize the physiologic basis of assessment and intervention and apply concepts to practice through the use of case studies and hands-on skill practice. Fetal monitoring would be taught within the nursing model as a component of overall childbirth knowledge and skills, not as an isolated technical skill.

The NAACOG Committee on Education appointed a National Steering Committee of member experts in fetal monitoring education from geographically diverse areas. This volunteer committee met regularly for 2 years and created a 2-day workshop (now the Intermediate Course) along with a printed manual, audio-visual material, and skill models (Schmidt, 2000). A train-the-trainer plan included preparing qualified NAACOG members to be workshop instructors and instructor-trainers to prepare additional instructors. The FHMPP workshop was piloted in 1992, an Instructor Enhancement Course was added in 1994, and an Advanced FHMPP course was added in 1998. A newsletter, *The Beat Goes On*, was launched in 1997 to provide periodic program updates for instructors and instructor-trainers. Progressive course revisions led to the current comprehensive Fetal Heart Monitoring Program Learning Pathway building introduction, intermediate, advanced, and case assessment levels using instructor-led courses, online education, and books and publications. More than 20 years after the first pilot, AWHONN educates over 15,000 health care professionals per year in FHM.

THE NURSING PROCESS AND THE FETAL HEART MONITORING PROGRAM

A systematic framework for providing patient care is useful for clinicians. The framework for the Fetal Heart Monitoring program and this textbook has transitioned from the original use of the nursing process (assessment, interpretation, diagnosis, intervention, and evaluation) to the Collaborative Fetal Monitoring Process. This process is a scientific problem-solving model for decision making about FHM, and is based on the critical-thinking skills of analysis, synthesis, and evaluation. Scientific problem-solving frameworks and critical-thinking skills are similarly used across professional disciplines (Figure 1-1).

FIGURE 1-1 The Collaborative Process and Fetal Heart Monitoring

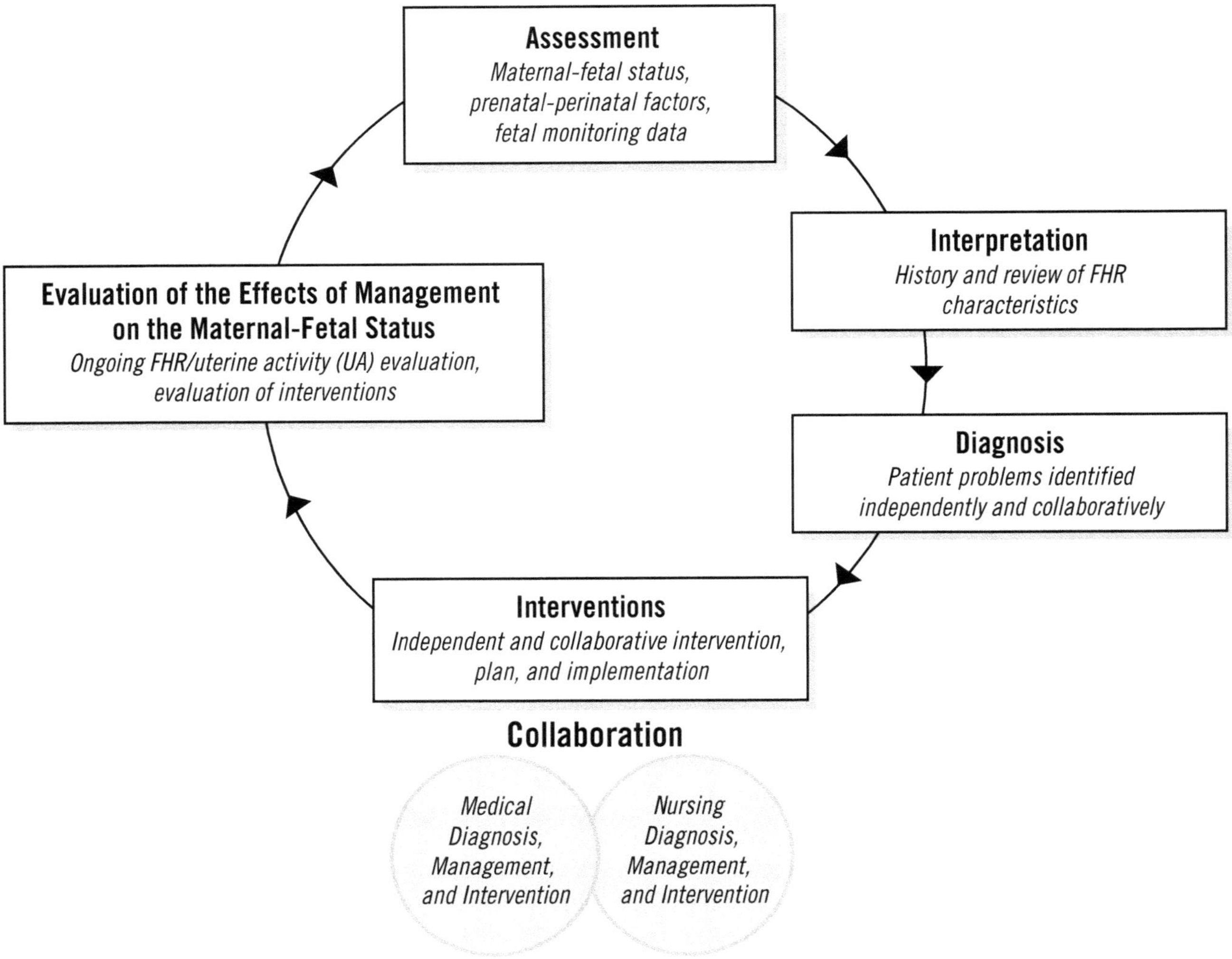

REFERENCES

Adelsperger, D. (1990). *Train the trainer program.* Santa Clara, CA: Hewlett Packard.

Afriat, C. I., Simpson, K. R., Chez, B. F., & Miller, L. A. (1994). Electronic fetal monitoring competency—to validate or not to validate: The opinions of experts. *Journal of Perinatal & Neonatal Nursing, 8*(3), 1–16.

American College of Obstetricians and Gynecologists. (1995). *Fetal heart rate patterns: Monitoring, interpretation, and management* (ACOG Technical Bulletin No. 207). Washington, DC: Author.

American College of Obstetricians and Gynecologists. (1998). *Inappropriate use of the terms fetal distress and birth asphyxia* (ACOG Committee Opinion No. 197). Washington, DC: Author.

American College of Obstetricians and Gynecologists. (2001). *Fetal pulse oximetry* (ACOG Committee Opinion No. 258). Washington, DC: Author.

American College of Obstetricians and Gynecologists. (2005a). *Inappropriate use of the terms fetal distress and birth asphyxia* (ACOG Committee Opinion No. 326). Washington, DC: Author.

American College of Obstetricians and Gynecologists. (2005b). *Intrapartum fetal heart rate monitoring* (ACOG Practice Bulletin No. 70). Washington, DC: Author.

American College of Obstetricians and Gynecologists. (2009). Intrapartum fetal heart rate monitoring: Nomenclature, interpretation and general management principles (ACOG Practice Bulletin No. 106). *Obstetrics and Gynecology, 114*(1), 192–202. doi: 10.1097/AOG.0b013e3181aef106

Association of Women's Health, Obstetric and Neonatal Nurses. (2000). *Written statement of AWHONN to Subcommittee on Health, Committee on Ways and Means on the Institute of Medicine Report on Medical Errors.* Washington, DC: Author.

Association of Women's Health, Obstetric and Neonatal Nurses. (2005, August). NICHD terminology transition. *AWHONN's FHMPP Program Newsletter,* p. 4.

Association of Women's Health, Obstetric and Neonatal Nurses. (2008). Fetal heart monitoring (Position Statement). Washington, DC: Author.

Ayres-de Campos, D., Bernardes, J., Garrido, A., Marques-de-Sá, J., & Pereira-Leite, L. (2000). SisPorto 2.0: A program for automated analysis of cardiotocograms. *Journal of Maternal-Fetal and Neonatal Medicine, 9*(5), 311–318.

Banta, D. H., & Thacker, S. B. (2001). Historical controversy in health technology assessment: The case of electronic fetal monitoring. *Obstetrical and Gynecological Survey, 56*(11), 707–719.

Benson, R. C., Shubeck, F., Deutschberger, J., Weiss, W., & Berendes, H. (1968). Fetal heart rate as a predictor of fetal distress. A report from the collaborative project. *Obstetrics and Gynecology, 32*(2), 259–266.

Blackwell, S. C., Grobman, W. A., Antoniewicz, L., Hutchinson, M., & Bannerman, C. G. (2011). Interobserver and intraobserver reliability of the NICHD 3-Tier Fetal Heart Rate Interpretation System. *American Journal of Obstetrics and Gynecology, 205*(4), 378.e1–378.e5. doi:10.1016/j.ajog.2011.06.086

Bloom, S. L., Spong, C. Y., Thom, E., Varner, M. W., Rouse, D. J., Weininger, S., . . . National Institute of Child Health and Human Development Maternal–Fetal Medicine Units Network. (2006). Fetal pulse oximetry and cesarean delivery. *New England Journal of Medicine, 355*(21), 2195–2202. doi:10.1056/NEJMoa061170

Chez, B. F., Skurnick, J. H., Chez, R. A., Verklan, M. T., Biggs, S., & Hage, M. L. (1990). Interpretations of nonstress tests by obstetric nurses. *Journal of Obstetric, Gynecologic and Neonatal Nursing, 19*(3), 227–232.

Clark, S. L., Gimovsky, M. L., & Miller, F. C. (1982). Fetal heart rate response to scalp blood sampling. *American Journal of Obstetrics and Gynecology, 144*(6), 706–708.

Clark, S. L., Gimovsky, M. L., & Miller, F. C. (1984). The scalp stimulation test: A clinical alternative to fetal scalp blood sampling. *American Journal of Obstetrics and Gynecology, 148*(3), 274–277.

Clark, S. L., & Paul, R. H. (1985). Intrapartum fetal surveillance: The role of fetal scalp blood sampling. *American Journal of Obstetrics and Gynecology, 153*(7), 717–720.

Devoe, L., Golde, S., Kilman, Y., Morton, D., Shea, K., & Waller, J. (2000). A comparison of visual analyses of intrapartum fetal heart rate tracings according to the new National Institute of Child Health and Human Development guidelines with computer analyses by an automated fetal heart rate monitoring system. *American Journal of Obstetrics and Gynecology, 183*(2), 361–366.

Devoe, L. D. (2011). Fetal ECG analysis for intrapartum electronic fetal monitoring: A review. *Clinical Obstetrics and Gynecology, 54*(1), 56–65. doi:10.1097/GRF.0b013e31820a0ee7

Dochterman, J. M., & Bulechek, G. M. (Eds.). (2004). *Nursing interventions classification (NIC)* (4th ed.). St. Louis, MO: Mosby.

Eganhouse, D. J., McCloskey, J. C., & Bulechek, G. M. (1996). How NIC describes MCH nursing. *MCN: American Journal of Maternal/Child Nursing, 21*(5), 247–252.

Elliott, C., Warrick, P., Graham, E., & Hamilton, E. (2010). Graded classification of fetal heart rate tracings: Association with neonatal metabolic acidosis and neurologic morbidity. *American Journal of Obstetrics and Gynecology, 202*(3), 258.e1–258.e8. doi:10.1016/j.ajog.2009.06.026

Feinstein, N. F., Sprague, A., & Trépanier, M. J. (2009). *Fetal heart rate auscultation* (2nd ed.). Washington, DC: Association of Women's Health, Obstetric and Neonatal Nurses.

Freeman, R. K. (1975). The use of the oxytocin challenge test for antepartum clinical evaluation of uteroplacental respiratory function. *American Journal of Obstetrics and Gynecology, 121*(4), 481–489.

Freeman, R. K., Garite, T. J., Nageotte, M. P., & Miller, L. (Eds.). (2012). *Fetal heart rate monitoring* (4th ed.). Philadelphia, PA: Lippincott Williams & Wilkins.

Gabbe, S. G., Niebyl, J. R., Galan, H. L., Jauniaux, E. R. M., Landon, M. B., Simpson, J. L., & Driscoll, D. A. (2012). *Obstetrics: Normal and problem pregnancies* (6th ed.). Philadelphia, PA: Elsevier-Saunders.

Garite, T. J. (2013). The search for an adequate back-up test for intrapartum fetal heart rate monitoring. *American Journal of Obstetrics and Gynecology, 208*(3), 163–164. doi:10.1016/j.ajog.2012.12.001

Goodlin, R. C. (1979). History of fetal monitoring. *American Journal of Obstetrics and Gynecology, 133*(3), 323–352.

Graham, E. M., Petersen, S. M., Christo, D. K., & Fox, H. E. (2006). Intrapartum electronic fetal heart rate monitoring and the prevention of perinatal brain injury. *Obstetrics and Gynecology, 108*(3, Pt. 1), 656–666.

Graham, I. D., Logan, J., Davies, B., & Nimrod, C. (2004). Changing the use of electronic fetal monitoring and labor support: A case study of barriers and facilitators. *Birth, 31*(4), 293–301.

Haggerty, L. A. (1996). Assessment parameters and indicators in expert intrapartal nursing decisions. *Journal of Obstetric, Gynecologic and Neonatal Nursing, 25*(6), 491–499.

Haggerty, L. A. (1999). Continuous electronic fetal monitoring: Contradictions between practice and research. *Journal of Obstetric, Gynecologic and Neonatal Nursing, 28*(4), 409–416.

Haggerty, L. A., & Nuttall, R. L. (2000). Experienced obstetric nurses' decision-making in fetal risk situations. *Journal of Obstetric, Gynecologic and Neonatal Nursing, 29*(5), 480–490.

Haverkamp, A. D., Thompson, H. E., McFee, J. G., & Cetrulo, C. (1976). The evaluation of continuous fetal heart rate monitoring in high-risk pregnancy. *American Journal of Obstetrics and Gynecology, 125*(3), 310–320.

Hillis, D. S. (1917). Attachment for the stethoscope. *Journal of the American Medical Association, 68*, 910.

Hon, E. (1958). The electronic evaluation of the fetal heart rate. *American Journal of Obstetrics and Gynecology, 75*(6), 1215–1230.

Kinnick, V. G. (1989). A national survey about fetal monitoring skills acquired by nursing students in baccalaureate programs. *Journal of Obstetric, Gynecologic and Neonatal Nursing, 18*(1), 57–58.

Kinnick, V. (1990). The effect of concept teaching in preparing nursing students for clinical practice. *Journal of Nursing Education, 29*(8), 362–366.

Kohn, L. T., Corrigan, J. M., & Donaldson, M. S. (Eds.). (2000). *To err is human: Building a safer health system.* Washington, DC: National Academy Press.

MacDonald, D., Grant, A., Sheridan-Pereira, M., Boylan, P., & Chalmers, I. (1985). The Dublin randomized controlled trial of intrapartum fetal heart rate monitoring. *American Journal of Obstetrics and Gynecology, 152*(5), 524–539.

MacEachin, S. R., Lopez, C. M., Powell, K. J., & Corbett, N. L. (2009). The fetal heart rate collaborative practice project: Situational awareness in electronic fetal monitoring. *Journal of Perinatal and Neonatal Nursing 23*(4), 314–323. doi:10.1097/JPN.0b013e3181a1bf07

Macones, G. A., Hankins, G. D., Spong, C. Y., Hauth, J., & Moore, T. (2008). The 2008 National Institute of Child Health and Human Development workshop report on electronic fetal monitoring: Update on definitions, interpretation, and research guidelines. *Obstetrics and Gynecology, 112*(3), 661–666, doi:10.1097/AOG.0b013e3181841395; and *Journal of Obstetric, Gynecologic and Neonatal Nursing, 37*(5), 510–515. doi:10.1111/j.1552-6909.2008.00284.x

Mahomed, K., Nyoni, R., Mulambo, T., Kasule, J., & Jacobus, E. (1994). Randomised controlled trial of intrapartum fetal heart rate monitoring. *British Medical Journal, 308*(6927), 497–500.

Manning, F. A., Platt, L. D., & Sipos, L. (1980). Antepartum fetal evaluation: Development of a fetal biophysical profile. *American Journal of Obstetrics and Gynecology, 136*(6), 787–795.

McCartney, P. R. (1999). Certification in fetal heart monitoring: Is it really worth the additional effort and expense for perinatal nurses? Con position. *MCN: American Journal of Maternal/Child Nursing, 24*(1), 10–11.

McCartney, P. R. (2000). Computer analysis of the fetal heart rate. *Journal of Obstetric, Gynecologic and Neonatal Nursing, 29*(5), 527–536.

McCartney, P. R. (2009). The American Recovery and Reinvestment Act: Health information technology stimulus. *MCN: The American Journal of Maternal/Child Nursing, 34*(4), 262. doi:10.1097/01.NMC.0000357923.48724.d5

McCartney, P. R. (2011). Computer fetal heart rate pattern analysis. *MCN: The American Journal of Maternal/Child Nursing, 36*(6), 397. doi:10.1097/NMC.0b013e31822e2883

McCartney, P. R. (2013). Meaningful Use stages 1 and 2. *MCN: The American Journal of Maternal/Child Nursing, 38*(1), 56. doi:10.1097/NMC.0b013e31827401f6

McCartney, P., & Barnes, J. (2012). *Perinatal nursing informatics guide for clinical health information technology.* Washington, DC: Association of Women's Health, Obstetric and Neonatal Nurses.

Miller, F. C., Pearse, K. E., & Paul, R. H. (1984). Fetal heart rate pattern recognition by the method of auscultation. *Obstetrics and Gynecology, 64*(3), 332–336.

Morrison, J. C., Chez, B. F., Davis, I. D., Martin, R. W., Roberts, W. E., Martin, J. N., Jr., & Floyd, R. C. (1993). Intrapartum fetal heart rate assessment: Monitoring by auscultation or electronic means. *American Journal of Obstetrics and Gynecology, 168*(1, Pt. 1), 63–66.

Murray, M. (1999). Certification in fetal heart monitoring: Is it really worth the additional effort and expense for perinatal nurses? Pro position. *MCN: The American Journal of Maternal/Child Nursing, 24*(1), 10–11.

Murray, M. L., & Higgins, P. (1996). Computer versus lecture: Strategies for teaching fetal monitoring. *Journal of Perinatology, 16*(1), 15–19.

National Institute of Child Health and Human Development Research Planning Workshop. (1997). Electronic fetal heart rate monitoring: Research guidelines for interpretation. *Journal of Obstetric, Gynecologic and Neonatal Nursing, 26*(6), 635–640. doi:10.1111/j.1552-6909.1997.tb02737.x

National Library of Medicine. (2013). *Medical subject headings.* Retrieved from http://www.nlm.nih.gov/mesh/2013/mesh_browser/MBrowser.html

Paine, L. L., Zanardi, L. R., Johnson, T. R., Rorie, J. A., & Barger, M. K. (2001). A comparison of two time intervals for the ausculated acceleration test. *Journal of Midwifery and Women's Health, 46*(2), 98–102.

Parer, J. T., & Hamilton, E. F. (2010). Comparison of 5 experts and computer analysis in rule-based fetal heart rate interpretation. *American Journal of Obstetrics and Gynecology, 203*(5), 451.e1–451.e7. doi:10.1016/j.ajog.2010.05.037

Parer, J. T., King, T., Flanders, S., Fox, M., & Kilpatrick, S. J. (2006). Fetal acidemia and electronic fetal heart rate patterns: Is there evidence of an association? *Journal of Maternal–Fetal and Neonatal Medicine, 19*(5), 289–294.

Pehrson, C., Sorensen, J. L., & Amer-Wåhlin, I. (2011). Evaluation and impact of cardiotocography training programmes: A systematic review. *BJOG: An International Journal of Obstetrics and Gynaecology, 118*(8), 926–935. doi:10.1111/j.1471-0528.2011.03021.x

Read, J. A., & Miller, F. C. (1977). Fetal heart rate acceleration in response to acoustic stimulation as a measure of fetal well-being. *American Journal of Obstetrics and Gynecology, 129*(5), 512–517.

Rochard, F., Schifrin, B. S., Goupil, F., Legrand, H., Blottiere, J., & Sureau, C. (1976). Nonstressed fetal heart rate monitoring in the antepartum period. *American Journal of Obstetrics and Gynecology, 126*(6), 699–706.

Sandelowski, M. (2000). Retrofitting technology to nursing: The case of electronic fetal monitoring. *Journal of Obstetric, Gynecologic and Neonatal Nursing, 29*(3), 316–324.

Sauer, P. (1993, June). *Interpretations of fetal heart rate tracings by obstetric nurses: Comparison of test scores with experience and education in electronic fetal heart rate monitoring*. Poster session presented at the annual meeting of the Association of Women's Health, Obstetric and Neonatal Nurses, Reno, NV.

Schmidt, J. V. (2000). The development of AWHONN's fetal heart monitoring principles and practices workshop. Association of Women's Health, Obstetric and Neonatal Nurses. *Journal of Obstetric, Gynecologic and Neonatal Nursing, 29*(5), 509–515.

Schmidt, J. V., & McCartney, P. R. (2000). History and development of fetal heart assessment: A composite. *Journal of Obstetric, Gynecologic and Neonatal Nursing, 29*(3), 295–305.

Schuit, E., Amer-Wahlin, I., Ojala, K., Vayssière, C., Westerhuis, M. E., Maršál, K., . . . Kwee, A. (2013). Effectiveness of electronic fetal monitoring with additional ST analysis in vertex singleton pregnancies at >36 weeks of gestation: An individual participant data metaanalysis. *American Journal of Obstetrics and Gynecology, 208*(3), 187.e1–187.e13. doi:10.1016/j.ajog.2013.01.028

Smith, C. V., Nguyen, H. N., Phelan, J. P., & Paul, R. H. (1986). Intrapartum assessment of fetal well-being: A comparison of fetal acoustic stimulation with acid-base determinations. *American Journal of Obstetrics and Gynecology, 155*(4), 726–728.

Society of Obstetricians and Gynaecologists of Canada. (1995). SOGC Policy Statement: Fetal health surveillance in labour. *Journal of Obstetrics and Gynaecology Canada, 17*, 865–901.

Society of Obstetricians and Gynaecologists of Canada. (2002). *Fetal health surveillance in labour* (SOGC Clinical Practice Guidelines No. 112). Ottawa, Ontario, Canada: Author.

Society of Obstetricians and Gynaecologists of Canada. (2007). Fetal health surveillance: Antepartum and intrapartum consensus guideline (SOGC Clinical Practice Guidelines No. 197). Ottawa, Ontario, Canada: Author.

Thacker, S. B., & Stroup, D. F. (1999). *Continuous electronic fetal monitoring versus intermittent auscultation for assessment during labor* (Cochrane Library, Vol. 2). Oxford, UK: Update Software.

Thacker, S. B., Stroup, D., & Chang, M. H. (2006). Continuous electronic heart rate monitoring for fetal assessment during labor. *Cochrane Database of Systematic Reviews*, Issue 3 (Article No. CD000063). doi:10.1002/14651858.CD000063.pub2

Trépanier, M. J., Niday, P., Davies, B., Sprague, A., Nimrod, C., Dulberg, C., & Watters, N. (1996). Evaluation of a fetal monitoring education program. *Journal of Obstetric, Gynecologic and Neonatal Nursing, 25*(2), 137–144.

Wood, S. H. (2003). Should women be given a choice about fetal assessment in labor? *MCN: American Journal of Maternal/Child Nursing, 28*(5), 292–298.

Wulf, K. H. (1985). History of fetal heart rate monitoring. In W. Künzel (Ed.), *Fetal heart rate monitoring: Clinical practice and pathophysiology* (pp. 3–15). New York: Springer-Verlag.

Yeh, S. Y., Jilek, J., & Hon, E. H. (1974). On-line diagnosis of ominous fetal heart rate patterns: A warning device. *American Journal of Obstetrics and Gynecology, 118*(4), 559–563.

CHAPTER 2

Physiologic Basis for Fetal Monitoring

Nancy O'Brien-Abel

Fetal monitoring is an ongoing indirect assessment of fetal oxygenation. Physiologic influences that are both extrinsic and intrinsic to the fetus impact fetal oxygenation and heart rate control. The fetus is dependent on uterine blood flow, placental exchange, umbilical blood flow, oxygen transport to tissue, and its innate compensatory factors to control fetal heart rate (FHR). When interruptions in fetal oxygenation occur, the fetus responds with detectable FHR changes.

Although the study of maternal and fetal physiology is an evolving science, research using animal models and ongoing clinical evaluations of associations observed between FHR tracings and fetal outcomes has led to progressive improvement in understanding the process of fetal homeostasis. Consideration of the potential underlying physiology is important for clinical decision making when the FHR characteristics or patterns are indeterminate (category II) or abnormal (category III). The presumed underlying physiology helps to guide the interventions and the need for further evaluation of fetal oxygenation.

This chapter reviews both extrinsic and intrinsic physiologic influences that impact fetal oxygenation and FHR. Extrinsic influences discussed include placental structure and function, uteroplacental and fetal–placental circulations, placental transfer, maternal oxygen transport, uterine blood flow, and umbilical cord and amniotic fluid structure and function. Intrinsic influences including fetal circulation, oxygenation of fetal tissues, and factors controlling FHR regulation are also presented. Finally, fetal homeostatic responses to normal and abnormal stresses of labor and birth are illustrated in a dynamic physiologic model of FHR adaptations.

PHYSIOLOGY UNDERLYING EXTRINSIC INFLUENCES ON THE FHR

Maternal–Fetal Exchange

Placenta

Although the mature placenta contains both maternal and fetal tissue, it is primarily a fetal structure responsible for the physiologic exchange of gases, nutrients, and substances between the mother and developing fetus. Other major functions of the placenta throughout gestation include metabolism (e.g., synthesis of glycogen, fatty acids, cholesterol, enzymes), endocrine secretion (e.g., human chorionic gonadotropin, human placental lactogen, estrogen, progesterone), and immunologic protection from pathogens and from physiologic maternal rejection of the "foreign" fetal tissue (Blackburn, 2013c).

Moore, Persaud, and Torchia's (2011) schematic drawing of a transverse section through a full-term placenta is displayed in Figure 2-1. The fetal surface of the placenta is covered by a thin, transparent amniochorionic membrane, beneath which the fetal chorionic villi lie. Chorionic villi are protrusions of fetal tissue exposed to circulating maternal blood within the intervillous space. On the maternal side of the placenta, the decidua basalis forms the outer layer, which attaches to the myometrium. Significant variations exist in placental size and shape, partially because of racial and ethnic differences, altitude, maternal habits such as smoking, and disease. The normal-term placenta is disc shaped, has a diameter of 18 × 20 cm, a thickness of approximately 2 cm, and weighs approximately 400–500 grams when the membranes and umbilical cord have been removed (Benirschke, 2009b).

FIGURE 2-1 Schematic Drawing of a Transverse Section through a Full-Term Placenta Showing Maternal and Fetal Placental Circulation

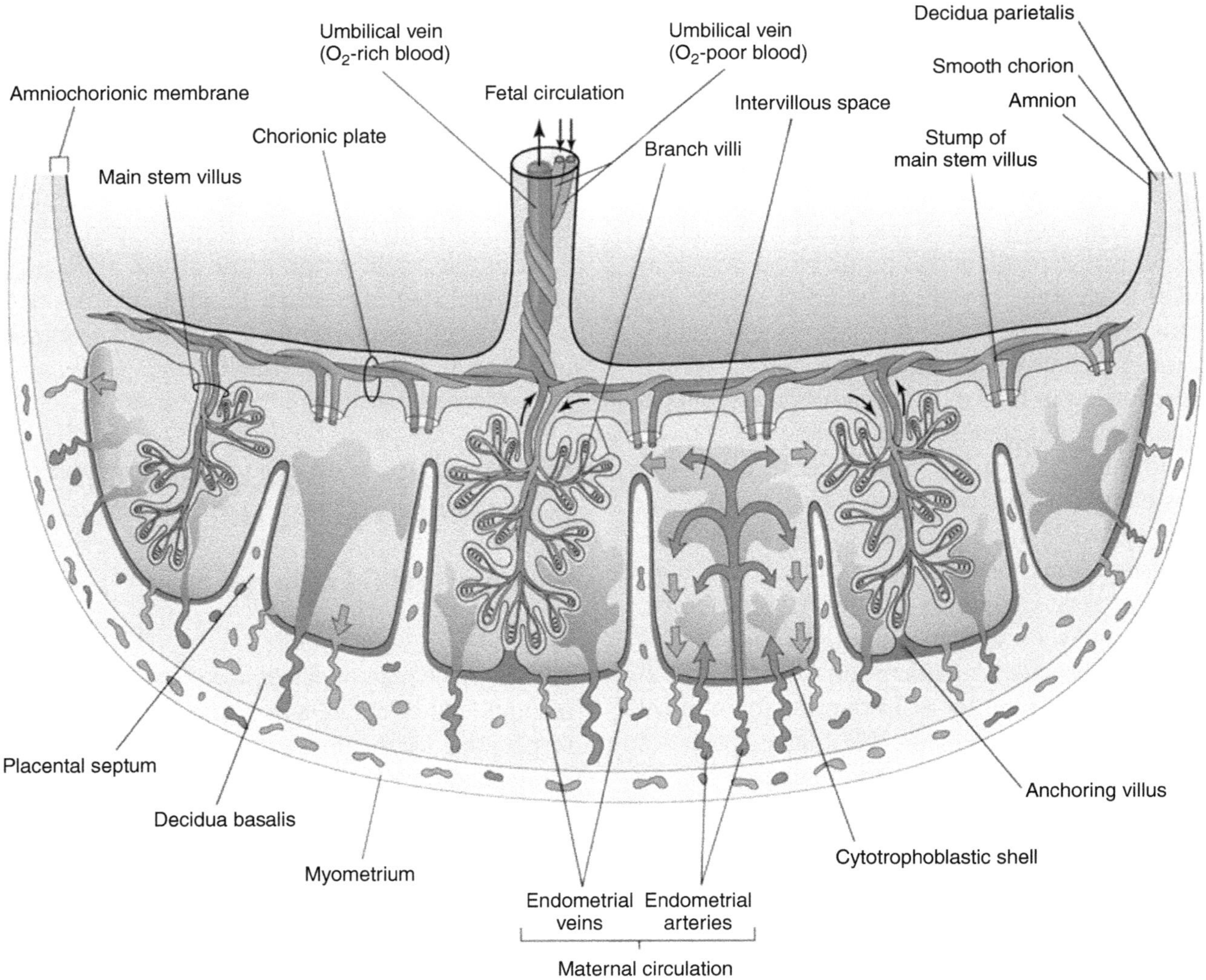

Note: From *The developing human: Clinically oriented embryology* (9th ed.). by K. L. Moore, T. V. N. Persaud, & M. G. Torchia. Copyright 2013 by Elsevier. Reprinted with permission.

Maternal Uteroplacental Circulation

Maternal blood enters the intervillous space of the placenta via spiral arteries, which traverse the endometrium. Here, oxygenated blood, propelled by maternal arterial blood pressure, spurts fountain-like toward the chorionic plate, which forms the roof of the placenta. As the pressure dissipates, maternal blood bathes the fetal chorionic villi, allowing for exchange of substances between the maternal and fetal circulations. Eventually, deoxygenated maternal blood returns through the endometrial veins to the maternal circulation.

Fetal oxygenation depends on well-oxygenated maternal blood flow to the placenta. Both adequate maternal oxygen saturation (percent of oxygen carried on the hemoglobin, SaO_2) and adequate oxygen tension in maternal arterial blood (PaO_2) are needed to promote fetal oxygenation. Maternal arterial oxygen tension depends on adequate maternal ventilation and pulmonary integrity (Zakowski & Ramanathan, 2013). While most pregnant women have adequate pulmonary function, maternal conditions that may impair oxygen delivery to the fetus include asthma, congestive heart failure, congenital cardiac defects, and severe anemia.

Fetal–Placental Circulation

Poorly oxygenated blood leaves the fetus and passes through the two umbilical arteries, which spiral around the umbilical vein to the placenta. As the umbilical cord enters the placenta, the umbilical arteries successively divide into smaller vessels, eventually creating an extensive arteriovenous system within each chorionic villus (Blackburn, 2013c). Within this arteriovenous system, fetal blood is extremely close to the maternal blood, facilitating exchange between the fetal and maternal circulations. This newly well-oxygenated fetal blood flows into veins that follow the chorionic arteries back to the site of umbilical cord attachment. Here the veins converge, forming the large, single umbilical vein in the umbilical cord that carries the well-oxygenated blood to the fetus.

Placental Transfer

The exchange of gases, nutrients, medications, waste products, and other substances is facilitated by the large surface area of the placental membrane separating the maternal and fetal blood (Figure 2-2). As pregnancy advances, transfer of substances across the placental membrane increases because of the decreased distance between maternal and fetal blood, increased maternal and fetal blood flow, and greater fetal physiologic and metabolic demands. However, uteroplacental exchange may be altered by decreased uterine blood flow, maternal diseases (e.g., hypertension, diabetes mellitus, infection), or decreased placental surface area or diffusing capacity. Only on rare occasions can the placental membrane act as a barrier to substances (e.g., heparin, IgM) (Moore et al., 2011).

Mechanisms by which substances transfer between fetal and maternal blood across the placental membrane include simple (passive) diffusion, facilitated diffusion, active transport, pinocytosis, bulk flow, capillary breaks or leaks, independent movement, and infection. Table 2-1 summarizes these transport mechanisms and provides examples of substances transported (Blackburn, 2013c; Moore et al., 2011; Zakowski & Ramanathan, 2013).

The ability of the fetus to cope with compromises in oxygen and nutrient exchange appears as percentages of reduced blood flow in Parer's (1983) representation of placental transfer capacity (Figure 2-3). When the placental transfer capacity is near 100%, the fetus is provided with approximately twice the resources it needs to grow and be well oxygenated. This is also known as *fetal reserve*. However, at less than approximately 75% of maximal transfer capacity, fetal nutrition is limited and intrauterine growth restriction may evolve. If placental function is reduced beyond approximately 50% of maximal exchange, oxygen and carbon dioxide transfer decrease and fetal compromise can result.

FIGURE 2-2 Transfer of Substances between the Mother and Fetus across the Placental Membrane

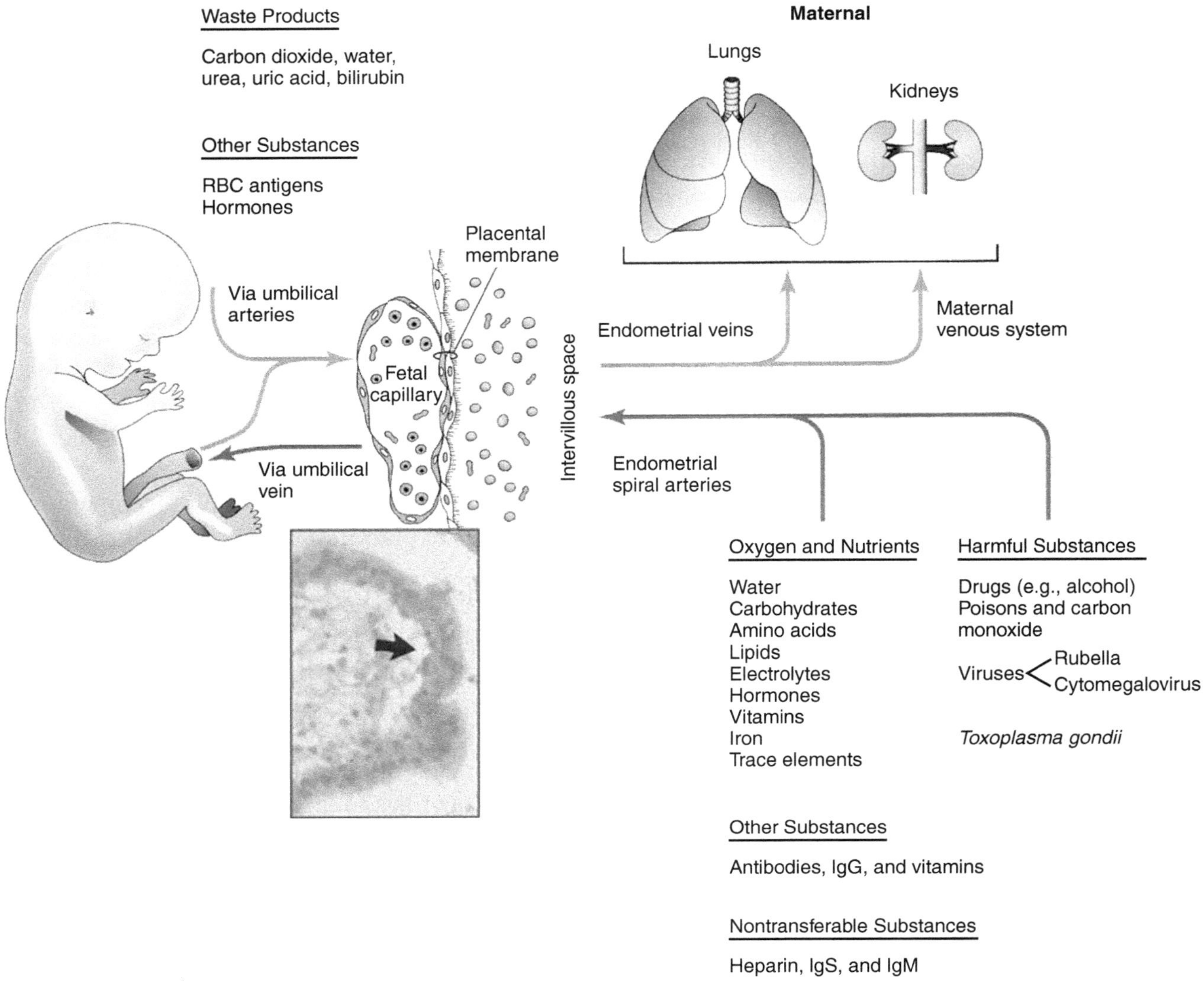

Note: From *The developing human: Clinically oriented embryology* (9th ed.)., by K. L. Moore, T. V. N. Persaud, & M. G. Torchia. Copyright 2013 by Elsevier. Reprinted with permission.

Maternal Oxygen Transport Physiology

The fetus depends on a constant supply of well-oxygenated maternal blood to maintain aerobic metabolism. Oxygen transport physiology involves four basic components: oxygen content, oxygen affinity, oxygen delivery, and oxygen consumption. Specifics relating to oxygen transport to fetal tissue are addressed later in this chapter.

Oxygen Content

Maternal oxygen content is defined as the total amount of oxygen in the maternal arterial blood and includes two components:

1. *The amount of oxygen dissolved in plasma (PaO_2), also known as the "partial pressure of oxygen" or "oxygen tension."* Because oxygen is relatively insoluble in water,

TABLE 2-1 Transport Mechanisms of Exchange Between Fetal and Maternal Blood

TRANSPORT MECHANISMS	EXAMPLE SUBSTANCES
Simple (passive) diffusion Transfer down concentration gradient (higher to lower concentration); no energy required	Water, oxygen, carbon dioxide, some electrolytes, urea, creatinine, fatty acids, steroids, fat-soluble vitamins, narcotics, barbiturates, anesthetic gases, antibiotics
Facilitated diffusion Transfer down concentration gradient involving protein transporters or carrier molecules	Glucose
Active transport Transfer against concentration gradient; carrier molecules and energy required	Amino acids, water-soluble vitamins, calcium, potassium, phosphate, iron, iodine
Pinocytosis Engulfing, and then suspending particles within small vesicles to transfer through cell (form of endocytosis)	Immunoglobulin G (IgG), phospholipids, lipoproteins, some viruses
Bulk flow Transfer resulting from changes in hydrostatic or osmotic gradient	Water, electrolytes
Breaks or leaks Transfer of substances through microscopic breaks in placental membrane	Intact blood cells
Independent movement Transfer of cells under their own power	Maternal leukocytes, microorganisms such as *Treponemapallidum* (syphilis)
Infection Transfer by creating lesions and then crossplacental membrane through defects	Some bacteria and protozoa such as *Toxoplasma gondii*

Blackburn (2013c); Moore et al. (2011); Zakowski and Ramanathan (2013).

FIGURE 2-3 Ability of the Placenta to Transport Substances (Placental Transfer Capacity) and Effects on the Fetus

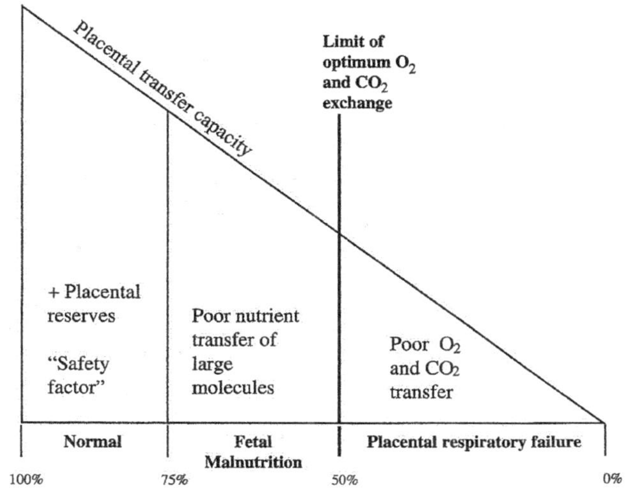

Note: From "Physiologic regulation of fetal heart rate," by J. T. Parer in *Journal of Obstetric, Gynecologic and Neonatal Nursing 5*, (p. 27S). Copyright 1976 by the Association of Women's Health, Obstretric and Neonatal Nurses.

only 1–2% of oxygen dissolves in the blood plasma. The PaO_2 helps bind oxygen molecules to hemoglobin. The amount of oxygen bound to the hemoglobin at any time is related, in large part, to the PaO_2 to which the hemoglobin is exposed. In the lungs, at the alveolar-capillary interface where the PaO_2 is typically high, oxygen binds readily to hemoglobin. As the blood circulates to other body tissues in which the PaO_2 is lower, the hemoglobin releases oxygen (Wagner, Powell, & West, 2010).

2. *Oxygen saturation or the percent of oxygen carried on the hemoglobin (SaO_2).* Approximately 98–99% of oxygen is transported by molecules of hemoglobin in red blood cells. One molecule of hemoglobin consists of four subunits, each with a heme group that has an iron atom at its center (Wagner et al., 2010). The iron binds to the oxygen; thus, each hemoglobin molecule can carry four molecules of oxygen. When a hemoglobin molecule is combined with oxygen, it is called *oxyhemoglobin*. The oxygen-carrying capacity is determined by the amount of hemoglobin present in the blood. Oxygen saturation is the ratio of oxyhemoglobin to the total amount of hemoglobin available, as illustrated in Figure 2-4.

Oxygen Affinity

The affinity of hemoglobin for oxygen is the means by which hemoglobin readily acquires and releases oxygen molecules. The dynamics of the uptake and release of oxygen by hemoglobin molecules is demonstrated in the sigmoid-shaped oxyhemoglobin dissociation curve, which relates oxygen saturation (SaO_2) and partial pressure of oxygen in the blood (PaO_2) (Figure 2-5).

At low PaO_2 levels (<50 mmHg), the oxyhemoglobin curve is steep and small changes in

FIGURE 2-4 Percent Saturation of Hemoglobin

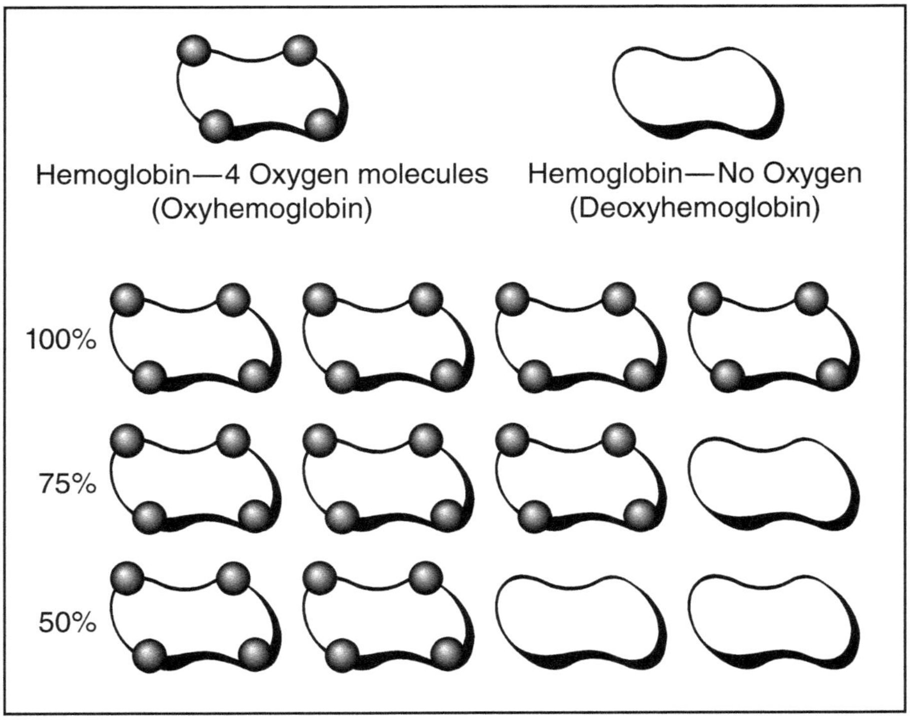

Note: From AWHONN's *high-risk and critical care obstetrics* (3rd ed., p. 34). Eds N. H. Troiano, C. J. Harvey, & B. F. Chez (2013). Copyright 2013 by the Association of Women's Health, Obstetric and Neonatal Nurses.

FIGURE 2-5 Maternal and Fetal Oxyhemoglobin Dissociation Curves

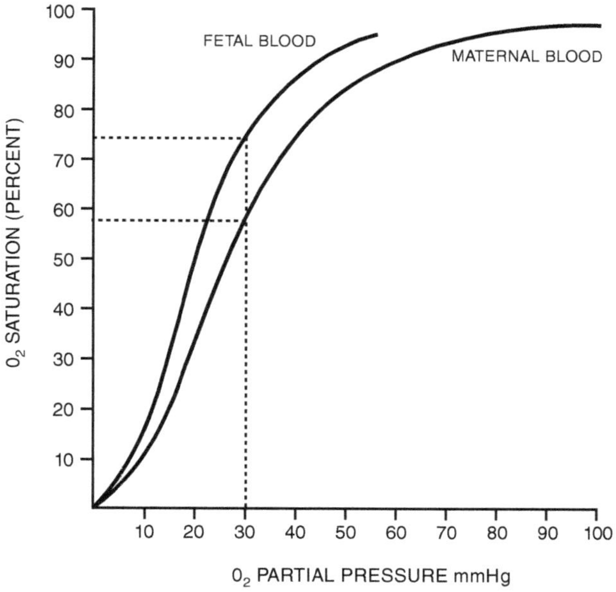

The vertical broken line illustrates the higher oxygen affinity of fetal blood. Fetal blood is more highly saturated with oxygen than maternal blood at the same oxygen partial pressure.
Note: From *Handbook of fetal heart rate monitoring* (2nd ed.). by J. T. Parer. p. 15. Copyright 1997 by W. B. Saunders. Reprinted with permission.

PaO_2 result in large changes in SaO_2 (Blackburn, 2013d). As blood circulates to other body tissue in which the PaO_2 is lower, hemoglobin readily releases oxygen into tissue as the affinity of hemoglobin for oxygen diminishes.

At the upper end of the curve where it appears relatively flat (>50 mmHg), increases in PaO_2 produce minimal increases in SaO_2 (Blackburn, 2013d). In this upper range, where the PaO_2 is typically high, oxygen binds readily to hemoglobin in the lungs.

The PaO_2 at which the hemoglobin is 50% saturated, known as the P_{50}, is typically about 26 or 27 mmHg for a healthy adult (Blackburn, 2013d; Wagner et al., 2010). In the presence of disease or other conditions that change the affinity of hemoglobin for oxygen and, consequently, shift the curve to the right or left, the P_{50} changes accordingly. An increased P_{50} indicates a rightward shift of the standard curve, implying a decreased oxygen affinity and lower saturation at any given PaO_2. This makes it more difficult for the hemoglobin to bind to oxygen (requiring a higher PaO_2 to achieve the same oxygen saturation), but it makes it easier for the hemoglobin to release bound oxygen (e.g., increase of temperature, hydrogen ion concentration, PCO_2, concentration of 2,3-diphosphoglycerate [2,3-DPG] in the red cell, or pregnancy) (Blackburn, 2013d; Bobrowski, 2010; Wagner et al., 2010). Conversely, conditions that lower P_{50} and shift the curve to the left (e.g., alkalosis, hypothermia, carbon monoxide, decreased 2,3-DPG, fetal hemoglobin) result in increased oxygen affinity, making it easier for the hemoglobin to pick up oxygen but harder to release it (Bobrowski, 2010; Wagner et al., 2010).

In pregnancy, the mother's oxyhemoglobin dissociation curve typically shifts to the right, enhancing the transfer of oxygen from the mother to the fetus (see Figure 2-5). At term, the P_{50} increases from approximately 26 to 30 mmHg (Blackburn, 2013d). Because the fetal hemoglobin has a higher affinity for oxygen compared with maternal hemoglobin, the fetal oxyhemoglobin curve shifts to the left of the mother's curve, thereby further enhancing oxygen uptake by the fetus.

Oxygen Delivery

The quantity of oxygen delivered to the tissues per unit of time is known as oxygen delivery (DO_2). Both cardiac output and arterial oxygen content (i.e., PaO_2 and SaO_2) affect the delivery of oxygen from the lungs to the tissues. Factors that increase maternal cardiac output (e.g., exercise, uterine contractions, increased metabolism, certain medications) or increase total arterial oxygen content (e.g., transfusion of packed red blood cells) increase oxygen delivery to the tissues (Troiano & Gaddipati, 2013). Factors that decrease either maternal cardiac output or oxygen content (e.g., hypovolemia, hypoxemia, anemia) may decrease oxygen delivery (Troiano, 1999; Troiano & Gaddipati, 2013).

Maternal hemoglobin and arterial oxygen content typically decrease as a result of the physiologic anemia of pregnancy. However, oxygen delivery is maintained at or above normal because maternal cardiac output increases 50% by the third trimester of pregnancy and an additional 20% during labor (Bobrowski, 2010). Thus, the pregnant woman, as compared with the nonpregnant patient, is more dependent on cardiac output for oxygen delivery. Because the healthy pregnant woman's oxygen delivery normally exceeds her oxygen consumption, even during labor, she is able to maintain adequate oxygen delivery to both herself and her fetus (Bobrowski, 2010). However, if the pregnant woman's oxygen delivery decreases, especially during labor, both she and her fetus can rapidly become seriously compromised (Bobrowski, 2010).

Oxygen Consumption

Oxygen consumption is a reflection of metabolic rate or the rate at which oxygen is consumed by the tissues each minute. Under normal conditions, the human body consumes approximately 25% of the total oxygen available (Troiano & Gaddipati, 2013). When the supply of oxygen is reduced, or if oxygen consumption is high (e.g., as a result of pregnancy, hyperthermia, stress), more oxygen is extracted from the blood so that oxygen consumption is maintained. During pregnancy, oxygen consumption increases 20% and an additional 10% in twin gestations due to increased metabolic demands (Bobrowski, 2010). During labor, oxygen consumption increases approximately 40–60% (Blackburn, 2013d; Bobrowski, 2010). If oxygen delivery is severely reduced and the tissues are unable to sustain aerobic metabolism, oxygen consumption decreases and the tissues begin to use anaerobic glycolysis, resulting in metabolic acidosis and, eventually, irreversible tissue damage and death (Zakowski & Ramanathan, 2013).

Uterine Blood Flow

Adequate uterine blood flow is critical for the passage of respiratory gases and substances across the placenta (Blackburn, 2013c; Parer, 1997; Zakowski & Ramanathan, 2013). The rate of uterine blood flow progressively increases throughout pregnancy from 50 mL/min to approximately 700 mL/min at term, representing 10% of maternal cardiac output (Zakowski & Ramanathan, 2013). Approximately 70–90% of the uterine blood flow circulates through the intervillous space, while the remainder of the blood primarily supplies the myometrium and endometrium (Ross, Ervin, & Novak, 2012; Zakowski & Ramanathan, 2013). Because the maternal spiral arteries carrying oxygenated blood to the intervillous space are maximally dilated and have lost some ability to "autoregulate" or constrict, decreased uterine blood flow can adversely affect the fetus. In clinical practice, there exist few useful means of increasing uterine blood flow after it becomes suboptimal (Zakowski & Ramanathan, 2013). However, clinicians can be aware of and manage clinical situations that have the potential to decrease uterine blood flow and uteroplacental perfusion. Box 2-1 lists clinical factors that have the potential to decrease uterine blood flow. Examples of interventions to maximize uterine blood flow during labor would include promoting adequately spaced uterine contractions, use of side lying positions or ambulation, and maintenance of maternal blood pressure with regional analgesia. See Chapter 6 for further discussion of supportive physiologic interventions.

Umbilical Cord

The umbilical cord is the vascular connection between the placenta and fetus. Normally, the umbilical cord contains three vessels—two arteries and one vein—that spiral within the cord. The single umbilical vein carries the oxygen-rich blood from the placenta to the fetus; the two arteries return from the fetus carrying deoxygenated blood. Wharton's jelly, a mucoid connective tissue, helps protect the umbilical cord from compression.

At term, the normal umbilical cord averages 55–60 cm in length (Benirschke, 2009b; Blackburn, 2013c). Cord length is influenced by amniotic fluid volume, fetal movement, and genetics (Blackburn, 2013c; Marino, 2004). Twisting and spiraling of the umbilical vessels

BOX 2-1 Factors That May Decrease Uterine Blood Flow

Excessive uterine activity
- Uterine tachysystole
- Uterine hypertonus
- Uterine stimulants (oxytocin, prostaglandins)
- Abruptio placenta

Maternal hypotension
- Supine hypotensive syndrome (vena caval compression)
- Regional analgesia/anesthesia (sympathetic block)
- Hypovolemia
- Low cardiac output

Maternal hypertension

Placental changes
- Decreased surface area (abruptio placenta)
- Degenerative (hypertension, prolonged pregnancy, diabetes)
- Calcifications (smoking)
- Infarction (abruptio placenta, prolonged pregnancy)
- Infection (chorioamnionitis)
- Edema (erythroblastosis fetalis)

Vasoconstriction, endogenous
- Sympathetic discharge
- Adrenal medullary activity

Vasoconstriction, exogenous
- Most sympathomimetics (alpha-adrenergic effects). Ephedrine is exception (primarily beta-adrenergic effect)

Adapted from Zakowski and Ramanathan (2013).

within the cord are thought to protect the cord against compression and entanglement (Blackburn, 2013c). These twists may form false knots, creating varicosities of umbilical vessels that may protrude on the cord surface and have no clinical significance (Benirschke, 2009b). Frequently, the umbilical cord becomes wrapped around fetal body parts, particularly the fetal neck (nuchal cord). While a single nuchal cord is usually an incidental finding, the presence of multiple nuchal cords has been associated with variable decelerations, meconium-stained amniotic fluid, need for neonatal resuscitation, and lower umbilical artery pH (Jauniaux, Ramsay, Peellaerts, & Scholler, 1995; Marino, 2004).

Attachment of the umbilical cord is usually near the center of the fetal surface. Cord insertion at the placental margin is sometimes referred to as "Battledore placenta." With a velamentous insertion, the umbilical vessels run between the amnion and chorion without the protection of Wharton's jelly. Vasa previa may occur when the unprotected vessels from a velamentous cord insertion pass over the cervical os or over the dividing membrane when the second twin's cord has a velamentous insertion on the dividing membrane (Benirschke, 2009a).

In antenatal testing, umbilical artery Doppler assessments may be used to assess growth-restricted fetuses. In normally growing fetuses, umbilical artery waveforms are characterized by high-velocity diastolic flow. However, in growth-restricted fetuses, umbilical artery diastolic flow is diminished, absent, or reversed in severe cases and associated with fetal hypoxia and increased perinatal morbidity and mortality (Signore, Freeman, & Spong, 2009). Doppler assessments are discussed further in Chapter 10.

Umbilical cord compression is the physiologic basis for FHR changes that are described as variable decelerations. In Lee, Di Loreto, and O'Lane's (1975) classic figure (Figure 2-6), FHR and fetal systemic blood pressure are shown in relationship to umbilical artery and umbilical vein compression occurring during a uterine contraction. Partial umbilical cord compression may cause occlusion of the low-pressure vein, leading to decreased return of blood to the fetal heart, decreased cardiac output, hypotension, and a compensatory FHR "acceleration" (Freeman, Garite, Nageotte, & Miller, 2012; James et al., 1976; Lee et al., 1975). With complete cord occlusion, the two umbilical arteries become occluded, resulting in sudden fetal hypertension, stimulation of the baroreceptors, and a sudden drop in FHR resulting in a variable deceleration (Freeman et al., 2012; Lee & Hon, 1963). Although Lee et al. described umbilical cord compression in relationship to uterine contractions, any etiology of umbilical cord compression may cause the same mechanism and subsequent variable decelerations.

FIGURE 2-6 FHR and Fetal Systemic Blood Pressure (FSBP) Occurring during a Uterine Contraction (UC) with Compression of Umbilical Vein (UV) and Umbilical Artery (UA)

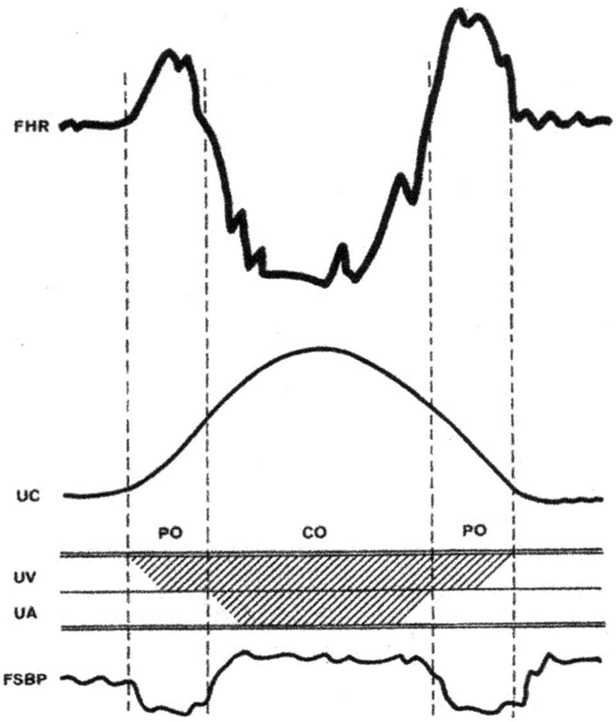

Note: From "A study of fetal heart rate acceleration patterns," by C. V. Lee, P. C. Di Loreto, and J. M. O'Lane, *Obstetrics and Gynecology*, *50*, p. 142. Copyright 1975 by the American College of Obstetricians and Gynecologists. Reprinted with permission.

Amniotic Fluid

Amniotic fluid provides several critical functions in the normal growth and development of the fetus (Box 2-2). Although wide variations exist, amniotic fluid volume normally increases from 10–20 mL at 10 weeks' gestation to approximately 800 mL at 24 weeks (Brace, 1997; Gilbert, 2012). Subsequently, increases in volume slow, and little change occurs until 36–38 weeks, after which volume begins to decrease progressively (Beall & Ross, 2012; Brace, 1997). Amniotic fluid volume is maintained by a balance of fetal fluid production (fetal urine and liquid lung secretions) and fluid reabsorption (fetal swallowing and flow across fetal membranes and placenta) (Gilbert, 2012). At term, a normal fetus can swallow 400 mL amniotic fluid per day (Moore et al., 2011).

BOX 2-2 Critical Functions of Amniotic Fluid

- Provides space for symmetric fetal growth
- Allows free fetal movement, aiding muscular development
- Permits normal fetal lung development
- Prevents adherence of amnion to fetus
- Maintains relatively constant temperature
- Protects and cushions fetus against impacts
- Distributes pressure from uterine contractions evenly
- Acts as barrier to infection
- Maintains homeostasis of fluids and electrolytes
- Provides access to fetal cells for fetal diagnoses

Beall & Ross (2009); Blackburn (2013c); Moore et al. (2011).

Estimation of amniotic fluid volume (AFV) is an integral part of both the biophysical profile (BPP) and the modified BPP tests of fetal health. The BPP combines real-time ultrasonography observations of amniotic fluid volume, fetal breathing movements, fetal movement, and fetal tone along with the NST to provide a composite score of 0–10. While fetal breathing, body movements, tone, and the NST assess acute signs of fetal hypoxia, amniotic fluid volume is the only marker for chronic hypoxia (Signore et al., 2009). The modified BPP combines amniotic fluid volume (indicator of long-term placental function) and the NST (short-term indicator of fetal status).

Recent data from several randomized control trials recommend amniotic fluid volume be estimated by the use of a single deepest vertical pocket (ACOG, 2014). A measurement of greater than 2 cm is evidence of adequate AFV whereas a measurement of 2 cm or less (not containing umbilical cord or fetal extremities) is used to diagnose oligohydramnios which should prompt further evaluation (ACOG, 2014). These assessments are discussed in further detail in Chapter 10.

Abnormalities in amniotic fluid volume often require further evaluation and can significantly impact perinatal outcome. The underlying etiology of the decrease or absence of amniotic fluid determines perinatal outcome. For example, with premature rupture of membranes and a significant loss of amniotic fluid, a low amniotic measurement is no longer valid for prediction of decreased placental function; rather neonatal outcome is determined by gestational age and the presence of intra-amniotic infection. If oligohydramnios (AFV <2 cm) is present with intact membranes, decision to proceed with expectant management or deliver should be individualized based on gestational age and maternal and fetal condition (ACOG, 2014). If the cause for oligohydramnios is renal agenesis (failure of kidney formation), approximately 100% of neonates will die as a result of pulmonary hypoplasia (Gilbert, 2012).

Hydramnios, or excessive amniotic fluid, complicates approximately 1% of all pregnancies (Gilbert, 2012; Marino, 2004). As with oligiohydramnios, the underlying etiology determines perinatal outcome. While many cases of hydramnios are idiopathic, when a cause is identified, almost 80% will have moderate to severe hydramnios (Panting-Kemp, Nguyen, Chang, Quillan, & Castro, 1999). Fetal gastrointestinal obstructions (e.g., esophageal atresia with or without tracheosophageal fistula or duodenal atresia) can result in early-onset severe hydramnios (Gilbert, 2012). Severe hydramnios in the second trimester is associated with a significant increase in aneuploidy, congenital malformations, preterm birth, and perinatal mortality (Gilbert, 2012). In contrast, mild hydramnios, especially when identified toward the end of the third trimester, is usually idiopathic, or related to diabetes mellitus, and has little impact on perinatal outcome (Gilbert, 2012).

PHYSIOLOGY UNDERLYING INTRINSIC INFLUENCES ON THE FHR

Fetal Circulation

Fetal circulation differs significantly from that of the adult. In the adult, respiratory gases exchange in the pulmonary vasculature and oxygenated blood returns via the pulmonary veins to the left ventricle to be ejected into the adult circulation. In the fetus, blood does not need to enter the lungs to become oxygenated; rather, oxygenation occurs in the placenta. Another difference is that the ventricles of the fetal heart work in parallel, not in a series as in the adult configuration. Well-oxygenated fetal blood enters the left ventricle, which supplies the heart and brain, and less-oxygenated blood enters the right ventricle, which supplies the rest of the body. This presence of oxygenated blood in the right and left atria and great vessels is unique to the fetus and made possible by several anatomic shunts (e. g., foramen ovale and ductus arteriosus). A third shunt, the ductus venosus, allows relatively well-oxygenated blood to enter the fetal heart directly, bypassing the liver. At birth, when circulation of fetal blood through the placenta ceases and the neonate's lungs expand, these anatomic shunts normally close rapidly and cease to function.

Fetal circulation is illustrated in Figure 2-7. Highly oxygenated, nutrient-rich blood returns from the placenta via the umbilical vein. As the umbilical vein approaches the liver, approximately 70–80% of the oxygen-rich blood enters the sinusoids of the liver, reflecting the increased demand of the fetal liver near term (Blackburn, 2013a; Kiserud, 2001). The blood then drains via the hepatic vein into the inferior vena cava, where it mixes with desaturated blood returning from the lower body. The remaining 20–30% of oxygen-rich blood in the umbilical vein is shunted via the ductus venosus directly into the inferior vena cava. This richly oxygenated blood from the umbilical vein has a greater oxygen content and kinetic energy, resulting in a distinct "stream" of blood as it enters the right atrium (Blackburn, 2013a; Edelstone & Rudolph, 1979; Fineman & Clyman, 2009; Kiserud, 2001).

As the well-oxygenated umbilical venous blood streams preferentially across the foramen ovale into the left atrium, it mixes with a small amount of pulmonary venous return, passes through the mitral valve, and is then ejected by the left ventricle into the ascending aorta. This preferential streaming allows the most highly oxygenated umbilical venous blood to supply the coronary circulation and vessels that supply the head, neck, and upper extremities (Edelstone &

FIGURE 2-7 Fetal Circulation

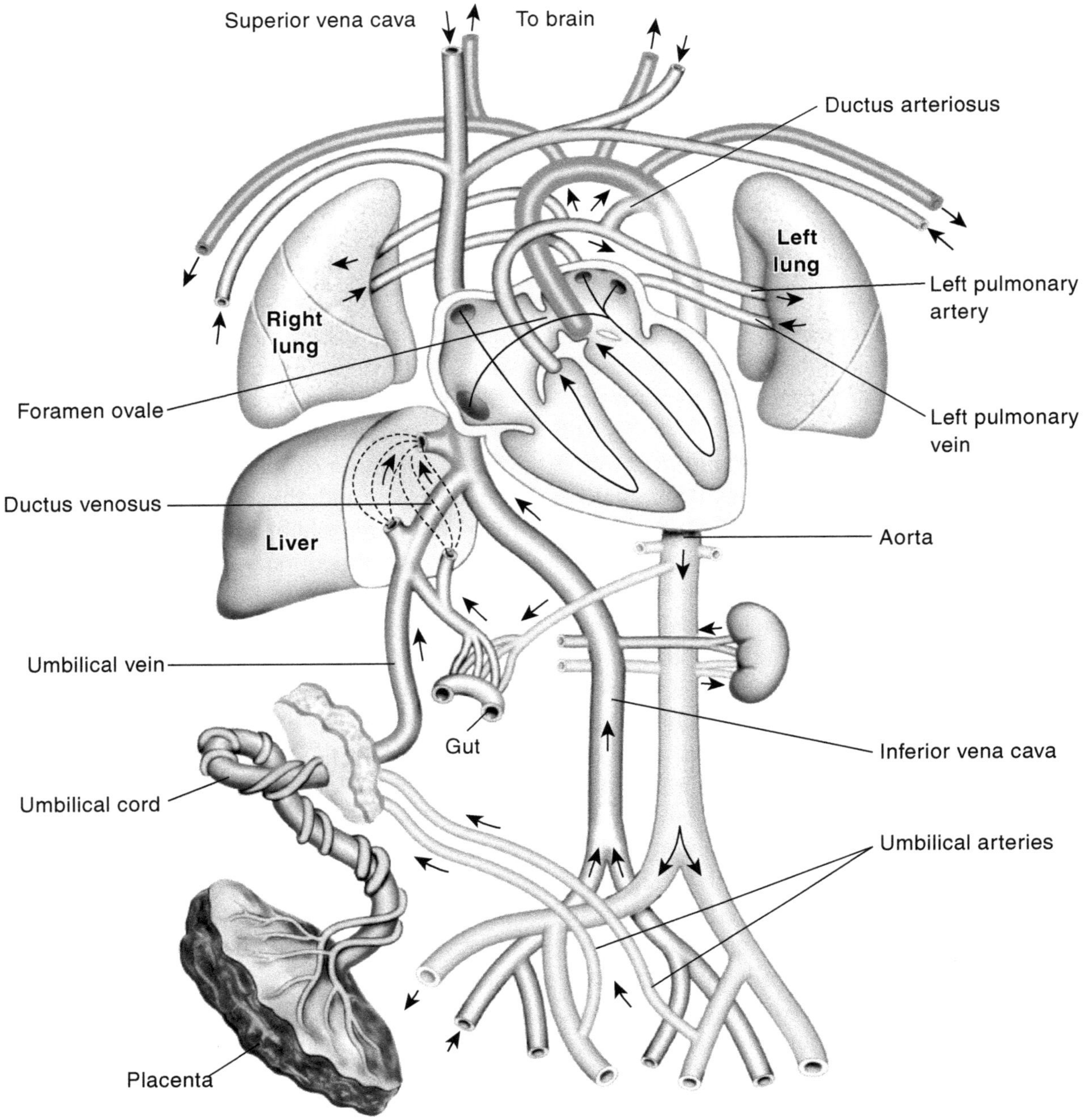

Rudolph, 1979; Fineman & Clyman, 2009). The second stream of blood, which consists of desaturated blood returning from the lower body, the liver, and some umbilical venous return, mixes in the right atrium with blood returning in the superior vena cava and coronary sinus. From here, a small amount enters the pulmonary artery and lung tissue. Most of the remaining second stream (that which does not go through the foramen ovale or to the lungs) is directed downward across the tricuspid valve, into the right ventricle, and is then shunted across the ductus arteriosus to enter the descending aorta. The descending aorta supplies the gut, kidneys, lower body, and umbilical circulation. This preferential streaming of blood returning from the superior vena cava and coronary sinus is advantageous to the fetus because it directs the desaturated blood toward the placenta for reoxygenation (Fineman & Clyman, 2009).

At birth, major physiologic and anatomic transitional events occur in the neonatal circulation. Oxygenation moves from the placenta to the neonate's lungs, resulting in a dramatic fall in pulmonary vascular resistance, increased pulmonary blood flow, and a rise in PO_2 levels (Blackburn, 2013a). Under normal circumstances, the neonate's ventricles begin working in sequence, as in the adult configuration, rather than in parallel. Finally, fetal shunts close and cease to function. The ductus venosus functionally closes within minutes of birth because of the cessation of blood flow. Pressure changes within the cardiac chambers close the flap of the foramen ovale that separates the two atria. The ductus arteriosus begins to constrict at birth yet may remain patent for several days.

Oxygen Transport to the Fetus

The fetal umbilical vein, which carries the well-oxygenated blood from the placenta to the fetus, has approximately the same amount of dissolved oxygen (partial pressure oxygen or PO_2) as in the maternal uterine vein (Meschia, 2009). Despite a low PO_2, the fetal blood transports large amounts of oxygen from the placenta to the body tissues. Several physiologic adaptations make this possible (King, 2013; King & Parer, 2000; Martin & Gingerich, 1976; Meschia, 2009; Parer, 1997):

- Fetal blood has a higher hemoglobin concentration than adult blood, allowing for greater oxygen-carrying capacity.
- Fetal hemoglobin has a higher affinity for oxygen compared with the mother's blood, an important adaptation to the low PO_2 at which the placenta oxygenates the fetus. The fetal oxyhemoglobin dissociation curve favors a higher saturation of the hemoglobin with oxygen at any given PO_2. As shown previously, Figure 2-5 compares the oxygen dissociation curves for the maternal and fetal blood. At a PO_2 of 30 mmHg and blood pH of 7.4, fetal blood is approximately 74% saturated with oxygen, whereas maternal blood is only 58% saturated.
- The fetus has a higher heart rate and cardiac output relative to its body size compared to the adult.

These adaptations support efficient exchange of respiratory gases and fetal aerobic metabolism. Aerobic metabolism appears to be maintained until the available oxygen in the intervillous space decreases to 50% of normal levels (King, 2013; Parer, 1997; Zakowski & Ramanathan, 2013). With transient hypoxemia, the normoxic fetus compensates with the following mechanisms to maintain oxygen supply to vital organs (Cohn, Sacks, Heymann, & Rudolph, 1974; King, 2013; Parer, 1997; Zakowski & Ramanathan, 2013):

- *Redistribution of fetal blood flow favoring vital organs.* Blood flow to the heart, brain, and adrenal glands is increased two- to three-fold; blood flow to the gut, spleen, kidneys and limbs is decreased (Figure 2-8).
- *Decrease in total O_2 consumption.* As the FHR slows in response to hypoxia, the myocardium consumes less oxygen. With moderate hypoxia, fetal oxygen consumption drops to 50% of the normal level.

If these temporary compensatory measures do not supply sufficient oxygen for fetal metabolic needs, anaerobic metabolism follows with accumulation of lactic acid, resulting in metabolic acidemia (accumulation of lactic acid in the blood) and metabolic acidosis (accumulation of lactic acid in the tissues). Without restoration of fetal oxygenation, metabolic acidosis will progress to asphyxia and arterial oxygenation will fall below critical levels (King, 2013; Parer, 1997). Decreases in fetal cardiac output, arterial blood pressure, and blood flow to the heart and brain are followed by myocardial depression, brain ischemia, and, ultimately, fetal death (Nageotte & Gilstrap, 2009; Parer, 1997).

Fetal Heart Rate Control

The source of integration for FHR control is the cardioregulatory center (CRC), a loosely defined collection of neurons in the ventral and lateral surface of the medulla oblongata (Blackburn, 2013a; Manning, 1995) (Figure 2-9). The CRC receives input from a variety of sources, and these signals interact with neurons to alter output. Output from the CRC radiates throughout

FIGURE 2-8 Schematic Illustration of the Redistribution of Blood Flow that Occurs during Fetal Hypoxia

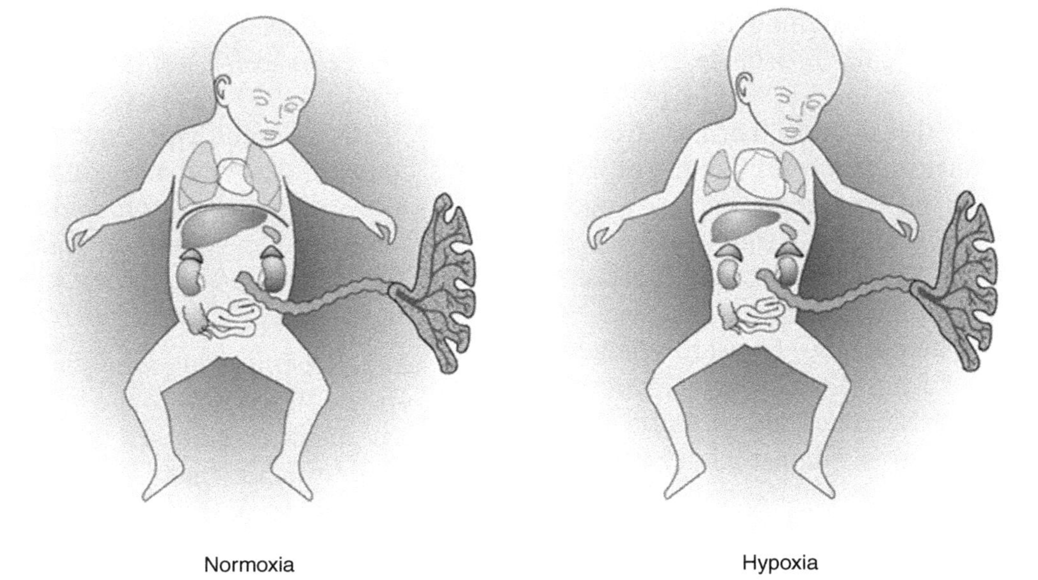

FIGURE 2-9 Cerebral Influences on Fetal Heart Rate

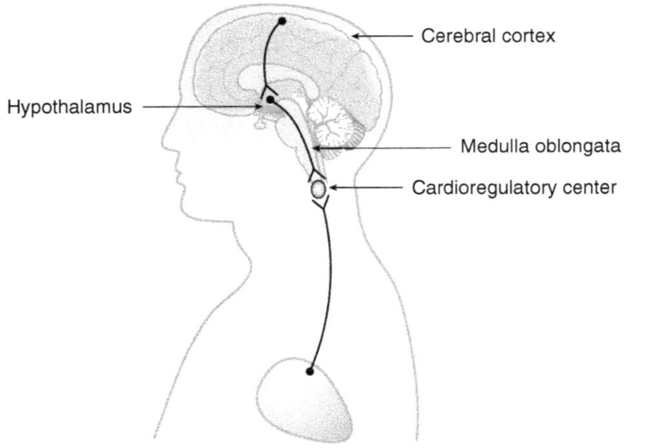

Note: From "Physiologic regulation of fetal heart rate," by J. T. Parer in *Journal of Obstetric, Gynecologic and Neonatal Nursing, 5,* (p. 27S). Copyright 1976 by the Association of Women's Health, Obstretric and Neonatal Nurses.

most organ systems and to adjacent higher centers within the fetal brain. The integration of these influences from the CRC exerts control over FHR. baseline rate, variability, and various FHR patterns provide indirect insights into the functioning of the central nervous system.

Parasympathetic and sympathetic branches of the autonomic nervous system, baroreceptors, chemoreceptors, fetal hormones, sleep–wake cycles, breathing movements, painful stimuli, sound and vibrations, and temperature interact with the CRC to influence FHR. Research using animal models, coupled with the ongoing clinical evaluation of associations observed between FHR tracings and fetal outcomes, has led to progressive improvement in our understanding of how these factors regulate heart rate in humans. Major factors believed to influence the integration of FHR control are outlined in Table 2-2.

Parasympathetic Nervous System

The parasympathetic branch of the autonomic nervous system is perhaps the most important controlling mechanism of the FHR. Parasympathetic supply to the heart travels from the CRC in the ventral surface of the fetal medulla via the vagus or 10th cranial nerve. The right and left branches of the vagus nerve innervate the sinoatrial (SA) and atrioventricular nodes within the fetal heart. Stimulation of the vagus nerve causes marked slowing of the FHR, an effect mediated by the release of acetylcholine from the nerve endings; this causes a decrease in the firing of

TABLE 2-2 Factors Influencing FHR Control

INFLUENCE	ACTION	FHR EFFECT
Cardioregulatory Center: • Collection of neurons in ventral and lateral surface of medulla oblongata	• Integrating source for control of FHR • Interacts with parasympathetic and sympathetic nervous systems, baroreceptors, chemoreceptors, fetal hormones, sleep–wake cycles, breathing movements, painful stimuli, sound, vibrations, and temperature to influence FHR	• Baseline heart rate, variability, and various FHR patterns provide indirect insights into functioning of central nervous system
Parasympathetic Branch of the Autonomic Nervous System: • Originates in medulla oblongata • Vagus nerve (10th cranial) innervates SA and AV nodes	• Stimulation releases acetylcholine • Pathway for transmission of variability	• ↓ FHR • Slow, gradual ↓ FHR with ↑ gestational age (approximately 10 bpm difference in baseline FHR between 28 weeks and term) • Maintains transmission of beat-to-beat variability • Moderate variability indicates absence of severe hypoxia or metabolic acidemia • Modulates baseline FHR with sympathetic branch
Sympathetic Branch of the Autonomic Nervous System: • At term, nerve fibers widely distributed throughout myocardium	• Stimulation releases catecholamines (e.g., norepinephrine, epinephrine) • Reserve mechanism to improve the heart's pumping ability during intermittent stress • Catecholamines can also cause fetal vasoconstriction and hypertension	• ↑ FHR • Blocking with propranolol results in ↓ FHR of approximately 10 bpm • Modulates baseline FHR with parasympathetic branch
• **Baroreceptors:** • Protective, stretch receptors • Located in aortic arch and carotid sinuses at bifurcation of external and internal carotid arteries	• When ↑ arterial BP, the baroreceptors quickly detect amount of stretch, sending impulses via vagus nerve to midbrain • Impulses return via vagus nerve, causing sudden ↓ FHR, ↓ CO, and ↓ blood pressure, thereby protecting fetus	• Abrupt ↓ FHR • Abrupt ↓ CO • Abrupt ↓ blood pressure • Variable decelerations with moderate variability are baroreceptor influenced
Chemoreceptors: • Central—located in medulla oblongata • Peripheral—in aortic arch and carotid sinuses	*In the adult:* • When arterial blood perfusing chemoreceptors contains ↑ PCO_2 or ↓ PO_2: – Central—chemoreceptors respond with reflex tachycardia and hypertension, most likely in an attempt to circulate blood and ↓ PCO_2 – Peripheral—chemoreceptors, respond with bradycardia	*In the fetus:* • Interaction of central and peripheral chemoreceptors poorly understood • Combined effect is slowing of FHR • Described in mechanisms of late decelerations and variable decelerations resulting from umbilical arterial occlusion coupled with hypoxemia • When blood flow is below threshold for normal respiratory gas exchange, ↑ PCO_2 stimulates chemoreceptors to slow FHR

(continued)

TABLE 2-2 (Continued)

INFLUENCE	ACTION	FHR EFFECT
Hormonal Regulation:		
• Epinephrine and norepinephrine secreted from the adrenal medulla	• In response to stressful situations, compensatory response shunts blood away from less vital organs and toward brain, heart, and adrenal glands	• ↑ FHR, ↑ strength of cardiac contractions, ↑ CO, ↑ arterial BP
• Arginine vasopressin secreted from posterior pituitary	• In adult, responds to ↓ plasma volume, ↑ plasma osmolarity • In fetal sheep, hypoxemia most potent stimulus; distributes blood flow	• ↑ FHR, ↑ cardiac output, ↑ arterial BP • Sinusoidal heart rate in experimental animal studies
• Renin–angiotensin–aldosterone secreted from kidneys	• Responds to ↓ plasma volume or ↓ BP; protects fetus from hemorrhagic stress by stimulating vasoconstriction	• ↑ FHR, ↑ cardiac output, ↑ arterial BP
Cardiac Output:		
• In the adult, CO = HR × SV • The Frank Starling mechanism dictates: ↑ inflow of blood into heart stretches cardiac muscle, thereby resulting in ↑ force of contraction and ↑ SV	• Compared to adult, fetal SV does not fluctuate significantly; fetal heart appears to operate near the top of its cardiac function curve	• Therefore, fetal CO ≈ HR • At extreme rates (e.g., tachycardia >240 bpm or bradycardia <60 bpm), CO can be significantly decreased

AV, atrioventricular; BP, blood pressure; bpm, beats per minute; CO, cardiac output; FHR, fetal heart rate; HR, heart rate; PCO_2, partial pressure of carbon dioxide; PO_2, partial pressure of oxygen; SA, sinoatrial; SV, stroke volume.

the SA node and slows the rate of transmission to the ventricles (King, 2013; Parer, 1997).

The slow, gradual decrease in FHR observed with advancing gestational age is due to the increased dominance of parasympathetic influence on the fetal heart (Dalton, Dawes, & Patrick, 1983; Renou, Newman, & Wood, 1969). The fetal heart is similar to the adult heart, with the SA node functioning as the intrinsic pacemaker, setting the rate in the normal heart. The average baseline FHR in the normal fetus at 20 weeks' gestation is 155 beats per minute (bpm); at 30 weeks, 144 bpm; and at term before labor, 140 bpm (normal range, 110–160 bpm) (Parer, 1997). Although resting FHR decreases with advancing gestational age because of increased parasympathetic tone, the difference in baseline FHR between 28 and 30 weeks' gestation and term is approximately 10 bpm. Therefore, any preterm fetus with a baseline FHR greater than 160 bpm should be evaluated further to rule out fetal compromise, rather than just assuming the tachycardia is secondary to prematurity (Freeman et al., 2012).

The second primary function of the vagus nerve is the transmission of beat-to-beat irregularity or variability resulting from the irregular fluctuations in time between consecutive fetal cardiac cycles. Blocking the vagus nerve with atropine (a substance that blocks the effects of acetylcholine) results in the disappearance of beat-to-beat variability (Dalton et al., 1983; Parer, 1997).

FHR variability is a reflection of neuromodulation of an active central nervous system (CNS) and normal cardiac responsiveness. The presence of FHR variability represents an intact nervous pathway through the cerebral cortex, the midbrain, the vagus nerve, and the normal cardiac conduction system (Parer, 1983, 1997). When the fetus is alert and active, the CNS responds with moderate FHR variability. If fetal brain function is reduced, FHR variability decreases. Potential causes of decreased variability include fetal sleep cycles, medications (e.g., narcotics, barbiturates, tranquilizers, general anesthesia), extreme prematurity, previous neurologic insult, or anatomic brain damage. Because severe hypoxia and metabolic acidosis will decrease CNS function, the presence of moderate FHR variability reliably indicates a well-oxygenated fetus without metabolic acidosis at the time it is observed (Freeman et al., 2012; Parer, 1997).

Sympathetic Nervous System

The sympathetic nervous system provides a reserve mechanism to improve the heart's pumping ability during intermittent stress (King, 2013). Nerve fibers from the sympathetic branch of the autonomic nervous system are widely distributed throughout fetal myocardium at term. Stimulation of these nerve fibers releases catecholamines (e.g., norepinephrine, epinephrine), causing an increase in FHR. Blocking the action of these sympathetic nerve fibers with propranolol results in a decrease in FHR of approximately 10 bpm (Parer, 1997). The effect of sympathetic stimulation in the fetus is not easily understood. Most observed FHR changes represent an integration of a variety of stimulant and inhibitory inputs. Although catecholamines have an accelerative effect on the FHR, these sympathetic agents also cause fetal vasoconstriction and fetal hypertension, which excite baroreceptor discharge and may cause reflex slowing of the FHR (Manning, 1995).

Although the parasympathetic and sympathetic nervous systems appear to work together to modulate baseline FHR, it is unclear whether they have a distinctly separate or combined role in the transmission of FHR variability (Parer, 1997). Animal research has demonstrated important species differences in the influence of the sympathetic nervous system on FHR variability. Parasympathetic stimulation appears to have a greater influence than sympathetic regulation on the transmission of FHR variability (Parer, 1997).

Baroreceptors

Baroreceptors are protective stretch receptors located in the aortic arch and the carotid sinuses at the bifurcation of the external and internal carotid arteries (Figure 2-10). When fetal arterial blood pressure increases, the baroreceptors

FIGURE 2-10 The Peripheral Chemoreceptors and Baroreceptors and Their Input to the Cardiac Regulating Center in the Medulla Oblongata

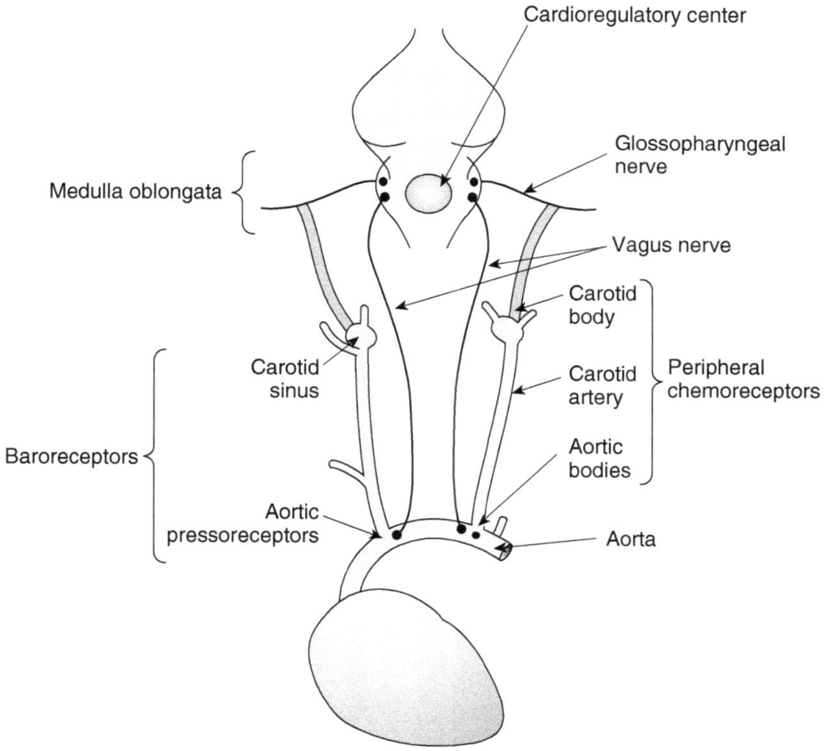

Note: From "Physiologic regulation of fetal heart rate," by J. T. Parer in *Journal of Obstetric, Gynecologic and Neonatal Nursing, 5,* (p. 28S) Copyright 1976 by the Association of Women's Health, Obstretric and Neonatal Nurses.

quickly detect the amount of stretch and send impulses via the vagus nerve to the midbrain. Returning impulses via the vagus nerve cause a sudden decrease in FHR, cardiac output, and blood pressure, thereby protecting the fetus from the deleterious effects of excessive arterial pressures.

Lee et al.'s (1975) classic illustration of a variable deceleration (see Figure 2-6) depicts the relationship between the variable deceleration, a uterine contraction, umbilical cord compression, and fetal blood pressure. As a contraction begins, partial umbilical cord compression causes occlusion of the low-pressure vein and decreased return of blood to the fetal heart, resulting in decreased cardiac output, hypotension, and a compensatory FHR "acceleration" (Freeman et al., 2012; James et al., 1976; Lee et al., 1975). With complete umbilical cord occlusion, the two umbilical arteries also become occluded, resulting in sudden fetal hypertension, stimulation of the baroreceptors, and a sudden drop in FHR (Freeman et al., 2012; Lee & Hon, 1963). As the contraction begins to dissipate, the umbilical arteries open first, and a transient increase in FHR (a "secondary acceleration") may be seen. Finally, the contraction subsides and all three umbilical vessels are open, returning the FHR to predeceleration values.

Chemoreceptors

Chemoreceptors primarily function to regulate respiratory activity and control circulation by responding to changes in arterial PO_2, partial pressure of carbon dioxide (PCO_2), and acid-base balance. Central chemoreceptors are located in the medulla oblongata, and peripheral chemoreceptors are found in the carotid sinuses and aortic arch (see Figure 2-10). The interaction of the central and peripheral chemoreceptors is better understood in the adult than in the human fetus.

In the adult, when arterial blood perfusing the central chemoreceptors contains increased PCO_2 or decreased PO_2, reflex tachycardia and hypertension occur, most likely in an attempt to circulate blood and decrease the PCO_2. In contrast, when increased PCO_2 or decreased PO_2 are detected by the peripheral chemoreceptors, bradycardia ensues (Parer, 1997).

In the fetus, the function of central and peripheral chemoreceptors is not well understood. Fetal chemoreceptor stimulation has been described in the mechanism of late decelerations and in the mechanism of variable decelerations resulting from umbilical arterial occlusion coupled with hypoxemia (Freeman et al., 2012; Parer, 1997). In both situations, when blood flow falls below the threshold for normal respiratory gas exchange, increased PCO_2 stimulates the chemoreceptors, resulting in activation of the CRC and slowing of the FHR.

Hormonal Influences

The release of hormones by the adrenal glands, sympathetic nerves, hypothalamus, pituitary gland, and other fetal organs is believed to play an important role in fetal hemodynamic compensatory responses to stressors. The fetus responds to stress by releasing hormones that play a role in fetal circulatory regulation, allowing maximal perfusion to vital organs, primarily the fetal brain, heart, and adrenal glands. Key hormones that influence fetal circulation and FHR control include epinephrine, norepinephrine, arginine vasopressin, and hormones in the renin-angiotensin-aldosterone system.

When the fetus is stressed, catecholamines (e.g., epinephrine, norepinephrine) are secreted from the adrenal medulla. Epinephrine and norepinephrine increase FHR, increase force of myocardial contractions, and increase arterial blood pressure, similar to sympathetic stimulation (Parer, 1997). This compensatory response shunts blood away from the less vital organs and toward the brain, heart, and adrenal glands.

In the adult, arginine vasopressin (antidiuretic hormone) is released from the posterior pituitary gland in response to decreases in plasma volume and increases in plasma osmolarity. In fetal sheep, hypoxemia is the most potent stimulus known for arginine vasopressin secretion (Ross et al., 2012).

Arginine vasopressin has been shown to affect the distribution of blood flow, thereby increasing FHR, cardiac output, and arterial blood pressure (Ross et al., 2012). Murata et al. (1985) implicated arginine vasopressin in the sinusoidal heart rate pattern after finding increased levels of vasopressin and the sinusoidal pattern in fetal sheep during hemorrhage.

The renin–angiotensin–aldosterone system is a complex hormone system that responds to decreases in plasma volume or blood pressure. In the fetus, angiotensin II and aldosterone levels do not increase in proportion to changes in the plasma renin, in contrast to what occurs in the newborn or adult. This uncoupling of the fetal renin–angiotensin–aldosterone system is most likely due to increased placental clearance of angiotensin II, limited angiotensin-converting enzyme available as a result of reduced pulmonary blood flow in the fetus, and the direct inhibition of aldosterone (Ross et al., 2012). The net effect of this hormone system is to protect the fetus from hemorrhagic stress by stimulating vasoconstriction (Parer, 1997).

FHR and Cardiac Output

In the adult, heart rate (HR) is related to cardiac output (CO) and stroke volume (SV) in the following equation: $CO = HR \times SV$. Stroke volume is influenced by the Frank-Starling mechanism, which states that an increased inflow of blood into the heart stretches the cardiac muscle, thereby resulting in a greater force of contraction and increased stroke volume. In the fetus, this mechanism has not been found to apply on the basis of studies involving fetal and adult lambs (Rudolph, 1985). The human fetal heart appears to normally operate near the top of its cardiac function curve (Fineman et al., 2012). Because stroke volume in the fetus does not fluctuate significantly, fetal cardiac output is essentially rate dependent (Fetal $CO \approx HR$). Normal FHR baseline variations have minimal effect on fetal cardiac output. However, at extreme rates (e.g., tachycardia $>$240 bpm or bradycardia $<$60 bpm), fetal cardiac output can be significantly decreased (Parer, 1997).

Fetal Sleep States

The FHR is also influenced by fetal sleep–wake cycles, which begin to emerge during the third trimester of pregnancy. Because sleep–wake cycles in the fetus and infant are qualitatively and quantitatively different than the adult, they are commonly referred to as "states" (Blackburn, 2013b). The duration of transitions into and out of a particular state are measures of neurophysiological development, integrity, and maturity (Van den Bergh & Mulder, 2012). Fetal states are most often defined by a specific combination of three variables: FHR variations, absence or presence of fetal generalized body movements, and absence or presence of rapid eye movements (REM).

In early pregnancy, fetal movement is largely continuous; however, with increasing maturation, periods of quiescence emerge. By 28 weeks' gestation, distinct periods of REM and respiratory movements begin alternating with periods of no REM and inactivity (Peirano, Algarin, & Uauy, 2003). Between 28 and 34 weeks' gestation, cyclic changes in FHR baseline oscillations begin to occur with alternating periods of REM and inactivity (Peirano, Algarin, & Uauy, 2003; Swartjes, van Geijn, Mantel, van Woerden, & Shoemaker, 1990). However, not all fetuses, even at 36–38 weeks' gestation, will demonstrate state organization with distinct cycles of sleep and wakefulness (Van den Bergh & Mulder, 2012). This sleep–wake cycle is credited with being the prenatal version of the alternation of quiet sleep (fetal state 1F) and REM (fetal state 2F) (Blackburn, 2013b).

In quiet or non-REM sleep (fetal state 1F), the fetus may be observed to have absent eye movements, infrequent or absent body movements, normal FHR baseline, minimal FHR variability, a nonreactive NST, and can respond to external stimuli (e.g., vibroacoustic stimulation) (Manning, 1995; Richardson & Gagnon, 2009). Active REM sleep (fetal state 2F) may be characterized by rapid darting eye movements, active body movements, moderate FHR variability, FHR accelerations, and a reactive NST (Manning, 1995; Richardson & Gagnon,

BOX 2-3 Characteristics of Fetal Sleep States

Fetal State 1F (quiet sleep):
- Eye movements absent
- Movements infrequent or absent
- Fetal tone present, but reduced
- Normal baseline FHR, minimal variability, accelerations absent
- Nonreactive NST
- Response to external stimuli (e.g., vibroacoustic stimulation)

Fetal State 2F (active REM sleep):
- Rapid darting eye movements
- Active body movements
- Fetal tone increased
- Moderate variability, accelerations present
- Reactive NST
- Unresponsive to external stimuli

FHR, fetal heart rate; NST, nonstress test; REM, rapid eye movement.

2009). Box 2-3 lists characteristics of fetal quiet sleep (1F) and active REM sleep (2F). The mean time period of cycling between active and quiet sleep is approximately 40 minutes (Blackburn, 2013b); however, the duration of a given behavioral state may last longer than 1 hour (Parer, 1997).

FETAL HOMEOSTATIC RESPONSES

Fetal monitoring is an ongoing indirect assessment of physiologic factors, both extrinsic and intrinsic to the fetus, that affect fetal oxygenation. The fetus depends on uterine blood flow, placental exchange, umbilical blood flow, oxygen transport to tissue, and, finally, innate compensatory factors to control FHR when challenged by labor and other stressors. With a decrease in PO_2 and an increase in PCO_2, the normoxic fetus initiates compensatory mechanisms that usually maintain physiologic integrity without damage to vital organs. Redistribution of fetal blood flow favoring the heart, brain, and adrenal glands is increased, whereas blood flow to the gut, spleen, kidneys, and limbs is decreased (see Figure 2-7). As the FHR slows, the fetal myocardium consumes less oxygen. Without restoration of fetal oxygenation, metabolic acidosis will progress to asphyxia and arterial oxygenation will fall below critical levels, resulting in myocardial depression, brain ischemia, and, ultimately, fetal death (King, 2013; Nageotte & Gilstrap, 2009; Parer, 1997). The fetal homeostatic responses to normal and abnormal stresses of labor and birth are illustrated in a dynamic physiologic model of FHR adaptations (Figure 2-11).

FIGURE 2-11 Dynamic Physiologic Response Model

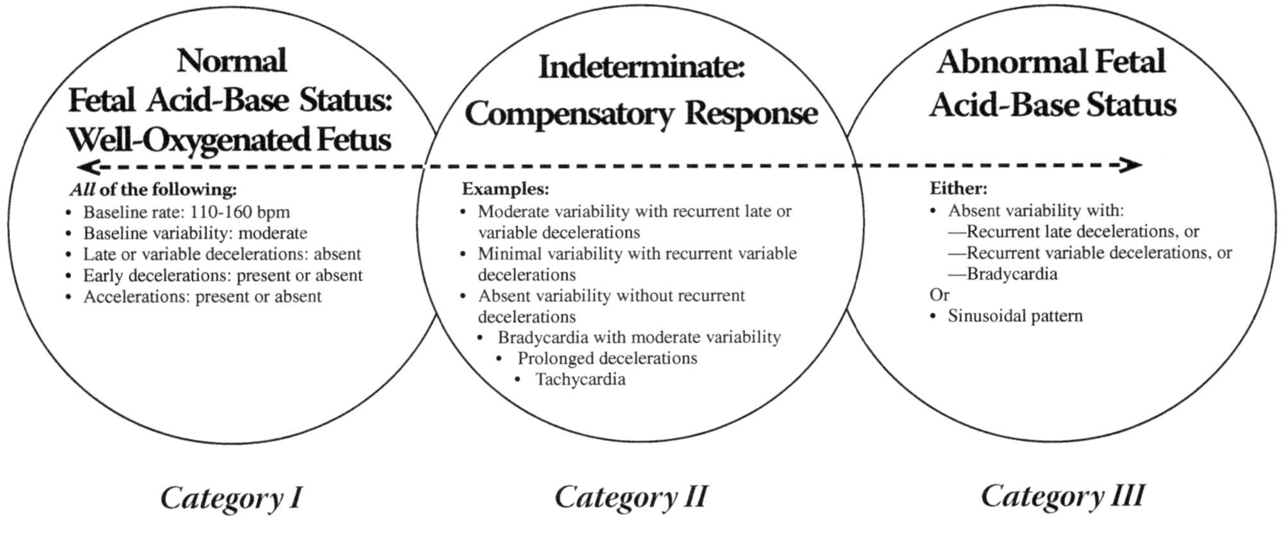

Note: This diagram is not meant to be all inclusive. All patterns must be treated with interventions that are based on suspected underlying physiologic causes and evaluation of individual patient presentation.

Interpretation of these physiologic responses to fetal oxygenation is reflected in an ongoing assessment of the continuum of FHR characteristics presented by the fetus (Figure 2-11). A normal FHR tracing (category I: moderate baseline variability, normal rate, and no late or variable decelerations) represents a well-oxygenated fetus, and is not associated with fetal acidemia. Accelerations and early decelerations may or may not be present in the tracing of a well-oxygenated fetus. At the other end of the continuum, an abnormal FHR tracing (category III: absent FHR variability combined with recurrent variable or late decelerations; absent variability combined with bradycardia; or sinusoidal pattern) conveys an increased risk for fetal acidemia at the time of observation. However, many fetuses will exhibit indeterminate FHR characteristics falling between these two extremes (Category II: any combination of characteristics that cannot be characterized as category I or category III). In summary, FHR interpretation requires an understanding of the evolution of FHR patterns in relation to fetal oxygenation, knowledge of extrinsic and intrinsic factors that influence fetal oxygenation, and ongoing assessment of FHR characteristics throughout labor and birth. FHR pattern interpretation is discussed in further detail in Chapter 5.

Case Study: Susan

Age:	41 years old
Gravidity/Parity:	G41112
Gestational Age:	28-2/7 weeks
Medical History:	Unremarkable
Surgical History:	Unremarkable
Psychosocial History:	Day care worker, married Smoker—one pack per day
Past Obstetric History:	Spontaneous vaginal birth at 38-3/7 weeks Spontaneous abortion at 13-1/7 weeks Preterm birth at 33 weeks (abruption)
Current Obstetric History:	Advanced maternal age: normal first trimester screening test Symmetric fetal growth restriction Primary cytomegalovirus (CMV) diagnosed on amniocentesis

Susan was admitted to the high-risk antepartum unit for severe fetal growth restriction with no interval growth between 25 and 28 weeks. The ultrasound revealed a fetus in the 3rd percentile for growth and an estimated fetal weight less than 575 grams. Doppler flow studies showed absent end diastolic flow, a worrisome finding. The amniotic fluid volume was 2 cm (oligohydramnios). A sterile speculum examination ruled out ruptured membranes. VE revealed a cervix that was closed and long. The fetus was in a breech presentation. A biophysical profile was 6 out of 10 with points being taken off for decreased amniotic fluid and a nonreactive nonstress test. Antenatal steroids were administered.

Susan: Second Inpatient Hospital Day; EFM Tracing at 1530 Using Ultrasound and Tocodynamometer

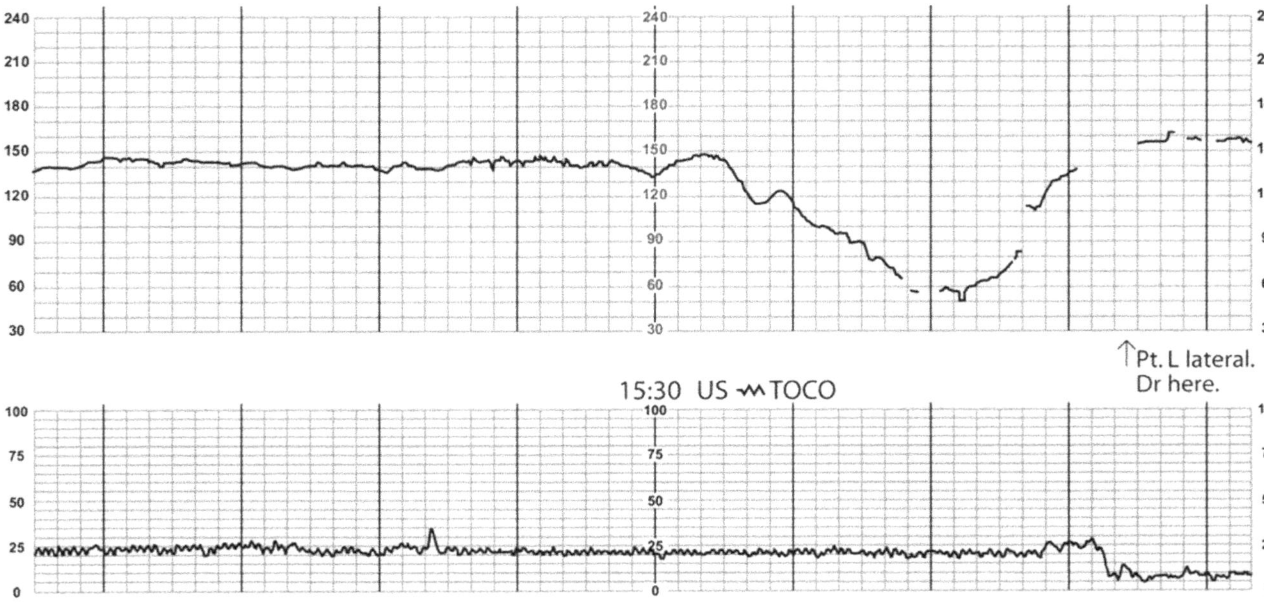

1. Baseline FHR:	**145 bpm**		
2. Variability	Absent (undetectable)	_____	
	Minimal (> 0 but ≤ bpm)	_____	
	Moderate (6–25 bpm)	_____	
	Marked (>25 bpm)	_____	
	Unable to determine	_____	
3. Contractions	Frequency:	**None**	
	Duration:	**Not applicable**	
	Intensity:	**Not applicable**	
	Resting tonus:	**Need to palpate**	

4. Accelerations and decelerations. When present, circle P if periodic or E if episodic.

Accelerations	P	E
Early decelerations	P	
Variable decelerations	P	E
Late decelerations	P	
Prolonged decelerations	P	**E**
None present		

5. Interpretation	Category I	________
	Category II	________
	Category III	________

6. List possible underlying physiologic mechanisms or rationales for observed patterns.

- **Cord compression related to oligohydramnios, fetal movement, or decreased Wharton's jelly**
- **Uteroplacental insufficiency related to the following:**
  - **Maternal smoking**
  - **Hypotension from supine maternal positioning during monitoring session**
  - **Placental abnormalities from CMV**
- **Associated with an indeterminate fetal acid-base status at present**

7. List in order of priority the physiologic goal(s) for observed patterns.

- **Maximize umbilical circulation.**
- **Maximize oxygenation.**
- **Maximize uteroplacental blood flow.**

8. List actions and interventions indicated based on overall interpretation (physiologic based, instrumentation based, and further assessments).

- **Position changes to promote uteroplacental blood flow and relieve cord compression.**
- **Palpate uterus to validate uterine monitoring data and adjust tocodynamometer to monitor contraction pattern if palpable.**
- **Assess maternal vital signs (blood pressure).**
- **Continue to assess deceleration pattern and variability.**
- **Provide reassurance to Susan and her family.**
- **Review previous tracings to evaluate variability and periodic/nonperiodic changes.**
- **Keep provider notified of FHR pattern (decelerations and variability), interventions, and maternal–fetal response.**

- **Evaluate maternal–fetal response to interventions.**
- **Continue routine assessments and interventions such as providing maternal comfort measures and keeping family informed of clinical situation.**
- **Prepare for birth if FHR pattern cannot be corrected.**
- **Alert neonatal team for possible birth.**

REFERENCES

American Academy of Pediatrics & American College of Obstetricians and Gynecologists. (2012). *Guidelines for perinatal care* (7th ed.). Elk Grove Village, IL: Authors.

American College of Obstetricians and Gynecologists (2014). Antepartum fetal surveillance. Practice bulletin no. 145. *Obstetrics and Gynecology, 124,* 182–92. doi: 10.1097/01.AOG.0000451759.90082.7b

Beall, M. H., & Ross, M. G. (2009). Amniotic fluid dynamics. In R. K. Creasy, R. Resnik, J. Iams, C. J. Lockwood, & T. R. Moore (Eds.), *Creasy and Resnik's maternal–fetal medicine: Principles and practice* (6th ed., pp. 47–54). Philadelphia, PA: Saunders Elsevier.

Benirschke, K. (2009a). Multiple gestation: The biology of twinning. In R. K. Creasy, R. Resnik, J. Iams, C. J. Lockwood, & T. R. Moore (Eds.), *Creasy and Resnik's maternal-fetal medicine: Principles and practice* (6th ed., pp. 55–68). Philadelphia, PA: Saunders Elsevier.

Benirschke, K. (2009b). Normal early development. In R. K. Creasy, R. Resnik, J. Iams, C. J. Lockwood, & T. R. Moore (Eds.), *Creasy and Resnik's maternal-fetal medicine: Principles and practice* (6th ed., pp. 37–45). Philadelphia, PA: Saunders Elsevier.

Blackburn, S. T. (2013a). Cardiovascular system. In S. T. Blackburn (Ed.), *Maternal, fetal, &neonatal physiology: A clinical perspective* (4th ed., pp. 252–296). Maryland Heights, MO: Elsevier Saunders.

Blackburn, S. T. (2013b). Neurologic, muscular, and sensory systems. In S. T. Blackburn (Ed.), *Maternal, fetal, & neonatal physiology: A clinical perspective* (4th ed., pp. 509–559). Maryland Heights, MO: Elsevier Saunders.

Blackburn, S. T. (2013c). The prenatal period and placental physiology. In S. T. Blackburn (Ed.), *Maternal, fetal, & neonatal physiology: A clinical perspective* (4th ed., pp. 61–114). Maryland Heights, MO: Elsevier Saunders.

Blackburn, S. T. (2013d). Respiratory system. In S. T. Blackburn (Ed.), *Maternal, fetal, & neonatal physiology: A clinical perspective* (4th ed., pp. 297–355). Maryland Heights, MO: Elsevier Saunders.

Bobrowski, R. A. (2010). Pulmonary physiology in pregnancy. *Clinical Obstetrics and Gynecology, 53*(2), 285–300. doi:10.1097/GRF.0b013e3181e04776

Brace, R. A. (1997). Physiology of amniotic fluid volume regulation. *Clinical Obstetrics and Gynecology, 40*(2), 280–289.

Cohn, H. E., Sacks, E. J., Heymann, M. A., & Rudolph, A. M. (1974). Cardiovascular responses to hypoxemia and acidemia in fetal lambs. *American Journal of Obstetrics and Gynecology, 120*(6), 817–824.

Dalton, K. J., Dawes, G. S., & Patrick, J. E. (1983). The autonomic nervous system and fetal heart rate variability. *American Journal of Obstetrics and Gynecology, 146*(4), 456–462.

Edelstone, D. I., & Rudolph, A. M. (1979). Preferential streaming of ductus venosus blood to the brain and heart in fetal lambs. *American Journal of Physiology, 237*(6), H724–H729.

Fineman, J. R., & Clyman, R. (2009). Fetal cardiovascular physiology. In R. K. Creasy, R. Resnik, J. Iams, C. J. Lockwood, & T. R. Moore (Eds.), *Creasy and Resnik's maternal–fetal medicine: Principles and practice* (6th ed., pp. 159–170). Philadelphia, PA: Saunders Elsevier.

Freeman, R. K., Garite, T. J., Nageotte, M. P., & Miller, L. A. (Eds.). (2012). *Fetal heart rate monitoring* (4th ed.). Philadelphia, PA: Lippincott Williams & Wilkins.

Gilbert, W. M. (2012). Amniotic fluid disorders. In S. G. Gabbe, J. R. Niebyl, J. L. Simpson, M. B. Landon, H. L. Galan, E. R. M. Jauniaux, & D. A. Driscoll. (Eds.), *Obstetrics: Normal and problem pregnancies* (6th ed., pp. 759–768). Philadelphia, PA: Elsevier Saunders.

James, L. S., Yeh, M. N., Morishima, H. O., Daniel, S. S., Caritis, S. N., Niemann, W. H., & Indyk, L. (1976). Umbilical vein occlusion and transient acceleration of the fetal heart rate. Experimental observations in subhuman primates. *American Journal of Obstetrics and Gynecology, 126*(2), 276–283.

Jauniaux, E., Ramsay, B., Peellaerts, C., & Scholler, Y. (1995). Perinatal features of pregnancies complicated by nuchal cord. *American Journal of Perinatology, 12*(4), 255–258.

King, T. L. (2013). Fetal assessment. In S. T. Blackburn (Ed.), *Maternal, fetal, and neonatal physiology: A clinical perspective* (4th ed., pp. 163–182). Maryland Heights, MO: Elsevier Saunders.

King, T., & Parer, J. (2000). The physiology of fetal heart rate patterns and perinatal asphyxia. *Journal of Perinatal and Neonatal Nursing, 14*(3), 19–39.

Kiserud, T. (2001). The ductus venosus. *Seminars in Perinatology, 25*(1), 11–20. doi:10.1053/sper.2001.22896

Lee, C. Y., Di Loreto, P. C., & O'Lane, J. M. (1975). A study of fetal heart rate acceleration patterns. *Obstetrics and Gynecology, 45*(2), 142–146.

Lee, S. T., & Hon, E. H. (1963). Fetal hemodynamic response to umbilical cord compression. *Obstetrics and Gynecology, 22*(5), 553–562.

Manning, F. A. (1995). *Fetal medicine: Principles and practice.* Norwalk, CT: Appleton & Lange.

Marino, T. (2004). Ultrasound abnormalities of the amniotic fluid, membranes, umbilical cord, and placenta. *Obstetrics and Gynecology Clinics of North America, 31*(1), 177–200.

Martin, C. B., Jr., & Gingerich, B. (1976). Uteroplacental physiology. *Journal of Obstetric, Gynecologic, and Neonatal Nursing, 5*(Suppl. 5), 16s–25s.

Meschia, G. (2009). Placental respiratory gas exchange and fetal oxygenation. In R. K. Creasy, R. Resnik, J. Iams, C. J. Lockwood, & T. R. Moore (Eds.), *Creasy and Resnik's maternal–fetal medicine: Principles and practice* (6th ed., pp. 181–191). Philadelphia, PA: Saunders Elsevier.

Moore, K. L., Persaud, T. V. N., & Torchia, M. G. (2011). *The developing human: Clinically oriented embryology* (9th ed.). Philadelphia, PA: Elsevier Saunders.

Murata, Y., Miyake, Y., Yamamoto, T., Higuchi, M., Hesser, J., Ibara, S., . . . Tyner, J. G. (1985). Experimentally produced sinusoidal fetal heart rate pattern in the chronically instrumented fetal lamb. *American Journal of Obstetrics and Gynecology, 153*(6), 693–702.

Nageotte, M. P., & Gilstrap, L. C. (2009). Intrapartum fetal surveillance. In R. K. Creasy, R. Resnik, J. Iams, C. J. Lockwood, & T. R. Moore (Eds.), *Creasy and Resnik's maternal–fetal medicine: Principles and practice* (6th ed., pp. 397–417). Philadelphia, PA: Saunders Elsevier.

Panting-Kemp, A., Nguyen, T., Chang, E., Quillan, E., & Castro, L. (1999). Idiopathic polyhydramnios and perinatal outcome. *American Journal of Obstetrics and Gynecology, 181*(5, Pt. 1), 1079 –1082.

Parer, J. T. (1976). Physiologic regulation of fetal heart rate. *Journal of Obstetric, Gynecologic and Neonatal Nursing, 5,* 26S–29S.

Parer, J. T. (1983). *Handbook of fetal heart rate monitoring*. Philadelphia, PA: Saunders.

Parer, J. T. (1997). *Handbook of fetal heart rate monitoring* (2nd ed.). Philadelphia, PA: Saunders.

Peirano, P., Algarin, C., & Uauy, R. (2003). Sleep-wake states and their regulatory mechanisms throughout early human development. *Journal of Pediatrics, 143*(Suppl. 4), S70–S79.

Renou, P., Newman, W., & Wood, C. (1969). Autonomic control of fetal heart rate. *American Journal of Obstetrics and Gynecology, 105*(6), 949–953.

Richardson, B. S., & Gagnon, R. (2009). Behavioral state activity and fetal health and development. In R. K. Creasy, R. Resnik, J. Iams, C. J. Lockwood, & T. R. Moore (Eds.), *Creasy and Resnik's maternal–fetal medicine: Principles and practice* (6th ed., pp. 171–179). Philadelphia, PA: Saunders Elsevier.

Ross, M. G., Ervin, M. G., & Novak, D. (2012). Placental and fetal physiology. In S. G. Gabbe, J. R. Niebyl, J. L. Simpson, M. B. Landon, H. L. Galan, E. R. M. Jauniaux, & D. A. Driscoll (Eds.), *Obstetrics: Normal and problem pregnancies* (6th ed., pp. 23–41). Philadelphia, PA: Elsevier Saunders.

Rudolph, A. M. (1985). Distribution and regulation of blood flow in the fetal and neonatal lamb. *Circulation Research, 57*(6), 811–821.

Signore, C., Freeman, R. K., & Spong, C. Y. (2009). Antenatal testing – a reevaluation: Executive summary of a Eunice Kennedy Shriver National Institute of Child Health and Human Development workshop. *Obstetrics and Gynecology, 113*(3), 687–701. doi:10.1097/AOG.0b013e318197bd8a

Swartjes, J. M., van Geijn, H. P., Mantel, R., van Woerden, E. E., & Schoemaker, H. C. (1990). Coincidence of behavioural state parameters in the human fetus at three gestational ages. *Early Human Development, 23*(2), 75–83.

Troiano, N. H. (1999). Invasive hemodynamic monitoring in obstetrics. In L. K. Mandeville & N. H. Troiano (Eds.), AWHONN's high –risk and critical care obstetrics (2nd ed., pp. 66–83). Philadelphia, PA: Wolters Kluwer, Lippincott Williams & Wilkins.

Troiano, N. H., & Gaddipati, S. (2013). Invasive hemodynamic monitoring and oxygen transport monitoring during pregnancy. In N. H. Troiano, C. J. Harvey, & B. F. Chez (Eds.), *AWHONN's high-risk and critical careobstetrics* (3rd ed., pp. 31–46). Philadelphia, PA: Wolters Kluwer, Lippincott Williams & Wilkins.

Van den Bergh, B. R., & Mulder, E. J. (2012). Fetal sleep organization: A biological precursor of self-regulation in childhood and adolescence? *Biological Psychology, 89*(3), 584–590. doi:10.1016/j.biopsycho.2012.01.003

Wagner, P. D., Powell, F. L., & West, J. B. (2010). Ventilation, blood flow, and gas exchange. In R. J. Mason, V. C. Broaddus, T. R. Martin, T. E. King, Jr., D. E. Schraufnagel, J. F. Murray, & J. A. Nadel (Eds.), *Murray and Nadel's textbook of respiratory medicine, Vol. 1,* (5th ed., pp. 53–88). Philadelphia, PA: Saunders Elsevier.

Zakowski, M. I. & Ramanathan, S. (2013). Uteroplacental circulation and respiratory gas exchange. In M. S. Suresh, B. S. Segal, R. Preston, R. Fernando, & C. L. Mason (Eds.), *Shnider and Levinson's anesthesia for obstetrics* (5th ed., pp. 18–45). Philadelphia, PA: Lippincott Williams & Wilkins.

SECTION TWO

Maternal–Fetal Assessment

CHAPTER 3

Maternal–Fetal Assessment

Kirsten Wisner
Dodi Gauthier

INTRODUCTION

The admission assessment of the woman, fetus, and her family by perinatal nurses is multidimensional, and includes physical exam; review of the woman's medical, surgical, and obstetric history; psychosocial assessment; and inquiry into her and her family's needs and desires related to their labor and birth experience. Along with continuous assessment of maternal–fetal physiologic stability and response to labor, a primary role for perinatal nurses is to support women and their families to achieve a safe, family-centered labor and birth. Treatment plans should align with normal physiologic labor processes, promote emotional well-being and family bonding, and minimize unnecessary interventions and the potential for iatrogenic harm.

HEALTH HISTORY

Overview

Maternal–fetal assessment is a collaborative, ongoing process that begins early in prenatal care and continues throughout the peripartum period (see Figure 3-1). An admission history and physical exam should be completed for all women who are admitted to the perinatal unit. The focus is on the woman's obstetric and medical history and associated risk factors, issues in the current pregnancy, and labor symptoms or progress. Details of the history collected and physical exam are partly guided by whether or not she has had prenatal care, and how recently she has been examined by her provider, as well as by the presence and severity of risk factors (American Academy of Pediatrics [AAP] & American College of Obstetricians and Gynecologists [ACOG], 2012). A sample guideline for an intrapartum maternal–fetal admission assessment is presented in Box 3-1. Components of the woman's health, surgical, medical, and obstetric history can be taken from the prenatal record, and updated or verified. Other information will be obtained via a nursing assessment and interview.

Many women will have had a complete history and physical examination by their provider during prenatal care. If a woman has received ongoing prenatal care, has had a recent medical exam, and no new risk factors are reported or identified, the admission assessment may be limited to an interval history and a physical exam directed at the presenting condition (AAP & ACOG, 2012). Risk factors identified previously should be recorded. For women presenting without prenatal care, when new risk factors are identified despite ongoing prenatal care, or documentation

Figure 3-1 The Collaborative Process and Fetal Heart Monitoring

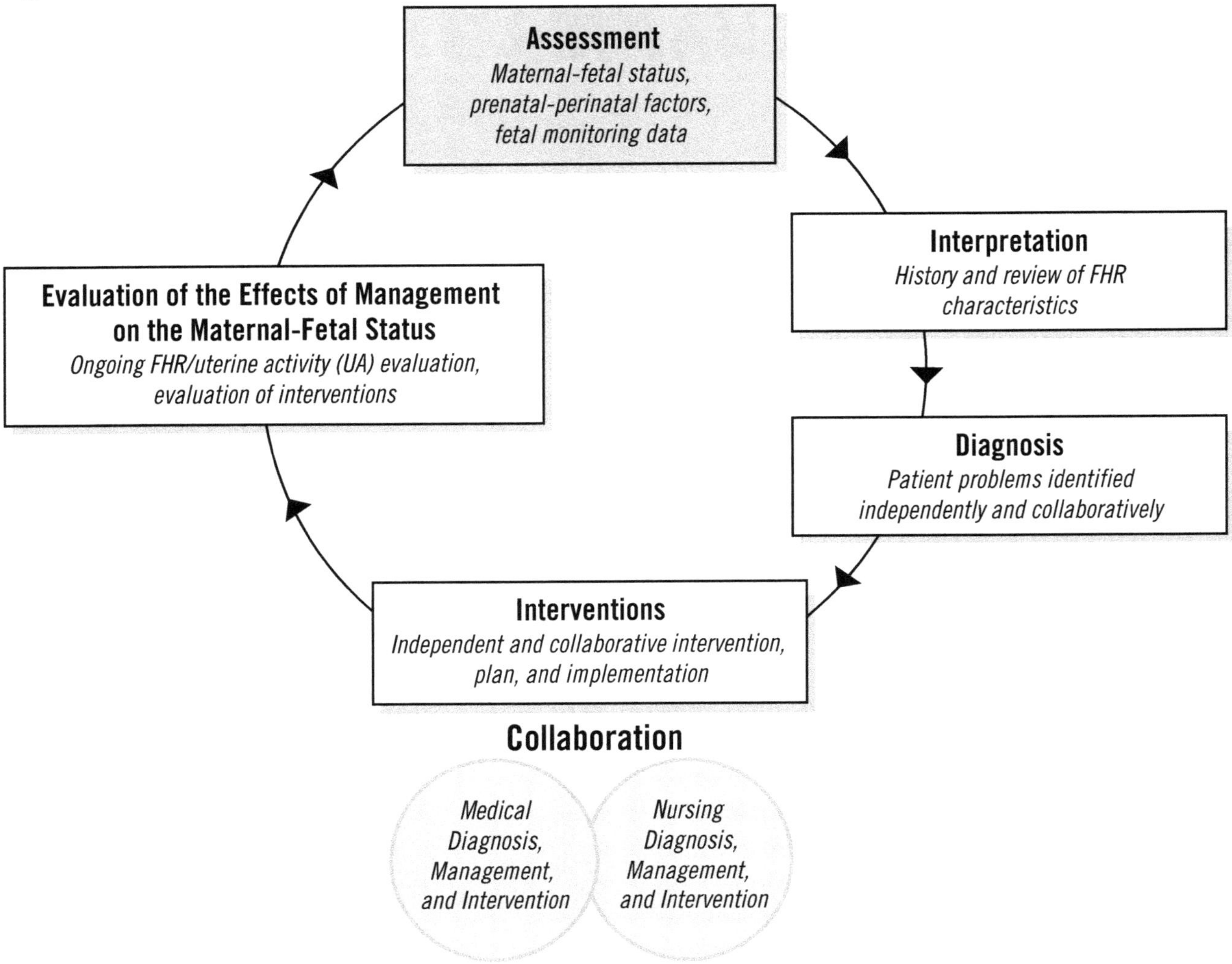

BOX 3-1 Outline of Maternal–Fetal Assessment for Intrapartum Admission

Initial Assessment:

1. Maternal physical status
2. Fetal status
3. Labor status
4. Review of prenatal records and health history
5. Demographic, socioeconomic, and psychosocial assessment
6. Physical exam

Further assessment is prioritized according to the patient's chief complaint and from information gathered during the initial evaluation, with a focus on achieving maternal–fetal stability if threats are detected. Assessment should include:

1. Maternal physical status:
    a. Chief complaint and associated concerns or symptoms
    b. Date/time of arrival
    c. GTPAL (gravidity, term, preterm, abortions, living)
    d. Vital signs

- e. Estimated date of delivery (EDD)
- f. Presence or absence of vaginal bleeding, including onset, duration, and associated bleeding characteristics or symptoms
- g. Pregnancy risk factors or complications
- h. Emotional/psychosocial status (supports available, adequacy of coping)

2. Fetal status
    - a. Estimated gestational age
    - b. Fetal movement
    - c. Fetal heart rate (FHR) by auscultation or electronic fetal monitoring (EFM)
    - d. Prenatal records review for fetal concerns, additional testing, or consults
3. Labor status
    - a. Uterine activity
        - i. Contraction onset, frequency, intensity, duration
        - ii. Resting tone
    - b. Membrane status
        - i. Subjective and clinical evaluation
            1. Patient subjective report
            2. Clinical exam via institutional policy
    - c. Cervical exam
        - i. Digital or speculum exam
        - ii. Dilation, effacement, position
        - iii. Fetal presentation and station
4. Prenatal records and review of health history
    - a. Obstetric history
    - b. Medical history
    - c. Surgical history
    - d. Review of laboratory data in prenatal record
    - e. Current and past medications
5. Demographic and socioeconomic risk factors evaluation
    - a. Demographic and socioeconomic assessment
        - i. Age-related, racial/ethnic, marital status, or socioeconomic risk factors
    - b. Psychosocial history/status
        - i. Threats to safety or health (intimate partner violence, smoking, substance abuse, adequacy/safety of housing)
        - ii. Barriers to health care
        - iii. Communication barriers
    - c. Labor plans/desires
    - d. Cultural needs/preferences
6. Physical Exam
    - a. Vital signs
    - b. Review of systems, or focused exam
        - i. Depends on how recently she was seen by primary provider, and presenting complaint
    - c. Review of current laboratory results

Note: From "Guidelines for the initial assessment and triage of obstetric patients," by N. Hess-Eggleston, N. H. Troiano, C. J. Harvey & B. F. Chez, 2013. *AWHONN high-risk and critical care obstetrics*. p. 371–372. Copyright 2013 by the Association of Women's Health, Obstetric and Neonatal Nurses.

is unavailable, a comprehensive examination by a physician or midwife and appropriate laboratory screening is advised (AAP & ACOG, 2012). For women being evaluated in triage for labor, or presenting with a nonobstetric complaint, the initial triage assessment may be adapted based on the presenting complaint and history of prenatal care. For any pregnant woman, the responsible provider should be notified immediately if any of the following findings are detected or suspected: vaginal bleeding, acute abdominal pain, temperature $\geq$ 100.4° F (38° C), preterm labor, preterm premature rupture of membranes, hypertension, or an indeterminate (category II) or abnormal (category III) fetal heart rate tracing (AAP & ACOG, 2012).

Prenatal Records

The prenatal record guides the primary provider in obtaining a complete physical assessment and health history, identifying risk factors, and performing baseline and ongoing assessments aimed at recognizing concerning trends or changes in maternal–fetal stability or well-being (Phelan, 2008). Assessments during prenatal visits are documented and monitored for the development of pregnancy-related disorders, as well as to track growth and development of the fetus. Laboratory data collected at recommended intervals are recorded, along with any follow-up treatment and teaching. The prenatal record is a critical form of communication between the primary provider and nursing and other clinicians in the inpatient setting and serves as a risk-based assessment aimed at triggering appropriate referral and follow-up care (Phelan, 2008). In facilities without an integrated electronic medical record, the prenatal record should be sent to the associated inpatient unit by 34–36 weeks' gestation. Regardless of the source (paper vs. electronic), most prenatal records contain similar content and reflect standard-based screening recommendations from professional organizations such as the American College of Obstetricians and Gynecologists and the American Academy of Pediatrics.

Medical, Surgical, and Obstetric History

While the medical, surgical, and obstetric histories are summarized in the prenatal record, the triage or admission process provides an opportunity for nurses to verify and update these aspects of the woman's health history as well as identify previously unrecognized medical or psychosocial risk factors or needs.

Profound physiologic changes occur during pregnancy, affecting all maternal organ systems. Women and their families also undergo psychological and emotional changes as they prepare for their baby's birth. Certain medical conditions may be exacerbated by the physiologic changes occurring in pregnancy. For example, as pregnancy progresses, women with cardiovascular disease are vulnerable to cardiac decompensation as blood volume and cardiac output increase by as much as 30–50%, heart rate increases, and systemic vascular resistance and serum colloid osmotic pressure decrease (Abbas, Lester, & Connolly, 2005; Curry, Swan, & Steer, 2009). The extreme hemodynamic shifts associated with labor, birth, and postpartum further increase the risk of adverse outcomes and death in these women (Small et al., 2012). Latent cardiac conditions may manifest for the first time during the peripartum course as the cardiovascular system is challenged by rapid hemodynamic alterations, highlighting the need for heightened surveillance in all women.

The obstetric history provides important information that can guide intrapartum treatment planning, surveillance, and teaching during and after birth. Pregnancy-related conditions such as preeclampsia, gestational diabetes, and preterm labor may recur in subsequent pregnancies (Barton & Sibai, 2008; Esplin et al., 2008; Kim, Berger, & Chamany, 2007; Mostello, Kallogjeri, Tungsiripat, & Leet, 2008). A number of pregnancy-associated disorders may lead to long-term sequelae; hence, women may benefit from education regarding prevention strategies as well as recognizing signs and symptoms of developing disease. Women with preeclampsia are at higher risk of developing hypertension and other cardiac conditions (Melchiorre, Sutherland, Liberati, & Thilaganathan, 2011), and women with gestational diabetes are at increased risk of developing type 2 diabetes (Bellamy, Casas, Hingorani, & Williams, 2009). A woman's surgical history can provide information about her reaction to anesthesia, as well as identify procedures that are contraindications to labor or vaginal birth. Finally, prior shoulder dystocia, operative vaginal birth, emergency cesarean, or hemorrhage are examples of conditions that have both clinical and psychological significance. Along with alerting caregivers to potential problems in the index pregnancy, the woman and family may have suffered extreme distress and require additional or tailored labor support (Verreault et al., 2012).

A thorough review of the maternal and fetal implications of risk factors inherent in the woman's medical, surgical, and obstetric history is beyond the scope of this chapter. However, it is important that perinatal nurses maintain current and evidence-based knowledge of the primary contributors to maternal and neonatal morbidity and mortality, the trajectory of relevant chronic and pregnancy-related health conditions, and knowledge of preventive and/or management strategies known to mitigate the development, progression, or severity of these conditions or outcomes. Such knowledge can help nurses target their assessments to detect concerning trends or changes in maternal–fetal stability, understand how certain risk factors relate or contribute to adverse outcomes, and inform teaching efforts aimed at long-term health promotion and disease prevention for women and their families. Table 3-1 reviews selected medical and obstetric conditions and their implications for maternal–fetal health.

TABLE 3-1 Selected Medical and Obstetric Risk Factors and Associated Maternal–Fetal Assessment Implications

MATERNAL RISK FACTOR OR CONDITION[a]	FETAL IMPLICATIONS	MATERNAL IMPLICATIONS	MATERNAL–FETAL ASSESSMENT/FHM CONSIDERATIONS	HEALTH PROMOTION
Preeclampsia (with severe features)	IUGR Oligohydramnios PTB Hypoxia-acidosis Neurologic injury Death Placental ischemia (Cudihy & Lee, 2009; Sibai, 2011)	Eclampsia Abruption DIC Renal or liver failure Intracerebral or hepatic hemorrhage Pulmonary edema Renal failure Retinal detachment Death (Sibai, 2011)	Notify MD: s/s of abruption—tachysystole, pain, bleeding, FHR decels, and of Category II or III FHR tracing Magnesium sulfate ↓ FHR baseline and ↑ incidence of absent to minimal variability (Duffy, Odibo, Roehl, Macones, & Cahill, 2012) ↓ Intravascular volumes, → compromised uteroplacental perfusion, and ↓ tolerance to blood loss (Sibai, 2011) Preeclamptic women w/BP ≥ 160 systolic or 110 diastolic should be treated promptly with antihypertensive medication (ACOG, 2011a, 2013), preferably within 15 minutes (Clark & Hankins, 2012)	Following preterm preeclampsia, most women exhibit stage B asymptomatic heart failure PP and 40% have essential HTN 1–2 years later (Melchiorre et al., 2011) Risk of recurrence 22–65%, influenced by gestational age at onset, pregnancy-related and medical risk factors Modifiable risk factors include obesity, glycemic and preconception BP control (Barton & Sibai, 2008) ↑ Risk of CVD warrants teaching regarding disease trajectory and prevention strategies (Smith, Pudwell, Walker, & Wen, 2012)

(continued)

TABLE 3-1 (Continued)

MATERNAL RISK FACTOR OR CONDITION[a]	FETAL IMPLICATIONS	MATERNAL IMPLICATIONS	MATERNAL–FETAL ASSESSMENT/FHM CONSIDERATIONS	HEALTH PROMOTION
Diabetes mellitus Gestational diabetes	Fetal malformations PTB Macrosomia 3× risk of stillbirth Hypoglycemia Hyperbilirubinemia RDS (Vitoratos, Vrachnis, Valsamakis, Panoulis, & Creatsas, 2010)	Hypertensive disorders Hydramnios Shoulder dystocia Type 1 DM: 7× ↑ PTL (Vitoratos et al., 2010)	Risk for severe hyperglycemia ↑ with infection, and administration of beta-mimetics or antenatal steroids (Inturrisi, Linter, & Sorem, 2013)	Women w/GDM have ≥ 7-fold risk of developing type 2 DM compared to controls. Higher risk associated with black or Asian race, family history, and ↑ BMI (Bellamy et al., 2009) Maintaining normal BMI, lipids, and BP may mitigate GDM→DM disease progression (Bellamy et al., 2009) Following GDM, screening at 6–12 weeks PP and q3 years (AAP & ACOG, 2012) GDM recurrence 30–84%; highest in nonwhite race/ethnicities (Kim et al., 2007)
Asthma	↑ Incidence of: PTB LBW, SGA PPROM IUGR Breech presentation (Mendola et al., 2013; Murphy et al., 2011)	↑ Concurrent incidence: Preeclampsia and superimposed preeclampsia GDM Abruption, previa Hemorrhage Pulmonary embolism ↑ rates CS and induction ICU admission (Mendola et al. 2013; Murphy et al., 2011)	Active management of asthma shown to ↓ PTB risk (Murphy et al., 2011) Most adverse maternal–fetal effects thought to be related to impaired placentation (immunologic), ↓ perfusion from altered vascular reactivity, and hypoxia (Mendola et al., 2013; Rocklin, 2011) Heightened surveillance for signs of deteriorating or impaired oxygenation, ↓ uteroplacental perfusion; maintain hydration, oxygenation (≥95%), and adequate pain control to ↓ risk bronchospasm (Dombrowski & Schatz, 2010) Medication considerations: • Maintain asthma meds during labor • PGE_1 or PGE_2 safe for cervical ripening • Carboprost, ergonovine, methylergonovine, indomethacin may → bronchospasm • Magnesium sulfate and terbutaline are bronchodilators • Lumbar anesthesia reduces O_2 consumption, ↓ risk of bronchospasm (Dombrowski & Schatz, 2010)	Effect of pregnancy on asthma in individual women highly variable Most asthma medications safe in pregnancy; provide reassurance to continue meds during pregnancy and breastfeeding Oral corticosteroids linked to congenital malformations and impaired fetal growth, ↑ risk preeclampsia, GDM, PTB; in severe asthma, benefits of asthma control thought to outweigh risks (Rocklin, 2011)

MATERNAL RISK FACTOR OR CONDITION[a]	FETAL IMPLICATIONS	MATERNAL IMPLICATIONS	MATERNAL–FETAL ASSESSMENT/FHM CONSIDERATIONS	HEALTH PROMOTION
Cardiovascular conditions[b]	Fetal outcomes depend on extent/severity of cardiovascular event and efficacy of resuscitative efforts/interventions Very high potential for fetal asphyxia in maternal cardiac arrest IUGR, prematurity, death affect approx. 30% of infants born to women with significant CVD; risk of cardiac anomalies increased in women with congenital disease (Simpson, 2012) Most cardiac meds considered safe for fetus (hydralazine, aspirin, digoxin, beta blockers, diuretics); ACE inhibitors teratogenic in first trimester, and cause ↓ fetal renal blood flow and hypotension in second/third trimesters (Gelson et al., 2009)	Ischemic heart disease most common cause of cardiac death in pregnancy in developed world (Gelson, Gatzoulis, Steer, & Johnson, 2009) ↑ in CVD in pregnancy thought to be related to ↑ comorbidities (obesity, hypertension, diabetes) delayed childbearing, and women with congenital heart disease surviving to childbearing age (Simpson, 2012) ↑ risk miscarriage (Simpson, 2012) Cardiovascular conditions (inclusive of cardiomyopathy) are the leading cause of pregnancy-related death in the U. S., with deaths from ischemic heart disease and cardiomyopathy ↑ (Berg et al., 2010).	Include cardiac syndromes in differential diagnosis for women presenting with severe chest or subscapular pain requiring opioid pain management (Nelson-Piercy, 2011) Appropriate screening includes chest X-ray and EKG (Nelson-Piercy, 2011; Wolff & Weitzel, 2011) When MI is suspected/diagnosed, catheterization with thrombolysis and/or coronary angioplasty should not be withheld (Gelson et al., 2009) Women particularly vulnerable to cardiac decompensation during: • Intrapartum—pain, anxiety, and contractions further ↑ maternal HR, SV, CO, BP • Second stage—↑ hemodynamic andoxidative cardiac stress • Immediate PP—500 mL autotransfusion occurring after third stage may not be tolerated by women with limited cardiac reserve (Simpson, 2012) Two key modifications to CPR in pregnancy: • Left uterine displacement (15–30° tilt) via complete tilt of backboard, blanket roll under right hip, or manual displacement[c] • Delivery via postmortem CS within 5 minutes if resuscitation not successful at 4 minutes (Raschke, 2011)	Normal complaints of pregnancy (fatigue, palpitations, orthopnea, dyspnea, pedal edema) mimic symptoms of worsening or new-onset cardiac disease, complicating its diagnosis and assessment (Martin, 2011) Optimal preconception control of hyperlipidemia, HTN, DM can improve pregnancy/birth outcomes; stabilization of comorbid conditions should be goal for long-term health outcomes Smoking cessation and weight loss strongly encouraged

(continued)

TABLE 3-1 (Continued)

MATERNAL RISK FACTOR OR CONDITION[a]	FETAL IMPLICATIONS	MATERNAL IMPLICATIONS	MATERNAL–FETAL ASSESSMENT/FHM CONSIDERATIONS	HEALTH PROMOTION
Obesity	↑ risk of: PTB Perinatal mortality Low Apgar scores IUGR LBW Macrosomia/LGA Post dates Shoulder dystocia Birth trauma NICU admission Childhood obesity Congenital anomalies (Perlow, 2011) Ultrasound imaging may be impaired, limiting accuracy of diagnosis of fetal anomalies (AAP & ACOG, 2012)	↑ risk of: Miscarriage CS birth Hypertensive disorders DM/GDM Infection Operative and postoperative complications VTE (AAP & ACOG, 2012; Perlow, 2011)	Cardiac and respiratory function compromised in obese laboring patient Careful attention to optimal oxygenation, uteroplacental perfusion, preventing aortocaval compression Consider continuous pulse oximetry. Epidural analgesia may ↓ respiratory demands, ↑ cardiac function (Perlow, 2011) Women with BMI ≥ 35 or have preexisting medical conditions should have cardiac evaluation Because of ↑ risk of CS, planning for extra blood products, larger operating room table, extra personnel, and pre-delivery anesthesia consult may be warranted (AAP & ACOG, 2012) If CS birth, consider thromboprophylaxis beyond pneumatic compression devices because of ↑ risk of VTE (AAP & ACOG, 2012)	Obesity places pregnant woman at high-risk, hence periconception counseling should emphasize modifiable risk factors (normalization of BMI, smoking cessation, nutritional status), as well as optimal control of comorbid conditions (HTN, diabetes) (Perlow, 2011)

Note: BMI, body max index; BP, blood pressure; CO, cardiac output; CPR, cardiopulmonary resuscitation; CS, cesarean section; CVD, cardiovascular disease; DIC, disseminated intravascular coagulation; DM, diabetes mellitus; FHM, fetal heart monitoring; FHR, fetal heart rate; GDM, gestational diabetes mellitus; HR, heart rate; HTN, hypertension; ICU, intensive care unit; IUGR, intrauterine growth restriction; LBW, low birthweight; MI, myocardial infarction; NICU, neonatal intensive care unit; PGE_1/PGE_2, prostaglandins 1 and 2; PP, postpartum; PPROM, preterm premature rupture of membranes; PROM, premature rupture of membranes; PTB, preterm birth; RDS, respiratory distress syndrome; SGA, small for gestational age; SV, stroke volume; VTE, venous thromboembolism.

[a] These categories are not inclusive of all medical and obstetric risk factors found in pregnancy. The intent is to emphasize the range and complexity of potential risk factors associated with the perinatal period, and the importance of a comprehensive and holistic assessment of each laboring woman.

[b] Focus of discussion is on recognizing new-onset cardiac disease and understanding its contribution to perinatal mortality rather than a review of preexisting cardiac disease.

[c] Tilting maternal trunk only may compromise efficacy of compressions.

Infectious Disease Evaluation

Routine screening of specified conditions and lab tests is recommended at designated intervals for all pregnant women during prenatal care (AAP & ACOG, 2012). These are outlined in Table 3-2 with recommended timing, treatment, and follow-up, along with implications for intrapartum nursing assessment. A broader definition of infectious disease includes those infections seen in all populations, such as influenza or tuberculosis, which have important implications in pregnancy. Each institution should develop infectious disease policies pertaining to pregnant women consistent with governmental and professional regulations or requirements.

TABLE 3-2 Prenatal Screening

PRENATAL SCREENING					
CONDITION AND/OR SCREENING/LAB TEST	**A, ALL WOMEN; I, IF INDICATED**	**TEST COMMENTS**	**TIMING**	**FOLLOW-UP OR TREATMENT**	**INTRAPARTUM IMPLICATIONS**
Human immunodeficiency virus (HIV)	A	EIA[a] State laws vary regarding testing, reporting, consent Testing should be strongly encouraged and objections addressed; however, respect woman's right to decline	First visit	High-risk[b] or in high-prevalence area, retest in third trimester (before 36 weeks)	Rapid HIV-antibody test if unknown on admission[a] Initiate antiretroviral prophylaxis while awaiting confirmatory test results
Hepatitis B virus (HBV)	A	Routine testing of all pregnant women for hepatitis B surface antigen (HBsAg), even if vaccinated Results require interpretation to identify if markers signify prior vaccination, or acute, resolved, or chronic disease	First visit or first trimester	Vaccinate during pregnancy in high-risk[c] women Women with clinical hepatitis, unknown status, or at high risk[c] should be tested on admission via shortened protocols to expedite infant immunoprophylaxis	If mother positive, infant requires hepatitis B vaccine + hepatitis B immune globulin (HBIG) within 12 hours of birth Reporting to state/local health department can ensure infant treatment
Rubella	A	Confirmed evidence of immunity, or Hemagglutination Inhibition (HI) test; titers vary by lab; expressed as ratio	First visit		If nonimmune or equivocal, give vaccine prior to discharge; measles–mumps–rubella (MMR) vaccine recommended
Chlamydia (*Chlamydia trachomatis*)	AAP and ACOG recommend screening all women USPSTF recommends all women $\leq$ age 24 and high-risk[d] women	Urine, endocervical, or vaginal specimen NAATs have high specificity and sensitivity Co-infection with *N. gonorrhoeae* common	First visit	If positive, treat, retest in 3 weeks, and again after 3 months, preferably third trimester Third-trimester screen for high-risk[d] women Treat sexual partner(s)	Most frequently reported infectious disease in U. S., highest in $\leq$ age 25 Perinatal infection associated with miscarriage, PROM, PTL, LBW, infant mortality, neonatal chlamydial infection, and postpartum endometritis Risk reduction teaching for vulnerable women

(continued)

TABLE 3-2 (Continued)

PRENATAL SCREENING					
CONDITION AND/OR SCREENING/LAB TEST	**A, ALL WOMEN; I, IF INDICATED**	**TEST COMMENTS**	**TIMING**	**FOLLOW-UP OR TREATMENT**	**INTRAPARTUM IMPLICATIONS**
Gonorrhea (*Neisseria gonorrhoeae*)	I – Low prevalence in general, low-risk population, hence screening recommended for high-risk[d] women only	Urine, endocervical or vaginal specimen Culture, nucleic acid hybridization tests, and NAATs	First visit	If positive, treat and retest within 3–6 months, preferably third trimester Test high-risk[d] women in third trimester Sexual partner(s) from past 60 days should be treated	Risk of PROM, PTL, and chorioamnionitis Perinatal transmission to infants can cause conjunctivitis, blindness, sepsis with associated meningitis, endocarditis,or arthritis
Syphilis (*Treponema pallidum*)	A	Definitive diagnosis via dark-field microscopy of T. *pallidum* in lesion exudates/tissue (primary syphilis) Typically screen via nontreponemal tests (VDRL, RPR) Positive requires confirmation with treponemal test (FTA-ABS, TP-PA assay, various EIAs, and chemiluminescence immunoassays)	First visit	Screen untested women, and retest high-risk[e] women early in third trimester (approx 28 weeks) and at delivery Disease divided into overlapping stages; parenteral penicillin G preferred drug for all stages Test for HIV	Infants should not be discharged unless documentation of maternal status confirmed Penicillin effective for preventing maternal–fetal transmission and treating fetal infection Any woman delivering a stillbirth after 20 weeks should be tested
Tuberculosis	I	Screen high-risk[f] women with Mantoux tuberculin skin test or interferon-gamma release assay	First visit	Indeterminate or positive test requires confirmation with chest X-ray or sputum culture	
Blood type	A	Informational purposes for emergency transfusion and to alert providers of ABO incompatibility	First visit		
RhD Type	A	Tests for D antigen in maternal blood and expressed as (−/+) for the antigen All RhD(−) women require testing (see Antibody screen) for sensitization to D antigen, which may have occurred during prior pregnancy or blood product transfusion	First visit	Repeat antibody test in unsensitized D(−) women at 28–29 weeks, and administer 300 mcg anti-D immune globulin Additional dose indicated following possible fetal–maternal bleeding (trauma, abruption, ectopic, abortion, amniocentesis, or chorionic villus sampling)	RhD(−) women at risk of alloimmunization to D antigen when bleeding occurs at maternal–fetal interface Repeat dose of anti-D immune globulin $\leq$ 72 hours after delivery if infant D(+)

PRENATAL SCREENING					
CONDITION AND/OR SCREENING/LAB TEST	**A, ALL WOMEN; I, IF INDICATED**	**TEST COMMENTS**	**TIMING**	**FOLLOW-UP OR TREATMENT**	**INTRAPARTUM IMPLICATIONS**
Antibody screen	A	Detects Rh, ABO, and other potentially incompatible antibodies in maternal blood Incidence of RhD alloimmunization has ↓, resulting in a relative ↑ in cases of non-RhD alloimmunization; most common in ↓ order are Kell, Duffy, MNS, Kidd, and anti-U	First trimester	Results dictate follow-up, may require paternal testing to identify potential fetal incompatibilities	Maternal antibody formation to fetal red cell antigens (red cell alloimmunization) Resulting hemolytic disease of the fetus and newborn (HDFN) can range from mild anemia with hyperbilirubinemia to major fetal damage with stillbirth If HDFN severe, fetal transfusions and plans for delivery at 32–38 weeks may be required
Complete blood count (CBC)	A		First trimester Repeat H&H in third trimester	Microcytic anemia requires further evaluation for ferrous sulfate deficiency. If treated, retest in 3–4 weeks Hemoglobin electrophoresis to rule out thalassemia or sickle cell in women of African American, Asian, or Mediterranean descent	Heightened surveillance for bleeding if low H&H or PLT count. Follow hemorrhage protocols for women with bleeding risks
Urine culture	I			Treat asymptomatic bacteriuria, follow-up test for cure	
Urine screen	A	Urine dipstick for proteinuria for baseline screen of renal status	First visit	Unless risk factors present for UTIs, renal disease or preeclampsia, routine/repeat urine screen not recommended	
Gestational diabetes mellitus (GDM)	A	50-g oral GCT test; threshold ≥ 130–140 mg/dL (varies per lab/protocol); if over threshold, requires 3-hour GTT	24–28 weeks for most women	100-g, 3-hour GTT	↑ Risk of shoulder dystocia, macrosomia Educate women regarding GDM→DM disease progression

(continued)

TABLE 3-2 (Continued)

PRENATAL SCREENING					
CONDITION AND/OR SCREENING/LAB TEST	**A, ALL WOMEN; I, IF INDICATED**	**TEST COMMENTS**	**TIMING**	**FOLLOW-UP OR TREATMENT**	**INTRAPARTUM IMPLICATIONS**

Group B streptococcus (GBS)	A	Vaginal/rectal microbial swab, speculum exam not required
		Recommended for planned cesarean
			35–37 weeks	Indications for intrapartum antibiotic prophylaxis:
				• GBS(+) women at labor onset for vaginal birth, or ROM for planned vaginal or CS births
				• GBS bacteriuria in index pregnancy
				• Prior infant with early-onset GBS
				• If GBS status unknown at labor onset and any of the following:
				  • $<$37 weeks
				  • ROM $\geq$ 18 hours
				  • Temp $\geq$ 100.4°F (38° C)
				If unknown status, test on admission
					Intrapartum prophylaxis with penicillin or ampicillin; if penicillin-allergic, use cefazolin (if not high risk for anaphylaxis)
					If high risk for anaphylaxis, antimicrobial sensitivity testing should be performed, and use clindamycin or vancomycin
					Erythromycin no longer recommended; GBS isolate resistance as high as 25–32% for erythromycin and 13–20% for clindamycin
					Vancomycin used in drug-resistant organism or if sensitivity[g] testing not performed

Note: AAP, American Academy of Pediatrics; ACOG, American College of Obstetricians and Gynecologists; DM, diabetes mellitus; EIA, enzyme immunoassay; FTA-ABS, fluorescent treponemal antibody absorbed tests; GCT, glucose challenge test; GTT, glucose tolerance test; H&H, hemoglobin and hematocrit; NAATs, nucleic acid amplification tests; PLT, platelet; PROM, premature rupture of membranes, PTL, preterm labor; LBW, low birth weight; RPR, rapid plasma reagin; TP-PA, *T. pallidum* passive particle agglutination assay; USPTF, U. S. Preventive Services Task Force; UTI, urinary tract infection; VDRL, Venereal Disease Research Laboratory.

[a]Positive result requires confirmation with Western blot or immunofluorescent assay (IFA). Results can take several days.

[b]Women who use illicit drugs, have STDs during pregnancy, have multiple sex partners during pregnancy, live in areas with high HIV prevalence, or have HIV-infected partners.

[c]Multiple sex partners, evaluation/treatment for STI, HBsAg positive sex partner, recent/current injection-drug use.

[d]High-risk factors generally defined as ‹ 25, new or multiple sexual partners, history of disease or other STI, sex workers, drug use, inconsistent condom use, local prevalence of disease. Consideration should also be given to local epidemiology of disease when developing screening criteria.

[e]Uninsured women, women living in poverty, sex workers, illicit drug users, and women in communities with high syphilis morbidity, presence of other STI.

[f]HIV, exposure to TB, comorbidities such as diabetes, lupus, cancer, alcoholism, drug addiction; born/emigrated from high-prevalance country, medically underserved, homeless, occupational exposure risk, living in LTC facility.

[g]Guidelines include sensitivity testing of organism to antibiotics in penicillin-allergic women.

References

American Academy of Pediatrics & American College of Obstetricians and Gynecologists. (2012). *Guidelines for perinatal care.* Elk Grove, IL: Authors.

American College of Obstetricians and Gynecologists. (2006). *Management of alloimmunization during pregnancy* (Practice Bulletin No. 75). Washington, DC: Author.

Association of Women's Health, Obstetric, and Neonatal Nurses. (2012). *HIV screening for pregnant women and infants* (AWHONN Position Statement). Washington, DC: Author.

Centers for Disease Control and Prevention. (2006). *Rapid HIV-1antibody testing during labor and delivery for women of unknown HIV status: A practical guide and model protocol.* Atlanta, GA: Author.

Centers for Disease Control and Prevention. (2010). Prevention of perinatal group B streptococcal disease: Revised guidelines from CDC, 2010. *Morbidity and Mortality Weekly Report, 59*(RR-10), 1–32.

Centers for Disease Control and Prevention. (2010). Sexually transmitted diseases treatment guidelines. *Morbidity and Mortality Weekly Report, 59*(RR-12), 1–110.

Moise, K. J. (2009). Hemolytic disease of the fetus and newborn. In R. K. Creasy, R. Resnick, J. D. Iams, C. J. Lockwood, & T. R. Moore (Eds.), *Creasy & Resnick's maternal–fetal medicine: Principles and practice* (pp. 477–503). Philadelphia, PA: Saunders.

U. S. Preventive Services Task Force. (2005). Screening for gonorrhea: Recommendation statement. *Annals of Family Medicine, 3*(3), 263–267. doi: 10.1370/afm.337

U. S. Preventive Services Task Force. (2007). Screening for chlamydial infection: U. S. Preventive Services Task Force Recommendation Statement. *Annals of InternalMedicine, 147*(2), 128–134.

Gestational Age Assessment

Accurate determination of the estimated due date (EDD) has both social and clinical significance. For the pregnant woman and her family, it signifies a key landmark in the pregnancy around which important planning and anticipation centers. For clinicians, it guides various assessment intervals and interventions, and allows for comparisons of the fetus's growth and development against established norms. The EDD is usually determined during the first prenatal visit, and documented as a final EDD on the prenatal record. Since the 1800s, clinical dating based on last menstrual period (LMP) has been achieved using Naegele's Rule, which estimates EDD by adding 7 days to the LMP and subtracting 3 months. Using LMP as a proxy for ovulation, Naegele's Rule assumes that ovulation occurs on day 14 of the menstrual cycle, and that a full-term gestation is 266 days from conception, or 280 days from LMP. The calculation has some inherent variation since months vary in length by a few days. More importantly, errors in maternal recall of LMP, history of an irregular cycle, recent hormonal contraception use, pregnancy, lactation, as well as individual variations in the luteal phase and ovulation among women, make it an imprecise estimator of EDD. Studies suggest that as few as 10% of women ovulate exactly on day 14, and only 30% are fertile from day 10–17 despite having a regular, 28-day cycle (Baird et al., 1995; Wilcox, Dunson, & Baird, 2000).

In most developed countries, the use of biometric ultrasound assessments in the first half of pregnancy has become a key part of determining EDD. The gold standard ultrasound measurement for determining EDD is first-trimester (≤13 6/7 weeks) crown–rump length (CRL) (ACOG, AIUM, & SMFM 2014). In the all but rare circumstances the best obstetric estimate of EDD obtained in the first trimester by LMP and ultrasound should not be adjusted on the basis of later ultrasound data. In situations where no first trimester ultrasound has been performed, second trimester ultrasound can be used to evaluate EDD using composite biometric variables such as bipariateal diameter, head circumference, femur length, and abdominal circumference. Parameters that may support adjustment of EDD based on the timing of the ultrasound and the degree of discrepancy between LMP and ultrasound dates are listed in Table 3-3. If pregnancy resulted from assisted reproductive technology then the ART-derived gestational age is used to assign EDD.

Symphysis–fundal height assessment is used as a screening tool for tracking fetal growth, and is obtained by measuring from the symphysis pubis to the top of the fundus using a flexible measuring

TABLE 3-3 Guidelines for Redating Based on Ultrasonography

GESTATIONAL AGE DATE RANGE*	METHOD OF MEASUREMENT	DISCREPANCY BETWEEN ULTRASOUND DATING AND LMP DATING THAT SUPPORTS REDATING
≤13 6/7 wk	CRL	
• ≤8 6/7 wk		More than 5 days
• 9 0/7 wk to 13 6/7 wk		More than 7 days
14 0/7 wk to 15 6/7 wk	BPD, HC, AC, FL	More than 7 days
16 0/7 wk to 21 6/7 wk	BPD, HC, AC, FL	More than 10 days
22 0/7 wk to 27 6/7 wk	BPD, HC, AC, FL	More than 14 days
†28 0/7 wk and beyond	BPD, HC, AC, FL	More than 21 days

Abbreviations: AC, abdominal circumference; BPD, biparietal diameter; CRL, crown-rump length; FL, femur length; HC, head circumference; LMP, last menstrual period.

*Based on LMP

†Because of the risk of redating a small fetus that may be growth restricted, management decisions based on third-trimester ultrasonography alone are especially problematic and need to be guided by careful consideration of the entire clinical picture and close surveillance.

Note: From "Method for estimating due date (Committee Opinion No. 611)", by American College of Obstetricians and Gynecologists, American Institute of Ultrasound Medicine, & Society for Maternal-Fetal Medicine, 2014, *Obstetrics and Gynecology, 124*, p. 864. Copyright 2014 by the American College of Obstetricians and Gynecologists. Reprinted with permission.

tape. The height of the uterine fundus, measured in centimeters, closely matches gestational age (in weeks) from 20 to 34 weeks. The fundus usually reaches the height of the umbilicus by 20 weeks' gestation, and increases by approximately 1 centimeter per week until reaching the xyphoid process at 34–36 weeks. Fundal height has utility as a screening tool only, and is best used as a serial measurement to track fetal growth, as its specificity in detecting small- or large-for-gestational-age fetuses is as low as 20% (Hargreaves, Cameron, Edwards, Gray, & Deane, 2011). Some conditions or situations can alter the measurement, such as the presence of uterine fibroids, a full bladder, and maternal obesity.

Demographic and Socioeconomic Factors Assessment

Demographic and socioeconomic factors, such as age, race, marital status, income, and education level, are known to affect pregnancy outcomes. Extremes of age (≤ 18 or ≥ 35) are associated with a host of adverse pregnancy and birth outcomes. While teen pregnancy rates have decreased overall by 45% since 1991, racial disparities persist, with black and Hispanic teen pregnancy rates more than double that of white teens, respectively (Martin et al., 2012). Infants born to teens are at greater risk of low birth weight (LBW), preterm birth (PTB), and death during infancy (Centers for Disease Control and Prevention [CDC], 2011). More women are delaying childbearing, and may enter pregnancy with age-related comorbidities such as hypertension, diabetes, coronary artery disease, or obesity. Since 1990, birth rates have declined for women age 15–29 years old, and have declined each year since 2007 for women in their 30s. Rates for women age 40–44 have doubled since 1990, and have risen 300% from 1997 until 2009 for women over age 50 (Martin et al., 2011, 2012). Women age 35 and older are at increased risk of miscarriage, gestational diabetes mellitus (GDM), placenta previa, and cesarean birth. Infants born to women in this age group are at increased risk for macrosomia, and of having chromosomal abnormalities or congenital anomalies. After age 40, women are at increased risk of placental abruption, LBW, and perinatal mortality (Cleary-Goldman et al., 2005). For women age 35–39, and over 39, pregnancy-related mortality rates are two- to five-fold higher, respectively, compared to women in their 20s and early 30s (Berg, Callaghan, Syverson, & Henderson, 2010).

Women from low-income neighborhoods have been found to have higher incidences of LBW, small for gestational age (SGA), PTB, low 5-minute Apgar scores, and stillbirth (Liu et al., 2010; Metcalfe, Lail, Ghali, & Sauve, 2011). Single mothers have higher rates of LBW and PTB when compared to married or cohabitating women (Sullivan, Raley, Hummer, & Schiefelbein, 2012). For reasons that remain poorly understood, significant racial disparities exist in many adverse pregnancy and birth outcomes, with the burden falling disproportionately on black women. Black women have higher incidences of fetal death, PTB, fetal growth restriction, pregnancy-related hypertensive disorders, and higher rates of maternal morbidity overall (Bryant, Worjoloh, Caughey, & Washington, 2010). Pregnancy-related mortality in Black women is nearly four-fold that of Hispanic and non-Hispanic White women. Asian/Pacific Islander and Hispanic women have the highest incidences of GDM, and neural tube defects are seen disproportionately in Hispanic births (Bryant et al., 2010).

Women from different age, socioeconomic, and cultural or racial backgrounds may have distinct needs and preferences for support and education during the labor process. Throughout the peripartum period, individuals may be particularly receptive to teaching regarding the impact of their lifestyle choices and behaviors on their own and their infant's health, offering a window of opportunity for nurses to meaningfully influence the health of women and their families through health promotion teaching (Edvardsson et al., 2011). Perinatal nurses can tailor care and supportive strategies using knowledge of risk factors, an understanding of different needs likely to occur in different age groups and social situations, and by maintaining an inquisitive and attentive attitude toward cultural and individual needs.

Psychosocial Assessment

All women should be screened for psychosocial risk factors regardless of race or ethnicity, education level, and social status (AAP & ACOG, 2012). Assessment should include (1) exposure to intimate partner violence (IPV) and other safety concerns; (2) stress; (3) history of depression; (4) past or current alcohol or other substance use; (5) tobacco use or exposure; (6) nutrition; (7) barriers to health care; (8) desire for the pregnancy; (9) unstable housing; and (10) communication barriers. While this screening should occur throughout prenatal care and findings communicated in the prenatal record, women may withhold or delay disclosing highly sensitive and personal information for a variety of reasons. Moreover, changes in relationships or in life circumstances may introduce such risk factors late in the pregnancy. As such, perinatal nurses may be the first to detect them.

When available, screening should be done via the use of validated, evidence-based screening tools. Studies suggest that the use of such tools can increase detection of psychosocial issues or vulnerabilities potentially leading to postpartum depression, identify women experiencing IPV, or recognize substance or alcohol abuse (Blackmore et al., 2006; Chasnoff et al., 2005; Norton, Peipert, Zierler, Lima, & Hume, 1995). Some of these tools are brief and suitable for incorporating into the admission assessment, thereby ensuring routine screening for risk factors in all women. Examples include, but are not limited to, the *Abuse Assessment Screen* for detecting IPV (Parker & McFarlane, 1991) and the *4Ps Plus*© for substance and/or alcohol use (Chasnoff, Wells, McGourty, & Bailey, 2007).

Regardless of the tool or screening method used, questions should be asked in private, with appropriate support for any identified communication barriers, such as translation services. Family members, friends, or the woman's spouse or significant other should not be used as a translator in these circumstances, as issues such as IPV, depression, or substance abuse may not be reported. Nurses should make every effort to suspend personal bias or judgment as health risks are identified. Positive screening results should never be used punitively; rather, they should guide appropriate referral and follow-up and be utilized to assist the woman in obtaining supportive treatment and care. If physical, sexual, or emotional abuse is reported, it is imperative to inquire about immediate threats to the woman or her baby, and plan for necessary referral and support to address them prior to discharge. Health care providers should know their state laws regarding reporting of IPV, since, unlike child abuse, which is always reportable, state laws governing IPV reporting vary. Similarly, some states consider *in utero* drug exposure a form of child abuse, and require reporting of positive drug tests to the local child protection agency.

Medication Review

A thorough review of the woman's medication use should be performed to assess for potential teratogen exposure and other fetal effects, dependency issues, and potential impact on maternal–fetal stability during labor and birth, and to allow for medication reconciliation. Medication reconciliation is the process of comparing a patient's medication orders to the medications they have been taking. It was designated a National Patient Safety Goal by The Joint Commission (TJC) in 2005, and streamlined in 2011 (TJC, 2012). It is done to avoid medication errors such as omissions, duplications, dosing errors, or drug interactions, as well as to identify medications that should be continued, and should be performed at every care transition where new medications are ordered or existing orders are rewritten (TJC, 2012). The term "medication" can include prescription and sample medications, herbal remedies, vitamins, nutraceuticals, vaccines, over-the-counter drugs, diagnostic and contrast agents, radioactive medications, respiratory therapy treatments, parenteral nutrition, blood derivatives, and intravenous solutions (Greenwald et al., 2010). The name, dose, route, frequency, purpose, and last dose should be recorded. While documentation of current medications is often done by nurses, the reconciliation process is also a physician or primary provider responsibility. Institutional policies should ensure that effective and accurate medication reconciliation is occurring.

PHYSICAL EXAMINATION

Maternal Assessment

A comprehensive physical examination assists in identifying the physiologic status of both the woman and her fetus as well as the progress of her labor. This information guides the plan for appropriate care and support for a successful birth. It includes maternal physical exam (vital signs, systems review), labor status (cervical exam, membrane status, presence or absence of vaginal bleeding), and laboratory evaluation (see Box 3-1). An understanding of the normal physiologic adaptations in pregnancy is essential for accurate evaluation of maternal status, and forms the basis for interpreting signs and symptoms indicating pathophysiologic change or disease progression in the pregnant woman. A review of the normal physiologic adaptations seen in pregnancy is presented in Table 3-4. The four essential forces of labor are also evaluated and include assessment of uterine contractions (power), vaginal/pelvic exam (passage), fetal assessment (passenger), and maternal emotional status (psyche).

Clinical Assessment of Maternal Vital Signs

Maternal vital signs should be assessed at least every 4 hours, with increased frequency as guided by patient condition or unit policy (AAP & ACOG, 2012). An appropriately sized blood pressure cuff should be used as well as ensuring correct maternal positioning for accurate measurement. Blood pressure assessed in a left lateral position with the cuff on the right arm falsely lowers systolic, diastolic, and mean pressures. Blood pressure should be taken in the sitting position, with the cuff on the left arm positioned at heart level (Pickering et al., 2005).

TABLE 3-4 Normal Physiologic Adaptations in Pregnancy

SYSTEM	MODIFICATIONS	IMPLICATIONS
Cardiovascular	• Heart displaced upward, forward and to the left, ↑ size of heart • Apex rotated laterally • Heart rate ↑ 15–20 beats/minute • Exaggerated split of first heart sound • Stroke volume and cardiac output ↑ 30% • ↑ Blood volume 30–50% with ↓ hematocrit • WBC ↑ to 15,000 • Blood pressure ↓ second trimester • Widening of pulse pressure • Hypercoaguable: ↑ procoagulant activity and ↓ fibrinolytic activity	• Point of maximal impulse slightly more left lateral • Heart is enlarged • Perfusion depends on heart rate • Benign systolic murmurs are common • Electrocardiogram changes: inverted P wave, small Q wave, tachyarrhythmias • Physiologic anemia • ↑ Risk for clot formation (venous thromboembolism, disseminated intravascular coagulation)
Respiratory	• pH ↑ 7.40–7.45 • $PaCO_2$ ↓ 27–32 mmHg • HCO_3 ↓ 18–21 mmHg • Diaphragm elevates • Tidal volume ↑ 30–40%	• Compensated respiratory alkalosis • Oxygen consumption ↑ • Shortness of breath is a common complaint
Renal	• Glomerular filtration ↑ 40–50% • Hypertrophy of kidneys due to ↑ blood volume • ↑ Fluid and sodium retention	• Proteinuria more common • Hydronephrosis • Increased risk of urinary tract infection • Edema
Uterine	• Receives 10–20% of cardiac output • 700–800 mL/minute perfusion rate	• Regulated by BP and SVR (systemic vascular resistance) • Supine position compresses inferior vena cava and aorta, ↓ blood flow

Torgerson and Curran (2006).

Measurement of blood pressure in the left lateral recumbent position, on the left arm, does not differ substantially from blood pressure obtained in the sitting position (Pickering et al., 2005).

Pain assessment should include information about acute and chronic sources of pain, effectiveness of coping techniques, and assessment of the woman's and her family's expectations regarding pain management during labor. Evaluation of the effectiveness of pain management strategies should be performed at regular intervals during labor and birth as the "fifth vital sign." Assessing pain on a continuum may detect potential threats to maternal–fetal well-being such as epigastric pain (worsening preeclampsia) or unremitting uterine contractions (tachysystole or abruption). Distinctive circumstances may influence the woman's experience of pain, as may prior surgical procedures, interventions, length of labor, efficacy of coping/support mechanisms, and fatigue.

Assessing the woman's goals for pain management should be incorporated into the admission assessment. For the woman who desires a medication-free labor and birth, the labor nurse can play a pivotal role in her success by providing primary coaching and support or augmenting that provided by her partner or other support persons. For those who choose analgesia or regional anesthesia, their preferred method should be provided if no contraindications exist (ACOG, 2004). Analgesia and anesthesia may produce both therapeutic and side effects, potentially altering maternal and fetal assessments; hence, reassessment and documentation of efficacy and side effects should occur within 30–60 minutes of such interventions.

Maternal Height, Weight, and Weight Gain

Assessment of maternal height and weight, weight of any prior infants, and current pregnancy weight gain may provide additional information signaling potential risks for the laboring woman. Because maternal weight (overweight or underweight) is associated with adverse pregnancy outcomes, and may influence fetal size, maternal height and weight should be measured at the first prenatal visit and a body mass index (BMI) calculated. Discussion of the woman's target pregnancy weight gain should be based on evaluation of the BMI (see Table 3-5), which is calculated as follows:

$$\left(\frac{\textit{weight in pounds divided by height in inches}}{\textit{height in inches}}\right) \times 703$$

Obesity is associated with multiple comorbidities in pregnancy. A large prospective population-based cohort study demonstrated that women who were "morbidly obese" (defined as a BMI > 40) were at increased risk of diabetes, preeclampsia, induction of labor, cesarean birth, postpartum hemorrhage, and shoulder dystocia when compared with normal-weight women (Ramsay, Greer, & Sattar, 2006). Electronic monitoring and ultrasound exam may be more difficult in overweight women. Adipose attenuates the ultrasound signal; the quality of the image is sacrificed for the quality of depth (Ramsey et al., 2006). Obesity may interfere with maternal awareness of fetal activity. Due to the safety risks associated with obesity, advanced planning regarding process and equipment is

TABLE 3-5 Recommended Total Weight Gain in Pregnancy

	RECOMMENDED WEIGHT GAIN	
PREPREGNANCY BMI	**SINGLETON GESTATION**	**TWIN GESTATION**
Underweight (BMI < 18.5)	28–40 pounds	Insufficient information
Normal weight (BMI 18.5–24.9)	25–35 pounds	37–54 pounds
Overweight (BMI 25–29.9)	15–25 pounds	31–50 pounds
Obese (BMI > 30)	11–20 pounds	25–42 pounds

Institute of Medicine andNational Research Council Committee to Reexamine IOM Pregnancy Weight Guidelines (2009).

recommended to ensure safe care for the woman and her caregivers (Simpson, 2008). This may include consultation with anesthesia, longer spinal needles, operating room bed extenders, larger/longer blood pressure cuff, internal fetal and uterine monitoring devices, and use of patient lifts.

Fetal Assessment

Assessment of fetal well-being is a key component of perinatal care. It begins at the first prenatal visit with gestational age determination and continues during subsequent visits to include fetal activity assessment, antenatal testing (as indicated by maternal or fetal needs), and assessment of the fetus during labor.

Antenatal Assessment

The primary objective of antenatal testing is to detect the fetus at risk for injury or death. The basis for antenatal testing relies on the premise that the fetus whose oxygenation *in utero* is compromised will respond with a series of physiologic, adaptive or decompensatory signs as hypoxemia develops (Signore, Freeman, & Spong, 2010). Antepartum testing may be indicated in any pregnancy where the risk of antepartum fetal demise is increased (ACOG, 2000). A variety of technologies are available and include fetal movement or kick counting, nonstress test (NST), contraction stress test (CST), ultrasound exams (biophysical profile [BPP], modified BPP, amniotic fluid volume [AFV]), and Doppler velocimetry (uterine artery, umbilical artery, middle cerebral artery, and fetal veins). An in-depth discussion of antepartum assessment methods is presented in Chapter 10.

Method of Fetal Monitoring

The method of fetal monitoring used to assess fetal status during labor (auscultation, external, or internal) should be identified and documented. Each method has benefits and limitations, as discussed in Chapter 4. When using auscultation, the clinician can assess the FHR, rhythm, and accelerations and decelerations of the FHR. On the basis of those findings, interventions are planned and responses to interventions are assessed and documented.

When using external and internal electronic fetal heart monitoring, the baseline FHR, variability, accelerations and decelerations, and evolution of the tracing over time can be assessed. When electronic monitoring is used, information regarding uterine activity should be validated by the clinician through palpation. Interpretation of the data obtained with auscultation or the electronic fetal monitor, coupled with ongoing assessment of maternal physical and emotional status, can be used to plan interventions and assess maternal–fetal responses. Chapter 6 includes a detailed discussion of interventions related to fetal assessment by auscultation and palpation and electronic fetal monitoring.

Fetal Activity

Nonperception of fetal movement coupled with a history of conditions that may affect placental well-being should heighten the suspicion of fetal physiologic compromise or demise. Clinicians should ascertain time and quality of the last perceived fetal movements. See Chapter 10 for a detailed discussion of fetal movement counting.

Leopold's Maneuvers

Leopold's maneuvers are an abdominal assessment technique used to determine the presentation, position, and lie of the fetus, which then may be confirmed by a vaginal examination. *Fetal lie* is the position of the long axis of the fetus and is described as being longitudinal, transverse, or oblique. *Fetal presentation* refers to the part of the fetus that is entering the pelvis and is described as cephalic, breech, or shoulder. *Fetal position* describes the relationship of the presenting part to the pelvis and is described as anterior, posterior, or transverse. Leopold's maneuvers include assessment of four components:

1. Fetal part in the fundus
2. Location of the fetal back

3. Presenting part (Pallach's maneuver)
4. Descent and attitude of the presenting part

These four maneuvers provide a systematic approach to identify the point of maximal sound intensity of the fetal heart (Box 3-2; Figure 3-2). Optimal fetal heart sounds are usually heard over the curved part of the fetus presenting closest to the anterior uterine wall. The initial physical contact of obtaining Leopold's maneuvers may also promote a positive clinician–patient relationship.

Box 3-2 Steps to Perform Leopold's Maneuvers

1. Use measures to make the woman comfortable.
   a. Wash hands and warm them.
   b. Encourage the woman to empty her bladder.
   c. Expose the woman's abdomen from the symphysis pubis to the xiphoid process.
   d. Drape the woman appropriately.
   e. Position the woman with a pillow under her head, flex her knees, and rest her arms at her sides.
   f. Place a small wedge under the woman's hip.
   g. Explain the purpose of the procedure (to determine fetal lie, presentation, position, and the site for auscultation of the FHR) and the steps of the Leopold's maneuvers.
   h. Place warmed hands on the woman's abdomen while explaining the procedure to assist her in relaxing her abdominal muscles.
2. Prepare to perform Leopold's maneuvers.
   a. Inspect the woman's abdomen for bulges (small parts), fetal movement, and the long axis of the fetus.
   b. Use the palmar surface of the hands with fingers together for a gentle but firm examination.
   c. Stand at the woman's right or left side (e.g., a right-handed examiner should stand at the woman's right side; a left-handed examiner should stand at the woman's left side).
3. Perform Leopold's maneuvers (Figure 3-2).
   a. Begin with the first maneuver. Face the woman and place your hands at the top and side of the fundus. Be attentive to the size, shape, and consistency of the fetal part that is in the fundus (note where the longitudinal axis of the fetus is located).
   b. For the second maneuver, remain standing at the woman's side, facing her, with hands placed on either side at the middle of the abdomen. One hand will push the contents of the abdomen toward the other hand to stabilize the fetus for palpation. The hand that is palpating begins at the middle of the abdomen near the fundus and moves posterior toward the woman's back. Continue this process, progressing downward to the symphysis pubis. Determine which part of the fetus lies at the side of the abdomen. If firm, smooth, and consistent, it is likely to be the back. If smaller, protruding, and irregular, it is likely to be the small parts. Note the location of the small parts and the back. Reverse the hands and repeat the maneuver.
   c. For the third maneuver, remain facing the woman. With the middle finger and thumb grasp the part of the fetus situated over the pelvic brim. With firm, gentle pressure, determine whether the head is the presenting part. This maneuver should confirm what was felt during the first two maneuvers. If the presenting part is moveable, it is not engaged in the pelvis. If the presenting part is fixed and difficult to move, it is likely to be engaged. The third maneuver also is known as "Pallach's maneuver" or "Pallach's grip."
   d. For the fourth maneuver, turn and face the woman's feet. Place your hands at the sides of the uterus, below the umbilicus, pointing toward the symphysis pubis. Press deeply, with fingertips toward the pelvic inlet, feeling for the cephalic prominence. If the cephalic prominence is felt on the same side as the fetus's back, it will be the occiput (crown), and the head will be slightly extended. If the cephalic prominence is felt on the same side as the small parts, it is likely to be the sinciput (forehead), and the fetus will be in a vertex or well-tucked position. If the cephalic prominence is felt equally on each side, the fetus's head may be in a military position, which is common when the fetus is in a posterior position. Finally, move the hands toward the pelvic brim. If the hands come together around the presenting part, the presenting part is floating. If the hands stay apart, the presenting part is either dipping or engaged in the pelvis.
4. Share the information obtained with the woman, and ask if she would like to feel her fetus through palpation, if appropriate.
5. Locate and verify the FHR, which generally can be heard over the curved part of the fetus closest to the anterior wall of the uterus.
6. Document the findings of Leopold's maneuvers, the FHR and rhythm, and appropriate nursing interventions.

Figure 3-2 The Four Steps in Performing Leopold's Maneuvers

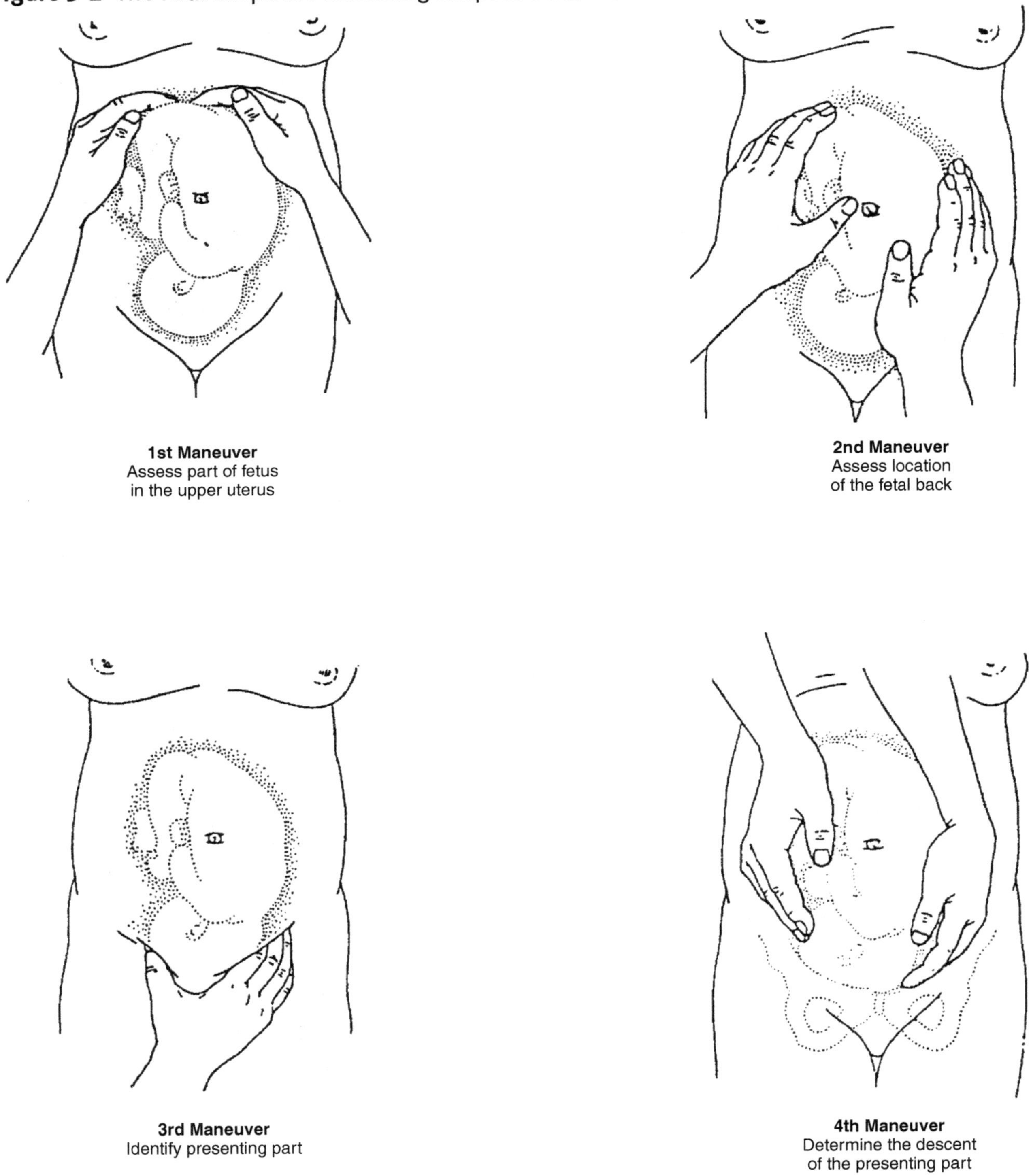

Assessment of Labor Status

Uterine Activity

Subjective and objective data are used to assess uterine contraction status. The woman should be asked about the onset, timing (frequency and duration), and intensity of her contractions. Clinicians should assess contraction frequency, duration, intensity, and resting tone via direct palpation and through electronic fetal monitoring (EFM) assessments. *Frequency* is measured from the beginning of one contraction to the beginning of the next described in minutes, and *duration* refers to contraction length and is described in seconds. *Intensity* refers to contraction strength and is described as mild, moderate, or strong by palpation, or in millimeters of mercury (mmHg) if internal monitoring is used. *Resting tone* is described as soft or firm by palpation, or in mmHg with internal monitoring.

Summary terms used to describe uterine activity are *normal* and *tachysystole* (Macones, Hankins, Spong, Hauth, & Moore, 2008). Normal uterine activity is defined as ≤ 5 contractions in 10 minutes averaged over 30 minutes, and tachysystole as > 5 contractions in 10 minutes averaged over 30 minutes. Excessive uterine activity has been associated with fetal acidosis at birth (Bakker, Kurver, Kuik, & Van Geijn, 2007). The goals in labor should be to identify and promote normal uterine activity and promptly correct any modifiable causes of tachysystole. For a more detailed discussion of uterine activity assessments, see Chapter 5.

Membrane Status

Membrane status is evaluated via history and/or objective assessment. Rupture of membranes (ROM) may present as a gush of fluid or a small leak. Assessment should include time of ROM, amniotic fluid color, amount, presence/absence of blood, and odor. Other methods may be used to confirm ROM, and are summarized in Table 3-6. A summary of the efficacy of certain tests for detecting ROM is presented in Table 3-7. Since the risk for infection and chorioamnionitis increases following ROM, vaginal examinations should be limited, and if stable, maternal temperature should be obtained every 2 hours if in labor. If being expectantly managed, temperature should be obtained every 4 hours. Attention to perineal hygiene may decrease the risk of infection (AAP & ACOG, 2012). Signs of chorioamnionitis may include (ACOG, 2007):

- Maternal fever (≥100.4° F [38° C])
- Maternal or fetal tachycardia
- Elevated maternal white blood cell count (nonspecific sign)
- Uterine tenderness
- Foul-smelling vaginal discharge

Intra-amniotic infection and decidual hemorrhage (abruption) occurring remote from term may release proteases into the choriodecidual tissues and amniotic fluid, leading to rupture of

TABLE 3-6 Clinical Tests to Confirm Rupture of Membranes

NAME OF TEST	METHOD	CONSIDERATIONS
Pooling	• Sterile speculum exam • Pooling of fluid in posterior fornix is visualized	• Other fluids may be mistaken for amniotic fluid
Nitrazine	• Sterile speculum exam • Litmus paper or swab • Alkalinity = blue	• False-positive may occur as a result of cervicitis, vaginitis, alkaline urine, blood, semen, or antiseptics
Ferning	• Sterile speculum exam • Fluidobtained from posterior fornix • Fluid swabbed onto a slide and allowed to dry • Crystallization of dry amniotic fluid in "fern-like" pattern is observed	• False-positive results may occur as a result of fingerprints on slide, blood, semen, or cervical mucus
Rapid Immunoassay for placental alpha microglobulin-1 (PAMG-1)	• Speculum not needed • "Kit" is needed from manufacturer	• Semen, urine, blood, or vaginal infectionsdo not affect results
Blue Dye	• Amniocentesis required • Dilute indigo carmine is instilled • Membranes are ruptured if the dye leaks into vagina within 20–30 minutes	• Invasive; may result in bleeding or infection

TABLE 3-7 Performance of Noninvasive Tests to Diagnose Rupture of the Fetal Membranes

TEST/REFERENCE	NAME OF TEST	CUTOFF	SENSITIVITY (%)	SPECIFICITY (%)	PPV (%)	NPV (%)
Nitrazine (pH)	—	Positive/negative	90–97	16–70	63–75	80–93
Ferning and/or pooling	—	Positive/negative	51–98	70–88	84–93	87–97
AFP	ROM Check® (Adeza Biomedical Corp., Sunnyvale, CA)	> 30/µg/l	90–94	95–100	94–100	91–94
Fetal fibronectin	—	> 50 ng/ml	97–98	70–97	74–93	98–100
IGFBP-1	PROM-TEST® (Medix Biochimica, Kauinianen, Finland), AMNI Check® (MAST Diagnostica, Reinfield, Germany)	> 3/µg/l	74–97	74–98	73–97	56–95
Prolactin	—	> 30–50/µIU/ml	70–95	76–78	72–84	75–93
Diamine oxidase	—	> 25 /µIU/test	83	90–100	100	89
β-hCG	—	> 40–65 /µIU/ml	68–95	70–95	73–91	78–97
Urea and creatinine	—	> 0.12–0.6 mg/dl	90–100	87–100	94–100	91–100
AmnioSense Absorbent pad	—	pH > 5.2	98.3	70	65–70	98
Lactate	Lac test®	≥ 4.5 mmol/1	79–86	88–92	88–92	78–87
PAMG-1	AmniSure® Test ROM (AmniSure International LLC, Cambridge, MA)	> 5.0 ng/ml	98–99	88–100	98–100	91–99

Abbreviations: AFP, alpha-fetoprotein; β-hCG, beta-subunit of human chorionic gonadotropin; IGFBP-1, insulin-like growth factor binding protein 1; NPV, negative predictive value; PAMG-1, placental alpha-microglobulin 1; PPV, positive predictive value.
Note: From "Guidelines for the management of spontaneous preterm labor: Identification of spontaneous preterm labor, diagnosis of preterm premature rupture of membranes, and preventive tools for preterm birth." By G. C. Di Renzo, L. Roura, F. Facchinetti, A. Antsaklis, G. Breborowicz, E. Gratacos, . . . Y. Ville, 2011, *Journal of Maternal-Fetal and Neonatal Medicine*, 24(5). p. 662. Copyright 2011 by Informa Healthcare. Reprinted with permission of Informa Healthcare.

membranes (Di Renzo et al., 2011). Invasive uterine procedures performed during pregnancy (amniocentesis, chorionic villus sampling, cervical cerclage, fetal surgery) can damage the membranes, causing them to leak. Early and accurate diagnosis of membrane rupture allows for gestational age-specific obstetrical interventions designed to optimize outcome and minimize complications (Di Renzo et al., 2011). Diagnosis is difficult when fluid leakage is small and/or intermittent. Noninvasive biochemical tests can assist in the diagnosis of rupture of membranes in these situations.

Vaginal Examination

Vaginal Bleeding or Discharge

Assessment should include evaluation of vaginal bleeding or discharge and identification of related potential risk factors in the patient's history. Vaginal bleeding may result from bloody show (blood-tinged mucus with mucous strands), which normally occurs with cervical dilation, or from more serious conditions, such as placenta previa, abruption, or uterine rupture. These conditions can alter uteroplacental perfusion and compromise maternal and fetal well-being.

Hemorrhage can occur during any stage of the perinatal period. If bleeding is present, vaginal examinations should be deferred until the source of bleeding is identified. Other information such as the onset, amount, color, and bleeding characteristics (presence or absence of clots), associated pain, and precipitating events should be assessed.

Since prompt recognition and treatment of hemorrhage is critical to preventing adverse maternal and fetal outcomes, it is imperative that perinatal nurses accurately quantify blood loss. Visual estimation may lead to underestimating the severity of maternal hemorrhage and contribute to treatment delays (Gabel & Weeber, 2012). Replacing estimated blood loss (EBL) derived from visual estimation and descriptors (scant, light, moderate, severe) with quantified blood loss (QBL) from actual measurement (1 gram = 1 milliliter) has been proposed as a more reliable method to assess and record blood loss (Gabel & Weeber, 2012).

The color and character of vaginal bleeding can be an important diagnostic indicator. Bright red, painless bleeding may indicate placenta previa, and dark red bleeding with clots or a board-like abdomen (typical of abruption) may indicate concealed blood loss. Overt placental abruption and uterine rupture may occur without bleeding. In those instances, maternal vital signs and FHR assessments will provide critical information (Ruth & Kennedy, 2011). Hypovolemia may result from excessive bleeding. The fetus is not protected from maternal blood loss because autoregulation of uterine perfusion does not occur, and the vasoconstrictive effects seen in hypovolemic shock exacerbate this problem. Maternal vital signs may remain unchanged until approximately 20% of blood volume is lost (Brown, 2009), at which point uteroplacental perfusion may be impaired. Fetal heart rate manifestations of decreased uteroplacental perfusion may include late decelerations, increasing baseline, and decreasing variability.

A narrowing of the pulse pressure occurs in Class 2 hemorrhage with a blood loss of 1000–1500 mL. Tachycardia is a hallmark sign of physiologic compensation for hypovolemia as the body attempts to increase cardiac output. Although tachypnea is a nonspecific response to volume loss, it is also a compensatory sign of volume deficit that is often overlooked (Ruth & Kennedy, 2011). Additional important signs of Class 2 hemorrhage are increasing maternal heart rate, orthostatic blood pressure changes, prolonged capillary refill (indicating decreased perfusion of extremities), and blanching or mottling of the extremities. Overt hypotension; marked tachycardia and tachypnea; and cold, clammy skin are signs of worsening hemorrhage (Class 3), with a blood loss of 1500–2500 mL (Ruth & Kennedy, 2011). The use of pulse oximetry may be helpful in assessment of maternal oxygenation, along with frequent vital signs, and ongoing FHR assessment.

Ultrasound evaluation by a qualified provider may be performed to assess the placenta and its location. A Kleihauer-Betke laboratory test is used to detect transplacental hemorrhage and can be helpful in predicting preterm labor following maternal trauma (Brown, 2009).

Near term, vaginal discharge normally increases. However, copious, malodorous, or discolored discharge may indicate infection and require further evaluation. The woman should be questioned about the onset, color, amount, and odor of vaginal discharge and about other unusual symptoms, such as vaginal pruritus, that may indicate a monilial or other infection.

Cervical Examination

A vaginal examination is performed to assess cervical status. The examination includes assessment of the cervix for dilation, effacement, position, and station of the presenting part. This is accomplished through gloved digital examination or by sterile speculum examination in the case of ruptured membranes without labor, premature ROM (PROM), or preterm PROM (PPROM). When contractions occur between 24 0/7 and 34 6/7 weeks' gestation, it may be of benefit to obtain a fetal fibronectin (fFN) sample prior to vaginal exam (Wax, Cartin, & Pinette, 2010).

After explaining the vaginal exam procedure to the woman and her support persons and allowing the woman to choose who will remain in the room, she should be draped for minimal exposure and positioned to maximize fetal oxygenation. Vaginal exams may be performed in positions other than lithotomy, such as sidelying or squatting, and may be more tolerable for the woman if she is coached to take slow, deep breaths during the procedure.

Cervical dilation is reported in a range between 0 and 10 cm, and effacement is reported as a percentage between 0% and 100%. The terms "complete" and "fully" are often used clinically for dilation of 10 cm and/or for 100% effacement. Cervical position is reported as posterior, midposition, or anterior; fetal station is reported numerically as a range from –5 cm (floating) to +5 cm (on the perineum), indicating the descent of the fetal head in relationship to the ischial spines. The presenting part is the part of the fetus that is presenting and felt through the cervix.

Maternal Assessment in Nonobstetric Setting

Assessment and care of pregnant women may occur outside the perinatal unit; most likely in the emergency department (ED), urgent care, operating room (OR) for nonobstetrical surgery, and intensive care unit (ICU). The focus of the assessment should not be on its location; rather, it should be on the obstetrical competency of the provider performing the assessment. Institution-specific policies should guide where pregnant women are evaluated based on the nature and severity of her presenting condition (primary survey), gestational age, and the type of care required to stabilize and treat her appropriately.

For antepartum evaluation, gestational age may drive where the woman is initially seen. Twenty weeks' gestation is often used as a parameter with pregnant women, with those < 20 weeks triaged through the ED, and those 20 weeks and over directed to the perinatal unit. However, gestational age should be only one aspect to use for decision making regarding where the pregnant woman is best evaluated and treated. A triage algorithm should be developed collaboratively by the perinatal, emergency, and perioperative departments, since interdepartmental cooperation is critical for best practice. For concerns that are clearly obstetric (contractions, vaginal bleeding, ROM, pelvic pressure, decreased fetal movement), the assessment is best accomplished in the perinatal area. With other complaints, many of which are confusing (abdominal pain, headache, nausea and vomiting, dizziness), the decision for the location of the assessment is not always well defined. Given that serious disorders, such as atypical preeclampsia, cardiac disease, and pulmonary embolism, may be associated with these and other symptoms, such complaints in pregnant women should be triaged with heightened concern. Ongoing interdepartmental communication may aid in determining the required expertise on a case-by-case basis.

When a pregnant woman presents to urgent care or the ED with cardiovascular, respiratory, trauma, surgical, or other nonobstetric concerns, she should initially be seen in the ED. Obstetric consultation is required, and should be defined by the institution. Information about fetal movement, cramping, contractions, pelvic pressure or backache, vaginal bleeding, or leaking of fluid should be obtained. An understanding of the normal physiologic adaptations in pregnancy is essential to interpreting lab values and other tests and for adapting certain interventions to accommodate pregnancy. To ensure fetal oxygenation, left uterine displacement is necessary at ≥ 20 weeks' gestation to prevent vena cava compression, promote maternal cardiac output, and prevent supine hypotension. For a summary of FHM considerations in nonobstetric surgery and trauma in pregnancy, see Table 9-7 in Chapter 9. Suggested management strategies aimed at optimizing maternal–fetal stability during evaluation of women presenting with trauma in the ED or other settings are summarized in Table 3-8.

The most common nonobstetrical surgeries in pregnant women are appendectomy and cholecystectomy (Gilo, Amini, & Landy, 2009). Fetal heart rate should be assessed before and after surgery in a woman with a previable (< 24 weeks) fetus. Sometimes, fetal monitoring

TABLE 3-8 Emergency Department Management Strategies for Trauma in Pregnancy

High-flow oxygen 10–15 liters/minute
Initiation of two large-bore IVs for rapid fluid replacement
Rapid treatment and transport
Rapid sequence intubation
Ultrasound to determine gestational age, placenta location, number of fetuses
Left uterine displacement and avoiding supine position to prevent aortocaval compression
Maintain compensatory respiratory alkalosis
Electronic fetal and uterine monitoring when > 24 weeks' gestation

Suresh, LaToya Mason, and Munnur (2010).

is recommended throughout the surgery since shunting of blood from the uterus to vital organs may compromise fetal oxygenation. Fetal tachycardia, late decelerations, and decreased variability may be observed before alterations in maternal vital signs manifest (Tweddale, 2006). Recommendations for pre- and intraoperative care of women ≥ 24 weeks requiring nonobstetrical surgery include:

- Preoperative cervical exam
- Preoperative medications including Zantac and sodium citrate
- Left uterine displacement in the OR and post anesthesia care unit (PACU)
- Oxygen saturation > 95%
- Mean arterial pressure (MAP) of > 65 mmHg
- Pre- and postoperative EFM
- Notification of woman's obstetrician prior to surgery (ACOG, 2011b)

Trauma is the leading non-obstetrical cause of maternal mortality and complicates an estimated 6–7% of pregnancies (Tweddale, 2006). Motor vehicle accidents (MVAs) are the most common type of trauma, followed by violence and assault (Brown, 2009). Trauma is associated with pregnancy loss, premature labor and birth, PROM, abruption, uterine rupture, and fetal injury or loss. Properly applied seat belts may reduce both maternal and fetal morbidity and mortality (Brown, 2009). Since fetal well-being depends on maternal stability, maternal resuscitation should be the first priority when caring for the injured pregnant woman (Brown & Mozurkewich, 2013; Mirza, Devine, & Gaddipati, 2010). Collaboration between the obstetrical and trauma teams can ensure an understanding of maternal physiologic changes in pregnancy, laboratory values, and comprehensive maternal–fetal assessment. Monitoring of uterine activity and fetal heart rate should occur until maternal–fetal stability is achieved. Delayed placenta abruption is less likely if uterine contraction frequency is less than every 10 minutes with normal fetal heart rate activity over a 4- to 6-hour period of observation. The observation also includes assessment for uterine tenderness, bleeding, and rupture of membranes (Brown, 2009). Fetal–maternal hemorrhage can be a complication of maternal trauma. A Kleihauer-Betke test for fetal–maternal hemorrhage is a standard maternal assessment for blunt trauma; it is most helpful in Rh-D negative women to determine the amount of anti-D immune globulin to be given to prevent maternal alloimmunization. The team providing care to the trauma victim must be prepared for an emergency cesarean birth when the gestational age is ≥ 24 weeks; however, in general stabilizing the mother will be more effective for promoting both maternal and fetal well-being than performing emergency cesarean.

SUMMARY

Maternal–fetal assessment begins at the first prenatal visit and continues through birth. Ongoing assessment of the physical and emotional condition of the mother and the physical condition of the fetus is key to ensuring appropriate care during the perinatal period. Gathering essential data assists the nursing and medical staff in formulating the plan of care for the family, anticipating potential problems, and intervening in a timely manner.

Each institution should address regulatory agency requirements for patient assessment through the development of interdisciplinary policy and procedure, provision of a means of communicating these requirements to its staff members, and planning for their implementation. Interdisciplinary and interdepartmental policies related to caring for pregnant women with nonobstetric conditions should also be developed. Emphasis should be on the severity and acuity of the presenting condition and ensuring that resources and personnel are utilized optimally within each institution to care for women in these circumstances (AAP & ACOG, 2012).

Care of women and their families should be evidence- and standards-based, and administered by physicians and nurses who maintain up-to-date information about the normal physiologic processes of labor and birth, maternal and family preferences, and complicating conditions and diseases most likely to affect the population they care for. This knowledge may be derived from the latest information from systematic reviews; morbidity and mortality data in pregnancy; evidence-based guidelines and position statements from professional organizations; current research on pregnancy-related diseases and disorders; and from clinical experiences enriched by feedback and outcomes from women and their families in each clinical setting.

Case Study: Margaret

Age:	23 years old
Gravidity/Parity:	G20010
Gestational Age:	37-4/7 weeks
Medical History:	Chronic hypertension requiring Labetolol 200 mg po bid
Surgical History:	Unremarkable
Psychosocial History:	Married; father of baby involved
Past Obstetric History:	Spontaneous abortion at 11 weeks
Current Obstetric History:	Twin gestation (dichorionic/diamniotic)
	Gestational diabetes mellitus A2 requiring insulin

Mild preeclampsia

Margaret was admitted to labor and delivery at 0500 for labor induction because of worsening blood pressures (140–150s/90s mmHg) and proteinuria (462 mg in 24-hour urine). VE on admission revealed a cervix that was 1 cm dilated and 50% effaced. The fetal vertex for twin A was at −1 station with Twin B in a transverse lie. Induction was started with a Foley bulb and low-dose oxytocin. Magnesium sulfate was started for seizure prophylaxis. Hourly fingerstick blood glucose samples were obtained, and values were within a normal range. Spontaneous rupture of membranes occurred at 1720. The fluid was clear, and the Foley bulb was removed.

The patient requested an epidural at 2100. VE after epidural placement revealed a cervix that was 4 cm dilated, 90% effaced, and a fetal vertex at 0 station. Oxytocin was infusing at 12 mU/minute. Margaret's vital signs were as follows: oral temperature, 97.8° F (36.5° C); blood pressure, 135–157/66–90 mmHg; pulse, 107–120 bpm; and respirations, 22 breaths per minute.

Margaret: Labor and Delivery EFM Tracing at 2135 Using Ultrasound and Tocodynamometer

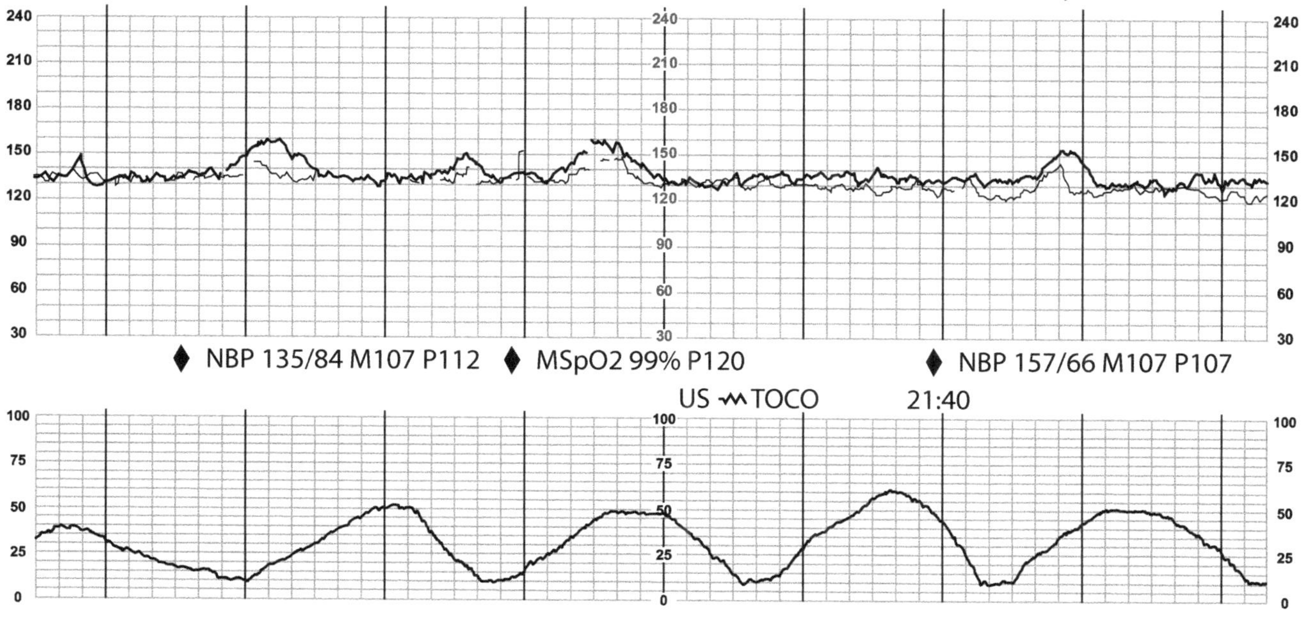

Case Study Exercise B: Margaret

1. Baseline FHR: **Twin A (dark line): 135 bpm**

   Twin B (light line): 130 bpm

2. Variability

Absent (undetectable)	_____	
Minimal (>0 but £5 bpm)	_____	
Moderate (6–25 bpm)	_____	**(Twin A & B)**____
Marked (>25 bpm)	_____	
Unable to determine	_____	

3. Contractions

Frequency:	**q 1½–2 min**
Duration:	**90–100 seconds**
Intensity:	**Palpate**
Resting tone:	**Palpate**

4. Accelerations and decelerations. When present, circle P if periodic or E if episodic.

Accelerations	P	**E (Twin A & B)**
Early decelerations	P	
Variable decelerations	P	E
Late decelerations	P	
Prolonged decelerations	P	E
None present		

5. Interpretation

Category I	________
Category II	________
Category III	________

6. List possible underlying physiologic mechanisms or rationales for observed patterns.
   - Associated with adequate oxygenation and a normal fetal acid-base status at present
   - Spontaneous fetal movement or in response to environmental stimulus
   - Uterine contraction
   - Direct sympathetic stimulation of the fetus
   - Autonomic regulation of FHR

7. List in order of priority the physiologic goal(s) for observed patterns.
   - Maintain appropriate levels of uterine activity.
   - Promote maternal comfort and labor progress.
   - Maximize oxygenation.
   - Maximize uteroplacental blood flow.
   - Maximize umbilical circulation.

8. List actions and interventions indicated based on overall interpretation (physiologic based, instrumentation based, and further assessments).

- Decrease oxytocin given adequate labor progress and contractions every 1½–2 minutes with less than 1 minute resting tone between them.
- Continue to observe FHR patterns.
- Maternal positioning to optimize oxygenation and maternal comfort.
- Monitor maternal vital signs.
- Palpate contractions to validate uterine monitoring data.
- Continue routine assessments and interventions for care of the high-risk labor patient to include blood sugar monitoring, magnesium sulfate management, blood pressure evaluation, and maternal comfort and support.
- Keep provider informed of FHR patterns (normal), interventions, and maternal–fetal response.

REFERENCES

Abbas, A. E., Lester, S. J., & Connolly, H. (2005). Pregnancy and the cardiovascular system. *International Journal of Cardiology*, *98*(2), 179–189. doi:10.1016/j.ijcard.2003.10.028

American Academy of Pediatrics & American College of Obstetricians and Gynecologists. (2012). *Guidelines for perinatal care* (7th ed.). Elk Grove, IL: Authors.

American Academy of Pediatrics & American College of Obstetricians and Gynecologists. (2012). *Guidelines for perinatal care*. Elk Grove, IL: Authors.

American College of Obstetricians and Gynecologists. (2000). Antepartum fetal surveillance. (Practice Bulletin No. 9, October 1999), Clinical management guidelines for obstetrician-gynecologists. *International Journal of Gynaecology and Obstetrics, 68*(2), 175–185.

American College of Obstetricians and Gynecologists. (2004). Pain relief during labor (ACOG Committee Opinion No. 295). *Obstetrics and Gynecology, 104*(1), 213.

American College of Obstetricians and Gynecologists. (2006). *Management of alloimmunization during pregnancy* (Practice Bulletin No. 75). Washington, DC: Author.

American College of Obstetricians and Gynecologists. (2009). ACOG Practice Bulletin No. 101: Ultrasonography in pregnancy. *Obstetrics and Gynecology, 113*(2, Pt. 1), 451–461. doi:10.1097/AOG.0b013e31819930b0

American College of Obstetricians and Gynecologists. (2011a). Emergent therapy for acute-onset, severe hypertension with preeclampsia or eclampsia (ACOG Committee Opinion No. 514). *Obstetrics and Gynecology, 118*(6), 1465–1468. doi:10.1097/AOG.0b013e31823ed1ef

American College of Obstetricians and Gynecologists. (2011b). Nonobstetric surgery during pregnancy (ACOG Committee Opinion No. 474). *Obstetrics and Gynecology, 117*(2, Pt. 1), 420–421. doi:10.1097/AOG.0b013e31820eede9

American College of Obstetricians and Gynecologists' Task Force on Hypertension in Pregnancy. (2013). Hypertension in pregnancy: Executive summary. *Obstetrics and Gynecology, 122*(5), 1122–1131. doi:10.1097/01.AOG.0000437382.03963.88

American College of Obstetricians and Gynecologists, American Institute of Ultrasound in Medicine, & Society for Maternal-Fetal Medicine. (2014). Method for estimating due date (ACOG Committee Opinion No. 611). *Obstetrics and Gynecology, 124*(4), 863–866. doi:10.1097/01.AOG.0000454932.15177.be http://www.acog.org/-/media/Committee-Opinions/Committee-on-Obstetric-Practice/co611.pdf?dmc=1&ts=20141025T1918278842

Association of Women's Health, Obstetric, and Neonatal Nurses. (2012). *HIV screening for pregnant women and infants* (AWHONN Position Statement). Washington, DC: Author.

Baird, D. D., McConnaughey, D. R., Weinberg, C. R., Musey, P. I., Collins, D. C., Kesner, J. S., . . . Wilcox, A. J. (1995). Application of a method for estimating day of ovulation using urinary estrogen and progesterone metabolites. *Epidemiology, 6*(5), 547–550.

Bakker, P. C., Kurver, P. H., Kuik, D. J., & Van Geijn, H. P. (2007). Elevated uterine activity increases the risk of fetal acidosis at birth. *American Journal of Obstetrics and Gynecology, 196*(4), 313.e1–313.e6.

Barton, J. R., & Sibai, B. M. (2008). Prediction and prevention of recurrent preeclampsia. *Obstetrics and Gynecology, 112* (2, Pt.1), 359–372. doi:10.1097/AOG.0b013e3181801d56

Bellamy, L., Casas, J. P., Hingorani, A. D., & Williams, D. (2009). Type 2 diabetes mellitus after gestational diabetes: Asystematic review and meta-analysis. *Lancet, 373*(9677), 1773–1779. doi:10.1016/S0140-6736(09)60731-5

Berg, C. J., Callaghan, W. M., Syverson, C., & Henderson, Z. (2010). Pregnancy-related mortality in the United States, 1998-2005. *Obstetrics and Gynecology, 116*(6), 1302–1309. doi:10.1097/AOG.0b013e3181fdfb11

Blackmore, E. R., Carroll, J., Reid, A., Biringer, A., Glazier, R. H., Midmer, D., . . . Stewart, D. E. (2006). The use of the Antenatal Psychosocial Health Assessment (ALPHA) tool in the detection of psychosocial risk factors for postpartum depression: Arandomized controlled trial. *Journal of Obstetrics and Gynaecology Canada, 28*(10), 873–878.

Brown, H. L. (2009). Trauma in pregnancy. *Obstetrics and Gynecology, 114*(1), 147–160. doi:10.1097/ACOG.0b013e3181ab6014

Brown, S., & Mozurkewich, E. (2013). Trauma during pregnancy. *Obstetrics and Gynecology Clinics of North America, 40*(1), 47–57. doi:10.1016/j.ogc.2012.11.004

Bryant, A. S., Worjoloh, A., Caughey, A. B., & Washington, A. E. (2010). Racial/ethnic disparities in obstetric outcomes and care: Prevalence and determinants. *American Journal of Obstetrics & Gynecology, 202*(4), 335–343. doi:10.1016/j.ajog.2009.10.864

Centers for Disease Control and Prevention. (2006). Rapid HIV-1antibody testing during labor and delivery for women of unknown HIV status: A practical guide and model protocol. Retrieved from www.cdc.gov/hiv/topics/testing/resources/guidelines/rt-labor&delivery_part2.htm.

Centers for Disease Control and Prevention. (2010). Prevention of perinatal group B streptococcal disease: Revised guidelines from CDC, 2010. *Morbidity and Mortality Weekly Report, 59*(RR-10), 1–32.

Centers for Disease Control and Prevention. (2010). Sexually transmitted diseases treatment guidelines. *Morbidity and Mortality Weekly Report, 59*(RR-12), 1–110.

Centers for Disease Control and Prevention. (2011). Vital signs: Teen pregnancy—United States, 1991–2009. *Morbidity and Mortality Weekly Report*, *60*(13), 414–420.

Chasnoff, I. J., McGourty, R. F., Bailey, G. W., Hutchins, E., Lightfoot, S. O., Pawson, L. L., . . . Campbell, J. (2005). The 4P's Plus screen for substance use in pregnancy: Clinical application and outcomes. *Journal of Perinatology*, *25*(6), 368–374. doi:10.1038/sj.jp.7211266

Chasnoff, I. J., Wells, A. M., McGourty, R. F., & Bailey, L. K. (2007). Validation of the 4P's Plus screen for substance use in pregnancy validation of the 4P's Plus. *Journal of Perinatology*, *27*(12), 744–748. doi:10.1038/sj.jp.7211823

Clark, S. L., & Hankins, G. D. (2012). Preventing maternal death: 10 clinical diamonds. *Obstetrics & Gynecology*, *119*(2, Pt. 1), 360–364. doi:10.1097/AOG.0b013e3182411907

Cleary-Goldman, J., Malone, F. D., Vidaver, J., Ball, R. H., Nyberg, D. A., Comstock, C. H., . . . D'Alton, M. (2005). Impact of maternal age on obstetric outcome. *Obstetrics and Gynecology*, *105*(5, Pt. 1), 983–990. doi:10.1097/01.AOG.0000158118.75532.51

Cudihy, D., & Lee, R. V. (2009). The pathophysiology of pre-eclampsia: Current clinical concepts. *Journal of Obstetrics and Gynaecology*, *29*(7), 576–582. doi:10.1080/01443610903061751

Curry, R., Swan, L., & Steer, P. J. (2009). Cardiac disease in pregnancy. *Current Opinion in Obstetrics and Gynecology*, *21*(6), 508–513. doi:10.1097/GCO.0b013e328332a762

Di Renzo, G. C., Roura, L. C., Facchinetti, F., Antsaklis, A., Breborowicz, G., Gratacos, E., . . . Ville, Y. (2011). Guidelines for the management of spontaneous preterm labor: Identification of spontaneous preterm labor, diagnosis of preterm premature rupture of membranes, and preventive tools for preterm birth. *Journal of Maternal–Fetal and Neonatal Medicine*, *24*(5), 659–667. doi:10.3109/14767058.2011.553694

Dombrowski, M. P., & Schatz, M. (2010). Asthma in pregnancy. *Clinical Obstetrics and Gynecology*, *53*(2), 301–310. doi:10.1097/GRF.0b013e3181de8906

Duffy, C. R., Odibo, A. O., Roehl, K. A., Macones, G. A., & Cahill, A. G. (2012). Effect of magnesium sulfate on fetal heart rate patterns in the second stage of labor. *Obstetrics and Gynecology*, *119*(6), 1129–1136. doi:10.1097/AOG.0b013e318257181e

Edvardsson, K., Ivarsson, A., Eurenius, E., Garvare, R., Nyström, M. E., Small, R., & Mogren, I. (2011). Giving offspring a healthy start: Parents' experiences of health promotion and lifestyle change during pregnancy and early parenthood. *BMC Public Health*, *11*(936), 1–13. doi:10.1186/1471-2458-11-936

Esplin, M. S., O'Brien, E., Fraser, A., Kerber, R. A., Clark, E., Simonsen, S. E., . . . Varner, M. W. (2008). Estimating recurrence of spontaneous preterm delivery. *Obstetrics and Gynecology*, *112*(3), 516–523. doi:10.1097/AOG.0b013e318184181a

Gabel, K. T., & Weeber, T. A. (2012). Measuring and communicating blood loss during obstetric hemorrhage. *Journal of Obstetric, Gynecologic, and Neonatal Nursing*. *41*(4), 551–558. doi:10.1111/j.1552-6909.2012.01375.x

Gelson, E., Gatzoulis, M. A., Steer, P., & Johnson, M. R. (2009). Heart disease – why is maternal mortality increasing? *BJOG: An International Journal of Obstetrics and Gynaecology*, *116*(5), 609–611. doi:10.1111/j.1471-0528.2008.02082.x

Gilo, N. B., Amini, D., & Landy, H. J. (2009). Appendicitis and cholecystitis in pregnancy. *Clinical Obstetrics and Gynecology*, *52*(4), 586–596. doi:10.1097/GRF.0b013e3181c11d10

Greenwald, J. L., Halasyamani, L. K., Greene, J., LaCivita, C., Stucky, E., Benjamin, B., . . . Williams, M. V. (2010). Making inpatient medication reconciliation patient centered, clinically relevant and implementable: A consensus statement on key principles and necessary first steps. *Journal of Hospital Medicine*, *5*(8), 477–485. doi:10.1002/jhm.849

Hargreaves, K., Cameron, M., Edwards, H., Gray, R., & Deane, K. (2011). Is the use of symphysis-fundal height measurement and ultrasound examination effective in detecting small or large fetuses? *Journal of Obstetrics and Gynaecology*, *31*(5), 380–383.doi:10.3109/01443615.2011.567343

Hess-Eggleston, N., Troiano, N. H., Harvey, C. J., & Chez, B. F. (2013). Guidelines for the initial assessment and triage of obstetric patients. In N. H. Troiano, C. J. Harvey, & B. F. Chez (Eds.), *AWHONN high-risk andcritical care obstetrics* (pp. 371–373). Philadelphia, PA: Wolters Kluwer, Lippincott, Williams & Wilkins.

Institute of Medicine and National Research Council Committee to Reexamine IOM Pregnancy Weight Guidelines. (2009). Rasmussen, K. M., & Yaktine, A. L. (Eds). *Weight gain during pregnancy: Reexamining the guidelines.* Washington, DC: National Academies Press.

Inturrisi, M., Linter, N. C., & Sorem, K. (2013). Diabetic ketoacidosis and continuous insulin infusion management in pregnancy. In N. H. Troiano, C. J. Harvey, & B. F. Chez (Eds.), *AWHONN high-risk and critical care obstetrics* (3rd ed., pp. 163–174). Philadelphia, PA: Lippincott, Williams & Wilkins.

The Joint Commission. (2012). National patient safety goals effective January 1, 2013: Hospital accreditation program. Retrieved from www.jointcommission.org/assets/1/18/NPSG_Chapter_Jan2013_HAP.pdf.

Kim, C., Berger, D. K., & Chamany, S. (2007). Recurrence of gestational diabetes mellitus: A systematic review. *Diabetes Care*, *30*(5), 1314–1319. doi:10.2337/dc06-2517

Liu, N., Wen, S. W., Katherine, W., Bottomley, J., Yang, Q., & Walker, M. C. (2010). Neighbourhood family income and adverse birth outcomes among singleton deliveries. *Journal of Obstetrics and Gynaecology of Canada, 32*(11), 1042–1048.

Macones, G. A., Hankins, G. D., Spong, C. Y., Hauth J., & Moore, T. (2008). The 2008 National Institute of Child Health and Human Development workshop report on electronic fetal monitoring: Update on definitions, interpretation, and research guidelines. *Journal of Obstetric, Gynecologic and Neonatal Nursing. 37*(5), 510–515. doi:10.1111/j.1552-6909.2008.00284.x

Martin, J. A., Hamilton, B. E., Ventura, S. J., Osterman, M. J. K., Kirmeyer, S., Mathews, T. J., & Wilson, E. C. (2011). Births: Final data for 2009. *National Vital Statistics Reports, 60*(1), 1–70.

Martin, J. A., Hamilton, B. E., Ventura, S. J., Osterman, M. J. K., Wilson, E. C., & Mathews, T. J. (2012). Births: Final data for 2010. *National Vital Statistics Reports, 61*(1), 1–72.

Martin, S. R. (2011). Cardiac disease in pregnancy. In M. R. Foley, T. H. Strong, Jr., & T. J. Garite (Eds.), *Obstetric intensive care manual* (3rd ed., pp. 91–116). New York, NY: McGraw-Hill.

Melchiorre, K., Sutherland, G. R., Liberati, M., & Thilaganathan, B. (2011). Preeclampsia is associated with persistent postpartum cardiovascular impairment. *Hypertension, 58*(4), 709–715. doi:10.1161/HYPERTENSIONAHA.111.176537

Mendola, P., Laughon, S. K., Männistö, T. I., Leishear, K., Reddy, U. M., Chen, Z., & Zhang, J. (2013). Obstetric complications among US women with asthma. *American Journal of Obstetrics & Gynecology, 208*(2), 127.e1–127.e8. doi:10.1016/j.ajog.2012.11.007

Metcalfe, A., Lail, P., Ghali, W. A., & Sauve, R. S. (2011). The association between neighbourhoods and adverse birth outcomes: A systematic review and meta-analysis of multi-level studies. *Paediatric and Perinatal Epidemiology, 25*(3), 236–245. doi:10.1111/j.1365-3016.2011.01192.x

Mirza, F. G., Devine, P. C., & Gaddipati, S. (2010). Trauma in pregnancy: A systematic approach. *American Journal of Perinatology, 27*(7), 579–586. doi:10.1055/s-0030-1249358

Moise, K. J. (2009). Hemolytic disease of the fetus and newborn. In R. K. Creasy, R. Resnick, J. D. Iams, C. J. Lockwood, & T. R. Moore (Eds.), *Creasy & Resnick's maternal–fetal medicine: Principles and practice* (pp. 477–503). Philadelphia, PA: Saunders.

Mostello, D., Kallogjeri, D., Tungsiripat, R., & Leet, T. (2008). Recurrence of preeclampsia: Effects of gestational age at delivery of the first pregnancy, body mass index, paternity, and interval between births. *American Journal of Obstetrics and Gynecology, 199*(1), 55.e1–55.e7. doi:10.1016/j.ajog.2007.11.058

Murphy, V. E., Namazy, J. A., Powell, H., Schatz, M., Chambers, C., Attia, J., & Gibson, P. G. (2011). A meta-analysis of adverse perinatal outcomes in women with asthma. *BJOG: An International Journal of Obstetrics and Gynaecology, 118*(11), 1314–23. doi:10.1111/j.1471-0528.2011.03055.x

Nelson-Piercy, C. (2011). Saving Mothers' Lives: Reviewing maternal deaths to make motherhood safer: 2006–2008. *BJOG: An International Journal of Obstetrics and Gynaecology, 118*(Suppl. 1), 109–118. doi:10.1111/j.1471-0528.2010.02847.x

Norton, L. B., Peipert, J. F., Zierler, S., Lima, B., & Hume, L. (1995). Battering in pregnancy: An assessment of two screening methods. *Obstetrics and Gynecology, 85*(3), 321–325.

Parker, B., & McFarlane, J. (1991). Identifying and helping battered pregnant women. *MCN, The American Journal of Maternal/Child Nursing, 16*(3), 161–164.

Perlow, J. H. (2011). Obesity in the obstetric intensive care patient. In M. R. Foley, T. H. Strong, Jr., & T. J. Garite (Eds.), *Obstetric intensive care manual* (3rd ed., pp. 61–72). New York, NY: McGraw-Hill.

Phelan, S. T. (2008). The prenatal medical record: Purpose, organization and the debate of print versus electronic. *Obstetrics and Gynecology Clinics of North America, 35*(3), 355–368. doi:10.1016/j.ogc.2008.06.001

Pickering, T. G., Hall, J. E., Appel, L. J., Falkner, B. E., Graves, J., Hill, M. N., . . . Roccella, E. J. (2005). Recommendations for blood pressure measurement in humans and experimental animals: Part 1: Blood pressure measurement in humans: A statement for professionals from the Subcommittee of Professional and Public Education of the American Heart Association Council on High Blood Pressure Research. *Hypertension, 45*(1), 142–161. doi:10.1161/01.HYP.0000150859.47929.8e

Ramsay, J. E., Greer, I., & Sattar, N. (2006). ABC of obesity: Obesity and reproduction. *British Medical Journal, 333*(7579), 1159–1162.

Raschke, R. A. (2011). Advanced cardiac life support of the pregnant patient. In M. R. Foley, T. H. Strong, Jr., & T. J. Garite (Eds.), *Obstetric intensive care manual* (3rd ed., pp. 199–211). New York, NY: McGraw-Hill.

Rocklin, R. E. (2011). Asthma, asthma medications and their effects on maternal/fetal outcomes during pregnancy. *Reproductive Toxicology, 32*(2), 189–197. doi:10.1016/j.reprotox.2011.05.023

Ruth, D., & Kennedy, B. B. (2011). Acute volume resuscitation following obstetric hemorrhage. *Journal of Perinatal and Neonatal Nursing, 23*(3), 253–260. doi:10.1097/JPN.0b013e31822539e3

Sibai, B. M. (2011). Hypertensive emergencies. In M. R. Foley, T. H. Strong, Jr., & T. J. Garite (Eds.), *Obstetric intensive care manual* (3rd ed., pp. 49–60). New York, NY: McGraw-Hill.

Signore, C., Freeman, R. K., & Spong, C. Y. (2009). Antenatal testing – A reevaluation: Executive summary of a Eunice Kennedy Shriver National Institute of Child Health and Human Development workshop. *Obstetrics and Gynecology*, *113*(3), 687–701. doi:10.1097/AOG.0b013e318197bd8a

Simpson, K. R. (2008). Extreme obesity as a patient safety risk during labor and birth. MCN, The *American Journal Maternal/Child Nursing*, *33*(3), 196. doi:10.1097/01.NMC.0000318365.54224.7b

Simpson, L. L. (2012). Maternal cardiac disease: Update for the clinician. *Obstetrics and Gynecology, 119*(2, Pt. 1), 345–359. doi:10.1097/AOG.0b013e318242e260

Small, M. J., James, A. H., Kershaw, T., Thames, B., Gunatilake, R., & Brown, H. (2012). Near-miss maternal mortality: Cardiac dysfunction as the principal cause of obstetric intensive care unit admissions. *Obstetrics and Gynecology, 119*(2, Pt. 1), 250–255. doi:10.1097/AOG.0b013e31824265c7

Smith, G. N., Pudwell, J., Walker, M., & Wen, S. W. (2012). Ten-year, thirty-year, and lifetime cardiovascular disease risk estimates following a pregnancy complicated by preeclampsia. *Journal of Obstetrics and Gynaecology of Canada*, *34*(9), 830–835.

Sullivan, K., Raley, R. K., Hummer, R. A., & Schiefelbein, E. (2012). The potential contribution of marital-cohabitation status to racial, ethnic, and nativity differentials in birth outcomes in Texas. *Maternal and Child Health Journal, 16*(4), 775–784. doi:10.1007/s10995-011-0801-1

Suresh, M. S., LaToya Mason, C., & Munnur, U. (2010). Cardiopulmonary resuscitation and the parturient. *Best Practice and Research Clinical Obstetrics and Gynaecology, 24*, 383–400. doi: 10.1016/j.bpobgyn.2010.01.002

Torgerson, K. L., & Curran, C. A. (2006). A systemic approach to the physiologic adaptations of pregnancy. *Critical Care Nursing Quarterly*, *29*(1), 2–19.

Tweddale, C. J. (2006). Trauma during pregnancy. *Critical Care Nursing Quarterly, 29*(1), 53–67.

U. S. Preventive Services Task Force. (2005). Screening for gonorrhea: Recommendation statement. *Annals of Family Medicine*, *3*(3), 263–267. doi: 10.1370/afm.337

U. S. Preventive Services Task Force. (2007). Screening for chlamydial infection: U. S. Preventive Services Task Force Recommendation Statement. *Annals of Internal Medicine, 147*(2), 128–134.

Verreault, N., DaCosta, D., Marchand, A., Ireland, K., Banack, H., Dritsa, M., & Khalifé, S. (2012). PTSD following childbirth: A prospective study of incidence and risk factors in Canadian women. *Journal of Psychosomatic Research*, *73*(4), 257–263. doi:10.1016/j.jpsychores.2012.07.010

Vitoratos, N., Vrachnis, N., Valsamakis, G., Panoulis, K., & Creatsas, G. (2010). Perinatal mortality in diabetic pregnancy. *Annals of the New York Academy of Sciences*, *1205*, 94–98. doi:10.1111/j.1749-6632.2010.05670.x

Wax, J. R., Cartin, A., & Pinette, M. G. (2010). Biophysical and biochemical screening for the risk of preterm labor. *Clinical Lab Medicine*, *30*(3),693–707. doi:10.1016/j.cll.2010.04.006

Wilcox, A. J., Dunson, D., & Baird, D. D. (2000). The timing of the "fertile window" in the menstrual cycle: Day specific estimates from a prospective study. *British Medical Journal, 321*(7271), 1259–1262.

Wolff, G. A., & Weitzel, N. S. (2011). Management of acquired cardiac disease in the obstetric patient. *Seminars in Cardiothoracic and Vascular Anesthesia*, *15*(3), 85–97. doi:10.1177/1089253211420302

Wu, F. S. Y., Hwu, Y. M., Lee, R. K., Li, S. H., Sun, F. J., Lin, M. H., & Lin, S. Y. (2012). First trimester ultrasound estimation of gestational age in pregnancies conceived after in vitro fertilization. *European Journal of Obstetrics andGynecology and Reproductive Biology, 160*(2), 151–155. doi:10.1016/j.ejogrb.2011.11.019

CHAPTER 4

Techniques for Fetal Heart and Uterine Activity Assessment

Molly M. Killion

INTRODUCTION

The goal of fetal surveillance is to assess how a fetus is responding to the intrauterine environment. This may be performed in the outpatient setting as a nonstress test or in the inpatient setting through intermittent auscultation (IA) or electronic fetal monitoring (EFM). When fetal surveillance is used in the intrapartum period, the goal is to assess fetal well-being and the fetal heart rate (FHR) response to labor in order to make appropriate, physiologically based clinical decisions and, ultimately, to identify those fetuses at risk for hypoxia and provide timely intervention to avoid adverse outcomes. Many factors should be taken into consideration when selecting methods of fetal monitoring. These may include maternal and fetal status, maternal preferences, institutional policies, and national guidelines. Regardless of the fetal heart monitoring (FHM) method selected for a given patient, the clinician is accountable for knowing how to recognize and respond to auditory and electronically obtained FHR data. This assessment is incomplete without also assessing uterine activity. Clinicians should be able to recognize and respond to uterine activity data obtained electronically and by palpation. The development of skills in these monitoring methods enables the clinician to select and combine the most appropriate techniques for each individual woman.

This chapter focuses on the varied techniques available for assessing the FHR and uterine activity and addresses the current state of the science for auscultation and EFM. Techniques, capabilities, limitations, procedures, and troubleshooting strategies for each monitoring method are also discussed.

ABDOMINAL ASSESSMENT

Determining the optimal location to place the instrument being used to listen to or record the FHR is the first step to fetal assessment. In general, the FHR is best heard over the curved part of the fetus that is closest to the anterior uterine wall. When the back is not facing the anterior side of the maternal abdomen, aiming near the fetal chest may allow for the strongest signal. For example, if the fetus is in a vertex or breech presentation with an anterior position, the fetal heart is generally heard by placing the monitoring device over the fetal back. When there is a face or brow presentation or the fetus is in a posterior position, the FHR is often heard by placing the device over the fetal chest or small parts. After the point of maximal sound intensity is identified, the auscultation device or the Doppler ultrasound (U/S) transducer can be placed in the optimal position for fetal heart assessment. Placement of the device also depends on the degree of descent of the fetal presenting part. Leopold's maneuvers can be performed to assess the details of fetal position to identify the fetal back and ideal location for application of the auscultation or the Doppler U/S device. This provides a systematic approach to identifying the point of maximal sound intensity of the FHR. (Detailed review of the technique for conducting Leopold's maneuvers can be found in Chapter 3, Figure 3-2 and Box 3-2.)

PALPATION

Identifying the point of maximal sound intensity of the FHR by using touch to determine fetal position can be helpful, but touch is a required component when assessing uterine tone and contractions. When the uterus contracts its musculature becomes more firm and tense. This can be felt when the fingertips are placed over the woman's abdomen, ideally at the uterine fundus. Palpation provides information regarding uterine tone at rest and during contractions to measure frequency, intensity, and duration. In addition, direct uterine palpation can provide information about uterine tenderness, fetal size, and fetal movement (Feinstein, Sprague, & Trépanier, 2008). Assessment of contractions provides important contextual data when considering FHR information during labor.

Palpation Technique

Palpation should be performed throughout an entire contraction and should include palpation of the resting tone of the uterus between contractions. It is also used to confirm and supplement findings gathered from electronic uterine activity monitoring. The following steps may be used when performing palpation:

- Place fingertips on the maternal abdomen over the area where changes in uterine firmness can be best felt (often this is near the fundus). Fingertips are generally more sensitive than the palm of the hand.
- Firmly but gently attempt to indent the uterus with fingertips during and between contractions. Avoid sharp, jabbing movements to prevent undue discomfort to the woman.
- Assess *frequency* of contractions from the beginning of one contraction to the beginning of the next contraction.
- Assess *duration* of the contraction from the beginning of uterine tightening to its ending.
- Assess *intensity* of contractions as mild, moderate, or strong. Although there is no standard measure for determining palpated contraction intensity (strength), the following comparison approach is used by many clinicians based on the degree to which the uterine muscle can be indented (Table 4-1).
- Assess uterine resting tone between contractions as palpating soft or firm.
- Assess maternal perception of and response to uterine activity.

Using a measurement device (from a timepiece with a second hand and a pen and paper to a formal marking device on a fetal monitor), the woman can note each time she feels a contraction starting to allow for frequency measurements and/or note when she feels the contraction beginning, and again when she feels it end, to allow for duration measurements.

TABLE 4-1 Comparison Model for Palpation of Uterine Activity

PALPATION OF UTERUS	FEELS LIKE	CONTRACTION INTENSITY
• Easily indented	• Tip of nose	• Mild
• Can slightly indent	• Chin	• Moderate
• Cannot indent	• Forehead	• Strong

Note: Contractions should be referred to using one of the above descriptive terms—mild, moderate, strong—rather than labeled as "good" or "satisfactory."
Adapted from Malinowski, Pedigo, & Phillips (1989).

TABLE 4-2 Uterine Palpation

Capabilities	
• Detect relative uterine resting tone • Detect relative frequency, duration, and strength of uterine contractions	
Benefits and Limitations	
BENEFITS	**LIMITATIONS**
• Noninvasive; hands-on assessment and care of patient • Not limited by access to equipment; widely used • Provides information regarding relative frequency, duration, strength, and resting tone • Allows mother freedom of movement and ambulation • Use of touch may be reassuring to some women	• Palpation cannot be used to detect actual intrauterine pressures • Maternal size, amount of adipose tissue, uterine size, etc. may limit ability to palpate contractions • Subjectivity may result in different interpretations of uterine activity characteristics • Maternal preference or comfort may limit touch during contractions
Troubleshooting/Corrective Actions	
PROBLEM	**ACTION**
• Uterine contractions are not readily felt over the fundal area	• Attempt palpation over a variety of areas on the uterus to find best location

Benefits, limitations, and troubleshooting strategies for uterine palpation are summarized in Table 4-2.

AUSCULTATION

Auscultation of fetal heart characteristics requires attention to the audible characteristics of the FHR. This can be accomplished through continuous EFM or through intermittent auscultation (IA) with a variety of different devices. For a comprehensive discussion of auscultation, refer to Feinstein, Sprague, and Trépanier (2008).

Auscultation Devices

A fetoscope or Pinard-type stethoscope are both nonelectric devices that utilize bone conduction to allow the practitioner to hear the actual fetal heart sounds, including opening and closing of the ventricular valves (Goodwin, 2000). In contrast, a Doppler U/S device uses ultrasound technology to detect the motion of the heart walls or valves and convert it to sound. Some models of hand-held Dopplers also give a paper printout. These methods obtain information differently, but both can be appropriate choices in most clinical auscultation situations (American College of Nurse-Midwives [ACNM], 2010; Feinstein et al., 2008). Either method allows for detection of FHR baseline, rhythm, and changes from the baseline. Baseline rhythm is assessed for regularity and is described as either regular or irregular. However, of these methods, only the fetoscope can reliably clarify the presence of an irregular fetal heart rhythm (Feinstein et al., 2008). When an irregular heart rate is audible by Doppler U/S, assessment with a fetoscope-type device is warranted to rule out artifact. A Doppler cannot be used reliably to verify the presence of an irregular rhythm because of its technical limitations in information processing. For example, in a fetus with supraventricular tachycardia, the Doppler device could halve FHR because the rapid rate is higher than the rate that the device can accurately detect (Freeman, Garite, Nageotte, & Miller, 2012). In this situation, using the fetoscope device allows the practitioner to hear the actual heart sounds and rate. If an arrhythmia is suspected, further evaluation by other methods may be required to determine the type of arrhythmia present. Although most arrhythmias are benign and often revert to a normal rhythm during or after birth, all irregular FHRs should be reported to the primary care provider. Further discussion regarding arrhythmias can be found in Chapter 11. To allow for consistent interpretation and maximize accuracy of data, it is important for the practitioner to evaluate the capabilities of each available device (Table 4-3).

Auscultation is also a useful method for assessing FHR prior to initiation of EFM and for validating EFM findings (Murray, 2004; Parer, 1997). Maternal and fetal heart rates can, and should, be differentiated by palpating the maternal pulse in tandem with auscultating the FHR. This is an important assessment regardless of the monitoring modality in use because both the U/S and the fetal spiral electrode can transmit the maternal heart rate (MHR) signal in the case of a fetal demise (Murray, 2004). Signal ambiguity between maternal and fetal heart rates is known to occur (Freeman et al., 2012), especially in cases of maternal tachycardia or fetal bradycardia when the fetal signal is difficult to obtain (VanVeen, Belfort, & Kofford, 2012). Auscultation along with verification of maternal pulse can clarify the source of the signal and may assist in ruling out artifact.

Although less commonly thought of for use in IA, the external U/S transducer of the fetal monitor may be used to listen to the FHR intermittently. It should be noted that some EFM computerized systems automatically archive any data obtained, even if the paper tracing is turned off. Although these brief and intermittent segments of EFM data may be retrievable, the data generated would be of too short a duration to be reliably interpreted. To minimize this potential issue, using a hand-held Doppler or fetoscope may be preferred. These issues should be addressed by institutional policies and procedures and by documenting the method of fetal monitoring being used (Feinstein et al., 2008).

Auscultation Techniques and Procedure

Auscultation of the FHR and palpation of the uterus are necessary to evaluate the fetal heart status when IA is used because both of these assessments are critical in all types of FHR monitoring to develop a comprehensive clinical picture. Abdominal palpation is used to assess the resting tone of the uterus and characteristics of uterine contractions as previously discussed. After uterine activity and fetal position have been assessed, the bell of the fetoscope or the Doppler transducer is placed over the fetal back (Feinstein et al., 2008). While the maternal pulse is being assessed, FHR is auscultated between uterine contractions to establish the FHR baseline. Palpation of the uterine contractions also assists the practitioner in clarifying the relationship between FHR and uterine activity.

TABLE 4-3 Capabilities of Auscultation Devices

THE FETOSCOPE CAN:	THE DOPPLER CAN:
• detect FHR baseline • detect FHR rhythm • verify the presence of an irregular rhythm • detect increases (accelerations) and decreases (decelerations) from FHR baseline • clarify double counting or half-counting by EFM	• detect FHR baseline • detect FHR rhythm • detect increases (accelerations) and decreases (decelerations)

Note: EFM, Electronic fetal monitor(ing); FHR, fetal heart rate.
Note: From *Fetal Heart Rate Auscultation* (p. 14), by N. F. Feinstein, A. Sprague, and M. J. Trépanier, 2008, Washington DC: Association of Women's Health, Obstetric and Neonatal Nurses. Copyright 2008 by the Association of Women's Health, Obstetric and Neonatal Nurses. Used with permission.

Listening and Counting: The Art of Auscultation

With IA, the practitioner is the data processing center for the sounds and information being generated. Auscultation requires both *listening* and *counting* and necessitates the ability to differentiate the sounds generated by the specific device being used (Feinstein et al., 2008). Erroneous conclusions about fetal status could be inferred if maternal blood flow sounds are incorrectly thought to be fetal heart sounds. Thus, palpation of maternal pulse is necessary when auscultating FHR to ensure differentiation of fetal and maternal heart rates (Feinstein et al., 2008).

Determining the Baseline Rate

To identify the baseline rate, the fetal heart rate should be auscultated and counted between contractions when the fetus is not moving for at least 30–60 seconds. Once the baseline rate has been established, the FHR is then auscultated and counted while palpating maternal pulse at prescribed intervals for 15–60 seconds in between contractions in the absence of fetal activity to monitor baseline rate and to determine changes to the baseline as labor progresses (ACNM, 2010).

It should be noted that because there is no clear evidence about the best method of counting to determine the baseline rate, the practitioner's preference often dictates the method used. For example, some practitioners count for one full minute and use that number as the baseline rate in beats per minute (bpm). Others count for 30 seconds and multiply by two, or count during a few consecutive 15-second intervals and multiply each by four. This allows the clinician to obtain an approximate baseline rate and to determine the presence of variations within that rate. None of these methods has been determined to be superior to the others, and different counting intervals may be appropriate for different conditions. For example, longer intervals may help establish the baseline, whereas repeated short sampling of the FHR may help differentiate accelerations and decelerations of the FHR (Feinstein et al., 2008).

Determining Changes from the Baseline

Once the baseline rate has been established, listening for accelerations and decelerations is the next component in evaluating FHR. This is often done by auscultating the FHR over 15–60 seconds and noting any increases or decreases in rate (ACNM, 2010). When these changes in FHR are heard during auscultation, a technique that may assist in clarifying the nature of the audible changes is to count for multiple, brief, consecutive periods. This method consists of counting for consecutive 6-second intervals and multiplying the number of beats for each interval by 10,which gives a rough estimate of the number of bpm for each interval. This gives additional information regarding the nature (increase or decrease) and amplitude of FHR change and may assist in the decision making regarding whether to initiate EFM for further evaluation and clarification (Feinstein et al., 2008). Similarly, listening to the FHR during a contraction and for a short period of time after the uterus has relaxed may allow the practitioner to recognize decreases or decelerations in the FHR (ACNM, 2010). A stepwise approach to the procedure for IA is offered in Table 4-4.

What Cannot Be Assessed via Intermittent Auscultation?

Calculating FHR baseline variability requires visualization of a tracing to identify cyclic fluctuations in the heart rate over minute long segments (Murray, Huelsmann, & Koperski, 2011). Categorizing FHR deceleration patterns requires visualization of a tracing to assess the characteristics of the decelerations. Evidence does not support the ability of an individual to accurately and reliably assess FHR baseline variability or discriminate FHR deceleration patterns through auscultation alone (Parer, 1997). Based on the available research, IA is appropriate to assess the FHR baseline rate, rhythm, and increases or decreases from the baseline but baseline variability and types of decelerations should not be assigned when using auscultation because these are based on visual interpretations of electronic FHR data. If auscultation of decreases in the

TABLE 4-4 Auscultation Procedure

PROCEDURE	RATIONALE
1. Explain the procedure to the woman and her support person(s).	1. Allays fears and anxiety; offers opportunity for emotional and informational support.
2. Assist the woman to a semi-Fowler's or wedged lateral position.	2. Decreases potential for supine hypotension and promotes comfort.
3. Palpate the maternal abdomen and perform Leopold's maneuvers.	3. Locates the fetal vertex, buttocks, and back and determines the optimal location for auscultation (fetal heart sounds are best heard over the fetal back).
4. Assess uterine contractions (frequency, duration, intensity) and uterine resting tone by palpation.	4. Determines the maternal and fetal response to uterine activity.
5. Apply conduction gel to underside of the Doppler device, if used.	5. Provides an airtight seal and aids in the transmission of U/S waves.
6. Position the bell of fetoscope or Doppler device on the area of maximal intensity of the fetal heart sounds (usually over the fetal back). Use firm pressure if using the fetoscope.	6. Obtains the strongest FHR signal.
7. Palpate the woman's radial pulse.	7. Differentiates maternal from fetal heart rate.
8. Count the FHR after uterine contractions for at least 30–60 seconds.	8. Identifies the baseline FHR (in bpm), the rhythm (regular or irregular), and the presence or absence of increases/accelerations or decreases/decelerations of the FHR between contractions.
9. In clarifying FHR changes, recounts for multiple, consecutive brief periods of 6–10 seconds (multiplied by 10 and 6, respectively) may be particularly helpful.	9. Clarifies the presence of FHR changes. Provides data about the nature and amplitude of FHR changes.
10. Interpret FHR findings and document per unit protocol.	10. Provides record of assessments.
11. Share findings with woman and support person(s) and answer questions as needed	11. Provides informational support.
12. Promote maternal comfort and fetal oxygenation.	12. Provides physical support and promotes fetal well-being.

Abbreivation: bpm, beats per minute; FHR, fetal heart rate.
Note: From "*Fetal Heart Rate Auscultation*" by N. F. Feinstein, A. Sprague, and M. J. Trépanier, 2008, (p. 20). Copyright 2008 by the Association of Women's Health, Obstetric and Neonatal Nurses. Used with permission.

fetal heart rate causes provider concern, a visual assessment of FHR information may be warranted and EFM may be initiated. Alternatively, other methods to assess fetal well-being, such as fetal stimulation (scalp or acoustic) or fetal capillary sampling (which is no longer commonly used in the United States), may be appropriate as adjunct assessments to IA.

Interpreting Auscultated FHR Characteristics

The guidelines for interpretation of EFM tracings as defined by the National Institute of Child Health and Human Development (NICHD) (Macones, Hankins, Spong, Hauth, & Moore, 2008; see Chapter 5) were designed to establish a set of common definitions to describe the interpretation of fetal heart rate monitoring and to establish a three-tiered system of categories for interpretation of fetal heart rate patterns. These definitions and categories also have implications for the interpretation and communication of FHR data obtained with IA. Using a common language for the discussion of fetal status is a key principle of effective clinical communication and has the potential to decrease communication errors. It would be confusing to have one set of terms for interpretation of IA and another set of terms for interpretation of EFM, especially when clinicians may at times use both methods of fetal assessment in the course of caring for the same patient. In the past, the terms "reassuring" and "nonreassuring" were used in interpreting auscultation findings but these are no longer recommended as they are not well defined. In order to maintain a consistent language for discussion of FHR findings, the two categories that contain data obtainable through IA for interpretation of the FHR are Category I and Category II (Box 4-1). The definitions of these categories are consistent with the terminology used to interpret EFM patterns, but refer only to auscultation.

Category I auscultated FHR characteristics are normal (Lyndon, O'Brien-Abel, Simpson, 2009) (Box 4-1). Normal IA findings include all of the following characteristics: FHR baseline between 110 and 160 beats per minute (bpm), regular rhythm, the presence or absence of FHR increases or accelerations, and the absence of FHR decreases or decelerations. Normal FHR characteristics are predictive of fetal well-being at the time they are observed and may be followed with routine supportive measures.

Category II auscultated FHR characteristics include all findings that are not classified as normal, or Category I (Box 4-1). Irregular rhythm, presence of decreases or decelerations from baseline, tachycardia, and bradycardia are all indeterminate IA findings. They cannot be classified as abnormal without information about FHR baseline variability, which cannot be reliably assessed through IA. Category II FHR characteristics require evaluation, ongoing surveillance, and reevaluation, consistent with the assessment of the overall clinical circumstances. This may include, but is not limited to continuous EFM, use of intrauterine resuscitation techniques, ruling out maternal heart rate, and assessment of the continuation of indeterminate findings.

There is no Category III classification for IA findings. To classify a pattern as Category III, there must be absent variability or a sinusoidal pattern. These determinations require a visual assessment of the FHR tracing, thus cannot be made with auscultation, and EFM is required to classify an FHR pattern as Category III. As with EFM, IA findings and management needs are interpreted in the context of the overall clinical picture. Preparations to expedite birth in emergent situations (e.g., apparent auscultated significant fetal bradycardia) should be undertaken simultaneously with efforts to ameliorate, verify, and determine the precise nature of the FHR findings.

BOX 4-1 Interpretation of Auscultation Findings

CATEGORY I

Category I FHR characteristics by auscultation include all of the following:

- Normal FHR baseline between 110 and 160 bpm
- Regular rhythm
- Presence or absence of FHR increases or accelerations from the baseline rate
- Absence of FHR decreases or decelerations from the baseline

CATEGORY II

Category II FHR characteristics by auscultation include any of the following:

- Irregular rhythm
- Presence of FHR decreases or decelerations from the baseline
- Tachycardia (baseline > 160 bpm > 10 minutes in duration)
- Bradycardia (baseline < 110 bpm < 10 minutes in duration)

Auscultation as Compared with EFM

Although IA has been used for many years, EFM has been the predominant method of intrapartum fetal surveillance since its pervasive introduction into clinical practice in the 1970s and 1980s (Devane, Lalor, Daly, McGuire, & Smith, 2012), even for women considered to be low risk. EFM was adopted into clinical practice prior to scientific validation of its presumed benefits (Banta & Thacker, 2001; Parer, 2003). A retrospective study looking at singleton births with no anomalies in the United States found an increase in the use of EFM from 73.4% in 1990 up to 85.7% in 2004 (Ananth, Chauhan, Chen, D'Alton, & Vintzileos, 2013). In a nationally representative survey of childbearing women in the United States released in 2013, 89% of women reported receiving EFM, with 80% reporting continuous monitoring and only 12% reporting intermittent monitoring (5% reporting EFM being used as a baseline assessment only) (Declercq, Sakala, Corry, Applebaum, & Herrlich, 2013). In a similar survey from Canada, women reported some amount of EFM in 90.8% of labors, with 62.9% reporting continuous monitoring and only 6.5% reporting IA exclusively (no use of EFM at any time during the labor) (Public Health Agency of Canada, 2009).

As discussed in Chapter 1, the expected improvements in neonatal outcomes (such as decreased incidence of cerebral palsy) have not been demonstrated despite the widespread use of EFM in labor. Continuous EFM has been shown to increase the incidence of cesarean and operative vaginal birth rates without generating a corresponding reduction in perinatal mortality or childhood morbidity (Alfirevic, Devane, & Gyte, 2013). Even when EFM was limited to an initial nonstress test (NST) (see Chapter 10) then converted to IA, investigators found an increased cesarean rate without a difference in neonatal outcomes (Devane et al., 2012). A meta-analysis found that when compared with IA, continuous EFM did not show significant difference with overall perinatal death rates but did show a reduction in neonatal seizures (Alfirevic et al., 2013). However, in the children who were followed long term, there was no difference in cerebral palsy rates between the two groups. There was a significant increase in instrumented vaginal births and in the rate of cesarean births in the EFM group. The increase in cesarean births is particularly concerning due to the association between cesarean and increased morbidity in both primary and repeat cesarean at the time of birth and in the immediate and delayed postpartum periods (Declercq et al., 2007; Liu et al., 2007; Lyndon, Lee, Gilbert, Gould, & Lee, 2012; Silver et al., 2006). Over 90% of women in the United States who have a primary cesarean section will have a repeat cesarean in subsequent pregnancies, with increased risk of complications with each additional surgery (Spong, Berghella, Wenstrom, Mercer, & Saade, 2012). Current evidence does not support the idea that the use of EFM is "safer" than IA in low-risk women, so practitioners should feel confident that they are practicing evidence-based care when obtaining auditory FHR data with IA, provided they are following recommended professional organizations and institutionally developed practice guidelines (Feinstein et al., 2008). Such guidelines should include the indications for IA and EFM and the appropriate monitoring methods, frequency of assessment, interpretation, and documentation.

The available evidence supports IA as an appropriate primary method of fetal heart rate surveillance during labor for women who have a low risk of developing uteroplacental insufficiency (AAP & ACOG, 2012; ACNM, 2010; ACOG, 2009; Feinstein et al., 2008; SOGC, 2007). Sources are conflicting on their position regarding use of IA in women with risk factors (AAP & ACOG, 2012; ACOG, 2008).

Benefits and Limitations of Auscultation

As with all monitoring modalities, auscultation has benefits and limitations. Depending on patients' and practitioners' preferences and viewpoints, some properties may fit into either category (Table 4-5). Auscultation may be less costly and less constricting than EFM. It increases freedom of movement and may also more easily permit assessments of FHR with the woman immersed in water in the absence of waterproof EFM transducers. At times clinicians may have difficulty hearing the FHR with auscultation, and some women may feel that the technique is more intrusive because of the

TABLE 4-5 Benefits and Limitations of IA over EFM

BENEFITS	LIMITATIONS
• Based on RCTs, neonatal outcomes are comparable to those monitored with EFM. • Lower cesarean birth rates have been associated with IA over EFM • The technique is noninvasive. • Widespread application is possible. • Freedom of movement and ambulation are increased. • The equipment is less costly than EFM equipment. • Hands-on time and one-to-one support are facilitated because the caregiver must be present at the bedside for frequent assessments.	• Use of a fetoscope may limit the ability to hear the FHR (e.g., in cases of obesity, increased amniotic fluid volume, maternal/fetal movement, and with uterine contractions). • Certain FHR characteristics associated with EFM (e.g., variability and types of decelerations) cannot be assessed. • Some women may feel that auscultation is more intrusive. • Documentation on paper or electronically is not automatic (as is the case with EFM, which may be perceived as an important component by some practitioners). • There is a potential need to increase or realign staff to meet the 1:1 nurse-to-patient ratio recommended on the basis of RCTs comparing IA to EFM. • Education, practice, and skill in auditory assessment are required.

Note: EFM, electronic fetal monitor(ing); FHR, fetal heart rate; RCT, randomized controlled trial.
Adapted from "*Fetal Heart Rate Auscultation*" by N. F. Feinstein, A. Sprague, and M. J. Trépanier, 2008, (p. 15). Copyright 2008 by the Association of Women's Health, Obstetric and Neonatal Nurses. Used with permission.

frequency of assessment and the need for the hands-on approach to IA (Feinstein et al., 2008). The results of one randomized controlled trial (RCT) comparing women's responses to IA versus EFM during labor revealed no difference between the two groups regarding their perceived labor experience (Killien & Shy, 1989). However, in the same study, the women's evaluations of their labor experiences were significantly affected by the level of perceived nursing support received during labor.

In a systematic review looking at pain and women's satisfaction with their childbirth experience, four factors were reported as being the most important in women's evaluation of their experience: personal expectations, support from caregivers, quality of the relationship between the patient and caregiver, and involvement in making decisions (Hodnett, 2002). In a more recent review, the identified themes were the severity and type of pain, pain relief received, perceived involvement in decision making, and level of control (Lally, Murtagh, Macphail, & Thomson, 2008). When IA is offered as an informed choice to low-risk women eligible for this modality of fetal monitoring and with the need for one-on-one caregiver support and presence to meet the frequency requirements of auscultation, IA could contribute to patient satisfaction and the perception of a more positive birth experience (ACNM, 2010) by meeting the needs that women self-identify as important (Hodnett, 2002; Lally et al., 2008).

IA does not provide a continuous record of FHR characteristics, and some devices (fetoscopes or Dopplers that do not provide a paper printout) do not produce any visual representation of FHR. From a legal perspective, some perceive this as a benefit, whereas others argue that this is a limitation (Feinstein et al., 2008).

Clinical Management

Clinical decision making is a complex process and a skill acquired over time. The process involves total assessment of a situation, development of a realistic plan of care based on the assessment, implementation of the plan, and evaluation of the effects. Haggerty (1999) advised that decisions about using fetal surveillance cannot be made by relying on simple algorithmic rules. Indeterminate (Category II) IA findings require ongoing evaluation, surveillance, and reevaluation. Other ancillary tests may or may not need to be performed, the need for a different monitoring modality may or may not be warranted, and intrauterine resuscitation techniques may or may not need to be initiated.

Making clinical decisions about auscultated FHR findings is similar to clinical decision making with EFM. As with any woman in labor, decision making begins with a review of the woman's medical and pregnancy history to determine her risk factors. Then all available aspects of the maternal and fetal status should be assessed. The plan of care is developed based on a synthesis of this information. The choice to change to a different monitoring modality may be warranted, depending on the overall clinical picture. Decisions to institute any of the above reveal the importance of having well-educated, well-trained practitioners at the bedside to evaluate the comprehensive clinical picture of the woman for whom they are providing care.

For example, if the FHR baseline is regular and within the defined normal range with audible increases, it is appropriate to continue to assess FHR using IA at the designated intervals while providing routine care and support for the laboring woman. When a change in the FHR baseline is auscultated, it is appropriate to reassess and confirm whether a change has occurred and/or if it persists. It is important to consider the potential physiologic reasons for the auscultated change (such as a maternal fever when fetal tachycardia is noted). When a decrease from the FHR baseline is audible, it may be appropriate to reassess with subsequent contraction(s) to confirm the finding. In addition, interventions to promote the physiologic goals of improving uterine blood flow, umbilical cord blood flow, and oxygenation (including the possibility of reducing uterine activity) are implemented as appropriate to the individual situation (Figure 4-1).

Staffing Issues and IA

The protocols in the RCTs comparing EFM and IA during the active and second stages of labor used a 1:1 (one-to-one) nurse–patient ratio. The AWHONN staffing guidelines recommend a 1:1 nurse–woman ratio when IA is used during the active phase and second stage of labor (AWHONN, 2010). These staffing guidelines were endorsed by ACNM, AAP, the National Association of Neonatal Nurses, and the American Nurses Association, among other organizations. Therefore, it is reasonable to recommend that a 1:1 nurse–woman ratio be maintained during the active and second stages of labor when IA is the method of fetal surveillance in use. This 1:1 ratio actually reflects a 1:2 nurse–patient ratio, given that both the mother and the fetus are being assessed (SOGC, 2007). Many other situations also call for 1:1 staffing (AWHONN, 2010), but in some cases staffing may need to be realigned to meet the 1:1 recommendation for IA (Feinstein et al., 2008; SOGC, 2007). Conversely, in a setting with more patients than providers, IA may prove to be challenging to achieve (ACNM, 2010). Due to this recommended staffing ratio, the use of IA as a primary method of fetal surveillance may raise concerns in some settings related to appropriate staffing levels required and the potential costs associated with the need for additional staff to meet the recommended ratios.

In Canada, the SOGC (2007) promotes the use of IA as the primary fetal surveillance method for women at low risk for complications during the active phase of labor. In conjunction with that view, the SOGC has recognized the need for appropriate education to prepare clinicians and support the implementation of IA. In addition to the learning materials in this text, the AWHONN FHM courses and AWHONN auscultation monograph (Feinstein et al., 2008), a Canadian self-learning manual focusing on the fundamentals of IA and EFM, are available (Canadian Perinatal Programs Coalition, 2009). Administrative and clinical support for the use of IA in a particular setting is helpful to make it a viable and accepted monitoring modality (Davies et al., 2002). Although further study is needed to demonstrate the cost-effectiveness of IA, there are known benefits of one-to-one labor support for women that can be used to support the need for altered staffing patterns (Hodnett, Gates, Hofmeyr, & Sakala, 2013). This information may be helpful to facilities investing in the use of IA during labor.

FIGURE 4-1 Fetal Heart Monitoring Decision Tree

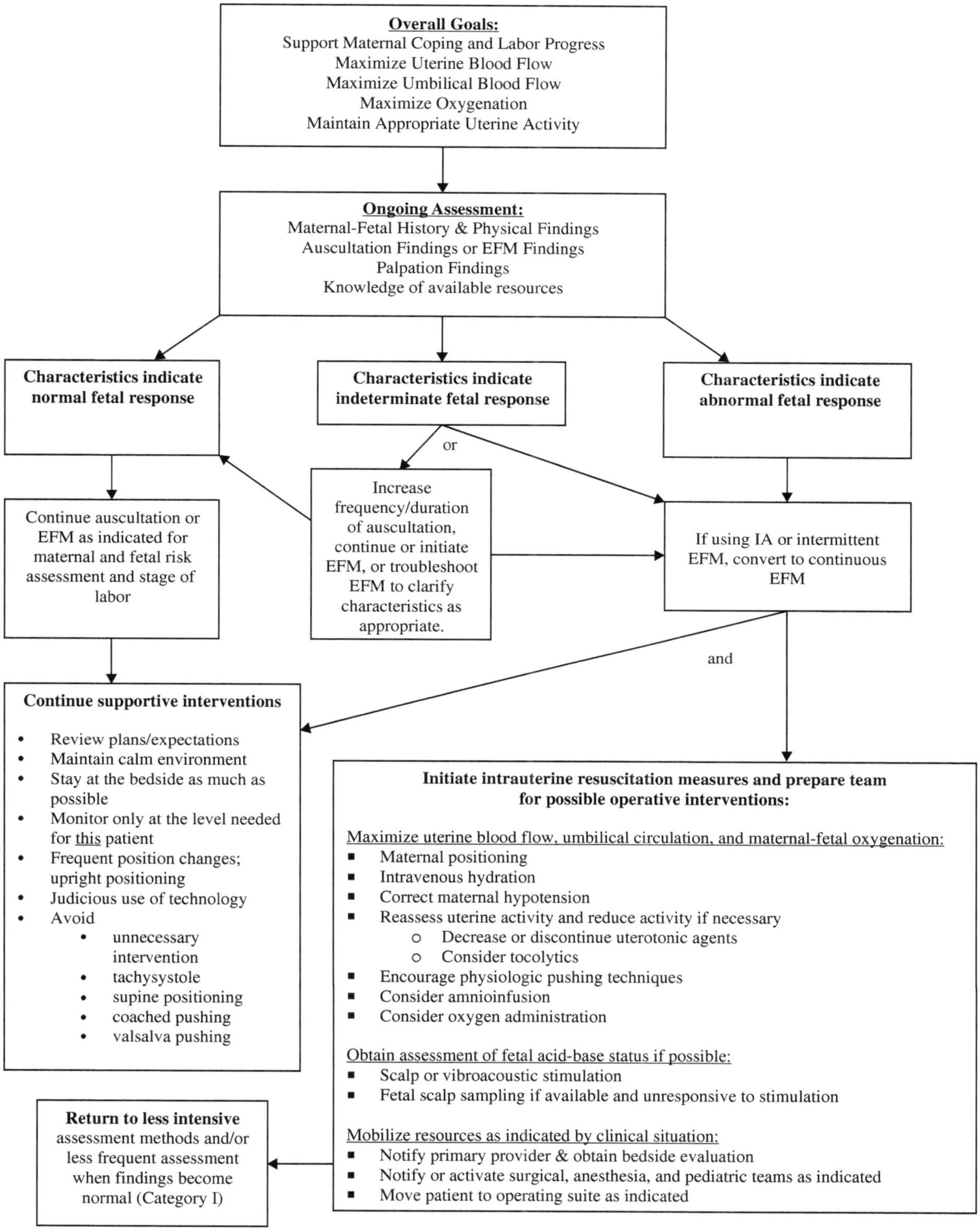

ELECTRONIC FETAL HEART RATE MONITORING

Doppler Ultrasound

The Doppler ultrasound (U/S) transducer is used to assess FHR characteristics and patterns. Multiple piezoelectric crystals within the U/S transducer generate sound waves that are transmitted toward the fetal heart and receive U/S waves reflected back from fetal heart movements (Figure 4-2). The sound waves returning from moving structures are altered in frequency from those sound waves originally transmitted toward the moving structure. This frequency shift, called the "Doppler shift," is detected and amplified to produce the waveform, which is then interpreted by the computer within the fetal monitor. From this interpretation, the monitor produces an audible sound and visual tracing to reflect the detected FHR.

First-Generation Monitors

In the evolution of the technology of Doppler FHR assessment, advances in the electronic processing of data have led to a distinction between two generations of equipment (Boehm, Fields, Hutchison, Bowen, & Vaughn, 1986). To compensate for the complexity and variation in waveforms, first-generation monitors employed two mechanisms: use of a refractory window and maximal peak detection. To prevent the

FIGURE 4-2 Linear Pictorial of Piezoelectric Effect

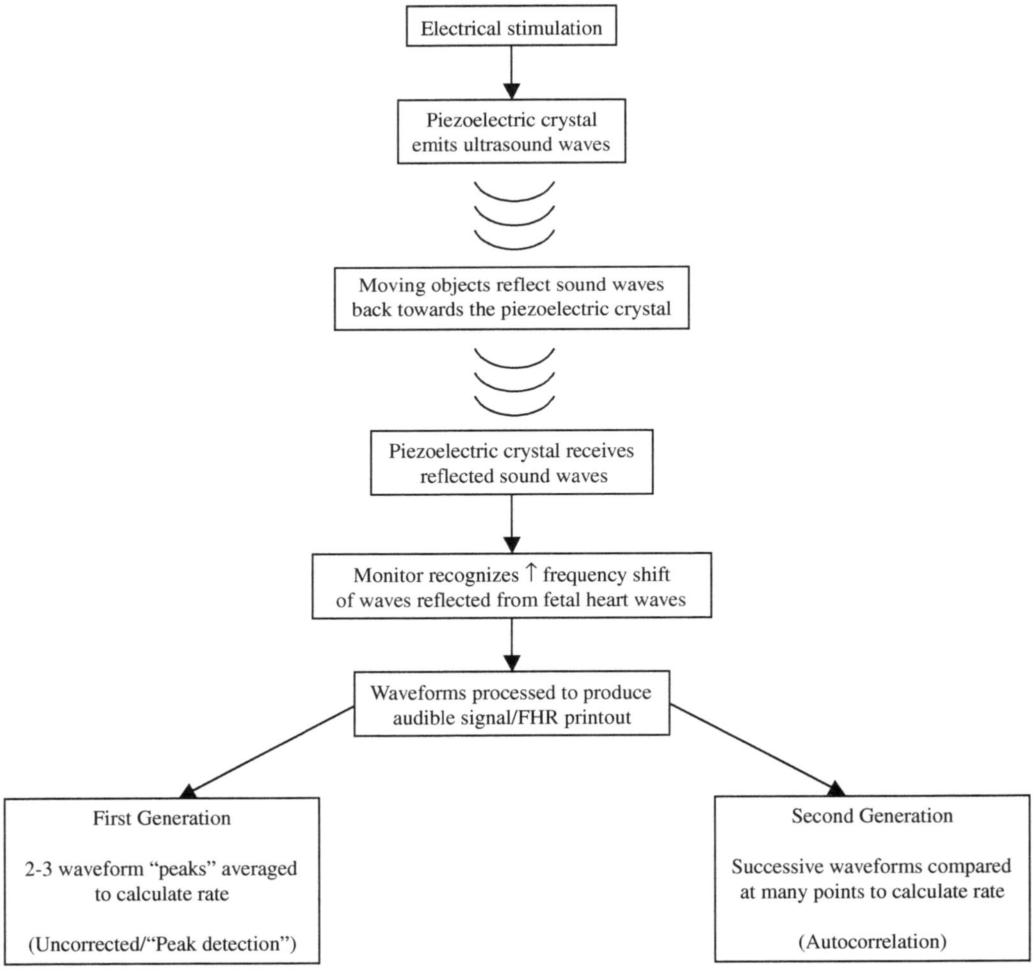

Note: This is a linear view, but in fact, the piezoelectric crystal is emitting and receiving sound waves continually. Adapted from Hon (1975) and Klavan, Laver, and Boscola (1977).

counting of both components of the fetal cardiac waveform as separate beats, a refractory window is used (Hutson & Petrie, 1986; Klapholz, 1978). This window of time is an inhibitory period in which the system does not attempt to count the incoming signal. This time period follows the moment of detection of the fetal cardiac waveform and is presumed to be the waveform's first component. The length of time of the refractory window, measured in milliseconds, is dynamic in that the time is set to vary according to the FHR. This variance, however, has limitations. Slow FHRs less than 90 bpm may cause the second component of the waveform to occur after the refractory window period. This action will produce double counting of a single waveform, leading to doubling on FHR tracing. Rapid FHRs may cause a second waveform to occur within the refractory window period and produce halving of FHR tracing because the second heart beat is not counted (Freeman et al., 2012).

The complexity and variability of first-generation Doppler-generated waveforms made accurate counting of the same point in the fetal cardiac cycle difficult. The mechanism that first-generation monitors used to compensate for this problem was maximal peak detection. When the movement of the fetal heart generates a waveform, the monitor detects its maximal peak and then counts the time interval between peaks. Problems with this technique are caused by Doppler signals from other anatomy, such as the umbilical cord, as well as variations in an early or late appearance of the peak in the waveform. These problems lead to false variability in the printed fetal heart tracing. Consequently, what was viewed on the tracing with first-generation monitors via the U/S transducer could not reliably be equated with the true FHR variability. Because of this, internal fetal monitors were often placed to get an accurate picture of FHR variability.

Second-Generation Monitors and Autocorrelation

The major alteration in Doppler signal processing associated with second-generation fetal monitors introduced in the 1980s is referred to as autocorrelation (Figure 4-2). This technique evolved from efforts to improve the quality of the processing of waveforms. Advancements in microprocessor technology facilitated the development of autocorrelation, which entails digitizing and analyzing the reflection of U/S waveforms. Autocorrelation was described by Schwartz and Young (2006) as computerized smoothing of waveforms. The internal computer averages three consecutive beat-to-beat intervals and then assigns the FHR. This averaging methodology minimizes artifact (Schwartz & Young, 2006). Autocorrelation works by matching each incoming waveform with the previous one by repetitively analyzing small segments of the waveforms. Important information will have regular form and repeat over time, whereas random noise is devoid of regularity and these artifactual waveforms are discarded (Freeman et al., 2012). The autocorrelation process of rejecting artifactual waveforms provides for a more accurate identification of the initiation of the fetal cardiac cycle than other techniques provide. Today, it is assumed that all ultrasound FHR signal processing uses autocorrelation techniques and interpretation of EFM data is based on this assumption (Macones et al., 2008).

Signal Ambiguity and Differentiation of Maternal and Fetal Heart Rates

Although second-generation technology is thought to provide more reliable determination of FHR, there have been reports of this technology producing erroneous data. Reported problems occurred most commonly during the second stage of labor and included halving of FHR, doubling of FHR, switching between fetal and maternal heart rates, an audible FHR output that differed from what was seen on the printed FHR tracing, and delayed FHR display when repositioning transducers. In 2009, the U.S. Food and Drug Administration (FDA) issued a "Dear Doctor" letter (an informational communication) regarding the Philips Avalon Fetal Monitors (models FM20, FM30, FM40, and FM50) in response to complaints received by the FDA about inaccuracy of FHR data related to the previously mentioned problems. These erroneous values were considered dangerous due to the possibility of not recognizing a tracing requiring intervention, or causing unnecessary interventions in response to a falsely worrisome tracing (FDA, 2009). In conjunction with the FDA's "Dear Doctor" letter, Philips issued a letter urging users to recognize the conditions as listed above and respond appropriately to avoid adverse outcomes. Philips has subsequently introduced new technology located within the tocodynamometer transducer (toco) to detect maternal heart rate anytime the toco is against the maternal abdomen (Koninklijke Philips Electronics N.V., 2011). This can prompt a maternal–fetal coincidence warning without needing a separate maternal electrocardiogram or pulse oximetery monitor to record the maternal heart rate.

All brands of electronic fetal monitors have been known to run the risk of the issues that prompted the FDA notification. The reminder to be aware of these possibilities and to take the appropriate steps to protect against misinterpreting data applies to all electronic monitors. Following the instructions for the particular monitor being used is important. Other steps to reduce risk include confirmation of fetal life before using the monitor; verification of the FHR with a fetoscope, hand-held Doppler, or ultrasound imaging; continued confirmation of fetal signal source for FHR (particularly if abrupt changes in FHR are noted) through monitoring of maternal heart rate or use of a fetal spiral electrode (although the FSE can also conduct maternal heart rate if there has been a fetal demise); and/or confirmation of maternal heart rate by palpation, auscultation, or electronic monitoring of maternal heart rate to aid in differentiation (Koninklijke Philips Electronics N.V., 2009).

Even though U/S transducers are designed to detect waveforms from the beating fetal heart, they may inadvertently detect and report signals from the MHR. When initiating placement of the U/S transducer or changing FHR modes, the clinician should palpate the mother's radial pulse and compare it with the audible signal and printed rate to rule out inadvertent recording of the MHR (Murray, 2004). The recorded MHR can mimic FHR patterns (Murray, 2004; Neilson, Freeman, & Mangan, 2008; Sherman et al., 2002), possibly resulting in the failure to diagnose fetal demise or deterioration. The MHR may be picked up by the external U/S transducer, especially if the fetus is active or the patient has a large body habitus (Schifrin, Harwell, Rubinstein, & Visser, 2001), a large maternal blood vessel is under the transducer (Sherman et al., 2002), or the MHR and FHR are similar (Neilson et al., 2008). An elevated MHR may be more easily confused with FHR, particularly during maternal pushing efforts in second-stage labor. It is recommended that sudden changes in recorded heart rate be investigated and that maternal pulse be assessed at times other than just when a recorded heart rate appears to be bradycardic, especially with noncontinuous tracings, to confirm whether the mother or the fetus is the signal source (Neilson et al., 2008; Schifrin et al., 2001; Sherman et al., 2002).

Today, many electronic fetal monitors allow for the monitoring and recording of both MHR and FHR patterns. This may be accomplished through maternal electrocardiogram (ECG) leads, a maternal pulse oximetry sensor, or sensors within the tocodynamometer that pick up maternal pulse. When these technologies are used through the fetal monitor, a tracing representing MHR will appear on the printout (paper or electronic) alongside the FHR for ease in differentiation. Some of the noted differing characteristics of the MHR and FHR are described below and include the following:

- Baseline MHR is significantly lower than the FHR baseline; MHR variability is significantly greater at all stages of labor; and a significant drop in maternal variability may be noted after the delivery of the placenta (Sherman et al., 2002).
- MHR accelerations have higher amplitude and longer duration, especially during second stage and pushing, and tend to increase in frequency as labor progresses while often coinciding with contractions and pushing efforts (Sherman et al., 2002).

- Where the FHR may show decelerations during contractions due to head or cord compression or uteroplacental insufficiency, the MHR may show accelerations due to increased cardiac output (Nurani, Chandraharan, Lowe, Ugwumadu, & Arulkumaran, 2012). In addition, MHR accelerations have been reported to be as high as 60 bpm above the baseline in the case of a fetal demise (Murray, 2004).
- MHR baseline as it approaches 140 bpm may flatten, especially if the patient is diabetic or hemodynamically or metabolically unstable. Artifact lines that move above and below the MHR may be the result of a weak signal, interruption of signal, or loss of signal (Murray, 2004).
- In situations of fetal death and transmission of the maternal ECG via the fetal spiralelectrode, a baseline bradycardic rate is often shown to be the most consistent finding (Sherman et al., 2002).

Artifact

"Artifact" is a term used to describe irregular variations or absence of the FHR on the fetal monitor record resulting from mechanical limitations of the monitor, electrical interference, or a weak signal, appearing on the tracing as gaps or dots (Murray et al., 2011). With the use of the Doppler U/S, gaps and dots may be noted on the tracing when the cardiac signal is either too weak to be continually traced or is undetected. When a fetal spiral electrode (FSE) is used, artifact may be present on the tracing in the form of irregular lines with varying lengths, unlike the regular lines seen with some arrhythmias (Figure 4-3).

A number of types of artifact can occur. These include, but are not limited to, increased variability on first-generation monitors, half-counting and double-counting of the FHR, and recording of the MHR. Half-counting of the FHR is most commonly seen when the FHR is rapid, such as with fetal supraventricular tachycardia. Double-counting may occur during periods of bradycardia. Troubleshooting efforts to improve the FHR signal include repositioning the U/S transducer, ensuring an adequate amount of coupling gel is used, and checking for proper placement of the fetal spiral electrode. Signal interference can also occur and cause artifact if the scalp electrode is intermittently

FIGURE 4-3 Example of Artifact on a Fetal Heart Rate Tracing

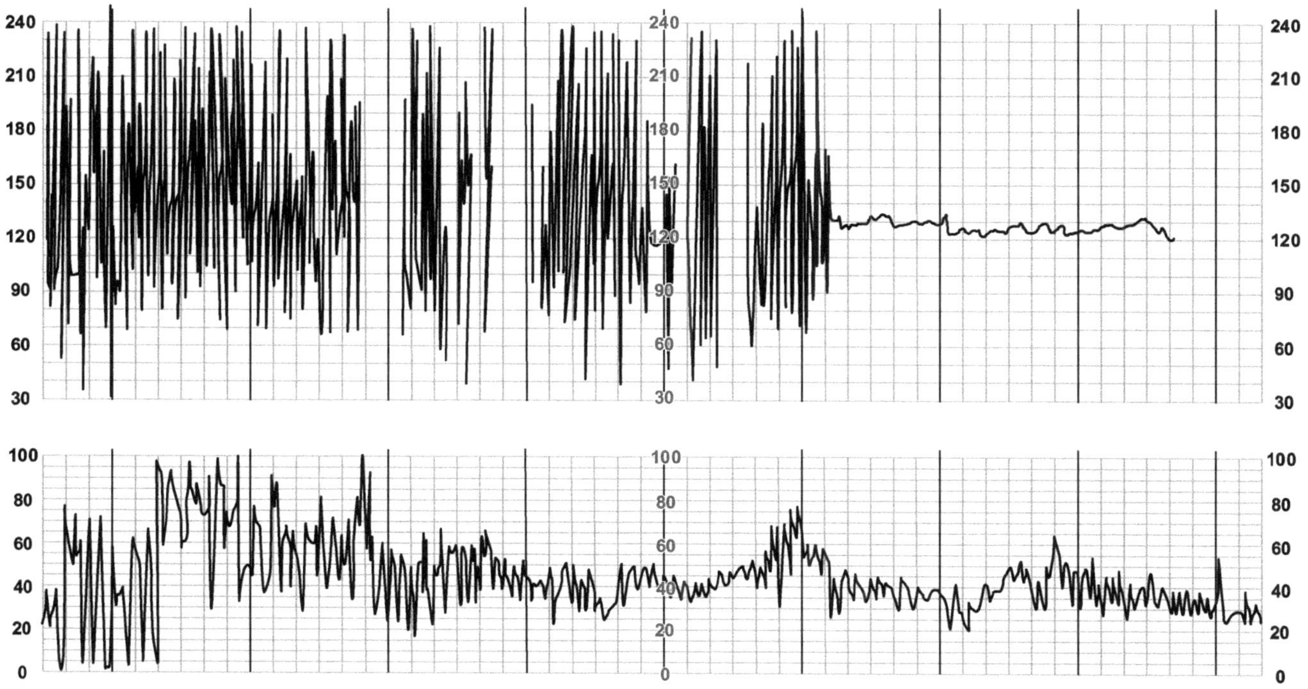

pushed against the vaginal wall, as can occur with maternal pushing efforts (Murray et al., 2011).

A summary of benefits, limitations, and troubleshooting actions to address common problems with U/S transducer use are included in Table 4-6.

Alarm Fatigue

Central fetal monitoring has allowed for multiple fetuses to be watched from a central location. As has been discussed previously, issues with electronic fetal monitors such as artifact, signal loss, and coincidence between maternal and fetal heart rates can trigger alarms in these monitoring systems in response to conditions that may not actually represent a worrisome fetal heart rate. While centralized monitoring was thought to contribute to patient safety by making fetal heart rate tracings available for team surveillance, it has been criticized for drawing nurses away from the bedside. The central monitor station has also become a place where alarms from call lights, ringing phones, and fetal monitors may be audible for extended periods of time. It has been estimated that between 85% and 99% of all medical alarm signals require

TABLE 4-6 Ultrasound (U/S) Transducer: Capabilities, Benefits, Limitations, and Troubleshooting/Corrective Actions

Capabilities	
• Detect FHR including variability, baseline rate and rhythm, accelerations, and decelerations	
Benefits and Limitations	
BENEFITS	**LIMITATIONS**
• Is noninvasive • Does not require rupture of membranes • Provides a permanent record either electronically archived or on paper (depending on storage conditions, heat can deteriorate paper over time)	• Signal transmission may be influenced by maternal obesity, occiput posterior fetal position, anterior placenta, and fetal movement (e.g., weak, absent, or false signal) • May restrict maternal movement • Maternal and fetal movement may interfere with continuous recording Monitor may half-count or double-count, especially in the presence of FHR tachycardia or bradycardia
Troubleshooting/Corrective Actions	
PROBLEM	**ACTIONS**

• Erratic recordings or gaps on the tracing paper
• Potential causes:
  • Inadequate conduction of U/S signal
  • Transducer may be displaced
  • Fetal or maternal movement
  • Arrhythmia
  • Paper not loaded correctly
  • Equipment malfunction
	• Evaluate potential causes
	• Assess whether sufficient ultrasonic gel is present under the transducer
	• Apply ultrasonic gel to the transducer as needed until a light seal is formed
	• Encourage maternal position changes to improve the signal
	• Determine whether the belt holding the transducer is snug around the abdomen; tighten as needed to improve contact and signal detection
	• Reposition the transducer over the fetal back (determined by Leopold's maneuvers), as necessary
	• Check maternal pulse; auscultate as needed
	• Check the connection to the power source as well as the connections to the monitor
	• Check paper for proper loading
	• Check equipment according to manufacturer's directions
	• Apply FSE if clinically indicated

Note: FHR, fetal heart rate; FSE, fetal spiral electrode.

no clinical intervention (The Joint Commission [TJC], 2013a). The concept of the sensory overload associated with the background noise of excessive alarms has been described as alarm fatigue (AACN, 2013).

Although alarm fatigue has not been studied specifically in relation to fetal monitoring, it has been studied in relation to alarms in critical care units, especially ECG alarms. The American Association of Critical-Care Nurses (AACN; 2013) cites several nursing actions related to managing alarms in an effort to reduce alarm fatigue and improve patient safety. Although many of these could be linked to perinatal nursing, the two that seem the most relevant are customizing the alarm parameters to meet the needs of the individual patient and reserving electronic monitoring for those patients with a clinical indication (AACN, 2013; Simpson, 2013). For example, if the default alarm parameters are not changed for a fetus with supraventricular tachycardia, that monitor will alarm constantly because of the higher fetal heart rate. Reserving continuous fetal monitoring for women with clinical indications or using intermittent monitoring for the majority of women would further reduce the incidence of erroneous central monitoring alarms and decrease unnecessary stimuli.

The Joint Commission (2013a) issued a *Sentinel Event Alert* regarding alarm safety that cited several tactics to help decrease alarm fatigue, such as establishing guidelines for alarm settings including the identification of when alarm signals are not clinically necessary, tailoring settings and limits for individual patients, and training all staff on processes for safe alarm management and response. As of January 1, 2014, TJC published a National Patient Safety Goal on Alarm Management to improve the safety of clinical alarm systems. This goal gives hospitals until 2016 to make alarm system safety a hospital priority, to identify the most important alarm signals, to establish policies and procedures for managing those alarms, and to educate staff on responsibilities and proper operation (2013b).

Fetal Spiral Electrode

Direct FHR monitoring with a fetal spiral electrode (FSE) uses electronic logic to detect and measure R-to-R wave intervals in consecutive QRS complexes to derive the FHR. The interval is recalculated with the detection of each new R wave. In addition to the direct measurement of the FHR, other benefits and limitations of the FSE are described in Table 4-7. To place the FSE, adequate cervical dilatation (usually at least 2 cm) and ruptured membranes (either before or at the time of placement) are needed. A sterile plastic sheath can then be inserted until in contact with the fetal presenting part (head or buttocks) and then the spiral electrode gently placed flush with the fetal skin and rotated clockwise one and a half times until the electrode is attached to the skin. The FSE should not be applied to the fetal face, fontanels, or genitalia nor should it be used with placenta previa, hemophilia, maternal HIV, herpes infections, or when the presenting part is not identifiable (Coviden, 2012). In the presence of extreme prematurity or maternal infections such as group B streptococcus, syphilis, gonorrhea, or hepatitis, use of an FSE is not recommended but may be placed if a clear benefit to the mother or fetus can be demonstrated by its use (Coviden, 2012). When an FSE is being used to assess FHR, a range of problems may require troubleshooting by the clinician to correct or improve the quality of monitor data. The EFM, like any instrument, is vulnerable to equipment malfunction, use of incorrect procedures, or human error. Common situations and suggestions for troubleshooting are included in Table 4-7. See Chapter 9 for discussion of documentation principles related to electronic modes of fetal monitoring.

TABLE 4-7 Fetal Spiral Electrode: Capabilities, Benefits, Limitations, and Troubleshooting/ Corrective Actions

Capabilities	
• Detect FHR including variability, baseline rate and rhythm, accelerations, and decelerations • Provide limited information about some types of arrhythmias	
Benefits and Limitations	
BENEFITS	**LIMITATIONS**
• Provides continuous detection of FHR when clinically necessary and not achievable by U/S transducer • Maternal position change does not alter ability to assess FHR or quality of tracing	• Invasive • Requires rupture of membranes, cervical dilation, and accessible/appropriate fetal presenting part • Contraindicated with placenta previa, herpes simplex virus, HIV, suspected or confirmed fetal hemophilia • Not recommended with maternal infection (such as hepatitis, GBS, etc.) or with extreme prematurity • Contraindicated to use with face presentations or other fetal parts (other than the scalp or buttocks) • Requires moist environment for detection of FHR • Potential risk for infection and fetal hemorrhage or injury • May record maternal heart rate in presence of fetal demise • Fetal arrhythmias may not be evident if logic or ECG button is engaged • Electronic interference and artifact may occur
Troubleshooting/Corrective Actions	
PROBLEM	**ACTIONS**

• Intermittent markings on the FHR tracing
  • Potential causes:
    • Artifact
    • Failure to detect electrical activity
    • Fetal arrhythmia
    • Monitor connections improperly attached
	• Evaluate potential causes
	• Confirm FHR with fetoscope
	• Check connections to the monitor, electrode and cable
	• Check circuitry of the monitor
	• Turn off the logic or ECG deactivation switch
	• Check FSE placement on presenting part, if possible
	• Apply new FSE as indicated

• Illegible FHR tracing
  • Potential causes:
    • Artifact
    • Faulty electronic connection or monitor placement
    • Faulty loading or feeding of monitor paper
• Abnormal rate on the tracing
  • Potential causes:
    • Doubling or halving of actual heart rate by monitor
    • Actual fetal tachycardia, bradycardia, or deceleration
    • Interference from maternal signal (e.g., fetal demise, FSE placement on maternal cervix)
    • Artifact
• FHR pattern compressed
  • Potential causes:
    • Paper speed or scaling errors
• INOP display
  • Potential causes:
    • Signal cannot be received
    • Leads not connected to leg plate
    • FSE may have a poor connection to the presenting part
    • Referencing electrode may not be operating
	• Press the test button; check the numerical value
	• Check the connection to the power source, check all lead connections, and/or replace cable
	• Check condition of monitor paper
	• Confirm "record" button is activated
	• Confirm/establish correct rate (e.g., auscultation with fetoscope)
	• Confirm maternal pulse simultaneously with FHR
	• Refer to manufacturer's instruction manual for procedure for separating or distancing the maternal signal from the fetal ECG signal
	• Replace the FSE if necessary
	• Verify paper speed (e.g., 3 cm/min in the United States)
	• Confirm that paper being used has the appropriate calibrations for the monitor in use
	• Check the lead connections to the monitor (gently remove the FSE wire), check the EFM circuitry, and/or replace cable
	• Vaginal secretions may be inadequate, and an external reference electrode, if available, may need to be applied
	• Palpate the maternal pulse and compare it with the audible signal and printed rate to rule out a recording of the maternal heart rate

Note: ECG, electrocardiogram; EFM, electronic fetal monitor; FHR, fetal heart rate; FSE, fetal spiral electrode; GBS, group B streptococcus; HIV, human immunodeficiency virus.

FETAL ECG MONITORING THROUGH ST-SEGMENT ANALYSIS

Overview

Assessment of the fetal ECG has been suggested as a promising adjunct to EFM. Similar to the adult ECG, the fetal ECG displays P, QRS, and T waves illustrating the electrical activity in the heart during each beat (Neilson, 2012). With fetal ECG, the most commonly studied waveforms are the PR to RR interval and the ST waveform (Neilson, 2012). Of these, ST segment analysis has been the most extensively tested through RCTs and is focused on in this discussion. For the fetal ECG to be recorded and assessed, placement of an internal fetal spiral electrode is required. The purpose of ST segment analysis (STAN, for ST ANalysis) is to identify cases of significant hypoxia and improve the timeliness and consistency of intervention (Norén et al., 2003; Rosén, 2005; Rosén, Amer-Wåhlin, Luzietti, & Norén, 2004). When multiple studies of EFM alone versus EFM plus ST waveform analysis were collected and analyzed together in both a Cochrane Review and an individual patient data meta-analysis, no significant differences between the two groups for cesarean births, newborns with severe metabolic acidosis at birth, or newborns with neonatal encephalopathy were found; but, the analyses did show a lower incidence of operative vaginal delivery and fetal scalp samples when EFM was used with ST analysis (Neilson, 2012; Schuit et al., 2013). As previously mentioned, few hospitals in the United States still perform scalp sampling, and furthermore FDA-approved fetal scalp sampling kits are not readily available, so it may be difficult to generalize these findings to areas that are not regularly performing that test (Schuit et al., 2013).

ST-Segment Pathophysiology

Theoretically, ST-segment analysis of the fetal ECG provides continuous information regarding the ability of the fetal heart to respond to stress in labor by providing information about intracardiac responses to intrapartum hypoxia (Kwee, Dekkers, van Wijk, van der Hoorn-van den Beld, & Visser, 2007; Rosén, 2005). ST-segment and T-wave changes occur with myocardial ischemia prior to permanent cell damage (Ross, Devoe, & Rosén, 2004). Analysis of the ST segment may permit detection of myocardial ischemia and the fetus's ability to respond to stress prior to peripheral organ and central nervous system damage (Amer-Wåhlin et al., 2002; Ross et al., 2004).

ST-segment and T-wave elevation are indicative of a fetus at risk for developing hypoxia but with some levels of reserves still present to respond to hypoxemia. These changes are the direct result of a catecholamine surge, beta-adrenoceptor activation, and myocardial glycogenolysis, which releases glycogen stores in the heart and acts as an extra source of energy (Norén et al., 2003; Olofsson, 2003; Rosén, 2005; Rosén et al., 2004). However, fetal ST-segment depression (biphasic ST) has been associated with the inability of the fetal heart to further respond to hypoxia, indicating that the fetus either had no time to respond or has exhausted compensatory mechanisms. ST depression is thought to reflect endocardial hypoxia (Amer-Wåhlin, Ingemarsson, Marsal, & Hearst, 2005; Kwee et al., 2007; Norén et al., 2003; Olofsson, 2003). ST depression has also been associated with infection, fetal heart malformation, and disturbances in the heart muscle function (Kwee et al., 2007) (Figure 4-4). Alternatively, the absence of alteration in the ST segment may aid in the determination of fetal well-being (Ross et al., 2004). Of note, fetal ST changes are thought to be clinically relevant only if they coincide with "intermediate" or "abnormal" FHR tracings because ST changes have occurred in the presence of normal FHR tracings (Kwee et al., 2007). A possible explanation for ST changes that have been observed with normal FHR tracings may be the catecholamine surge in response to the physical and stress forces of labor. A fetus with the ability to compensate will display an otherwise normal FHR tracing. Thus, the ST changes associated with a normal FHR tracing are more likely due to nonhypoxemic fetal stress and the surge of stress hormones (Kwee et al., 2007).

FIGURE 4-4 Fetal Electrocardiogram: ST-Segment and T-Wave Changes Associated with Intrapartum Hypoxia

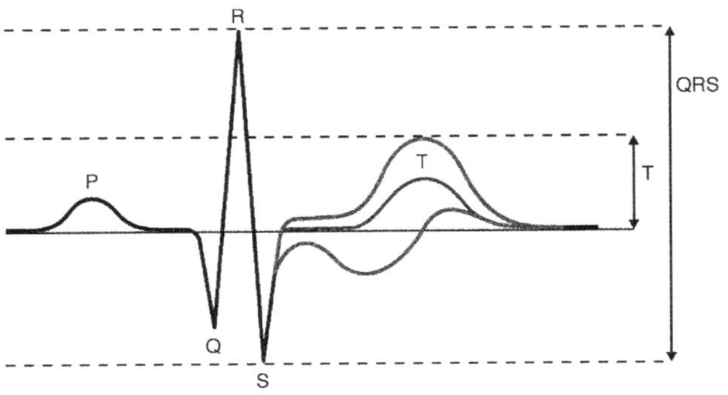

Note: M. G. Ross, L. D. Devoe, & K. G. Rosén, *Journal of Maternal-Fetal and Neonatal Medicine, 15*: 181–185, Copyright © 2004 Informa Healthcare. Reproduced with permission of Informa Healthcare.

A high-quality ECG signal is necessary to evaluate and interpret ST analysis (Rosén et al., 2004). FSE placement and use of a STAN monitor are required to retrieve the ECG data. ST analysis requires close observation of the quality of the fetal ECG signal. If the electrode is applied improperly, signal disturbance may still allow the FHR to be recorded but not allow adequate signals for ST analysis (Rosén, 2005).

Future Research and Implications for Practice

Adequate research did not occur prior to the introduction and dissemination of EFM technology in the 1960s. This has proved to be a significant disadvantage today. A Cochrane Systematic Review of the STAN methodology provides some support for the use of the ST waveform analysis when the decision has been made to perform continuous fetal monitoring during labor and a FSE is being placed (Neilson, 2012). Inclusion criteria for all but one study was gestation greater than 36 weeks. Thus, further research with preterm fetuses would be beneficial. In addition, information regarding long-term neurologic development of the newborns included in the trials would also be valuable (Neilson, 2012). At the time of publication, the NICHD is recruiting participants from several hospitals throughout the United States for a randomized trial to study the use of STAN in labor (ClinicalTrials.gov, 2012). Whether the technology will be adopted widely for clinical use is unknown at this time.

ELECTRONIC UTERINE ACTIVITY MONITORING

Tocodynamometer Transducer (Toco)

The contour of the uterus and abdomen changes somewhat with contractions. The toco is the part of the EFM that externally detects skin tightening or contour changes resulting from uterine contractions. Specifically, it is a form of strain gauge that detects changes in the shape of the abdomen resulting from uterine tension (Euliano et al., 2013; Euliano, Skowronski, Marossero, Shuster, & Edwards, 2006). The pressure sensor, usually a button-like device, should be placed on the abdomen over the uterine fundus at the point of maximal contraction intensity. The specific location is determined by abdominal palpation and is ideally a smooth part of the uterus where no fetal small parts are felt. The optimal location varies from woman to woman and may change during labor. Occasionally moving the location of the toco on the maternal abdomen may help maintain skin integrity and avoid buildup of pressure over one area of skin. Computer technology translates the degree of pressure detected by the sensor into an electrical signal that is displayed numerically on the monitor and graphically on the tracing paper. When the sensor is placed correctly, this mode of assessment is useful in determining the following:

- Approximate contraction frequency
- Approximate duration (length) of contractions
- Relative changes in abdominal pressure between uterine resting tone (tonus) and contractions

The effectiveness of monitoring contractions with a toco is often dependent on maternal habitus. On a slender patient whose gravid abdomen is taut, even mild contractions may be easy to trace and appear large. On a patient with greater abdominal adiposity, monitoring the skin tightening may prove challenging and strong contractions may appear small. Regardless of the appearance of the size of the contraction measured with a toco, it is important to note that use of the external toco transducer does not allow for determination of the actual contraction strength (intensity), another key element of contraction assessment. Palpation of the uterus during and between contractions and input from the laboring woman are essential for developing a complete and accurate picture of contraction quality at any given time. Palpation is used in conjunction with electronic uterine activity monitoring to validate uterine contraction intensity and uterine resting tone and to confirm findings from electronic monitoring. Palpation is also used to assess uterine activity when the toco is removed for ambulation, during procedures such as epidural placement, and to validate findings from intrauterine pressure catheter (IUPC) readings.

Caldeyro-Barcia and Poseiro (1960) described contractions as being abdominally palpable at a pressure of 10 mmHg, which is slightly below the point at which the laboring woman feels the pain of contractions (15 mmHg). Parer (1997) stated that women may often be aware of the contraction before the toco detects it. In most cases, toco transducers, in concert with palpation, provide satisfactory data to adequately assess uterine contraction patterns (LaCroix, 1968) (Figure 4-5). The uterine activity portion of the tracing paper is vertically marked

FIGURE 4-5 Comparison of Uterine Contraction Assessment by Palpation, External Tocodynamometer, and Intrauterine Pressure Catheter

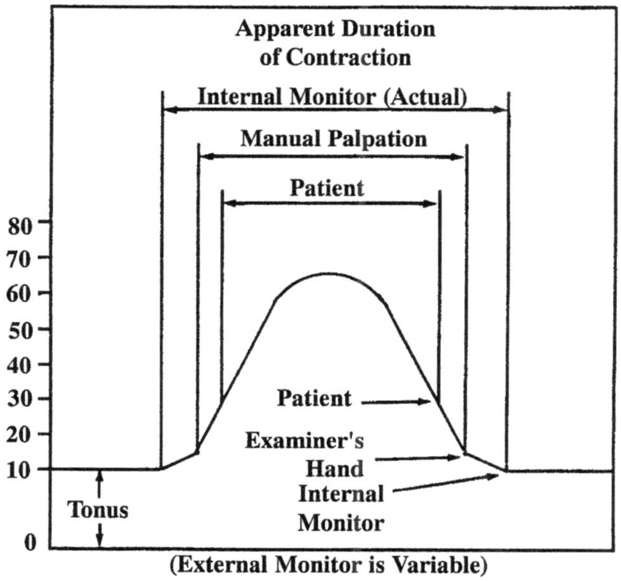

Note: From Freeman, R. K., Garite, T. J., & Nageotte, M. P. (2003). *Fetal heart rate monitoring* (3rd ed., p. 54). Philadelphia: Lippincott Williams & Wilkins. Copyright 2003 by Lippincott Williams & Wilkins. Reprinted with permission.

in specific units of measure. Millimeters of mercury (mmHg) are the units of measure used in North America. Kilopascals are considered the standard measure for contraction strength in some other parts of the world. These quantitative measures have utility only when an IUPC is used and are discussed in the next section.

When the external toco transducer is in use, the numbers that represent uterine contraction pressures on the uterine activity channel of the EFM are arbitrary. The uterine activity (UA) resting tone should be adjusted to approximately 10–20 mmHg between contractions in order to obtain the most readable tracing. A uterine activity transducer from the EFM (toco or IUPC) should be used when the U/S transducer or FSE is in use. This simultaneous assessment of UA ensures that FHR patterns and responses can be considered in relation to the timing, frequency, duration, and presence or absence of contractions.

When contractions are not being reliably recorded with a toco transducer, using a contraction marker may aid the practitioner in gathering data about uterine activity. The marker may be a hand-held device that is attached to the EFM and places a mark on the monitor paper and/or the electronic recording each time the button is pressed. This can be done as one press/one mark each time the woman feels a contraction starting which will give the *frequency* of contractions. It can also be one press/one mark each time she feels a contraction starting and again when it has ended to give *duration* of contractions. A limitation of this method is the unreliability of the degree of uterine activity that women with epidurals are able to feel. Similarly, marks to the tracing can be accomplished as previously discussed using palpation by the bedside practitioner who presses the button to mark the record or uses a pen to place a mark on the uterine activity section of the monitor paper (however, if the pen and paper method is used, the marking will not archive into the electronic system if one is in use).

Benefits, limitations, and troubleshooting strategies for using the toco are summarized in Table 4-8. Variations in the recording of uterine contractions with a toco are illustrated in Figure 4-6.

Intrauterine Pressure Catheter

Internal monitoring with an IUPC is used in the management of laboring women in the United States today at an approximate rate of one in every five women (Sciscione et al., 2005). Inserted internally into the uterine cavity via the vagina (transcervical insertion), the IUPC allows for greater quantitative measurement of uterine contraction frequency, duration, intensity or peak intrauterine pressure, and resting tone. There are currently three types of IUPCs in use: fluid-filled catheter systems, transducer-tipped catheters, and air-coupled (sensor-tipped) catheters.

Routine use of IUPCs is not supported by evidence and the decision to use one should be based on the clinical need for additional uterine activity information (ACOG, 2003; Bakker et al., 2010). Indications for IUPC placement include, but are not limited to, the need for amnioinfusion, titration of oxytocin for induction or augmentation when external methods of assessing uterine activity are not producing an interpretable uterine activity tracing, and lack of progress of labor when quantitative analysis of uterine activity is indicated for clinical decision making (ACOG, 2003) (such as contractions that appear strong on an external monitor but are not producing cervical change).

IUPC placement is invasive and requires consideration of the potential risks and benefits prior to placement (Table 4-9). IUPCs have been linked to an increase in the risk of maternal fever before or after birth (Harper, Shanks, Tuuli, Roehl, & Cahill, 2013). A physician, midwife, or registered nurse can place the catheter; however, state and provincial guidelines and hospital policies governing placement of IUPCs by registered nurses vary. The sterile, flexible catheter is inserted into the amniotic cavity of the uterus with the use of a guide. The catheter should be placed only after rupture of membranes has occurred and when adequate cervical dilatation (usually at least 2 cm) has been achieved.

TABLE 4-8 Toco Transducer: Capabilities, Benefits and Limitations, Troubleshooting/Corrective Actions

Capabilities	
• Detect relative changes in uterine resting tone and contractions • Detect relative frequency and duration of uterine contractions	
Benefits and Limitations	
BENEFITS	**LIMITATIONS**
• Is noninvasive • Is easily placed • Does not require ruptured amniotic membranes • Generates a tracing for future assessment and for a permanent medical record	• Is subjective • Is unable to detect actual uterine contraction intensity and resting tone • May be unable to accurately detect exact contraction frequency and duration, particularly if a woman has a large body habitus or is having preterm labor • Toco is location sensitive; poor placement can lead to false information • Sensitive to maternal or fetal movements that may be superimposed on the waveform • Transducer presence or position may be uncomfortable for the mother • May limit potential for maternal movement and ambulation during labor
Troubleshooting/Corrective Actions	
PROBLEM	**ACTIONS**
• Contractions not recording on the tracing • Contractions appear inverted	• Use manual palpation to validate presence of contractions • Confirm toco transducer is applied against the abdomen and connected to monitor • Ensure that placement of the toco is firm, but not tight, on the maternal abdomen • Test calibration of the toco system by pushing firmly on the abdominal transducer button; digital monitor display should show a particular numeric display (see operating manual for the monitor type you are using to confirm what the specific number should be) • Palpate the uterus for the area of strongest contraction and reposition the toco over that point • When the uterus is relaxed, set the UA dial or button to 10–20 mmHg • Reposition toco over the area the contraction feels strongest • Ensure toco is not positioned over the maternal umbilicus

• Recording only portions of contractions
• Other problems
  • Position
  • Pushing
  • Vomiting
	• Consider IUPC placement, if clinically indicated
	• Re-zero baseline resting tone with the uterus relaxed to ensure it is not set at a falsely high starting range
	• Palpate the uterus for the area of strongest contraction intensity; reposition the toco over that area
	• When the uterus is relaxed, set the uterine activity dial or button to 10–20 mmHg
	• Encourage position change as needed
	• Palpate to verify uterine activity
	• If necessary, note uterine contractions on tracing using the event marker
	• Note clinical events (e.g., vomiting, pushing)

Note: IUPC, intrauterine pressure catheter.

FIGURE 4-6 Tocodynamometer Variations

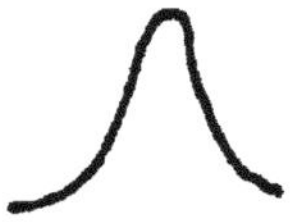

Normal

1. Uterine contraction wave form.

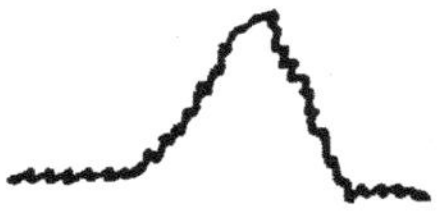

Respirations

2. Respiration may produce an undulating overlay.

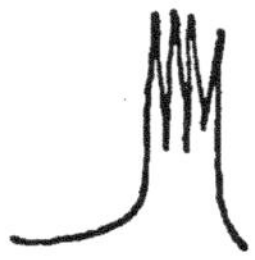

Pushing

3. Valsalva maneuver with pushing effects during the second state of labor may produce blunted spikes.

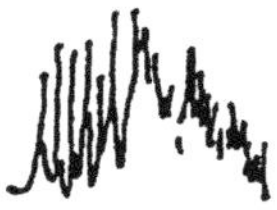

Vomiting seizures

4. Extreme maternal activity such as vomiting or a seizure may produce a series of sharp spikes.

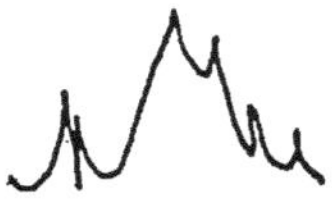

Fetal activity

5. Fetal movement may produce sharp isolated spikes.

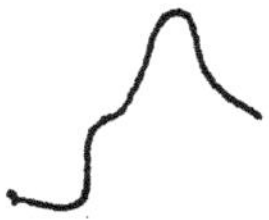

Sudden baseline shift

6. Sudden baseline shifts may be produced by maternal position change.

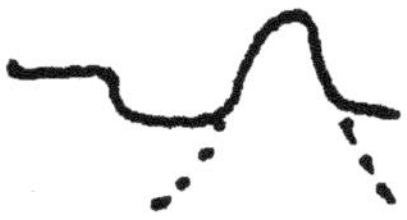

Obscured

7. Incorrect baseline setting may obscure all but tip of contractions.

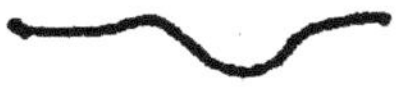

Inverted

8. Certain placements of tocodynamometer may produce reversed waveform when uterus contracts away from the tocodynamometer.

Adapted from information in Wagner and Cabaniss (unpublished).

TABLE 4-9 Intrauterine Pressure Catheters: Capabilities, Benefits and Limitations, Troubleshooting/Corrective Actions

Capabilities	
Intrauterine pressure catheters can be used to: • Detect uterine resting tone • Detect strength/intensity of uterine contractions • Detect frequency and duration of uterine contractions • Withdraw amniotic fluid for testing • Perform amnioinfusion	
Benefits and Limitations	
BENEFITS	**LIMITATIONS**
General • Objective method of assessing uterine contraction frequency, duration, and measurable intensity/resting tone • May provide a more accurate assessment of uterine activity when an accurate tracing cannot be obtained externally including the timing of FHR changes with contractions • Generates a tracing that is a permanent part of the medical record	General • Requires rupture of membranes and adequate cervical dilation • Invasive • Limits potential for maternal ambulation during labor • May be contraindicated with infections where rupture of membranes is discouraged to prevent maternal–fetal transmission (e.g., herpes, GBS, HIV, hepatitis) • May be contraindicated in presence of vaginal bleeding • Contraindicated with placenta previa • Has increased risk of uterine perforation (rupture), placental abruption or perforation, infection, or umbilical cord prolapse (Usta, Mercer, & Sabai, 1999) • Produces differences in readings between fluid-filled, sensor-tipped, and transducer-tipped catheters
Solid-state IUPC (transducer and sensor-tipped) • Easily zeroed to atmospheric pressure; most can be re-zeroed • Allows for amnioinfusion and aspiration of amniotic fluid (with most models) • Designed to avoid pressure artifacts that may be caused by a catheter that contains air or becomes kinked	Solid-state IUPC (transducer and sensor-tipped) • Maternal position may change hydrostatic pressure within the uterus and may alter readings including resting tone • Pressure readings may be higher than with fluid-filled catheters
Fluid-filled IUPC • Provides means for aspiration of amniotic fluid • Provides means for amnioinfusion	Fluid-filled IUPC • Catheter tip may become wedged against the uterine wall or fetal part and prevent the production of any pressure data; may produce a distorted or dampened waveform • Catheter tip in relation to external pressure transducer position may affect pressures • Maternal position changes require re-zeroing or recalibration • Catheter may become obstructed with particulate matter such as meconium or blood • Although not a true limitation, pressure readings may be lower than sensor-tipped (or solid) transducers
Troubleshooting/Corrective Actions	
PROBLEM	**ACTIONS**

No contractions recorded
• Potential causes
  • Displacement of IUPC
  • Obstructed catheter
  • Incorrectly zeroed catheter
  • Uterine perforation
Abnormal uterine contraction waveform appearance on tracing
• Potential causes
  • The IUPC tip may be lodged against the uterine wall, placenta, or a fetal body part
  • Fluid-filled IUPC may be dry or incompletely filled with sterile water, thus permitting air to dampen the waveform
	Evaluate potential causes
	• Ask patient to cough or perform Valsalva's maneuver to verify the position of the IUPC; a spike should appear if the IUPC is positioned properly
	• Palpate to confirm presence of contractions
	• Check monitor for loose connections
	• Flush fluid-filled catheter
	• Verify calibration per detailed instructions in transducer manufacturer's operating manual (run monitor's self-test)
	• Zero/re-zero the transducer according to manufacturer's operating manual and verify the position of the IUPC
	• In addition to troubleshooting for placement of IUPC, observe for signs of maternal or fetal compromise

(continued)

TABLE 4-9 (Continued)

• Catheter tip is above the diaphragm transducer level, creating higher pressure readings; or, if below, the reading may be artificially low • Inadvertent insertion of the IUPC between the wall of the uterus and the membranes (extraovular) • Uterine perforation, placental abruption, or perforation	Evaluate potential causes • Palpate uterus for contractions • Flush the IUPC, if applicable • Try rotating the IUPC 180 degrees; this may change the relationship of the pressure-sensing device to the fetus and uterus
Inverse tracing of uterine contractions • Potential causes • Uterine perforation	• Withdraw and reposition catheter if blood returned through catheter • In addition to troubleshooting for placement of IUPC, observe for signs of maternal or fetal compromise
Uterine resting tone or baseline tonus is elevated or not tracing • Potential causes • Fluid-filled IUPC is sensitive to hydrostatic pressure and changes in hydrostatic pressure • Pressures may vary in different maternal positions	Evaluate potential causes • In addition to troubleshooting for placement of IUPC, observe for signs of maternal or fetal compromise • Palpate uterine resting tone • Re-zero IUPC according to manufacturer's instructions • Record the uterine resting tone in all positions on insertion, especially when using IUPCs that cannot be re-zeroed after insertion

Note: FHR, fetal heart rate; GBS, group B streptococcus; HIV, human immunodeficiency virus; IUPC, intrauterine pressure catheter.

As previously mentioned, the most common North American unit of IUPC measurement for contraction intensity is millimeters of mercury (mmHg). Uterine baseline resting tone and peak intrauterine pressure intensity are usually described using the mmHg measurement from the monitor tracing. Alternative methods of describing uterine activity strength include determining the contraction amplitude by subtracting the difference in mmHg between the uterine contraction peak and baseline. Using this definition of amplitude, contraction strength tends to vary across a given labor from 25 to 75 mmHg and beyond (ACOG, 2003; Caldeyro-Barcia & Poseiro, 1959).

Another approach to quantify uterine contraction strength is use of Montevideo units (MVUs), a measurement defined in 1952 by Caldeyro-Barcia and colleagues from Montevideo, Uruguay. These units are calculated by measuring the peak intensity, or amplitude, in mmHg for each contraction occurring in a 10-minute period of time and adding these numbers together (Caldeyro-Barcia, Pose, & Alvarez, 1957). Contraction amplitude is the difference between the resting tone and the peak of the contraction (in mmHg). For example, if there are three contractions in 10 minutes, peaking 70, 80, and 75 mmHg of intrauterine pressure, and a baseline uterine tone of 10 mmHg, this would be calculated as $(70 - 10 = 60) + (80 - 10 = 70) + (75 - 10 = 65) = 195$ MVUs. It is important to note that these calculations are dependent on the accuracy of IUPC data. A contraction pattern totaling at least 200 MVUs per 10-minute period has long been considered as adequate labor (ACOG, 2003) and normal spontaneous labor activity is generally less than 280 MVUs (Caldeyro-Barcia & Poseiro, 1959), although MVUs can vary widely across spontaneous laboring women (Caldeyro-Barcia & Poseiro, 1960).

There is a wide range of variation of uterine forces from one labor to the next. Contraction amplitude in normal labor can vary from 25 to 75 mmHg and MVUs can vary from as low as 95 to as high as 395 per 10 minutes (ACOG, 2003). ACOG and the Society for Maternal Fetal Medicine (SMFM) recommend safe prevention of primary cesarean births can be achieved, in part, by using criteria for diagnosis of arrest of labor as outlined in Table 4-10 when other parameters of maternal and fetal status are reassuring.

TABLE 4-10 ACOG & SMFM Criteria for Diagnosis of Arrest of Labor When Other Maternal-Fetal Assessment Parameters are Reassuring

FIRST STAGE	SECOND STAGE
In spontaneous labor: • ≥ 6 cm dilation with ruptured membranes AND either: • ≥ 4 hours of adequate contractions OR • ≥ 6 hours of oxytocin administration with inadequate contractions and no cervical change In induced labor: • Allow latent phase ≥ 24 hours • Administer oxytocin ≥ 12–18 hours after rupture of membranes before declaring failure of induction	At least 2 hours of pushing in multiparous women At least 3 hours of pushing in nulliparous women • Longer duration of pushing may be appropriate as long as there is some documented labor progress. For example individualized assessment of continued pushing may be appropriate with epidural analgesia or fetal malposition. • "A specific absolute maximum length of time spent in the second stage of labor beyond which all women should undergo operative delivery has not been identified." (ACOG & SMFM, p. 185) • Chorioamnionitis is not an indication for cesarean birth

Source: ACOG & SMFM, (2014).

Fluid-Filled Intrauterine Pressure Catheter

The fluid-filled, or water column method, IUPC was the first type of intrauterine pressure–measuring catheter available and was widely used in the measurement of uterine contraction intensity until 1987 when use dramatically decreased after the introduction of the transducer-tipped catheter (Dowdle, 2003). The fluid-filled catheter works by transmitting the intrauterine pressure generated by a contraction through a water column to a transducer located away from the source of pressure, typically at the monitor site. This displaced fluid exerts pressure against a diaphragm in the transducer, generating changes in the electrical resistance of a series of wires. These electrical changes are converted to measures of pressure and displayed on the EFM uterine activity channel.

Technical problems with fluid-filled catheters include cumbersome setup and maintenance; catheter occlusion with solids (e.g., meconium or vernix) requiring intermittent flushing; kinking and entrapment of the catheter between the uterus and fetus; artifact resulting from catheter manipulation and maternal movement; and the need to recalibrate or re-zero the catheter with maternal position changes. These problems produce dampened uterine waveforms and inaccurate measurement of contractions (Devoe, Smith, & Stoker, 1993; Hutson & Petrie, 1986; Klapholz, 1978). See Table 4-9 for an overview of capabilities, benefits, limitations, and troubleshooting issues regarding the use of the fluid-filled IUPC.

Transducer-Tipped Intrauterine Pressure Catheters

The transducer-tipped IUPC was introduced in the 1980s as an alternative to the fluid-filled catheter systems (Strong & Paul, 1989). This technology was developed to include both the pressure sensor and transducer at the catheter tip, which is placed directly into the uterus (Beeson & Martens, 2005). The force exerted by a uterine contraction is converted to an electrical signal that is transmitted through a wire system to the fetal monitor where the uterine activity is displayed graphically on the fetal monitor tracing. This catheter offers the option of a dual-lumen version that enables simultaneous amnioinfusion or sampling of amniotic fluid and may be re-zeroed after insertion.

The baseline reading of resting tone from a transducer-tipped IUPC can be affected both by changes in maternal position and by the hydrostatic pressures exerted on the catheter. The position of the IUPC tip in relation to the position of the patient may affect the amount of pressure exerted by the fluid above the catheter. Intrauterine hydrostatic pressure readings can be altered by maternal position changes. Obtaining baseline pressure readings in the left, right, and supine with lateral tilt positions demonstrates these alterations and should be completed and

FIGURE 4-7 Baseline Reading of Transducer-Tipped IUPC after Insertion

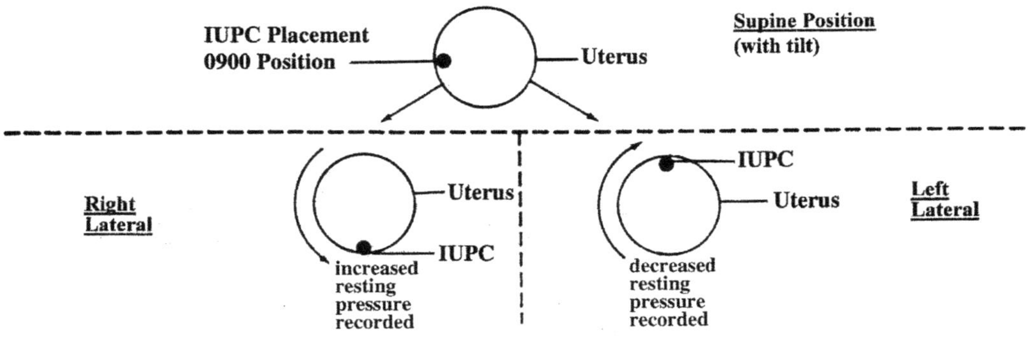

Note: From "*Intran® Plus User Guidelines*", by Utah Medical Products. Copyright 2006 Utah Medical Products. Adapted with permission. www.utahmed.com

documented after initial insertion (Figure 4-7). This in turn may prevent potential misinterpretations of changes to resting tone pressures following maternal position changes during labor. Knowing these baseline differences may prevent erroneous conclusions regarding induction or augmentation management.

Air-Coupled Intrauterine Pressure Catheters (Sensor-Tipped)

Air-coupling technology, which is a newer method of intrauterine pressure monitoring, uses a distally mounted flexible balloon in the uterus connected to an external reusable transducer in the monitor cable. Similar to the technology of noninvasive blood pressure monitors, this catheter consists of a membrane sensor at the tip of the catheter that communicates pressures through a microcolumn of air to a transducer located outside the body (Clinical Innovations, 2001). This type of IUPC has a smaller catheter tip with multiple holes transmitting the amniotic fluid pressure to the transducer (Dowdle, 1997). It also has the capability to zero the catheter *in utero* and increased flexibility in the tubing (Dowdle, 1997).

Transducer-Tipped versus Sensor-Tipped

The decision regarding what catheter type to use may depend on physician or nurse preference, hospital contractual agreements, budget, or study results. The ease and reliability of the various re-zeroing features of the IUPC may also affect decision making regarding the type of catheter selected by an institution. An industry-sponsored study conducted by Dowdle (2003) found that the two most common catheter types, transducer-tipped and sensor-tipped, yielded similar quantitative measurement of uterine activity including baseline tone, peak pressure readings, and the timing of contractions. In addition, both systems were found to function equally well in the display of abnormal uterine activity. This was studied by binding the two catheters together at the tip and placing them into the uterus as one unit for a side by side comparison.

Sciscione et al. (2005) found in a study of 249 women that the transducer-tipped catheters were significantly more likely to have an extraovular placement. Extraovular placement occurs when the catheter is inadvertently placed outside the amniotic membranes between the chorion and the decidua in the extra membranous space of the lower uterine segment. Placement in this space (as opposed to the fluid-filled amniotic cavity) is believed to be due to the rigidity of the transducer-tipped catheter and may increase the risk for abruption, especially in the presence of an amnioinfusion. Sciscione et al. also reported that IUPCs may function normally if placed in the extramembranous space so the true rate of these extraovular placements is unknown. Clear catheter lumens, now available in both types of catheters, can assist in determining proper placement (blood is usually seen in the catheter with extraovular placement) in addition to assessing for the presence of meconium-stained amniotic fluid.

Electrohysterography

Electrohysterography (EHG) is a noninvasive way of monitoring the uterine muscle electrical activity from the surface of the maternal abdomen, similar to using an electrocardiogram to monitor cardiac electrical currents instead of observing intracardiac pressures (Euliano et al., 2013). EHG was developed over 50 years ago but did not enter into clinical use at that time. Interest in EHG is currently increasing due to technical improvements and indications that it might be able to differentiate between efficient and inefficient contractions, which could prove beneficial within the context of suspected preterm labor (Jacod, Graatsma, Van Hagen, & Visser, 2010). In addition, because it monitors uterine muscle electrical activity, it may have utility as an external monitor for use in patients with a high body mass index (BMI).

Euliano et al. (2013) conducted a study of 73 women in labor and simultaneously monitored uterine activity with toco, IUPC, and EHG. IUPC was considered the "gold standard" of uterine monitoring and EHG and toco were compared against it. When compared directly with IUPC, EHG was found to correlate well with monitored contractions. The study showed a superiority of EHG over toco (when compared with IUPC) in laboring women for monitoring uterine activity regardless of body habitus. However, the authors noted that using EHG to infer intrauterine pressure remains an area of research. There are several mathematical algorithms in use to convert the electrical activity as monitored by the EHG into MVUs to determine intrauterine pressure, but a uniform approach has yet to be agreed upon (Jacod et al., 2010). Similarly, there is no uniform way of acquiring and processing the electrical signal from the uterus. Jacod et al. (2010) showed that EHG accurately detects uterine contractions in laboring women compared with IUPC, but correlation between these methods with regard to the characteristics of amplitude and duration of the contractions was moderate.

The suggestion that EHG may be able to differentiate between efficient and inefficient contractions without the need for invasive uterine monitoring may hold promise for integration into widespread use, but standardization in data collection and processing may be needed first (Euliano et al., 2013; Jacod et al., 2010). Whether this technology will be adopted widely for clinical use is unknown at this time.

COMBINED EXTERNAL INTEGRATED MONITORING

Maternal ECG, Fetal ECG, and Uterine EMG

Currently, there is one FDA-approved device for use in term, singleton pregnancies that has an integrated system that concurrently monitors maternal ECG, fetal ECG, and uterine EMG (electromyography, similar to electrohysterography, as discussed above) (Monica Healthcare Ltd., 2011). This device uses five cutaneous ECG electrodes applied to the maternal abdomen to detect electric voltage signals and then calculate the fetal ECG, maternal ECG, and uterine contractility in real time (Cohen et al., 2012; Reinhard et al., 2013). It has been reported to allow for easier external monitoring in the presence of high BMI and to maximize patient positioning and movement. It has been noted to decrease the ambiguity between maternal and fetal heart rates during the first and second stages of labor (Reinhard et al., 2013). This system uses Bluetooth technology to send the signal from the accessory (worn by the patient) to the base. The base plugs into commercial electronic fetal monitors to allow for archiving and central monitoring. The system does not replace the need for traditional monitors if internal monitoring of FHR or uterine activity were needed. Whether this technology will be adopted widely for clinical use is unknown at this time.

MONITOR TRACING ISSUES

Although the focus of this chapter is techniques for monitoring FHR and uterine activity, it is important to address tracing and paper speed technology when EFM is in use. Changes in paper speed can substantially alter the appearance of the tracing (Freeman et al., 2012), which could inherently provide for differences in interpretation of FHR data. Fetal monitor technology provides the capacity to set the tracing paper speed as well as the visual tracing display at various settings. On the commonly used paper in the United States, markings on the vertical scale range from 30 to 240 bpm, with dividing lines at 10-bpm intervals. On European-scaled paper, which is also used in South America and certain centers in the United States, markings range from 50 to 210 bpm with dividing lines at 5-bpm intervals. Paper speeds also vary throughout the United States, Canada, and Europe. Paper speed in the United States and Canada usually runs at 3 cm per minute on the horizontal scale, whereas paper speed in Europe, South America, and some centers in the United States and Canada runs at a range of 1 or 2 cm/minute. The FHR pattern at a slower paper speed will appear compressed with variability accentuated and periodic/episodic changes appearing more abrupt in nature (Freeman et al., 2012). The current date and time should be automatically printed by most monitors; however, the clinician should verify it on the tracing at regular intervals to ensure that the time is accurately and correctly shown on the EFM tracing.

Regardless of the paper speed being used, standardization of paper speed within and across practice settings is essential for optimal interpretation by professional care providers (SOGC, 2007), and switching paper speeds during individual labors is not recommended. Despite the recommendations for a consistent paper speed, there are geographic differences regarding paper speed practices even across North American and Canadian centers. These differences may be related to historical tradition, the country or location in which particular nurses and physicians previously trained and practiced, and/or the argument that slower paper speeds save paper and maximize storage efficiency.

Lack of consistency in paper speed settings may make interpretation and communication more challenging. This inconsistency may set the stage for misinterpretation of EFM data or miscommunication of those data. Because team communication is a key issue in cases with poor outcomes as discussed in The Joint Commission's *Sentinel Event Alert* (2004), each institution should define uniform paper speed standards and individual clinicians should use the defined paper speed consistently. Clinicians should also know where the paper speed switch is located on the monitors in his or her practice setting and document changes in paper speed if they occur. To date, scientific study of possible clinical influences of differences in paper speed has not yet been published.

FETAL SURVEILLANCE AND THE NURSE'S ROLE

Patient Education

Patient education regarding available and approved or recommended methods of fetal assessment should be customized for each woman and is essential for women to make fully informed decisions about their health care. Advances in technological capabilities and the technological society in which we live and practice often affect provider preference with regard to monitoring modality but also may influence patients' preferences for IA or EFM. More current studies regarding patient preferences or feelings about monitoring methods are warranted, although patients have already reported that they prefer to have support from caregivers and involvement in decision making during labor, including associated risks of accepting or declining a test or treatment (Declercq et al., 2013; Hodnett, 2002; Killien & Shy, 1989; Lally et al., 2009). Wood (2003) described the ethical decision-making models used to assist nurses to better delineate their role as patient advocates, such as with the use of IA versus EFM in labor.

Labor Support

All women benefit from receiving labor support. Hodnett (2002) found that the positive influence of supportive caregiver attitudes and behaviors had a stronger effect on women's satisfaction with childbirth than did any perceived negative influence from pain or medical interventions. Continuous labor support has been associated with increased spontaneous vaginal births and decreased operative births (both vaginal and cesarean), as well as reduction in the use of intrapartum pain medications and regional analgesia/anesthesia, and reduced likelihood of reports of negative birth experiences (Hodnett et al., 2013; Sakala & Corry, 2008). All women should have support throughout the labor and birth process as it has positive effects on clinical outcomes with no known harm (Hodnett et al., 2013).

It remains unclear as to which type of caregiver is most efficacious in achieving these labor support outcomes. It has been suggested that the most effective labor support may be that which is provided by someone who is neither a part of the hospital staff nor a member of the woman's immediate social network but who does have some training or experience in supporting women through labor (Hodnett et al., 2013). Although continuous labor support appears to be more effective if provided by support persons other than nurses, these findings may be related to constraints and other responsibilities placed on nurses by institutional policies and routine practices limiting the ability of nurses or hospital staff to provide continuous support (Hodnett et al., 2013). A randomized clinical trial of nurse-provided labor support in North America concluded that nursing care alone was not associated with reductions in cesarean birth rates or psychosocial outcomes for laboring women giving birth in environments characterized by high rates of routine intervention (Hodnett et al., 2002). Despite these findings, every effort should be made to provide women in labor with continuous support, because the birth experience can have a lifelong impact on women's psychological well-being (Goodman, Mackey, & Tavakoli, 2004; Simkin, 1991). Many professional organizations also advocate that women should ideally receive one-to-one nursing care and support in labor (AWHONN, 2010, 2011a, 2011b; Health Canada, 2000; NICE, 2007; SOGC, 2007).

Providing supportive care during labor is not dependent on the method of fetal surveillance used but rather on the philosophy, attitudes, and values of care providers. Although women undergoing EFM during labor can definitely benefit from all aspects of supportive care practices, women being monitored using IA may be more likely to receive close continuous presence of a caregiver because of the continual need for bedside assessment and palpation.

Clinicians and researchers have long cautioned against nursing activities becoming more heavily focused on monitors and other machinery, rather than on the woman in labor (Hoerst & Fairman, 2000; McNiven, Hodnett, & O'Brien-Pallas, 1992; Sandelowski, 1998). EFM technology does not replace the need for care by experienced providers (AWHONN, 2008). The NICE guidelines (UK) state that women who are in labor should have supportive one-to-one care and not be left alone unless requested or for a short period of time (NICE, 2007). This recommendation for labor support is not differentiated based on which mode of monitoring is being used. In Canada, SOGC (2007) strongly supports one-to-one nurse–patient ratios in labor so that patients may receive adequate supportive care. Although IA may necessitate a stronger presence at the bedside, women desire and deserve supportive care throughout labor and birth regardless of the method of monitoring being used.

Institutional Policies

Individual facilities should develop interdisciplinary policies and procedures for IA, uterine palpation, and EFM that are consistent with their appropriate state, provincial, or national guidelines or regulations. Inclusion of key nursing and obstetric providers and development of collaborative teams are suggested for planning and implementing evidence-based practices (AWHONN,

2011; Simpson, 2008; Smith & Onstad, 2005). Policies should address when it is appropriate to use IA and EFM, the frequency of assessment, and documentation of findings (AAP & ACOG, 2012).

Professional Education Regarding Monitoring Methods

It is valuable for professionals to receive training and preparation prior to implementing fetal monitoring, which includes the benefits and limitations of various techniques, the physiologic interpretation of data, and its implications for care (AWHONN, 2008; SOGC, 2007). Being able to select appropriate methods of fetal heart rate and uterine activity monitoring based on the specific clinical situation is an important clinical competency. Using a common language for discussion and documentation of fetal monitoring is another critical step that speaks to uniform training (Macones et al., 2008). Steps to implementing evidence-based practice include education preparation, resources, and support (Davies et al., 2002). Whether new skills are being taught or existing skills reinforced, the level of the learner (novice to expert) should be considered (Benner, 1984). Educational programs that employ adult learning principles with attention to the levels of the learners can assist care providers in increasing their skills in IA and EFM and aid in building their overall skill and confidence. Team-based training that includes integration of all disciplines can aid in care providers speaking the same language from within the same conceptual framework (MacEachin, Lopez, Powell, & Corbett, 2009).

According to The Joint Commission *Sentinel Event Alert* (2004), many risk-reduction strategies have been identified based on the examination of multiple root cause analyses. Included in these strategy recommendations are the development of clear guidelines for fetal monitoring interpretation; interdisciplinary FHM education for nurses, residents, nurse midwives, and physicians; and the use of standardized terminology to communicate fetal heart rate findings. The Joint Commission also recommends team training in perinatal areas to teach staff to work together and communicate more effectively. In order to successfully accomplish this goal, the discontinuation of long-practiced segregated educational models and the creation (or continuation) of joint education programs with all team clinical team members, nurses, residents, nurse-midwives, and physicians must be a priority.

Future Research

Additional research on methods of monitoring will continue to inform us regarding use of these monitoring methods, including identifying which women may be appropriately monitored with EFM or IA, and how frequently assessments should occur. With the endorsed support and recommended implementation of the NICHD terminology by ACOG, AWHONN, and ACNM, further research studies have the potential to be more widely generalizable with the use of this common language in describing fetal heart rates and patterns.

SUMMARY

Fetal surveillance methods allow data to be gathered for assessment of fetal well-being and uterine activity. High-quality data are vital for accurate interpretation, diagnosis, and subsequent interventions. Educated, appropriately trained clinicians are of paramount importance for this to be accomplished. As labor progresses, depending on the quality of information received for interpretation, the need for changes in methods may be required for adequate assessment, interpretation, clinical interventions, and evaluation. Understanding the methods, benefits, limitations, and troubleshooting measures for fetal surveillance is critical for informed decision making and skill in the use of these methodologies.

REFERENCES

Alfirevic, Z., Devane, D., & Gyte, G. M. (2013). Continuous cardiotocography (CTG) as a form of electronic fetal monitoring (EFM) for fetal assessment during labour. *Cochrane Database of Systematic Reviews*, Issue 5

(Article No. CD006066). doi:10.1002/14651858.CD006066.pub2

American Academy of Pediatrics & American College of Obstetricians and Gynecologists. (2012). *Guidelines for perinatal care* (7th ed.). Elk Grove Village, IL: Authors.

American Association of Critical-Care Nurses. (2013). Alarm management. *AACN Practice Alert*. Aliso Viejo, CA: Author. Retrieved from http://www.aacn.org/wd/practice/docs/practicealerts/alarm-management-practice-alert.pdf

American College of Nurse-Midwives. (2010). Intermittent auscultation for intrapartum fetal heart rate surveillance (replaces ACNM Clinical Bulletin #9, March 2007). *Journal of Midwifery and Women's Health, 55*(4), 397–403. doi:10.1016/j.jmwh.2010.05.007

American College of Obstetricians and Gynecologists. (2003). Dystocia and augmentation of labor (Practice Bulletin No. 49). Washington, DC: Author.

American College of Obstetricians and Gynecologists. (2009). Intrapartum fetal heart rate monitoring: Nomenclature, interpretation, and general management principles (Practice Bulletin No. 106). Washington, DC: Author.

American College of Obstetricians and Gynecologists and Society for Maternal-Fetal Medicine. (2014). Safe prevention of the primary cesarean delivery (Obstetric Care Consensus Series No. 1). *Obstetrics and Gynecology, 123*, 693–711. Retrieved from: http://www.acog.org/Resources-And-Publications/Obstetric-Care-Consensus-Series/Safe-Prevention-of-the-Primary-Cesarean-Delivery

Amer-Wåhlin, I., Bördahl, P., Eikeland, T., Hellsten, C., Norén, H., Sörnes, T., & Rosén, K. G. (2002). ST analysis of the fetal electrocardiogram during labor: Nordic observational multicenter study. *Journal of Maternal-Fetal and Neonatal Medicine, 12*(4), 260–266.

Amer-Wåhlin, I., Ingemarsson, I., Marsal, K., & Herbst, A. (2005). Fetal heart rate patterns and ECG ST segment changes preceding metabolic academia at birth. *BJOG: An International Journal of Obstetrics and Gynaecology, 112*(2), 160–165.

Ananth, C. V., Chauhan, S. P., Chen, H. Y., D'Alton, M. E., & Vintzileos, A. M. (2013). Electronic fetal monitoring in the United States: Temporal trends and adverse perinatal outcomes. *Obstetrics and Gynecology, 121*(5), 927–933. doi:10.1097/AOG.0b013e318289510d

Association of Women's Health, Obstetric and Neonatal Nurses. (2008). Fetal heart monitoring. Position Statement. Washington, DC: Author.

Association of Women's Health, Obstetric and Neonatal Nurses. (2010). *Guidelines for professional registered nurse staffing for perinatal units*. Washington, DC: Author.

Association of Women's Health, Obstetric and Neonatal Nurses. (2011a). *Antepartum and intrapartum fetal heart monitoring: Clinical competencies and education guide* (5th ed.). Washington, DC: Author.

Association of Women's Health, Obstetric & Neonatal Nurses. (2011b). Professional nursing support of laboring women. *Journal of Obstetric, Gynecologic and Neonatal Nursing, 40*(5), 665–666. doi:10.1111/j.1552-6909.2011.01288.x

Bakker, J. J. H., Verhoeven, C. J. M., Janssen, P. F., van Lith, J. M., van Oudgaarden, E. D., Bloemenkamp, K. W. M., . . . van der Post, J. A. M. (2010). Outcomes after internal versus external tocodynamometry for monitoring labor. *New England Journal of Medicine, 362*(4), 306–313. doi:10.1056/NEJMoa0902748

Banta, D. H., & Thacker, S. B. (2001). Historical controversy in health technology assessment: The case of electronic fetal monitoring. *Obstetrical and Gynecological Survey, 56*(11), 707–719.

Beeson, J., & Martens, M. (2005, February). *Variable intrauterine pressure catheter (IUPC) tracings with two catheters*. Paper presented at the annual meeting of the Society of Maternal-Fetal Medicine, Reno, NV.

Benner, P. (1984). *From novice to expert. Excellence and power in clinical nursing practice.* Menlo Park, CA: Addison-Wesley.

Boehm, F. H., Fields, L. M., Hutchison, J. M., Bowen, A. W., & Vaughn, W. K. (1986). The indirectly obtained fetal heart rate: Comparison of first- and second-generation electronic fetal monitors. *American Journal of Obstetrics and Gynecology, 155*(1), 10–14.

Caldeyro-Barcia, R., Pose, S. V., & Alvarez, H. (1957). Uterine contractility in polyhydramnios and the effects of withdrawal of the excess of amniotic fluid. *American Journal of Obstetrics and Gynecology, 73*(6), 1238–1254.

Caldeyro-Barcia, R., & Poseiro, J. J. (1959). Oxytocin and contractility of the pregnant human uterus. *Annals of the New York Academy of Sciences, 75*, 813–830. doi:10.1111/j.1749-6632.1959.tb44593.x

Caldeyro-Barcia, R., & Poseiro, J. (1960). Physiology of the uterine contraction. *Clinics in Obstetrics and Gynecology, 3*, 386.

Canadian Perinatal Programs Coalition. (2009). *Fundamentals of fetal health surveillance: A self-learning manual* (4th ed.). Ottawa, Ontario, Canada: Author.

Clinical Innovations. (2001). *Koala® IPC 5000, What is soft, sensitive, and great for measuring intrauterine pressure?* [Brochure]. Murray, UT: Author.

ClinicalTrials.gov. (2012). Fetal ST segment and T wave analysis in labor. ClinicalTrials. gov identifier: NCT01131260. Retrieved from http://clinicaltrials.gov/ct2/show/NCT01131260

Cohen, W. R., Ommani, S., Hassan, S., Mirza, F. G., Solomon, M., Brown, R., . . . & Hayes-Gill, B. R. (2012).

Accuracy and reliability of fetal heart rate monitoring using maternal abdominal surface electrodes. *Acta Obstetricia et Gynecologica Scandinavica, 91*(11), 1306–1313. doi:10.1111/j.1600-0412.2012.01533.x

Covidien. (2012). Kendall fetal spiral electrode system contraindications. Retrieved from http://www.kendallhq.com/pageBuilder.aspx?contentID=150595&webPageID=0&topicID=149607&breadcrumbs=0:121623,143502:0

Davies, B., Hodnett, E., Hannah, M., O'Brien-Pallas, L., Pringle, D., Wells, G., & Perinatal Partnership Program of Eastern and Southeastern Ontario and the Society of Obstetricians and Gynaecologists of Canada. (2002). Fetal health surveillance: A community-wide approach versus a tailored intervention for the implementation of clinical practice guidelines. *Canadian Medical Association Journal, 167*(5), 469–474.

Declercq, E., Barger, M., Cabral, H. J., Evans, S. R., Kotelchuck, M., Simon, C., . . . Heffner, L. J. (2007). Maternal outcomes associated with planned primary cesarean births compared with planned vaginal births. *Obstetrics and Gynecology, 109*(3), 669–677.

Declercq, E. R., Sakala, C., Corry, M. P., Applebaum, S., & Herrlich, A. (2013). *Listening to mothers III: New mothers speak out.* New York, NY: Childbirth Connection. Retrieved from http://transform.childbirthconnection.org/wp-content/uploads/2013/06/LTM-III_MSO.pdf

Devane, D., Lalor, J. G., Daly, S., McGuire, W., & Smith, V. (2012). Cardiotocography versus intermittent auscultation of fetal heart on admission to labour ward for assessment of fetal well being. *Cochrane Database of Systematic Reviews,* Issue 2 (Article No. CD005122). doi:10.1002/14651858.CD005122.pub4

Devoe, L. D., Smith, R. P., & Stoker, R. (1993). Intrauterine pressure catheter performance in an in vitrouterine model: A stimulation of problems for intrapartum monitoring. *Obstetrics and Gynecology, 82*(2), 285–289.

Dowdle, M. (1997). Evaluating a new intrauterine pressure catheter. *Journal of Reproductive Medicine, 42*(8), 506–513.

Dowdle, M. (2003). Comparison of two intrauterine pressure catheters during labor. *Journal of Reproductive Medicine, 48*(7), 501–505.

Euliano, T. Y., Nguyen, M. T., Darmanjian, S., McGorray, S. P., Euliano, N., Onkala, A., & Gregg, A. R. (2013). Monitoring uterine activity during labor: A comparison of 3 methods. *American Journal of Obstetrics and Gynecology, 208*(1), 66.e1–66.e6. doi:10.1016/j.ajog.2012.10.873

Euliano, T., Skowronski, M., Marossero, D., Shuster, J, & Edwards, R. (2006). Prediction of intrauterine pressure waveform from transabdominal electrohysterography. *Journal of Maternal–Fetal and Neonatal Medicine, 19*(12), 811–816.

Feinstein, N. F., Sprague, A., & Trépanier, M.-J. (2008). *Fetal heart rate auscultation* (2nd ed.). Washington, DC: Association of Women's Health, Obstetric and Neonatal Nurses.

Freeman, R. K., Garite, T. J., Nageotte, M. P., & Miller, L. A. (2012). *Fetal heart rate monitoring* (4th ed.). Philadelphia, PA: Lippincott Williams & Wilkins.

Goodman, P., Mackey, M. C., & Tavakoli, A. S. (2004). Factors related to childbirth satisfaction. *Journal of Advanced Nursing, 46*(2), 212–219.

Goodwin, L. (2000). Intermittent auscultation of the fetal heart rate: A review of general principles. *Journal of Perinatal and Neonatal Nursing, 14*(3), 53–61.

Haggerty, L. A. (1999). Continuous electronic fetal monitoring: Contradictions between practice and research. *Journal of Obstetric, Gynecologic and Neonatal Nursing, 28*(4), 409–416.

Haverkamp, A. D., Orleans, M., Langendoerfer, S., McFee, J., Murphy, J., & Thompson, H. E. (1979). A controlled trial of the differential effects of intrapartum fetal monitoring. *American Journal of Obstetrics and Gynecology, 134*(4), 399–412.

Haverkamp, A., D., Thompson, H. E., McFee, J. G., & Cetulo, C. (1976). The evaluation of continuous fetal heart rate monitoring in high-risk pregnancy. *American Journal of Obstetrics and Gynecology, 125*(3), 310–320.

Harper, L. M., Shanks, A. L., Tuuli, M. G., Roehl, K. A., & Cahill, A. G. (2013). The risks and benefits of internal monitors in laboring patients. *American Journal of Obstetrics and Gynecology, 209*(1), 38.e1–38.e6. doi:10.1016/j.ajog.2013.04.001

Health Canada. (2000). *Family-centred maternity and newborn care: National guidelines*. Ottawa, Ontario, Canada: Minister of Public Works and Government Services.

Hodnett, E. D. (2002). Pain and women's satisfaction with the experience of childbirth: A systematic review. *American Journal of Obstetrics and Gynecology, 186*(5, Suppl.), S160–S172.

Hodnett, E. D., Gates, S., Hofmeyr, G. J., & Sakala, C. (2013). Continuous support for women during childbirth. *Cochrane Database of Systematic Reviews,* Issue 7. doi: 10.1002/14651858.CD003766.pub5

Hodnett, E. D., Lowe, N. K., Hannah, M. E., Willan, A. R., Stevens, B., Weston, J. A., . . . Nursing Supportive Care in Labor Trial Group. (2002). Effectiveness of nurses as providers of birth labor support in North American hospitals: A randomized controlled trial. *Journal of the American Medical Association, 288*(11), 1373–1381.

Hoerst, B. J., & Fairman, J. (2000). Social and professional influences of the technology of electronic fetal monitoring on obstetrical nursing. *Western Journal of Nursing Research, 22*(4), 475–491.

Hon, E. H. (1975). *An introduction to fetal heart rate monitoring* (2nd ed.). Los Angeles: USC School of Medicine.

Hutson, J. M., & Petrie, R. H. (1986). Possible limitations of fetal monitoring. *Clinical Obstetrics and Gynecology, 29*(1), 104–113.

Jacod, B. C., Graatsma, E. M., Van Hagen, E., & Visser, G. H. A. (2010). A validation of electrohysterography for uterine activity monitoring during labour. *Journal of Maternal–Fetal & Neonatal Medicine, 23*(1), 17–22. doi:10.3109/14767050903156668

Kelso, I. M., Parsons, R. J., Lawrence, G. F., Arora, S. S., Edmonds, D. K., & Cooke, I. D. (1978). An assessment of continuous fetal heart rate monitoring in labor. A randomized trial. *American Journal of Obstetrics and Gynecology, 131*(5), 526–532.

Killien, M. G., & Shy, K. (1989). A randomized clinical trial of electronic fetal monitoring in preterm labor: Mother's views. *Birth, 16*(1), 7–12.

Klapholz, H. (1978). Techniques of fetal heart rate monitoring. *Seminars in Perinatology, 2*(2), 119–129.

Klavan, M., Laver, A. T., & Boscola, M. (1997). *Clinical concepts of fetal heart rate monitoring*. Andover, MA: Hewlett-Packard Company.

Koninklijke Philips Electronics N. V. (2009). Important device safety alert. (Letter to consumers in response to The FDA Safety Information and Adverse Event Reporting Program). Retrieved from http://www.healthcare.philips.com/pwc_hc/main/shared/Assets/Documents/patient_monitoring/avalon/FSN86201075_AVALON_LETTER_FINAL.pdf.pdf

Koninklijke Philips Electronics N.V. (2011, September 8). *Philips introduces unique backup fetal and maternal monitoring solution during pregnancy, labor and delivery* [Press release]. Retrieved from http://www.newscenter.philips.com/main/standard/about/news/press/2011/20110908smart_pulse.wpd

Kwee, A., Dekkers, A. H., van Wijk, H. P., van der Hoorn-van den Beld, C. W., & Visser, G. H. (2007). Occurrence of ST-changes recorded with STAN® S21-monitor during normal and abnormal fetal heart rate patterns during labour. *European Journal of Obstetrics, Gynecology and Reproductive Biology, 135*(1), 28–34.

LaCroix, G. E. (1968). Monitoring labor by an external tocodynamometer. *American Journal of Obstetrics and Gynecology, 101*(1), 111–119.

Lally, J. E., Murtagh, M. J., Macphail, S., & Thomson, R. (2008). More in hope than expectation: A systematic review of women's expectations and experience of pain relief in labour. *BMC Medicine, 6*(7), 1–10. doi:10.1186/1741-7015-6-7

Liu, S., Liston, R. M., Joseph, K. S., Heaman, M., Sauve, R., & Kramer, M. S. (2007). Maternal mortality and severe morbidity associated with low-risk planned cesarean delivery versus planned vaginal delivery at term. *Canadian Medical Association Journal, 176*(4), 455–460.

Luthy, D. A., Shy, K. K., van Belle, G., Larson, E. B., Hughes, J. P., Benedetti, T. J., Brown, Z. A., Effer, S., King, J. F., & Stenchever, M. A. (1987). A randomized trial of electronic fetal monitoring in preterm labor. *Obstetrics and Gynecology, 69*(5), 687–695.

Lyndon, A., Lee, H. C., Gilbert, W. M., Gould, J. B., & Lee, K. A. (2012). Maternal morbidity during childbirth hospitalization in California. *Journal of Maternal – Fetal and Neonatal Medicine, 25*(12), 2529–2535. doi: 10.3109/14767058.2012.710280

Lyndon, A., O'Brien-Abel, N., & Simpson, K. R. (2009). Fetal heart rate interpretation. In A. Lyndon & L. U. Ali (Eds.), *Fetal heart monitoring principles and practices* (4th ed., pp. 101–134). Dubuque, IA: Kendall Hunt.

MacDonald, D., Grant, A., Seridan-Pereira, M., Boylan, P., & Chalmers, I. (1985). The Dublin randomized controlled trial of intrapartum fetal heart rate monitoring. *American Journal of Obstetrics and Gynecology, 152*(5), 524–539.

MacEachin, S. R., Lopez, C. M., Powell, K. J., & Corbett, N. L. (2009). The fetal heart rate collaborative practice project: Situational awareness in electronic fetal monitoring—a Kaiser Permanente Patient Safety Program initiative. *Journal of Perinatal and Neonatal Nursing, 23*(4), 314–323. doi: 10.1097/JPN.0b013e3181a1bf07

Macones, G. A., Hankins, G. D., Spong, C. Y., Hauth, J. D., & Moore, T. (2008). The 2008 National Institute of Child Health Human Development workshop report on electronic fetal monitoring: Update on definitions, interpretations, and research guidelines. *Obstetrics* and *Gynecology, 112*, 661–666. doi:10.1097/AOG.0b013e3181841395; and *Journal of Obstetric, Gynecologic and Neonatal Nursing, 37*, 510–515.

Malinowski, J. S., Pedigo, C. G., & Phillips, C. R. (1989). *Nursing care during the labor process* (3rd ed.). Philadelphia, PA: F.A. Davis.

McNiven, P., Hodnett, E., & O'Brien-Pallas, L. L. (1992). Supporting women in labor: A work sampling study of the activities of labor and delivery nurses. *Birth, 19*(1), 3–8.

Monica Healthcare Ltd. (2011, February 8). *Monica Healthcare gains FDA clearance for groundbreaking wireless fetal monitor* [Press release]. Retrieved from: http://www.monicahealthcare.com/news_archive.php?id=36

Murray, M. L. (2004). Maternal or fetal heart rate? Avoiding intrapartum misidentification. *Journal of Obstetric, Gynecologic and Neonatal Nursing, 33*(1), 93–104.

Murray, M. L., Huelsmann, G., & Koperski, N. (2011). *Essentials of fetal monitoring* (4th ed.). New York, NY: Springer.

National Institute of Child Health and Human Development Research Planning Workshop. (1997). Electronic fetal heart rate monitoring: Research guidelines for interpretation. *American Journal of Obstetrics and Gynecology, 177*(6), 1385–1390 and *Journal of*

Obstetric, Gynecologic, and Neonatal Nursing, 26, 635–640.

National Institute for Health and Care Excellence. (2007). Intrapartum care: Care of healthy women and their babies during childbirth (NICE Clinical Guideline 55). Retrieved from http://www.nice.org.uk/Guidance/CG55

Neilson, D. R., Jr., Freeman, R. K., & Mangan, S. (2008). Signal ambiguity resulting in unexpected outcome with external fetal heart rate monitoring. *American Journal of Obstetrics and Gynecology, 198*(6), 717–724. doi:10.1016/j.ajog.2008.02.030

Neilson, J. P. (2012). Fetal electrocardiogram (ECG) for fetal monitoring during labour. *Cochrane Database of Systems Reviews,* Issue 4 (Article No. CD000116), doi:10.1002/14651858.CD000116.pub3

Neldam, S., Osler, M., Hansen, P. K., Nim, J., Smith, S. F., & Hertel, J. (1986). Intrapartum fetal heart rate monitoring in a combined low- and high-risk population: a controlled clinical trial. *European Journal of Obstetrics, Gynecology, and Reproductive Biology, 23*(1–2), 1–11.

Norén, H., Amer-Wåhlin, I., Hagberg, H., Herbst, A., Kjellmer, I., Marsål, K., . . . Rosén, K. G. (2003). Fetal electrocardiography in labor and neonatal outcome: Data from the Swedish randomized controlled trial on intrapartum fetal monitoring. *American Journal of Obstetrics and Gynecology, 188*(1), 183–192.

Nurani, R., Chandraharan, E., Lowe, V., Ugwumadu, A., & Arulkumaran, S. (2012). Misidentification of maternal heart rate as fetal on cardiotocography during the second stage of labor: The role of the fetal electrocardiograph. *Acta Obstetricia et Gynecologica Scandinavica, 91*(12), 1428–1432. doi:10.1111/j.1600-0412.2012.01511.x

Olofsson, P. (2003). Current status of intrapartum fetal monitoring: Cardiotocography versus cardiotocography + ST analysis of the fetal ECG. *European Journal of Obstetrics, Gynecology and Reproductive Biology, 110*(Suppl. 1), S113–S118.

Parer, J. T. (1997). *Handbook of fetal heart rate monitoring* (2nd ed.). Philadelphia, PA: W.B. Saunders.

Parer, J. T. (2003). Electronic fetal heart rate monitoring: A story of survival. *Obstetrical and Gynecological Survey, 58*(9), 561–563.

Public Health Agency of Canada. (2009). *What mothers say: The Canadian maternity experiences survey.* Ottawa, Ontario, Canada: Author. Retrieved from http://www.phac-aspc.gc.ca/rhs-ssg/surveyeng.php

Reinhard, J., Hayes-Gill, B. R., Schiermeier, S., Hatzmann, H., Heinrich, T. M., & Louwen, F. (2013). Intrapartum heart rate ambiguity: A comparison of cardiotocogram and abdominal fetal electrocardiogram with maternal electrocardiogram. *Gynecologic and Obstetric Investigation, 75*(2), 101–108. doi:10.1159/000345059

Renou, P., Chang, A., Anderson, I., & Wood, C. (1976). Controlled trial of fetal intensive care. *American Journal of Obstetrics and Gynecology, 126*(4), 470–476.

Rosén, K. G. (2005). Fetal electrocardiogram waveform analysis in labour. *Current Opinion in Obstetrics and Gynecology, 17*(2), 147–150.

Rosén, K. G., Amer-Wåhlin, I., Luzietti, R., & Norén, H. (2004). Fetal ECG waveform analysis. *Best Practice and Research Clinical Obstetrics & Gynaecology, 18*(3), 485–514.

Ross, M. G., Devoe, L. D., & Rosén, K. G. (2004). ST-segment analysis of the fetal electrocardiogram improves fetal heart rate tracing interpretation and clinical decision making. *Journal of Maternal–Fetal and Neonatal Medicine, 15*(3), 181–185.

Rouse, D. J., Owen, J., & Hauth, J. C. (1999). Active-phase labor arrest: Oxytocin augmentation for at least 4 hours. *Obstetrics and Gynecology, 93*(3), 323–328.

Rouse, D. J., Owen, J., Savage, K. G., & Hauth, J. C. (2001). Active phase labor arrest: Revisiting the 2-hour minimum. *Obstetrics & Gynecology, 98*(4), 550–554.

Sakala, C., & Corry, M. P. (2008). *Evidenced-based maternity care: What it is and what it can achieve.* New York, NY: Childbirth Connection, The Reforming States Group, and Milbank Memorial Fund. Retrieved from http://www.milbank.org/uploads/documents/0809MaternityCare/0809MaternityCare.html

Sandelowski, M. (1998). Looking to care or caring to look?: Technology and the rise of spectacular nursing. *Holistic Nursing Practice, 12*(4), 1–11.

Schifrin, B., Harwell, R., Rubinstein, T., & Visser, G. (2001). Maternal heart rate pattern: A confounding factor in intrapartum fetal surveillance. *Prenatal and Neonatal Medicine, 6*(1), 75–82.

Schuit, E., Amer-Wahlin, I., Ojala, K., Vayssiére, C., Westerhuis, M. E., Maršál, K., . . . Kwee, A. (2013). Effectiveness of electronic fetal monitoring with additional ST analysis in vertex singleton pregnancies at >36 weeks of gestation: An individual participant data metaanalysis. *American Journal of Obstetrics and Gynecology, 208*(3), 187.e1–187.e13. doi:10.1016/j.ajog.2013.01.028

Schwartz, N., & Young, B. K. (2006). Intrapartum fetal monitoring today. *Journal of Perinatal Medicine, 34*(2), 99–107.

Sciscione, A. C., Duhl, A., Pollock, M. A., Hoffman, M. K., Rhee, A., & Colmorgen, G. H. (2005). Extramembranous placement of an air-coupled vs. transducer-tipped intrauterine pressure catheter. *The Journal of Reproductive Medicine, 50*(8), 578–584.

Sherman, D. J., Frenkel, E., Kurzweil, Y., Padua, A., Arieli, S., & Bahar, M. (2002). Characteristics of maternal heart rate patterns during labor and delivery. *Obstetrics and Gynecology, 99*(4), 542–547.

Silver, R. M., Landon, M. B., Rouse, D. J., Leveno, K. J., Spong, C. Y., Thom, E. A., . . . National Institute of Child Health and Human Development Maternal–Fetal Medicine Units Network. (2006). Maternal morbidity associated with multiple repeat cesarean deliveries. *Obstetrics & Gynecology, 107*(6), 1226–1232.

Simkin, P. (1991). Just another day in a woman's life?: Women's long-term perceptions of their first birth experience. Part I. *Birth, 18*(4), 203–210.

Simpson, K. R. (2008). Perinatal patient safety and professional liability issues. In K.R. Simpson & P. Creehan (Eds.), *Perinatal nursing* (3rd ed., pp. 1–28). Philadelphia, PA: Lippincott Williams & Wilkins.

Simpson, K. R. (2013). Alarm fatigue. *MCN: The American Journal of Maternal/Child Nursing, 38*(6), 397. doi:10.1097/NMC.0b013e3182a537c6

Smith, J., Jr., & Onstad, J. H. (2005). Assessment of the fetus: Intermittent auscultation, electronic fetal heart rate tracing, and fetal pulse oximetry. *Obstetrics and Gynecology Clinics of North America, 32*(2), 245–254.

Society of Obstetrics and Gynaecologists of Canada & British Columbia Perinatal Health Program. (2007). Fetal health surveillance: Antepartum and intrapartum consensus guideline. Clinical Practice Guideline No. 197. *Journal of Obstetrics and Gynaecology in Canada, 29*(9, Suppl. 4), S3–S56.

Spong, C. Y., Berghella, C., Wenstrom, K. D., Mercer, B. M., & Saade, G. R. (2012). Preventing the first cesarean delivery: Summary of a joint Eunice Kennedy Shriver National Institute of Child Health and Human Development, Society for Maternal–Fetal Medicine, and American College of Obstetricians and Gynecologists workshop. *Obstetrics and Gynecology, 120*(5), 1181–1193. doi:http://10.1097/AOG.0b013e3182704880

Strong, T. H., Jr., & Paul, R. H. (1989). Intrapartum uterine activity: Evaluation of an intrauterine pressure transducer. *Obstetrics and Gynecology, 73*(3), 432–434.

The Joint Commission. (2013a, April 8). Medical device alarm safety in hospitals. *Sentinel Event Alert, 50*. Retrieved from http://www.jointcommission.org/assets/1/18/sea_50_alarms_4_5_13_final1.pdf

The Joint Commission. (2013b). National patient safety goal on alarm management (Prepublication requirements). Oakbrook Terrace, IL: Author.

The Joint Commission. (2004, July 21). Preventing infant death and injury during delivery. *Sentinel Event Alert, 30*. Retrieved from http://www.jointcommission.org/assets/1/18/SEA_30.PDF

U.S. Food and Drug Administration. (2009). Safety alerts for human medical products: Philips Avalon fetal monitors. Retrieved from http://www.fda.gov/Safety/MedWatch/SafetyInformation /SafetyAlertsforHumanMedicalProducts/ucm181505.htm

Usta, I. M., Mercer, B. M., & Sibai, B. M. (1999). Current obstetrical practice and umbilical cord prolapse. *American Journal of Perinatology, 16*(9), 479–484.

Utah Medical Products Inc. (2006). Intrans® plus user guidelines [Brochure]. Midvale, UT: Author.

VanVeen, T. R., Belfort, M. A., & Kofford, S. (2012). Maternal heart rate patterns in the first and second stages of labor. *Acta Obstetricia et Gynecologica Scandinavica, 91*(5), 598–604. doi:10.1111/j.1600-0412.2012.01371.x

Vintzileos, A. M., Antsaklis, A., Varvarigos, I., Papas, C., Sofatzis, I., & Montgomery, J. T. (1993). A randomized trial of intrapartum electronic fetal heart rate monitoring versus intermittent auscultation. *Obstetrics and Gynecology, 81*(6), 899–907.

Wood, S. H. (2003). Should women be given a choice about fetal assessment in labor? *MCN: The American Journal of Maternal/Child Nursing, 28*(5), 292–298.

SECTION THREE

Fetal Monitoring: Diagnosis and Intervention

CHAPTER 5

Fetal Heart Rate Interpretation

Audrey Lyndon
Nancy O'Brien-Abel
Kathleen Rice Simpson

INTRODUCTION

The purpose of this chapter is to discuss current concepts in fetal heart rate (FHR) interpretation, including points of both consensus and dissent about interpretation in the FHR monitoring literature. A review of the assumptions of the 2008 National Institute of Child Health and Human Development (NICHD) framework and definitions is followed by discussion of parameters for interpretation of FHR characteristics. The interpretation, presumed physiology and clinical significance, and general management of various FHR findings are discussed in this chapter. The underlying physiologic basis for fetal monitoring is discussed in Chapter 2. Physiologic goals and more detail on interventions for management of FHR tracings are discussed in Chapter 6. For a detailed discussion of the development of fetal monitoring techniques and the historical research base for fetal monitoring, refer to the first chapter of this book as well as the comprehensive summaries presented by Freeman, Garite, Nageotte, and Miller (2012) and Parer (1997).

Synthesis of the literature on FHR monitoring is challenging because of the lack of comparability of variables and outcome measures across documents. Comparison is hindered by both inconsistent definitions of FHR characteristics across studies (which NICHD [Macones, Hankins, Spong, Hauth, & Moore, 2008; NICHD, 1997] attempts to remedy) and lack of consistent definition of "acidemia" across studies and guidelines. Clinically significant metabolic acidemia is associated with an arterial umbilical blood pH value of less than 7.00 and a base excess below -12 mmol/L (American College of Obstetricians and Gynecologists [ACOG], 2006; Andres et al., 1999; Low, Lindsay, & Derrick, 1997; MacLennan, 1999). However, studies of relationships between FHR characteristics and fetal or newborn acidemia use values ranging from 7.00 to 7.20 to define "acidemia."

For the purposes of the Association of Women's Health, Obstetric and Neonatal Nurses (AWHONN) Fetal Heart Monitoring Program (FHMP) courses and this chapter, the physiologic threshold for avoiding significant acidemia at birth is an umbilical artery pH greater than 7.10 and a base excess greater than or equal to –12 mmol/L (i.e., between 0 and –12) (Andres et al., 1999; Fox, Kilpatrick, King, & Parer, 2000; Low et al., 1997). The absence of significant acidemia at birth may also be inferred by the presence of a 5-minute Apgar score of 7 or greater (Parer, King, Flanders, Fox, & Kilpatrick, 2006).

The goal of fetal heart monitoring is to prevent the development of significant acidemia while simultaneously minimizing unnecessary intervention and promoting a satisfying, family-centered birth experience.

Fetal heart monitoring is a complex skill requiring knowledge of maternal-fetal physiology, clinical judgment, and specialized education in the use of intermittent auscultation (IA) and electronic fetal monitoring (EFM) techniques. Professional registered nurses are the primary bedside provider of intrapartum FHM in most settings in the United States and Canada and are qualified to perform this ongoing assessment independently as well as in collaboration with a physician or midwife. It is inappropriate to delegate auscultation of the FHR, application of FHR transducers, or initial and ongoing assessment of maternal-fetal status, including interpretation of auscultation and electronic FHR findings to unlicensed assistive personnel (AWHONN, 2009a, 2009b).

Registered nurses, physicians, and midwives should work together with women and their families using a collaborative problem-solving framework to achieve an effective, integrated, patient-centered plan for ongoing maternal-fetal assessment and intervention in support of a family-centered birth. Within this framework, interpretation of FHR findings flows directly from the systematic analysis of maternal and fetal assessment data for the independent and collaborative diagnosis of patient problems, as indicated in Figure 5-1. Systematic use of a standardized language for interpreting and discussing FHR findings promotes understanding among clinicians, thereby promoting safe and effective care of laboring women.

Assumptions of the NICHD Terminology

The consensus reached by the Research Planning Workshop on Electronic Fetal Monitoring included the following set of assumptions about the interpretation of fetal monitoring data (NICHD, 1997), which were reaffirmed and updated at the 2008 meeting (Box 5-1) (Macones et al., 2008).

Definitions of Terms

The definitions of the FHR characteristics discussed in this chapter are presented in Table 5-1. Clinicians should be familiar with these definitions and use them consistently in the AWHONN FHM courses and in clinical practice.

Systematic Assessment of FHR Data

Appropriate interventions require an accurate interpretation of the characteristics of both the FHR and uterine activity. Although there may be disagreement among experts about the interpretation of some combinations of FHR characteristics, there is consensus on what constitutes a normal FHR tracing (Figure 5-2): normal baseline rate, moderate variability, and the absence of late or variable decelerations. Accelerations and early decelerations may or may not be present in a normal (category I) FHR tracing (Macones et al., 2008). Tracings exhibiting these normal characteristics are highly predictive of a well-oxygenated, nonacidotic fetus (ACOG, 2009, 2010; Berkus, Langer, Samueloff, Xernakis, & Field, 1999; Krebs, Petres, & Dunn, 1981; Krebs, Petres, Dunn, Jordaan, & Segreti, 1979; Low, Victory, & Derrick, 1999; Macones et al., 2008). Likewise, normal intermittent auscultation findings (normal baseline rate and rhythm, presence or absence of increases [accelerations] in FHR, absence of decreases [decelerations] in FHR) are predictive of fetal well-being (Paine, Benedict, Strobino, Gregor, & Larson, 1992; Paine, Zanardi, Johnson, Rorie, & Barger, 2001).

Attention should be given to the overall clinical picture and stability of, or changes in, FHR characteristics over time. Although the experienced clinician may assess individual characteristics such as rate and rhythm of the FHR simultaneously, a detailed and thorough evaluation of each component may be useful when planning appropriate interventions. Developing a structured approach to assessment and analysis of FHR findings is also helpful in developing skill in interpretation. A systematic fetal monitoring assessment includes the data outlined in Table 5-2.

FIGURE 5-1 The Collaborative Process and Fetal Heart Monitoring

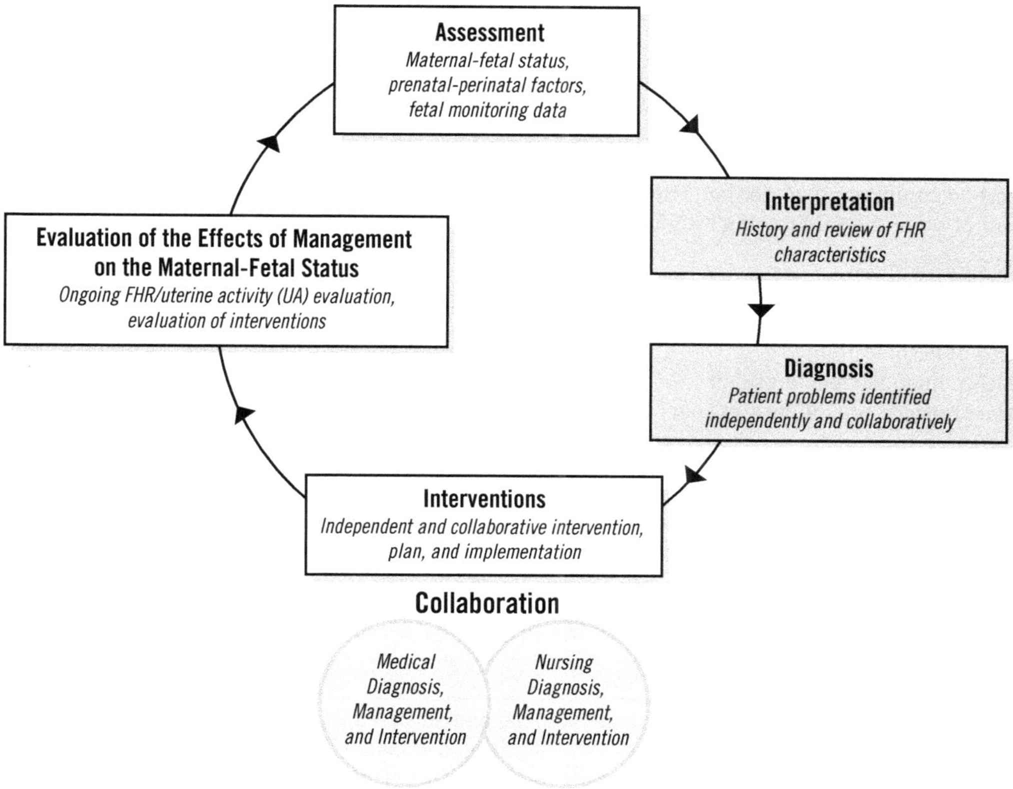

BOX 5-1 NICHD Consensus Assumptions about the Interpretation of Electronic Fetal Monitoring Data

A. The definitions are primarily developed for visual interpretation of FHR patterns. However, it is recognized that computerized interpretation is being developed and the definitions must also be adaptable to such applications.
B. The definitions apply to the interpretations of patterns produced from either a direct fetal electrode detecting the fetal electrocardiogram or an external Doppler device detecting the FHR events with use of the autocorrelation technique.
C. The record of both the FHR and uterine activity should be of adequate quality for visual interpretation.
D. The prime emphasis in the [2008 NICHD] report is on intrapartum patterns. The definitions may also be applicable to antepartum observations.
E. The characteristics to be defined are those commonly used in clinical practice and research communications.
F. The features of FHR patterns are categorized as either baseline, periodic, or episodic. Periodic patterns are those associated with uterine contractions, and episodic patterns are those not associated with uterine contractions.
G. The periodic patterns are distinguished on the basis of waveform, currently accepted as either "abrupt" or "gradual" onset.
H. Accelerations and decelerations are generally determined in reference to the adjacent baseline FHR.
I. No distinction is made between short-term variability (or beat-to-beat variability or R-R wave period differences in the electrocardiogram) and long-term variability because in actual practice they are visually determined as a unit. Hence, the definition of variability is based visually on the amplitude of the complexes, with exclusion of the sinusoidal pattern.

(continued)

BOX 5-1 (Continued)

J. There is good evidence that a number of characteristics of FHR patterns are dependent upon fetal gestational age and physiologic status as well as maternal physiologic status. Thus, FHR tracings should be evaluated in the context of many clinical conditions including gestational age, prior results of fetal assessment, medications, maternal medical conditions, and fetal conditions (e.g., growth restriction, known congenital anomalies, fetal anemia, arrhythmia, etc.).

K. The individual components of defined FHR patterns do not occur independently and generally evolve over time.

L. A full description of the EFM tracing requires a qualitative and quantitative description of

1. Uterine contractions
2. Baseline FHR
3. Baseline FHR variability
4. Presence of accelerations
5. Periodic or episodic decelerations
6. Changes or trends of FHR patterns over time

Note: From "The 2008 National Institute of Child Health Human Development Workshop Report on Electronic Fetal Monitoring: Update on Definitions, Interpretations, and Research Guidelines," by G. A. Macones, G. D. Hankins, C. Y. Spong, J. D. Hauth, & T. Moore, 2008, *Journal of Obstetric, Gynecologic and Neonatal Nursing, 37*, 510–515; *Obstetrics and Gynecology, 112*, p. 662.

TABLE 5-1 2008 NICHD Descriptive Terms for FHR Characteristics

TERM	DEFINITION
Baseline rate	Approximate mean FHR rounded to increments of 5 bpm during a 10-minute window excluding accelerations and decelerations and periods of marked variability. There must be ≥2 minutes of identifiable baseline segments (not necessarily contiguous) in any 10-minute window, or the baseline for that period is indeterminate. In such cases, one may need to refer to the previous 10-minute window for determination of the baseline.
Bradycardia	Baseline rate of < 110 bpm.
Tachycardia	Baseline rate of > 160 bpm.
Baseline variability	Determined in a 10-minute window, excluding accelerations and decelerations. Fluctuations in the baseline FHR that are irregular in amplitude and frequency and are visually quantified as the amplitude of the peak-to-trough in bpm.
— Absent variability	Amplitude range undetectable.
— Minimal variability	Amplitude range visually detectable but ≤ 5 bpm (greater than undetectable but ≤ 5 bpm).
— Moderate variability	Amplitude range 6–25 bpm.
— Marked variability	Amplitude range > 25 bpm.
Acceleration	Visually apparent **abrupt** increase in FHR. *Abrupt* increase is defined as an increase from onset of acceleration to peak in < 30 seconds. Peak must be ≥15 bpm, and the acceleration must last ≥15 seconds from the onset to return. Acceleration lasting ≥10 minutes is defined as a baseline change. Before 32 weeks of gestation, accelerations are defined as having a peak ≥10 bpm and a duration of ≥ 10 seconds.
Prolonged acceleration	Acceleration ≥ 2 minutes but < 10 minutes in duration.
Early deceleration	Visually apparent, usually symmetrical, **gradual** decrease and return of the FHR associated with a uterine contraction. A *gradual* FHR decrease is defined as one from the onset to the FHR nadir of ≥30 seconds. The decrease in FHR is calculated from the onset to the nadir of the deceleration. The nadir of the deceleration occurs at the same time as the peak of the contraction. In most cases, the onset, nadir, and recovery of the deceleration are coincident with the beginning, peak, and ending of the contraction, respectively.
Late deceleration	Visually apparent, usually symmetrical, **gradual** decrease and return of the FHR associated with a uterine contraction. A *gradual* FHR decrease is defined as from the onset to the FHR nadir of ≥30 seconds. The decrease in FHR is calculated from the onset to the nadir of the deceleration. The deceleration is delayed in timing, with nadir of the deceleration occurring after the peak of the contraction. In most cases, the onset, nadir, and recovery of the deceleration occur after the beginning, peak, and ending of the contraction, respectively.

TERM	DEFINITION
Variable deceleration	Visually apparent **abrupt** decrease in FHR. An *abrupt* FHR decrease is defined as from the onset of the deceleration to the beginning of the FHR nadir of < 30 seconds. The decrease in FHR is calculated from the onset to the nadir of the deceleration. The decrease in FHR is ≥15 bpm, lasting ≥15 seconds, and < 2 minutes in duration. When variable decelerations are associated with uterine contractions, their onset, depth, and duration commonly vary with successive uterine contractions.
Prolonged deceleration	Visually apparent decrease in FHR from the baseline that is ≥15 bpm, lasting ≥ 2 minutes, but < 10 minutes. A deceleration that lasts ≥ 10 minutes is baseline change.
Recurrent	Occurring with ≥ 50% of contractions in any 20-minute window.
Intermittent	Occurring with < 50% of contractions in any 20-minute window.
Sinusoidal pattern	Visually apparent, smooth, sine wave–like undulating pattern in FHR baseline with cycle frequency of 3–5/minute that persists for ≥ 20 minutes.

Adapted from Macones, G. A., Hankins, G. D., Spong, C. Y., Hauth, J. D., & Moore, T. (2008).

FIGURE 5-2 Visual Representation of Normal (Category I) FHR Characteristics by EFM

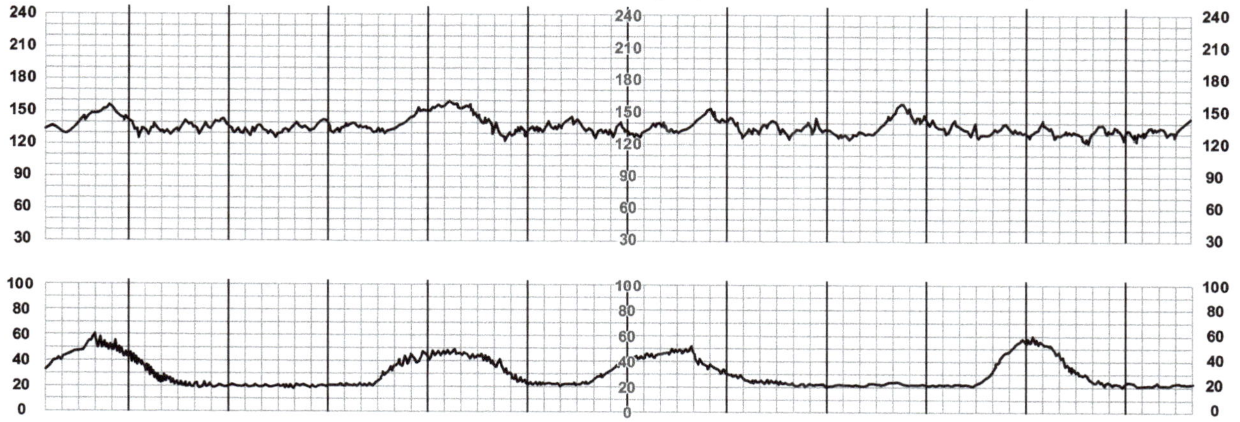

TABLE 5-2 Systematic Assessment of Fetal Monitoring Data

Baseline rate	Is the rate normal, tachycardic, or bradycardic?
Rhythm in intermittent auscultation (IA)	Is the rhythm regular or irregular?
Variability (EFM)	Is the FHR variability moderate, or is it absent, minimal, marked, or unable to be determined (e.g., poor signal quality)?
Periodic and episodic changes	Presence or absence of increases in FHR (IA) or accelerations (EFM) Presence or absence of decreases in FHR (IA) or decelerations (EFM) Are decelerations early, late, variable, or prolonged? (EFM) Are there other unusual characteristics such as sinusoidal or arrhythmic FHR? (EFM)
Uterine activity	What are the frequency, duration, and intensity of contractions? What is the uterine resting tone?
Evolution of the FHR over time	How has the FHR changed over time? What features of the FHR are stable?
Integration of findings with the overall clinical picture	How do the FHR findings fit with the overall clinical picture, including maternal medical history, current pregnancy history and fetal condition, gestational age, and other physical and laboratory findings? How does the overall clinical history guide interpretation of the fetal monitoring findings? What does the team need to prepare for? Are there potential complications the team needs to be especially vigilant for? Who needs to be aware of current maternal–fetal status? What parameters indicate the need for review of the current plan? Within what time frame is reevaluation or escalation of planning needed?

CHARACTERISTICS OF THE FHR AND UTERINE ACTIVITY

Baseline Fetal Heart Rate

The normal range for the baseline FHR is 110–160 beats per minute (bpm) (Macones et al., 2008). With IA the baseline is established by counting the FHR at repeated intervals for at least 30–60 seconds after uterine contractions (Feinstein, Sprague, & Trepanier, 2009) (see also Chapter 4). With EFM the baseline is determined by evaluating the tracing over a time frame of at least 10 minutes to determine the approximate mean rate rounded to the closest 5-bpm interval. Thus, if the FHR varies between 120 and 130 bpm over a 10-minute period, the baseline is reported at 125 bpm. Determination of the baseline by EFM requires at least 2 minutes of interpretable FHR data in any 10-minute period and excludes areas recording periodic or episodic changes and marked variability. The sections of tracing used to determine the baseline do not necessarily need to be contiguous, but if there are not at least 2 minutes of interpretable baseline within a 10-minute period, the baseline is classified as indeterminate. When this occurs, the clinician may need to review other recent sections of the tracing to determine the baseline. Regardless of monitoring method, a baseline rate less than 110 bpm for 10 minutes or longer is a bradycardia, and a baseline greater than 160 bpm for 10 minutes or longer is a tachycardia.

The baseline rate reflects integration of the many physiologic influences on the FHR but is predominantly controlled by the autonomic nervous system. The baseline rate is generated by the sinoatrial node of the fetal heart, which has an intrinsic pacemaker. The intrinsic rate in early gestation is under primary influence of the sympathetic nervous system and is therefore slightly higher in the preterm fetus. As the fetus matures, parasympathetic influence becomes stronger, and the intrinsic rate decreases incrementally (Nageotte & Gilstrap, 2009). However, the difference in baseline FHR between 28–30 weeks' gestation and term is approximately 10 bpm. Therefore, any preterm fetus with a baseline FHR greater than 160 bpm should be evaluated further to rule out fetal compromise, rather than assuming that the tachycardia is secondary to prematurity (Freeman et al., 2012).

Further discussion of the physiologic influences on the FHR, the fetal cardiac conduction system, and aberrations in conduction may be found in Chapters 2 and 11.

Tachycardia

Tachycardia represents increased sympathetic or decreased parasympathetic autonomic tone. Physiologic conditions that cause tachycardia may originate from the mother or the fetus, as illustrated in Table 5-3. A number of causes of tachycardia do not reflect a risk of acidemia, including the most common causes of fetal tachycardia in labor: maternal fever and medications affecting the heart rate (Garite, 2012; Nageotte & Gilstrap, 2009). Maternal fever raises core temperature, and fetal tachycardia in the setting of maternal fever is believed to be a response to an increase in the fetal metabolic rate rather than an indicator of sepsis. The FHR is estimated to increase by 10 bpm for every 1-degree increase in maternal temperature and may also be mildly elevated in response to beta-sympathomimetics, atropine, scopolamine, and phenothiazines (Garite, 2012). Other maternal causes of tachycardia include hyperthyroidism (Garite, 2012)

TABLE 5-3 Potential Causes of Fetal Tachycardia

MATERNAL	FETAL
Fever	Increased metabolic rate
Infection (chorioamnionitis, pyelonephritis)	Anemia
Beta-synpathomimetic drugs (terbutaline, epinephrine)	Acute blood loss
Parasympatholytic drugs (scopalomine, atropine, phenothiazines, hydroxyzine)	Hyperthyroidism
Dehydration	Heart failure
Hyperthyroidism	Hypoxemia
Cocaine	Infection or sepsis
	Tachyarrhythmia

ACOG (2010); Freeman, Garite, Nageotte, & Miller (2012); Garite (2012).

and dehydration. Premature fetuses may have baseline heart rates at or near the upper limits of the normal range (Freeman et al., 2012). Fetal tachyarrhythmias are discussed in Chapter 11.

Brief periods of tachycardia may be seen as a normal fetal compensatory or recovery response from acute hypoxia or acidosis, such as prolonged decelerations (Parer, 1997). This response is probably due to a transient rise in catecholamine levels following sympathetic nervous or adrenal stimulation (King, 2012; Parer, 1997). Fetal tachycardia is not believed to indicate fetal hypoxia when it occurs in the setting of moderate variability without recurrent decelerations (ACOG, 2010; Freeman et al., 2012; Parer, 1997). However, tachycardia does increase myocardial oxygen demand, potentially taxing fetal reserve.

As with other FHR characteristics, assessment and management of fetal tachycardia is based on the associated baseline FHR variability and the presence or absence of accelerations and decelerations. Efforts should be taken to determine the underlying etiology, including evaluation of maternal temperature, hydration status, and medication history (ACOG, 2010). Maximizing uteroplacental perfusion and avoiding excessive uterine activity are appropriate. The primary provider should be notified of fetal tachycardia, as it is important to differentiate sinus tachycardia from supraventricular tachycardia (Freeman et al., 2012). If tachycardia is observed in combination with recurrent late or variable decelerations or in combination with absent variability, a bedside evaluation by a physician is indicated.When tachycardia is observed in preterm fetuses, a bedside evaluation by a physician may also be indicated because preterm fetuses appear to have lower tolerance for stress as a result of the immaturity of their compensatory responses (Freeman et al., 2012).

Bradycardia

Fetal bradycardia may be due to normal physiologic variation, a change in maternal-fetal condition interrupting blood flow or gas exchange (e.g., a prolapsed cord, uterine rupture, abruptio placentae, maternal hypotension), or medication, hypoglycemia, hypothermia, and fetal bradyarrhythmias. An important issue in assessment of bradycardia is distinguishing it from a prolonged deceleration, which lasts at least 2 minutes but less than 10 minutes. While an established baseline bradycardia is usually innocuous, an acute prolonged deceleration may indicate significant fetal hypoxia (Garite, 2012).

Fetal bradycardia within the range of 80–110 bpm with moderate variability is associated with an oxygenated, nonacidemic fetus, as bradycardias in this range are generally vagally mediated and nonasphyxial (Freeman et al., 2012; Parer, 1997). A baseline FHR of 40–80 bpm, especially with minimal or absent variability, may indicate complete heart block. Complete heart block (discussed in Chapter 11) is a rare fetal bradyarrhythmia in which the fetus is not hypoxic (Garite, 2012).

When a bradycardia is observed on admission, differentiation of maternal and fetal heart rates is essential to rule out the possibility of fetal demise with a maternal rate being transmitted through dead fetal tissue. Recording of maternal heart rate can occur with either the external ultrasound transducer or direct fetal spiral electrode (Garite, 2012). During FHR auscultation, misinterpretation of maternal heart rate may also occur if maternal heart sounds are mistaken for fetal heart sounds. Real-time ultrasound may be used, especially during the antepartum period, to determine whether the bradycardia is fetal in origin (Freeman et al., 2012; see also Chapter 4).

Bradycardias occurring during the second stage of labor following a previously normal FHR pattern may be due to increased vagal tone related to head compression during descent (Parer, 1997) or, occasionally, umbilical cord occlusion. However, prolonged deceleration or bradycardia may reflect a progressive decrease in fetal oxygenation. Fetal cardiac output is presumed to fail at rates below 60 bpm (Ball & Parer, 1992; Parer, 1997). If the variability remains moderate or minimal and the FHR does not fall below 90–100 bpm, expediting birth may not be warranted (Ball & Parer, 1992; Gull et al., 1996; Parer, 1997). In this situation, efforts to alleviate the bradycardia should be taken and maternal pushing should be modified to allow the fetus to recover (see Chapter 6 for discussion of physiologic management of the second stage of labor).

Sudden profound bradycardia is a medical emergency and may result from an acute drop in maternal oxygenation (maternal respiratory depression, apnea, or seizure), acute impairment of uteroplacental exchange (maternal hypotension, excessive uterine activity, or loss of placental area with uterine rupture or abruptio placentae), prolonged occlusion of the umbilical cord, or profound vagal stimulation (Parer, 1997). In clinical practice, intervention is often necessary before the distinction can be made between a new onset of true bradycardia and a prolonged deceleration (see Table 5-1). These terms are therefore often used interchangeably when discussing emergent response to a profound drop in FHR in the clinical setting. Immediate vaginal examination to rule out cord prolapse and rapid descent as causes of the bradycardia is indicated, as is mobilization of the team in preparation to expedite birth, if necessary. The clinical picture at the onset of the bradycardia and the depth, duration, and FHR variability are critical factors in assessing fetal condition and determining the need to proceed with emergent cesarean birth.

Several clinical factors affect the potential impact of bradycardia on fetal outcome. Studies comparing decision-to-incision times for emergency cesarean birth have shown that there is a time-dependent relationship between the onset of the bradycardia, the depth of the bradycardia, the presence or absence of variability, and the development of metabolic acidosis (Korhonen & Kariniemi, 1994). Because the fetus has minimal capacity to increase stroke volume, very low heart rates result in inadequate cardiac output for sustaining oxygenation and fetal life. Bradycardias with rates of less than 60 bpm, those accompanied by late or variable decelerations, and those with minimal or absent variability are most often associated with adverse outcome (Berkus et al., 1999; Low et al., 1999; Parer, 1997).

The onset of a fetal bradycardia when a woman is laboring after a prior cesarean birth should cause concern for the onset of uterine rupture, signaling provider attendance at the bedside and preparation for an emergent cesarean birth. While variable, late, or prolonged decelerations may be seen initially, bradycardia is the FHR pattern most commonly associated with uterine rupture (Ridgeway, Weyrich, & Benedetti, 2004). Leung, Leung, and Paul (1993) evaluated the fetal consequences of catastrophic uterine rupture when the diagnosis was made at the onset of a fetal bradycardia. All infants with a previously normal FHR pattern born within 17 minutes following the onset of a prolonged deceleration that progressed to bradycardia survived without significant perinatal morbidity. However, perinatal asphyxia could occur as early as 10 minutes after the onset of bradycardia when these events were preceded by other signs of fetal stress, specifically "severe" late and variable decelerations. Similarly, Kamoshita et al. (2010) reviewed a retrospective case series of 19 women who demonstrated sudden bradycardias that were sustained at rates <100 bpm following a previously "reassuring" tracing. All cases were determined to be associated with significant events such as uterine rupture, cord prolapse, or abruptio placentae. The infants were followed up until 2 years of age and found to have normal neurologic outcomes when cesarean birth was achieved within 25 minutes of the onset of the bradycardia.

Baseline Fetal Heart Rate Variability

The term "variability" refers to the fluctuations in the FHR over time and is considered the most important predictor of adequate fetal oxygenation during labor (Clark et al., 2013; Dellinger, Boehm, & Crane, 2000; Martin, 1982; Parer et al., 2006). Variability is present when there are irregular fluctuations in the baseline FHR. Because the fluctuations in FHR are irregular in both amplitude and frequency, they are quantified by visual assessment of the amplitude of variation in FHR, as described in Table 5-1 and illustrated in Figure 5-3. Clinically, variability is visually determined as a unit without separating short- and long-term components (Macones et al., 2008). This single visual

FIGURE 5-3 Visual Variability Scale

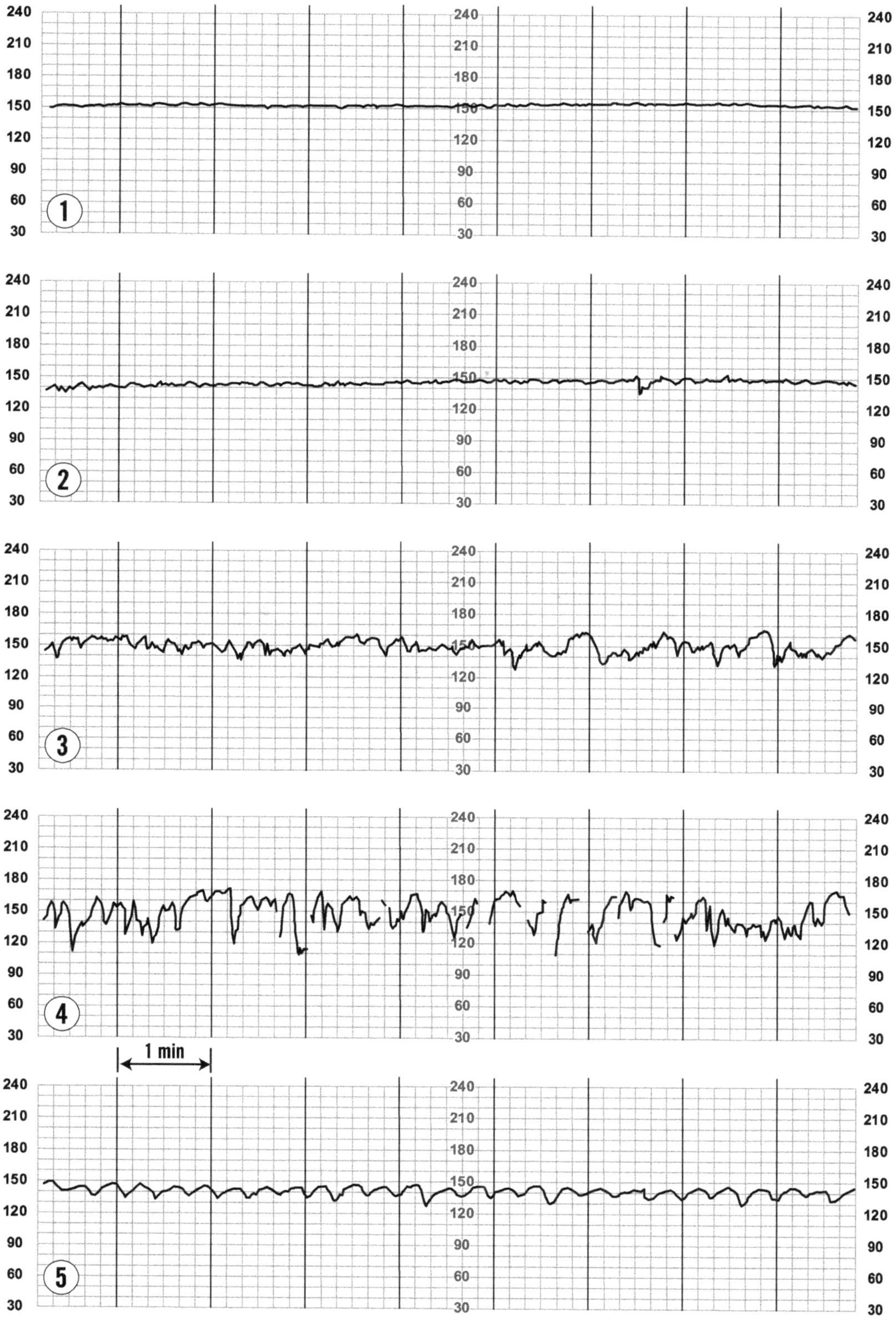

Varying degrees of FHR variability: (1) undetectable; (2) minimal; (3) moderate; (4) marked; and (5) sinusoidal pattern. Original scaling, 30 bmp per cm vertical axis, and paper speed 3 cm-min^{-1} horizontal axis.

From "Electronic Fetal Heart Rate Monitoring: Research Guidelines for Interpretation," National Institutes of Child Health and Human Development Research Planning Workshop, 1997, *Journal of Obstetric, Gynecologic and Neonatal Nursing, 26*, 635–640.

assessment captures both the long-term cycling and short-term R-R interval changes in the fetal QRS cycle that contribute to overall variability in FHR. By definition, FHR variability is a baseline FHR characteristic and therefore is assessed during the baseline FHR, not during decelerations or accelerations. The sinusoidal FHR pattern does not fall into the standard classification of variability (Macones et al., 2008).

Moderate Variability

The normal FHR tracing demonstrates moderate variability with an amplitude range of 6–25 bpm (Macones et al., 2008). Moderate variability presents visually as a rough line that is jagged and unpredictable (Fox et al., 2000; Parer, 1997). As discussed in Chapter 2, FHR variability is a reflection of neuromodulation of an active central nervous system and normal cardiac responsiveness. The parasympathetic influence is the predominant determinant of variability. When the fetus is alert and active, the central nervous system responds with moderate FHR variability. The presence of moderate variability is one of the FHR characteristics that predict adequate fetal oxygenation; another is the presence of accelerations (Berkus et al., 1999). However, decreases in variability and absence of accelerations are not necessarily predictive of fetal hypoxemia. Fetal quiet sleep, some maternal medications or substance use, congenital neurologic abnormalities, and cardiac conduction defects can also depress FHR variability (Parer, 1997). Because severe hypoxia and metabolic acidosis will decrease central nervous system function, the presence of moderate FHR variability reliably indicates a fetus that remains physiologically compensated at the time of observation (Freeman et al., 2012; Parer, 1997).

Alterations in Fetal Heart Rate Variability

Minimal Variability

Minimal variability has an amplitude greater than undetectable but less than or equal to 5 bpm (Macones et al., 2008). During the course of labor, baseline variability often transitions between moderate and minimal with fetal activity cycles (ACOG, 2010). While moderate variability reliably predicts the absence of fetal acidemia at the time of observation, minimal or absent variability alone does not reliably predict fetal hypoxemia or metabolic acidemia (Freeman et al., 2012; Macones et al., 2008).

Minimal variability without concomitant decelerations is almost always unrelated to fetal acidemia (Freeman et al., 2012; Parer & Livingston, 1990). The most common causes of a decrease in variability not associated with a risk for acidemia are centrally acting medications such as opioids, tranquilizers, magnesium sulfate, and other analgesics administered to women during labor. Minimal (but not absent) variability is also seen in premature gestations and during fetal sleep cycles (ACOG, 2010; Freeman et al., 2012). During quiet sleep, a fetus may demonstrate minimal FHR variability and no accelerations. At term, studies suggest that the mean length of the fetal quiet sleep is 23 minutes, but this behavioral state may persist for as long as 75 minutes (Patrick, Campbell, Carmichael, Natale, & Richardson, 1982; Timor-Tritsch, Dierker, Hertz, Deagan, & Rosen, 1978). If persistent minimal variability is observed in labor, the clinician should review the preceding hour or two of FHR tracing for the presence of accelerations and FHR variability and absence of late or variable decelerations and bradycardia.

When a woman first presents to the birth suite with minimal or absent FHR variability and there is no prior tracing to review, a prompt assessment of fetal well-being is indicated. In such situations it is not known whether the decrease in variability was preceded by other FHR changes indicative of hypoxic stress. Interviewing the mother about perceived fetal movement over the past several hours and days or performing vibroacoustic stimulation per unit protocol may provide additional information to differentiate between normal sleep cycles versus insufficient fetal oxygenation. FHR tracings presenting minimal or absent variability without other FHR abnormalities may reflect a preexisting (antepartum) fetal neurologic insult or the presence of a major neurologic or cardiac congenital abnormality (Clark et al., 2013; Freeman et al.,

2012; MacLennan, 1999). ACOG (2010) recommends considering a tracing with persistent minimal variability without accelerations and no response to scalp or vibroacoustic stimulation as possibly associated with fetal acidemia.

Absent Variability

Absent variability has an amplitude change that is undetectable. The FHR tracing with absent variability is smooth, blunted, and flat in appearance. Absent variability in conjunction with variable or late decelerations or bradycardia is presumed to reflect a significant risk for fetal metabolic acidemia (ACOG, 2010; Parer et al., 2006; Paul, Suidan, Yeh, Schifrin, & Hon, 1975) and requires prompt evaluation (Macones et al., 2008). Despite low positive predictive value, this combination of characteristics is the most sensitive indicator of metabolic acidemia in a fetus (ACOG, 2010; Beard et al., 1971; Clark, Gimovsky, & Miller, 1984; Low et al., 1999; Parer et al., 2006). Intrauterine resuscitation and interventions to expedite birth are warranted if fetal well-being cannot be rapidly confirmed (ACOG, 2010; Parer & Ikeda, 2007). A tracing with absent FHR variability in the context of a normal baseline rate and the absence of decelerations may represent a preexisting neurologic insult to the fetus (MacLennan, 1999).

Marked Variability

Marked variability, with an amplitude range greater than 25 bpm and a chaotic appearance, is a rare pattern, occurring in approximately 2% of FHR tracings (O'Brien-Abel & Benedetti, 1992). The etiology of marked variability is unclear; the increase in variability is presumed to result from an increase in alpha-adrenergic activity, which causes selective vasoconstriction of certain vascular beds. Marked variability was first described by Hammacher, Huter, Bokelmann, and Werners (1968), who found the pattern associated with low Apgar scores and poor neonatal outcome; however, it is unclear whether the pattern was present immediately before birth or whether it preceded an evolution to a more serious pattern (Hammacher et al., 1968).

In fetal sheep and monkeys, marked variability has been observed with episodes of acute hypoxemia or hypoxia (Dalton, Dawes, & Patrick, 1977; Martin, 1978; Parer et al., 1980). Other studies of human fetuses have associated marked variability with prolonged pregnancies (Cibils, 1975; O'Brien-Abel & Benedetti, 1992), maternal ephedrine administration (O'Brien-Abel & Benedetti, 1992; Wright, Shnider, Levinson, Rolbin, & Parer, 1981), fetal breathing (Dawes, Visser, Goodman, & Levine, 1981), and decreased uteroplacental perfusion or umbilical cord compression (Leveno et al., 1984; O'Brien-Abel & Benedetti, 1992).

In the absence of abnormal FHR heart rate changes, marked variability is not associated with acidemia as judged by fetal blood pH or Apgar scores (O'Brien-Abel & Benedetti, 1992; Wright et al., 1981) and should be interpreted in conjunction with the other FHR characteristics observed. Interventions to eliminate marked variability aim to promote placental blood flow and fetal oxygenation (Nagoette & Gilstrap, 2009; Parer, 1997). Strategies may include maternal lateral positioning, correcting maternal hypotension or excessive uterine activity, administering IV fluid bolus, or administering oxygen at 10L/min via nonrebreather mask (Garite & Simpson, 2011; Simpson, 2007).

Periodic and Episodic Changes

Characteristic changes from the FHR baseline are classified as either periodic (occurring in association with uterine contractions) or episodic (not associated with uterine contractions). These changes include accelerations and decelerations, both of which may occur in a periodic or episodic fashion. In EFM, periodic and episodic changes are classified on the basis of waveform, which is described as either "abrupt" or "gradual" in onset (Macones et al., 2008; see Table 5-1). The difference between abrupt and gradual onset is quantified by whether the onset to nadir or peak of the FHR change occurs in less than 30 seconds (abrupt) or takes 30 seconds or longer (gradual) (Macones et al., 2008). Accelerations and decelerations are determined in reference to the adjacent baseline FHR (Macones et al., 2008). With both IA and EFM, any FHR change with a duration of 10 minutes or longer is classified as a change in baseline rate rather than a periodic or episodic change (Macones et al., 2008), although in practice clinicians do not necessarily wait to make this differentiation, especially in the case of prolonged decelerations.

Accelerations

Accelerations are audible (IA) or visually apparent (EFM) abrupt increases in the FHR above baseline. In fetuses 32 weeks' gestation or greater, an acceleration's peak is at least 15 bpm above the baseline, and the acceleration lasts at least 15 seconds, but less than 2 minutes, from the onset to the point at which the FHR returns to baseline (Macones et al., 2008) (see Table 5-1 and Figure 5-4). Before 32 weeks of gestation, accelerations are defined as peaking at least 10 bpm above baseline and lasting at least 10 seconds (Macones et al., 2008). Accelerations, whether spontaneous or induced, are predictive of adequate central fetal oxygenation (Parer, 1997) and a fetal pH of at least 7.19; therefore, they rule out acidemia at the time they are observed (Porter & Clark, 1999; Williams & Galerneau, 2003). While the presence of accelerations is predictive of normal fetal acid-base status, the absence of accelerations during labor is not a reliable predictor of fetal acidemia (Macones et al., 2008). Accelerations lasting between 2 and 10 minutes are termed prolonged. A change in rate lasting 10 minutes or more is considered a change in baseline.

Decreases in Fetal Heart Rate

When auscultation is used to monitor the FHR, audible decreases in rate may be noted, and these are interpreted in the context of the overall clinical picture. There is no established nomenclature for describing FHR decreases noted with IA. When decreases in FHR are auscultated, interventions to promote maternal-fetal oxygenation are indicated, as is ongoing or additional assessment to clarify FHR findings and establish fetal well-being (Feinstein et al., 2009).

FIGURE 5-4 Accelerations

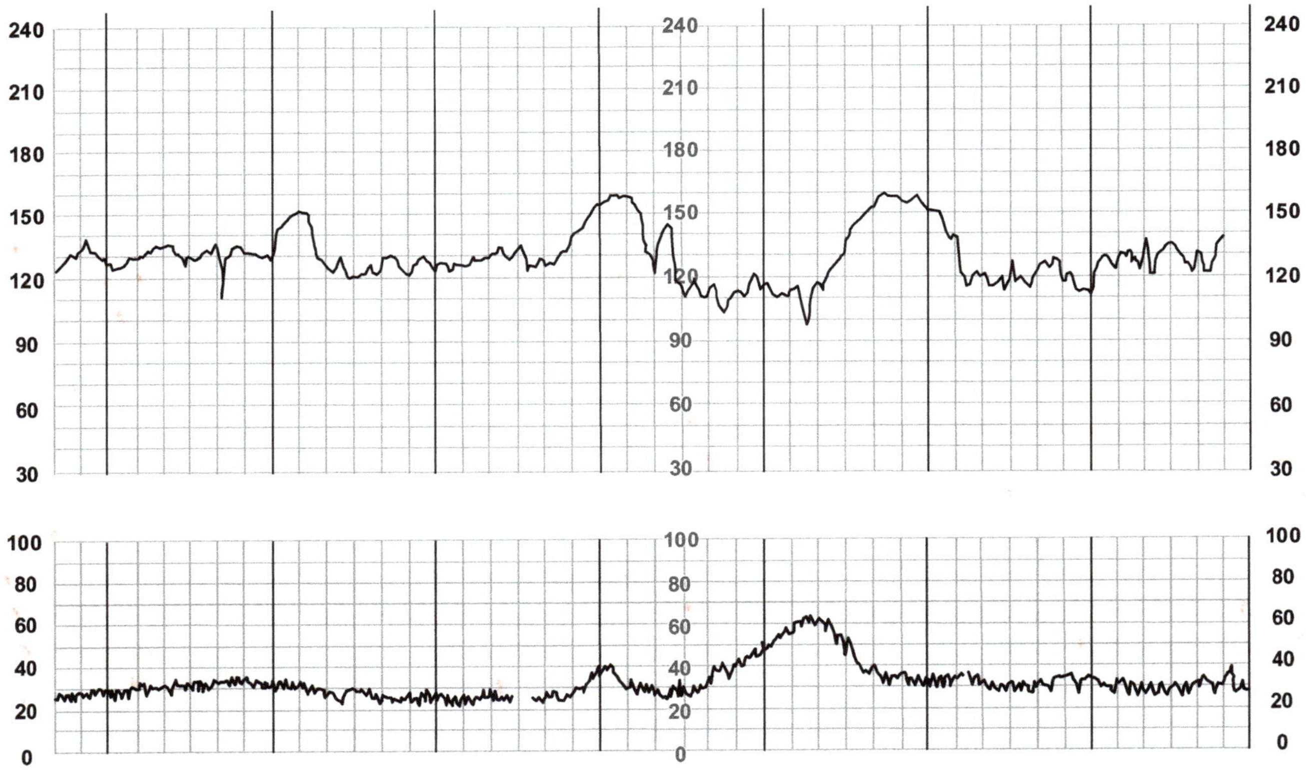

Decelerations

FHR decelerations are described as early, late, variable, and prolonged decelerations (see Table 5-1). Decelerations are distinguished by the shape of their onset and their relationship to the timing of uterine contractions. Decelerations are defined as *recurrent* when they occur with at least 50% of the contractions in a 20-minute period, and *intermittent* when they occur with less than 50% of contractions in a 20-minute period (Macones et al., 2008).

Early Decelerations

Early decelerations are visually apparent gradual decreases in the FHR (onset to nadir ≥30 seconds) (Figure 5-5). The onset, nadir, and recovery of early decelerations generally occur coincident with the onset, peak, and recovery of uterine contractions. Early decelerations are typically symmetrical in shape (Macones et al., 2008).

Early decelerations are believed to represent a vagal response to a cerebral redistribution of blood flow caused by compression of the fetal head (Freeman et al., 2012; Garite, 2012). When the contraction occurs, the fetal head is subjected to pressure, which stimulates the vagus nerve. The heart rate begins to drop at the onset of the contraction when the head compression begins and returns to the baseline rate at the end of the contraction when the head is no longer compressed. Early decelerations are often said to "mirror" the contraction causing them. Early decelerations may be present in a normal FHR pattern (Macones et al., 2008), and are not associated with fetal hypoxia, acidosis, or low Apgar scores (Freeman et al., 2012). No intervention is needed.

Late Decelerations

Late decelerations are visually apparent, gradual decreases in the FHR (onset to nadir ≥30 seconds) that are associated with uterine contractions (Figure 5-6). Late decelerations are delayed in timing, meaning the deceleration reaches its nadir

FIGURE 5-5 Early Decelerations

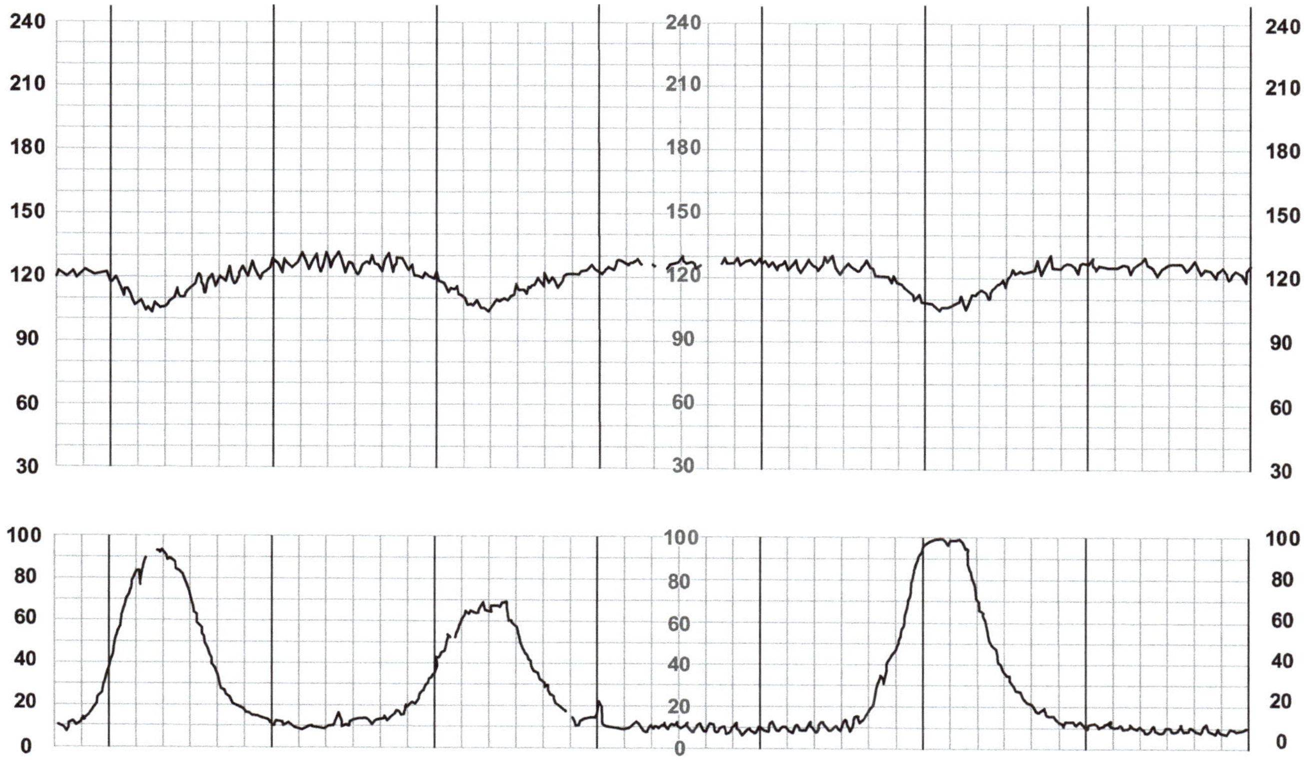

FIGURE 5-6 Late Decelerations

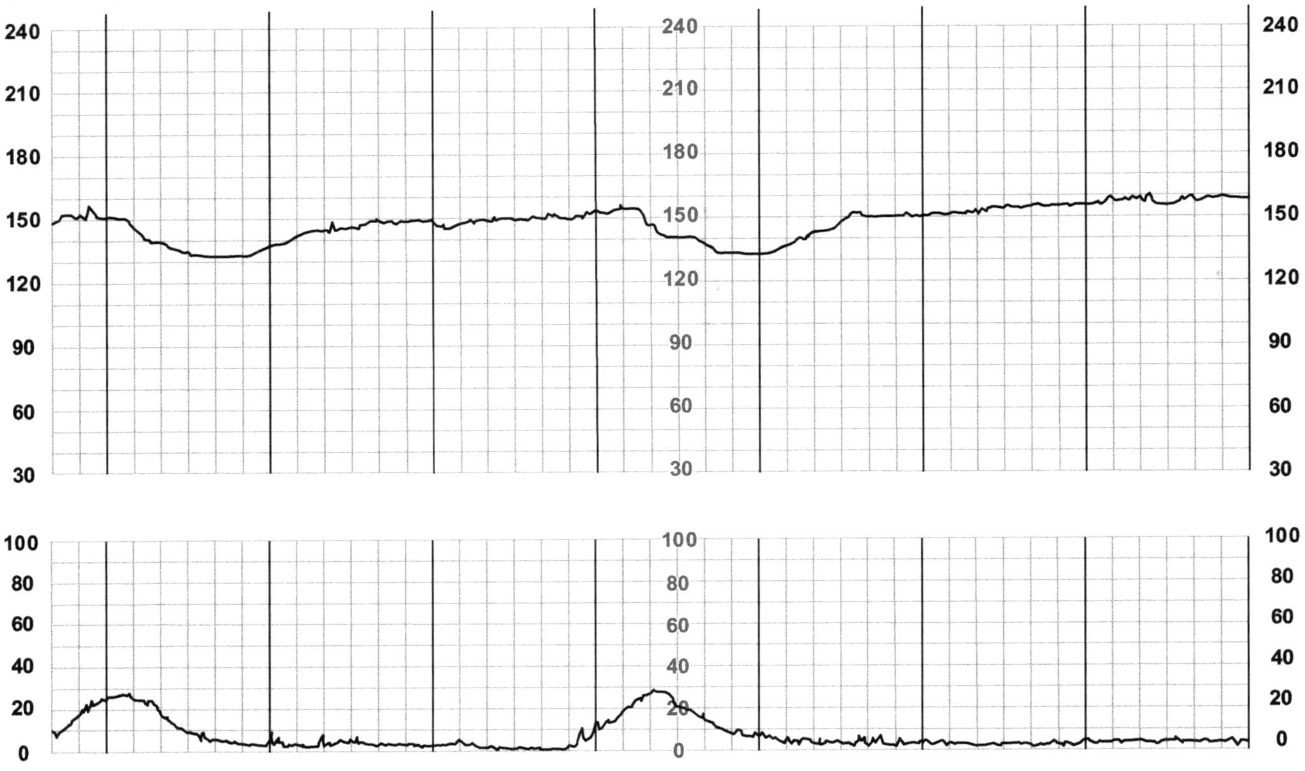

(lowest point) after the peak of the contraction. In most cases the onset, nadir, and recovery of the deceleration occur after the respective onset, peak, and resolution of the contraction. Late decelerations are typically symmetrical in shape (Macones et al., 2008). Late decelerations are believed to reflect the fetal response to transient or chronic uteroplacental insufficiency (ACOG, 2010; Freeman et al., 2102; Martin, 1978; Nageotte & Gilstrap, 2009).

Late decelerations occur on a continuum from those seen in conjunction with moderate baseline variability to those presenting with minimal and absent variability, and thus are evaluated in the context of FHR variability and the overall clinical picture. Late decelerations with moderate baseline variability, a stable baseline, and accelerations warrant less concern than late decelerations in the presence of an abnormal baseline rate, minimal or absent variability, and absence of accelerations. If the FHR pattern was normal prior to the onset of decelerations, an iatrogenic cause, such as maternal hypotension, can frequently be determined. Because late decelerations are believed to reflect the fetal response to transient or chronic uteroplacental insufficiency (ACOG, 2010; Freeman et al., 2012; Martin, 1978; Nageotte & Gilstrap, 2009), evaluation of maternal history for risk factors for uteroplacental insufficiency and evaluation of uterine activity are essential. Potential causes of both transient and chronic uteroplacental insufficiency are discussed in Chapters 2 and 4.

When late decelerations are accompanied by moderate variability, this is believed to reflect a chemoreceptor-mediated response to a transient hypoxemic event such as a reversible reduction in uterine blood flow (Freeman et al., 2012; Parer, 1997). In this situation, the decelerations are thought to occur when uterine blood flow decreases from baseline, resulting in decreased oxygenation of the fetal blood. The resulting hypoxemia is detected by chemoreceptors and ultimately results in firing of the vagus nerve and slowing of the fetal heart. Because the detection of hypoxemia by the chemoreceptors takes time and is not triggered until a threshold of low oxygen tension is reached, the deceleration is delayed in timing relative to the uterine contraction (Parer, 1997).

Moderate variability is predictive of adequate fetal oxygenation *at that moment in time* (Low et al., 1999; Macones et al., 2008; Nageotte & Gilstrap, 2009; Parer et al., 2006; Williams & Galerneau, 2003). Thus, late decelerations in the context of moderate variability do not suggest significant fetal acidemia at the time such a pattern is observed (ACOG, 2009; Parer et al., 2006). However, close surveillance is warranted and intrauterine resuscitation measures oriented toward maximizing uterine blood flow are appropriate (ACOG, 2010). Such decelerations are likely to resolve when the source of hypoxemia (e.g., maternal hypotension or excessive uterine activity) is resolved (Garite, 2012; Parer, 1997), as illustrated in the dynamic physiologic response model (Figure 5-7). Efforts should therefore be taken to eliminate the cause and prevent progression to patterns that are associated with significant acidemia (Clark et al., 2013; Freeman et al., 2012; Parer, 1997). Interventions are discussed in detail in Chapter 6.

If uteroplacental insufficiency cannot be corrected (e.g., in the setting of intrauterine growth restriction or other condition impairing placental function), hypoxemia continues, oxygen debt may accumulate, and the deoxygenated blood from the placenta may be insufficient to support myocardial metabolism. In this situation, direct depression of the myocardium occurs in conjunction with the vagal slowing of the heart rate (Garite, 2012; Nageotte & Gilstrap, 2009; Parer, 1997). Late decelerations with minimal variability may be associated with acidemia (Beard, Filshie, Knight, & Roberts, 1971; Berkus et al., 1999; Clark et al., 1984; Parer et al., 2006). Although considered an indeterminate tracing in relation to fetal acid-base status, this type of Category II pattern warrants intrauterine resuscitation, reevaluation, and consideration for expediting birth if no improvement with intrauterine resuscitation (ACOG, 2010).

Recurrent late decelerations with absent variability are associated with abnormal fetal acid-base status (Category III) (Macones et al., 2008), and warrant preparation for birth while simultaneously implementing intrauterine resuscitation measures (ACOG, 2010; Fox et al., 2000; Parer & Ikeda, 2007). Consideration for birth is indicated if such patterns cannot be resolved expeditiously (ACOG, 2010).

FIGURE 5-7 Dynamic Physiologic Response Model

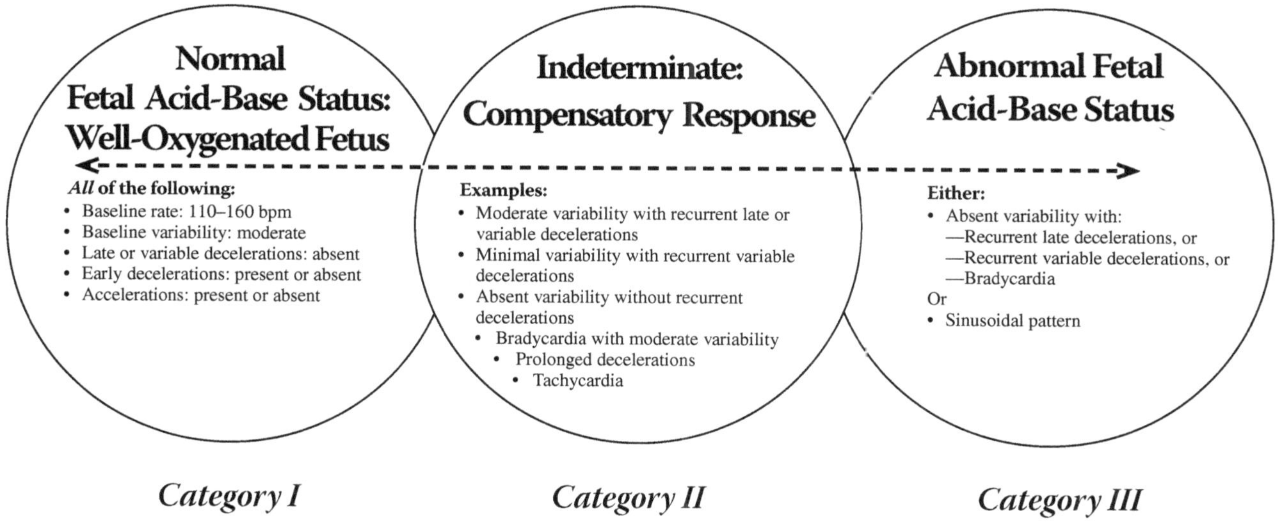

This diagram is not intended to be all inclusive. All patterns must be treated with interventions that are based on the suspected underlying physiologic causes and ongoing evaluation of individual patient presentation.

Variable Decelerations

Variable decelerations are visually apparent, abrupt decreases in the FHR (onset to beginning of nadir < 30 seconds) that may occur with or without relationship to uterine contractions (Figure 5-8). Variable decelerations decrease at least 15 bpm below baseline and last for at least 15 seconds but less than 2 minutes (Macones et al., 2008). They tend to vary in shape, depth, and duration and in their timing in relation to uterine contractions. Variable decelerations are the most frequently seen FHR deceleration pattern in labor (Freeman et al., 2012; Garite, 2012).

The abrupt FHR change characteristic of variable decelerations is most commonly caused by occlusion of umbilical blood flow. Interruption of umbilical blood flow can occur in any circumstances that allow compression of the cord, including oligohydramnios; cord prolapse or impingement; knots in the cord; and short, bandolier, or nuchal cord (Freeman et al., 2012). When the umbilical cord is compressed, the cessation of blood flow generates an increase in systemic vascular resistance and an increase in blood pressure that is detected by the fetal baroreceptors, triggering a vagal response and protective slowing of the FHR. Because the primary response is baroreceptor mediated rather than chemoreceptor mediated, the change in the heart rate is rapid (Lee & Hon, 1963).

Lee, Di Loreto, and O'Lane's (1975) classic illustration of a variable deceleration (Figure 5-9) depicts the relationship between the variable deceleration, uterine contraction, umbilical cord compression, and fetal blood pressure. As a contraction begins, partial umbilical cord compression causes occlusion of the low-pressure vein and decreased return of blood to the fetal heart, resulting in decreased cardiac output, hypotension, and a compensatory FHR acceleration (James et al., 1976; Lee et al., 1975). With complete umbilical cord occlusion, the two umbilical arteries also become occluded, resulting in sudden fetal hypertension, stimulation of the baroreceptors, and a sudden drop in FHR (Lee & Hon, 1963). As the contraction begins to dissipate,

FIGURE 5-8 Variable Decelerations

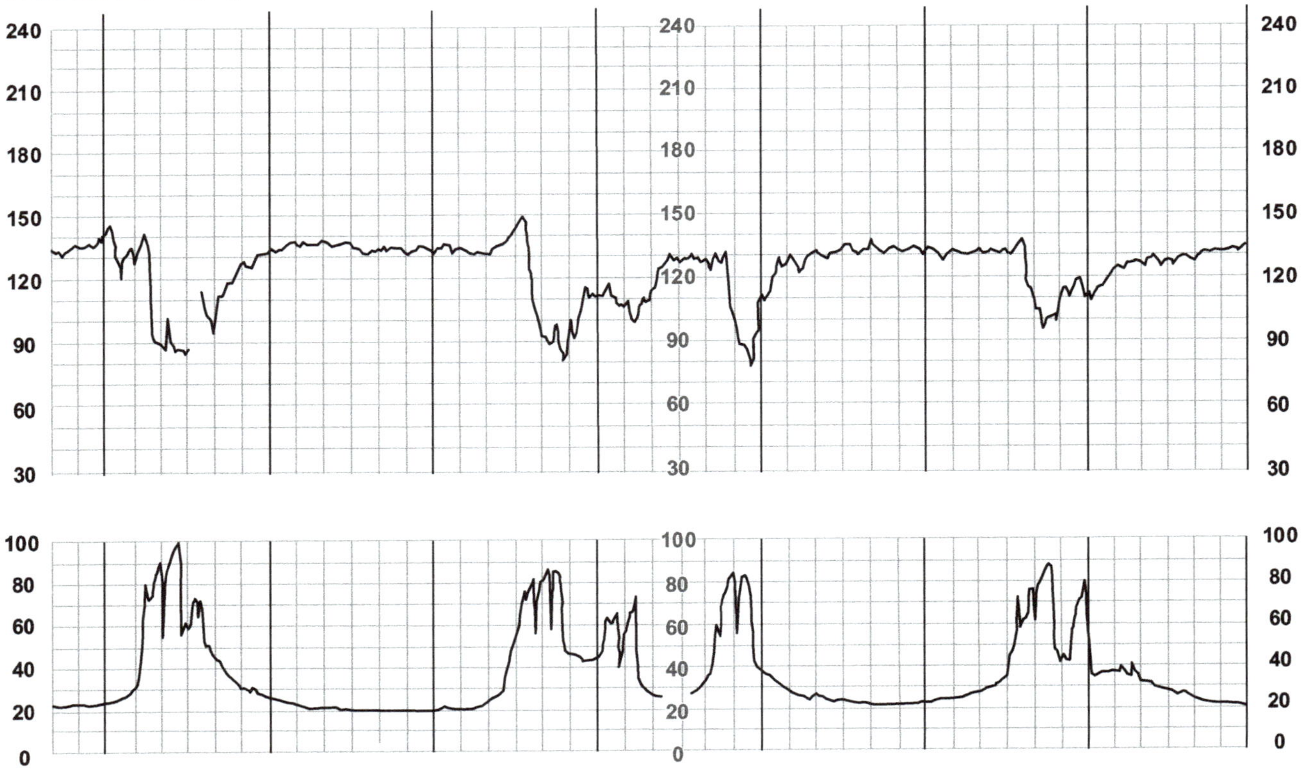

FIGURE 5-9 Fetal Heart Rate (FHR) and Fetal Systemic Blood Pressure (FSBP) Occurring during a Uterine Contraction (UC) with Compression of Umbilical Vein (UV) and Umbilical Artery (UA)

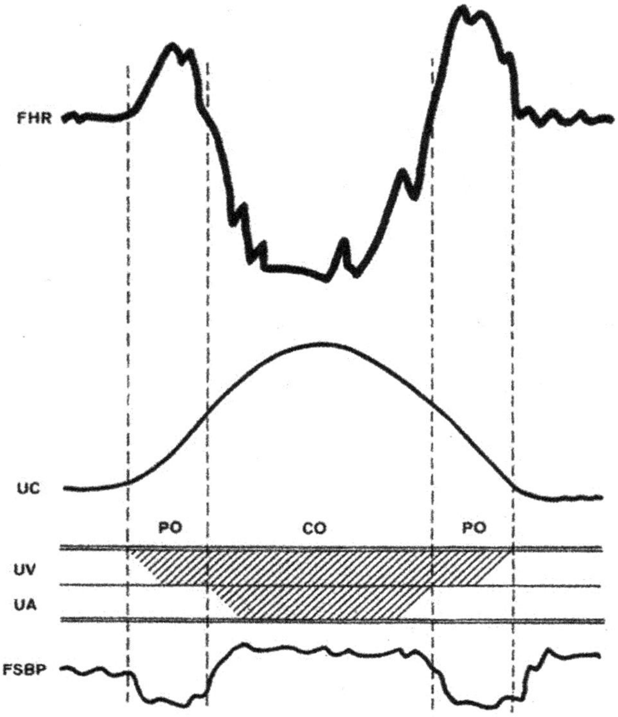

From "A study of fetal heart rate acceleration patterns," by C. V. Lee, P. C. Di Loreto, and J. M. O'Lane, *Obstetrics and Gynecologgy, 50*, p. 142. Copyright 1975 by the American College of Obstetricians and Gynecologists. Reprinted with permission.

the umbilical arteries open first, and a transient increase in FHR (a "secondary acceleration") may be seen. Finally, the contraction subsides and all three umbilical vessels are open, returning the FHR to predeceleration values. When variable decelerations occur during the second stage of labor, they may also be caused by the marked head compression and resultant intense vagal stimulation that occurs during rapid descent (Ball & Parer, 1992). Variable decelerations vary in all aspects of their appearance except one: the initial FHR change is abrupt.

As with late decelerations, interpretation of tracings with recurrent variable decelerations hinges on the assessment of the accompanying baseline FHR variability and the evolution of the tracing over time in the context of the overall clinical picture. When evaluating FHR tracings with recurrent variable decelerations the presence of moderate variability or a spontaneous or induced acceleration suggests the fetus is not currently acidemic (ACOG, 2010; Clark et al., 2013). In this context the decelerations represent a physiologic response to intermittent fetal stress (see Figure 5-7) and it may be reasonable to follow this pattern with close observation as long as the baseline FHR is within normal range, moderate variability is maintained (Freeman et al., 2012; Parer & Ikeda, 2007; Parer et al., 2006), labor is progressing (Clark et al., 2013), there is adequate recovery time for fetal oxygenation between contractions (Bakker, Kurver, Kuik, & Van Geijn, 2007), and resources are available to respond rapidly to any deterioration in fetal condition (Freeman et al, 2012). Recurrent variable decelerations that become deeper and last longer are more likely to be associated with fetal acidemia (ACOG, 2010; Clark et al., 2013; Parer et al, 2006).

Over the years, some clinicians and investigators have afforded significance to a variety of so-called "atypical" features of variable decelerations such as slow return to baseline, variations in rate during the deceleration, accelerations at the beginning and end of the deceleration, and longer accelerations following the deceleration ("overshoots") (Krebs, Petres, & Dunn, 1983). However, more recent studies have not supported an association between acidemia and "atypical features" of variable decelerations (Cahill, Roehl, Odibo, & Macones, 2012; Macones et al., 2008; Spong, Rasul, Collea, Eglinton, & Ghidini, 1998). A recent 5-year retrospective cohort study of FHR tracings 30 minutes before birth found no difference in atypical features between neonates with acidemia and without. No association between "shoulders" or slow returns and acidemia were found. Similarly, when compared with moderate variability within deceleration nadirs, neither minimal nor marked variability was significantly associated with acidemia (Cahill et al., 2012).

It is important to keep in mind that although variable decelerations are common in labor and especially in the second stage, the underlying conditions producing the decelerations can tax fetal reserve. It is appropriate to modify or eliminate these stressors whenever possible with measures such as maternal position changes, amnioinfusion, decreasing or discontinuing oxytocin infusion, and modified pushing (ACOG, 2010; Clark et al., 2013; Simpson, 2007) (see Chapter 6 for further discussion of interventions).

Prolonged Decelerations

Prolonged decelerations are visually apparent decreases in the FHR that drop at least 15 bpm below baseline and last at least 2 minutes but less than 10 minutes from their onset to the return to baseline (Macones et al., 2008) (Figure 5-10). The decrease in FHR is calculated from the adjacent baseline. During a prolonged deceleration, the FHR drops abruptly and stays down for several minutes. Prolonged decelerations may occur in the presence or absence of contractions and may have either an abrupt or slow return to the baseline rate.

Prolonged decelerations can be caused by more sustained instances of any of the previously discussed deceleration mechanisms (uteroplacental insufficiency, umbilical cord compression, or head compression), resulting in a profound response of a more sustained deceleration. Prolonged decelerations may occur in association with factors affecting uteroplacental perfusion or gas exchange, umbilical blood flow, or stimulation of the vagus nerve, as illustrated in Table 5-4.

Key factors in assessing prolonged decelerations include the baseline variability immediately preceding and following the decelerations, frequency of occurrence, duration of decelerations, and the individual characteristics of the overall clinical picture as well as institutional capacity to expedite birth should variability decrease or a prolonged deceleration evolve to frank bradycardia. Prolonged decelerations that are not recurrent and are preceded and followed by an FHR with a normal baseline and moderate variability are not associated with fetal hypoxemia of clinical significance. Management considerations are similar to those discussed previously in relation to fetal bradycardia, and in clinical practice clinicians typically do not wait to differentiate between the two before initiating intrauterine resuscitation measures and mobilizing a team response. Prompt birth is indicated in cases of prolonged decelerations with minimal or absent variability ACOG (2010).

Quantification of Decelerations

A number of experts have identified parameters they use to quantify the "severity" of variable and/or late decelerations (Clark et al., 2013; Freeman et al., 2012; Parer et al., 2006; Parer & Ikeda, 2007). Clark et al. (2013) define significant variable decelerations as having a duration of greater than 60 seconds and a nadir that is either below 60 bpm or is more than 60 bpm below the baseline FHR. Consensus has not been reached to date on parameters for the interpretation of depth and duration of late decelerations. Although the NICHD report discusses quantification of decelerations, it does not specify how depth and duration of decelerations should be interpreted (Macones et al., 2008). For documentation purposes it is sufficient to report the type of decelerations observed and the clinician's overall assessment of fetal status without a written description of depth or duration of decelerations when this information is already recorded by an EFM tracing (see Chapter 9 for further discussion of documentation issues). In verbal communication regarding FHR findings, inclusion of more detail regarding depth and duration may be needed, particularly if applying management algorithms that define significant decelerations (Clark et al., 2013).

Uterine Activity

During the intrapartum period, FHR is interpreted in relation to uterine activity, and the degree of uterine activity is a central component of the overall clinical picture. Therefore, interpretation of FHR patterns cannot occur in isolation of evaluation of uterine activity, which includes a complete assessment of four components of the uterine contractions: (1) frequency, (2) duration, (3) intensity, and (4) uterine resting tone between contractions. These assessments can be made by either palpation alone, or by palpation in

FIGURE 5-10 Prolonged Deceleration

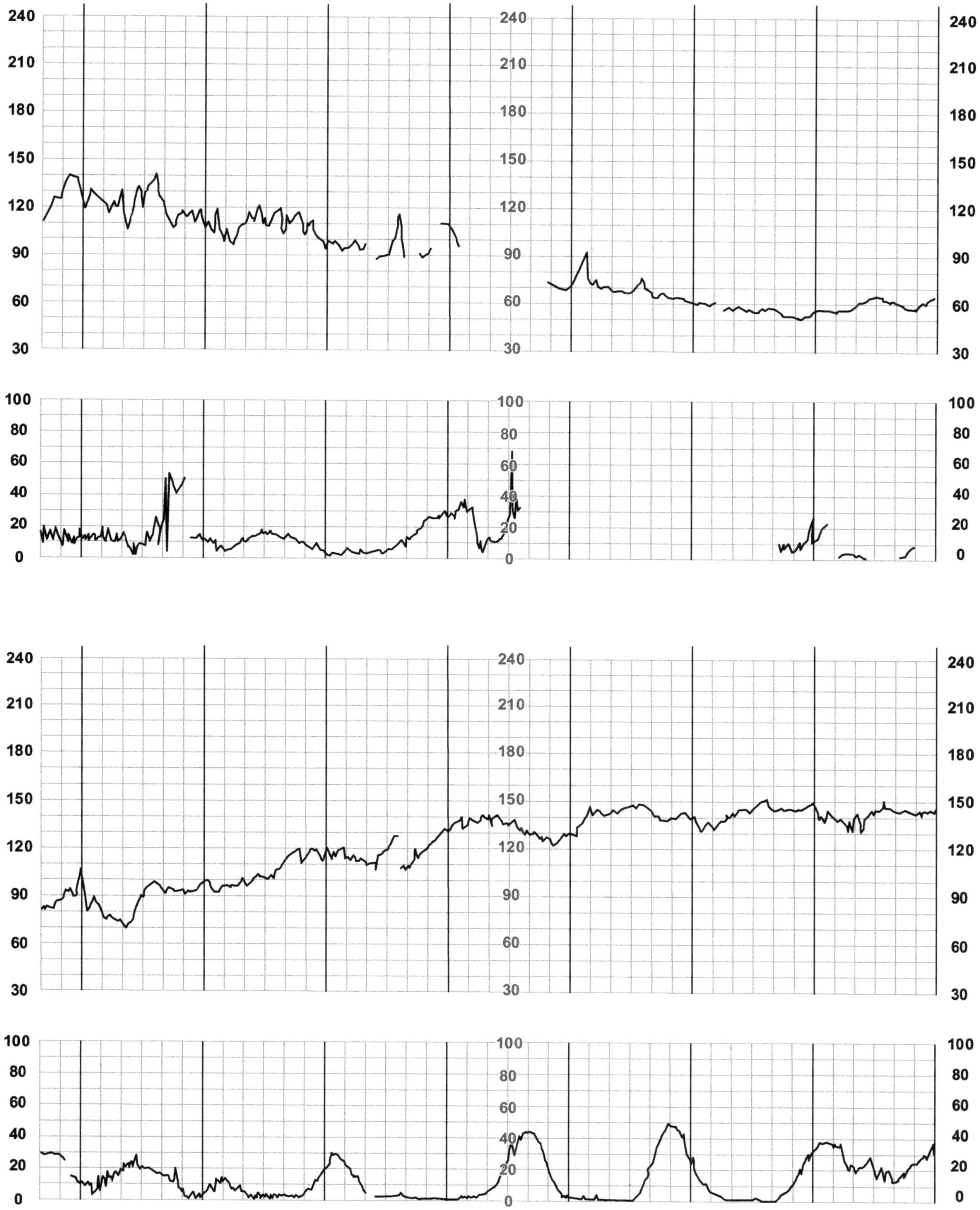

TABLE 5-4 Potential Causes of Prolonged Decelerations

INTERRUPTION OF UTEROPLACENTAL PERFUSION OR EXCHANGE	INTERRUPTION OF UMBILICAL BLOOD FLOW	VAGAL STIMULATION
Uterine tachysystole	Cord compression	Profound head compxression
Acute maternal hypotension	Cord prolapse	Rapid fetal descent
Acute maternal hypoxia (e.g., seizure, respiratory, or cardiac arrest)	Ruptured vasa previa	
Abruptio placentae		
Uterine rupture		

conjunction with an external tocodynamometer or intrauterine pressure catheter (IUPC), as discussed in Chapter 4.

Contraction frequency is measured from the beginning of one contraction to the beginning of the next and is described in minutes. Duration is the length of the contraction and is described in seconds. Intensity refers to the strength of the contraction. Intensity is described as mild, moderate, or strong by palpation or in millimeters of mercury (mmHg) if an IUPC is used. Uterine resting tone is assessed in the absence of contractions or between contractions. By direct palpation, resting tone is described as soft or hard, and via IUPC it is measured in mmHg. As with any procedure, the least invasive approach is preferred unless there is a clear maternal-fetal indication for internal monitoring.

After the frequency, duration, intensity, and resting tone have been determined, one can assess the adequacy of the uterine activity. Normal contraction frequency in the active phase of labor is every 2–3 minutes (ACOG, 2003). Some uterine activity patterns are dysfunctional or inadequate for generating progress in labor (Figure 5-11). Assessments of maternal pain, coping, and uterine tenderness also contribute to the interpretation of uterine activity, labor progress, and the overall clinical picture.

Uterine activity is classified by the number of contractions present in a 10-minute period, averaged over 30 minutes (Macones et al., 2008):

- Normal: ≤5 contractions in 10 minutes.
- Tachysystole: >5 contractions in 10 minutes. Tachysystole is further qualified by the presence or absence of associated FHR decelerations.

This definition of tachysystole is primarily based on expert opinion, as there are only a few published studies in the literature evaluating the effects of uterine activity on fetal well-being. Some evidence suggests that less than five contractions in 10 minutes may be optimal for supporting fetal well-being (Bakker et al., 2007; Simpson & James, 2008). Although tachysystole (Figure 5-12) can be spontaneous as a result of endogenous maternal oxytocin or prostaglandins, it is more often seen during exogenous stimulation with agents used in cervical ripening and induction and augmentation of labor (Crane, Young, Butt, Bennett, & Hutchens, 2001). The 2008 NICHD recommendations indicate that hyperstimulation and hypercontractility are not defined and both terms should be abandoned (Macones et al., 2008).

It is important to recognize that tachysystole increases the amount of time that blood in the intervillous spaces is in stasis, reducing the potential for maternal-fetal exchange of respiratory gases. These conditions result in physiologic stress for the fetus, whether or not associated FHR decelerations are present, and should be avoided. Although data on the effects of uterine activity are limited, increased uterine activity in labor has been linked to an increased risk for a progressive decrease in fetal oxygen saturation and umbilical artery acidemia at birth (Bakker et al., 2007; Simpson & James, 2008). If tachysystole occurs during oxytocin administration and the FHR is normal, the infusion should be managed as suggested in the protocol discussed in Chapter 6. If the FHR is not normal during oxytocin administration, the infusion should be discontinued until the FHR and uterine

FIGURE 5-11 Regular and Dysfunctional Uterine Activity Tracings

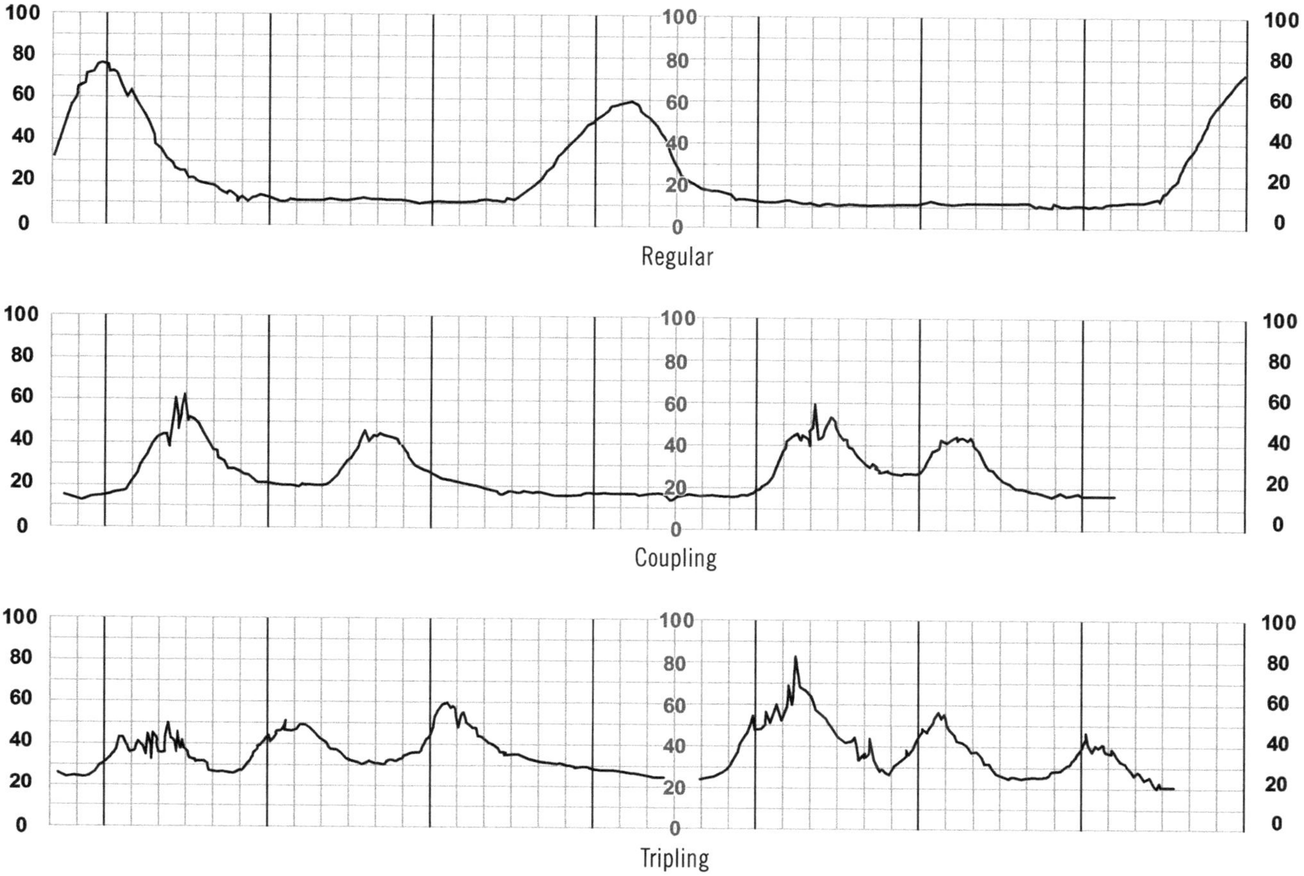

FIGURE 5-12 Tachysystole

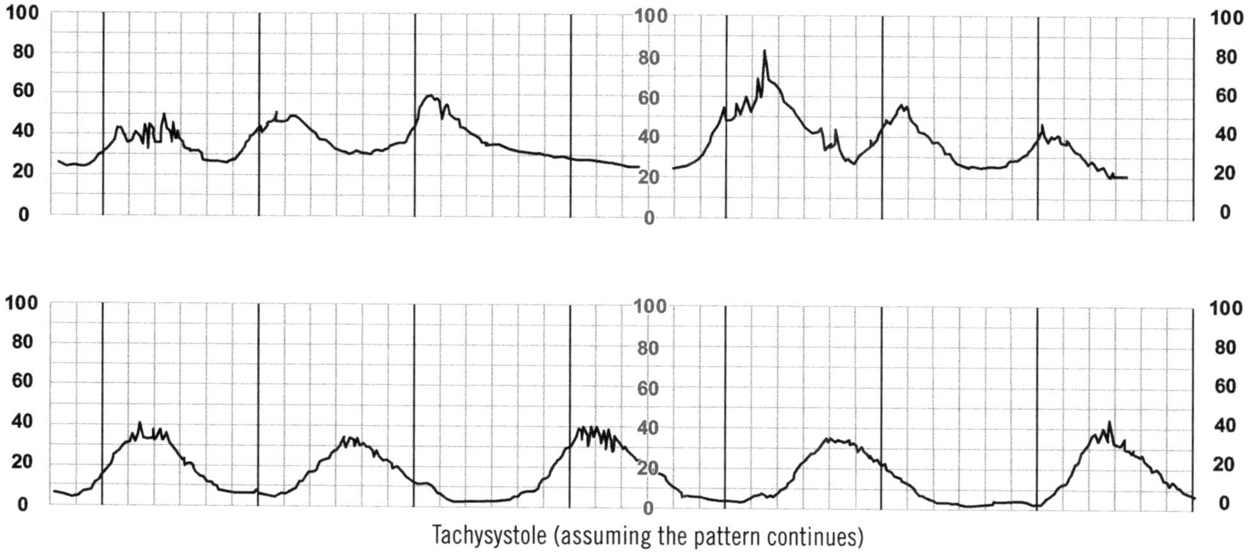

contraction pattern return to normal. Similarly, in the event of excessive uterine activity, additional doses of other uterotonic agents (e.g., dinoprostone [Cervidil, Prepidil] or misoprostol) should be delayed until the FHR is normal and the uterine contraction pattern returns to normal frequency, duration, and resting tone (Simpson, 2013). Lateral maternal positioning and an intravenous fluid bolus may be additional interventions to resolve uterine tachysystole (Simpson & James, 2008). A comprehensive protocol for the management of oxytocin-induced tachysystole is presented in Chapter 6.

"Coupling" or "tripling" refers to a pattern of two or three contractions with little or no interval followed by a regular interval of approximately 2–5 minutes (see Figure 5-11). This pattern may be indicative of a dysfunctional labor process and saturation or down-regulation of uterine oxytocin receptor sites in response to excess exposure to oxytocin (Dawood, 1995; Phaneuf, Rodriguez Linares, TambyRaja, MacKenzie, & Lopez Bernal, 2000; Zeeman, Khan-Dawood, & Dawood, 1997). Therefore, interventions to resolve the dysfunctional labor pattern do not include further increases in the oxytocin rate. Instead, an oxytocin rate decrease or discontinuation along with an intravenous fluid bolus may be therapeutic in creating conditions in which oxytocin receptor sites are again responsive to exogenous oxytocin for labor induction or augmentation.

Unusual Fetal Heart Rate Characteristics

Whenever an unusual tracing is observed from the beginning of EFM, the possibility of a previously unobserved hypoxic insult or the presence of a congenital fetal anomaly should be considered. An initial tracing with minimal or absent variability without accelerations or with other unusual characteristics should prompt an urgent assessment of fetal well-being. This may include fetal stimulation, an ultrasound evaluation, or other assessments as indicated by the overall clinical picture. Although most fetuses with congenital anomalies have normal FHR tracings (Nageotte & Gilstrap, 2009), hydrocephalic and anencephalic fetuses may present with unusual FHR patterns that do not fit any category or definition (Freeman et al., 2012). If possible, an ultrasound examination may be performed to rule out gross anomalies as the cause of the pattern, although results may be inconclusive. An anomaly that affects the fetal central nervous system most likely will have an impact on FHR variability or on the ability of the fetal cardiac system to accelerate and decelerate. Unusual decelerations with a flat, fixed rate may be seen.

Sinusoidal Heart Rate Pattern

A sinusoidal fetal heart rate pattern is a visually apparent, undulating, smooth sine wave-like pattern in the FHR baseline with a cycle frequency of 3–5 per minute that persists for at least 20 minutes (Macones et al., 2008) (Figure 5-13). There are no accelerations and no FHR responses to uterine contractions, fetal movement, or stimulation (Modanlou & Freeman, 1982).

A true sinusoidal FHR pattern is a rare occurrence. First identified in 1972, the sinusoidal FHR pattern was described as an undulating wave alternating with a flat or smooth baseline FHR in severely affected, Rh-sensitized, and dying fetuses (Manseau, Vaquier, Chavinie, & Sureau, 1972). The FHR pattern was named "sinusoidal" because of its sine waveform. The etiology of the sinusoidal heart rate includes severe fetal anemia as a result of Rh isoimmunization, massive feto-maternal hemorrhage, twin-to-twin transfusion syndrome, ruptured vasa previa, and fetal intracranial hemorrhage (Modanlou & Murata, 2004; Reddy, Moulden, & Redman, 2009). Other fetal conditions that have been reported to be associated with sinusoidal heart rate patterns include fetal hypoxia or asphyxia, fetal infection, fetal cardiac anomalies, and gastroschisis. Whatever the pathogenesis, a true sinusoidal heart rate pattern is indicative of a compromised fetus and requires immediate attention (Modanlou & Murata, 2004; Reddy et al., 2009).

A sinusoidal-appearing FHR pattern has been noted to follow the maternal administration of some opioids (especially butorphanol and fentanyl), fetal sleep cycles, and thumbsucking or rhythmic movements of the fetal mouth (Modanlou & Murata, 2004). As the medication is excreted or the fetus awakens or stops

FIGURE 5-13 Sinusoidal Fetal Heart Rate Pattern

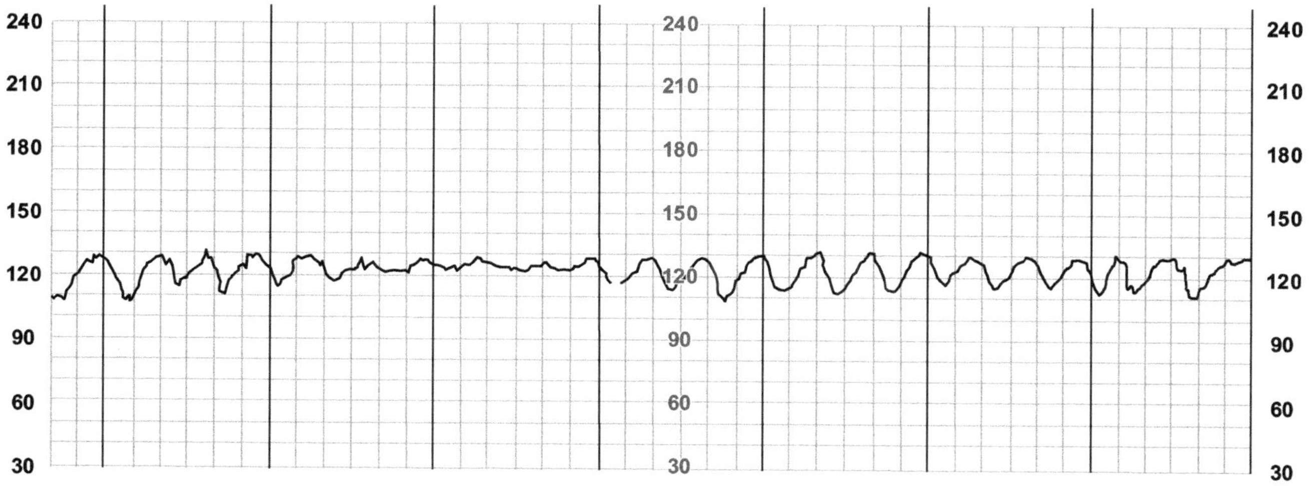

sucking, the sinusoidal-appearing FHR resolves, thus giving it the name of "pseudosinusoidal" or "medication-induced sinusoidal." Usually this undulating FHR pattern is of short duration and is both preceded and followed by an FHR with normal characteristics (Modanlou & Murata, 2004). No treatment is indicated for these sinusoidal-appearing patterns when history of maternal opioid administration is clearly related to the subsequent FHR pattern.

Fetal Arrhythmias

Fetal cardiac arrhythmias occur in approximately 1% of all pregnancies and are usually benign (Reed, 1989). Of those, approximately 90% are due to irregular rhythm and less than 10% are due to sustained brady- or tachyarrhythmias with clinical significance to the fetus (Kleinman & Nehgme, 2004; Reed, 1989). Fetal cardiac arrhythmias due to irregular rhythm have been recognized with increasing frequency at routine prenatal visits. The most common finding is the impression that the fetal heart is intermittently "skipping" beats. In most cases, this represents either a pause following an extrasystole that has not reset the sinus node pacemaker or an extrasystole occurring early in the cardiac cycle with a stroke volume that is inadequate to produce a detectable Doppler signal (Kleinman & Nehgme, 2004; Sklansky, 2009). Although the extrasystoles may be a source of anxiety for the parents, they usually resolve spontaneously later during pregnancy or during the first few days after birth.

Sustained fetal tachyarrhythmias or bradyarrhythmias are rare. However, when detected during routine prenatal visits, they require multidisciplinary evaluation. The most common important tachyarrhythmia is supraventricular tachycardia (SVT); the most severe bradyarrhythmia is complete heart block. Typically, SVT occurs in the range of 240–260 bpm with minimal or absent variability in a fetus with a structurally normal heart (Copel, Friedman, & Kleinman, 1997; Kleinman & Nehgme, 2004; Sklansky, 2009). Initially, SVT may manifest as an intermittent, nonsustained arrhythmia; however, sustained SVT may develop.

In complete heart block atrial electrical impulses are unable to pass through the conduction system to the ventricles. This typically results in the ventricles depolarizing at their own intrinsic rate, resulting in a sustained FHR of 40–70 bpm after 18 weeks' gestation (Friedman, 1992; Sklansky, 2009). Approximately 50% of fetuses with complete heart block have structurally normal hearts, and if they can maintain their heart rate greater than 55 bpm, generally tolerate the arrhythmia (Kleinman & Nehgme, 2004; Sklansky, 2009). Physiology, evaluation, and management of fetal arrhythmias are discussed further in Chapter 11.

INTERPRETATION OF ELECTRONIC FETAL MONITORING FINDINGS ACROSS THE CONTINUUM

FHR patterns present on a continuum from those displaying the classic characteristics of a normal tracing predictive of a normally oxygenated fetus, through tracings that suggest some degree of relative hypoxemia or hypoxia, to those tracings that experts agree are predictive of significant risk for fetal compromise resulting from inadequate tissue oxygenation and metabolic acidosis.

The 2008 NICHD guidelines suggest a three-tiered system for interpretation of FHR patterns: category I (normal), category II (indeterminate), and category III (abnormal) (Box 5-2).

A normal (category I) FHR tracing exhibits a baseline rate of 110–160 bpm, moderate baseline FHR variability, and no late or variable

BOX 5-2 2008 Three-Tier Fetal Heart Rate Interpretation System

CATEGORY I

Category I fetal heart rate (FHR) tracings include **all** of the following:

- Baseline rate: 110–160 beats per minute (bpm)
- Baseline FHR variability: moderate
- Late or variable decelerations: absent
- Early decelerations: present or absent
- Accelerations: present or absent

CATEGORY II

Category II FHR tracings include all FHR tracings not categorized as Category I or Category III. Category II tracings may represent an appreciable fraction of those encountered in clinical care. Examples of Category II FHR tracings include any of the following:

Baseline Rate

- Bradycardia not accompanied by absent baseline variability
- Tachycardia

Baseline FHR Variability

- Minimal baseline variability
- Absent baseline variability not accompanied by recurrent decelerations
- Marked baseline variability

Accelerations

- Absence of induced accelerations after fetal stimulation

Periodic or Episodic Decelerations

- Recurrent variable decelerations accompanied by minimal or moderate baseline variability
- Prolonged deceleration $\geq$ 2 minutes but $<$ 10 minutes
- Recurrent late decelerations with moderate baseline variability
- Variable decelerations with other characteristics, such as slow return to baseline, "overshoots," or "shoulders"

CATEGORY III

Category III FHR tracings include either

- Absent baseline FHR variability **and** any of the following:
  - Recurrent late decelerations
  - Recurrent variable decelerations
  - Bradycardia
- Sinusoidal pattern

Note: From "The 2008 National Institute of Child Health Human Development Workshop Report on Electronic Fetal Monitoring: Update on Definitions, Interpretations, and Research Guidelines," by G. A. Macones, G. D. Hankins, C. Y. Spong, J. D. Hauth, & T. Moore, 2008, *Journal of Obstetric, Gynecologic and Neonatal Nursing, 37*, 510–515; *Obstetrics & Gynecology, 112*, p. 665. Copyright 2008 by the American College of Obstetricians and Gynecologists. Reprinted with permission.

decelerations. Normal tracings may or may not exhibit accelerations or early decelerations. Experts generally agree that this type of FHR tracing is strongly predictive of normal fetal acid-base status at the time of observation (Macones et al., 2008). Normal FHR tracings may be followed with routine measures to support labor progress, maternal coping, and fetal oxygenation as discussed in Chapter 6 (ACOG, 2010). At the other end of the continuum from a completely normal tracing are abnormal (category III) FHR patterns predictive of abnormal fetal acid-base status at the time of observation. Category III FHR tracings are those exhibiting a sinusoidal pattern or exhibiting *absent variability* in conjunction with bradycardia or recurrent late or variable decelerations (Macones et al., 2008). These patterns require prompt evaluation and preparation for birth in conjunction with attempts to expeditiously resolve the abnormal findings. Prompt birth may be indicated when such patterns cannot be resolved (ACOG, 2010). True category III tracings appear to be extremely rare (Jackson, Holmgren, Esplin, Henry, & Warner, 2011).

All FHR tracings that do not meet criteria for category I or III classification are considered indeterminate with respect to fetal acid-base status and fall into category II (Macones et al., 2008). Category II includes (but is not limited to) tracings with *moderate or minimal variability* and recurrent late or variable decelerations, baseline tachycardia, marked variability, prolonged decelerations, and the absence of an acceleration response to fetal stimulation. Indeterminate tracings minimally require heightened surveillance and ongoing reevaluation. In most cases supportive actions to promote maternal and fetal adaptation to labor are also indicated, as described in Chapter 6. Proposed algorithms for management of indeterminate FHR tracings are displayed in Figure 5-14 (ACOG, 2010) and Figure 5-15 (Clark et al., 2013).

Electronic FHR Patterns and Fetal Acid-Base Status

Many fetuses have FHR findings that are classified as category II, and thus lie somewhere on the continuum between normal (normal baseline rate with moderate variability and no late or variable decelerations) and abnormal (absent variability with recurrent late or variable decelerations or bradycardia). In a retrospective review of FHR tracings from 48,444 laboring women, investigators found that 83% of women demonstrated more than one category of FHR tracing during labor, while only 16% of women had exclusively normal FHR tracings in labor (Jackson et al., 2011).

Virtually all women in the Jackson study (>99%) had normal FHR tracings for at least some portion of their labor, but most women (86%) also had segments of category II FHR patterns during labor. Category III tracings were observed in only 54 women (0.1% of the sample). Looking at the total FHR monitoring for all the women in the sample, the FHR pattern was classified as category I 78% of the time and category II 22% of the time. Category III was extremely rare, occurring in only 0.004% of the total FHR time monitored. The investigators also evaluated the final 2 hours of monitoring prior to birth. During this period, the percentage of time FHR tracings were normal decreased to 61% and category II tracings increased to 39%. Again, category III tracings were very rare, comprising 0.006% of time monitored. As the percentage of the last 2 hours of labor spent in category II exceeded 50%, there was a statistically significant increase in NICU admission and 1- or 5-minute Apgars < 7. Almost 10% of newborns with >75% of the last 2 hours of labor in category II FHR patterns were admitted to the NICU; however, these newborns were also generally vigorous at birth: 1.3% of these newborns had 5-minute Apgar < 7 (Jackson et al., 2011).

While indeterminate FHR tracings are identified in many labors, category II represents a heterogeneous group of fetal heart rate patterns. Historically there has not been general agreement among experts on clinical management of these tracings (Clark et al., 2013; Macones et al., 2008; NICHD, 1997). Parer and colleagues (Clark et al., 2013; Fox et al., 2000; Parer, 1997) have suggested that when moderate variability is present, these tracings are not associated with fetal morbidity because although they reflect

FIGURE 5-14 Algorithm for Management of Intrapartum FHR Tracing Categories Suggested by ACOG

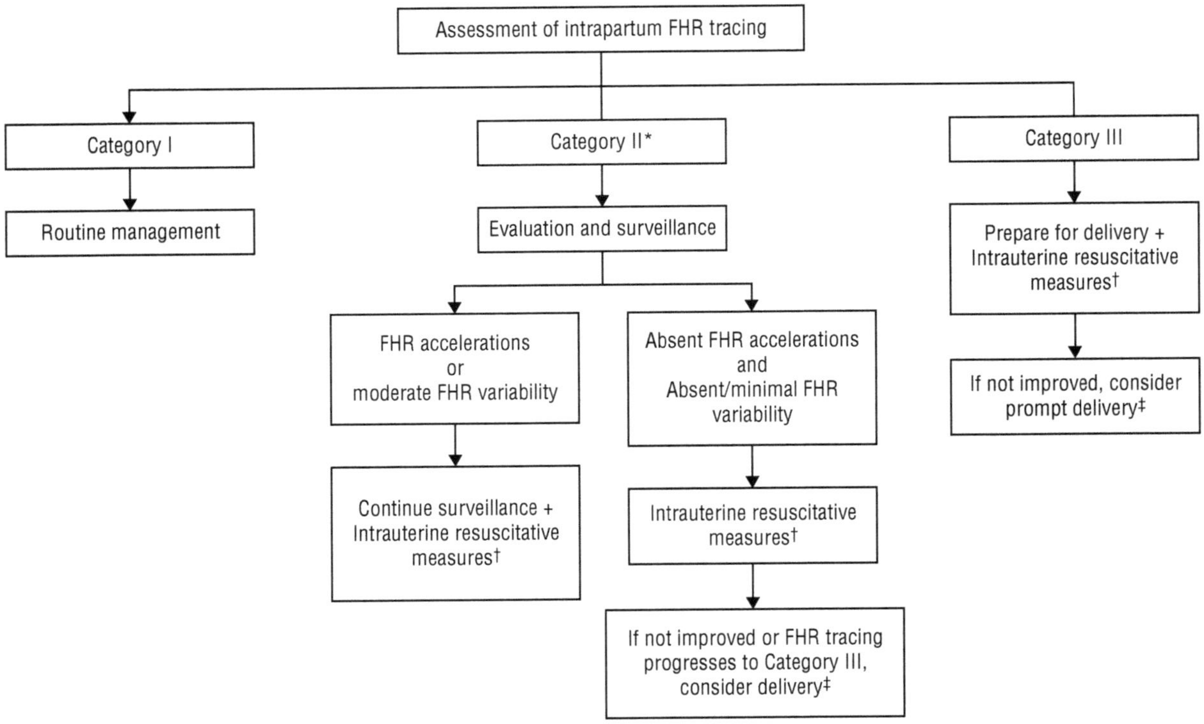

*Given the wide variation of FHR tracings in Category II, this algorithm is not meant to represent assessment and management of all potential FHR tracings, but provide an action template for common clinical situations.

†See Chapter 6 for intrauterine resuscitative measures.

‡Timing and mode of delivery based on feasibility and maternal-fetal status

Note: From "Management of intrapartum fetal heart rate tracings (Practice Bulletin No. 116)" by American College of Obstetricians and Gynecologists, *Obstetrics and Gynecology, 116*, p. 1232. Copyright 2010 by the American College of Obstetricians and Gynecologists. Reprinted with permission.

the presence of fetal stress, the maintenance of moderate variability indicates appropriate mobilization of compensatory mechanism and maintenance of adequate central oxygenation.

A 2006 review of the published literature on the association between FHR patterns and fetal acidemia found moderate FHR variability was strongly (98%) associated with an umbilical pH greater than 7.15 or newborn vigor (5-minute Apgar score of 7 or higher) (Parer et al., 2006). In this review the most consistent predictor of newborn metabolic acidemia was absent or minimal FHR variability with recurrent late or variable decelerations (although the association was only 23%), and there was a positive relationship between the degree of acidemia and the depth of decelerations or bradycardia. The authors therefore conclude that in the absence of a catastrophic event or a sudden profound bradycardia, newborn metabolic acidemia (expressed as decreasing variability in combination with decelerations) develops over a period of time approximating 1 hour (Parer et al., 2006), suggesting that there is usually time for attempting to improve fetal oxygenation through intrauterine resuscitation measures. A proposed "consensus" approach to managing such observation with an emphasis on fetal safety versus potential overuse of intervention was recently delineated (Clark et al., 2013; see Figure 5-15).

FIGURE 5-15 Algorithm for Management of Category II FHR Tracings Suggested by Clark et al. (2013)

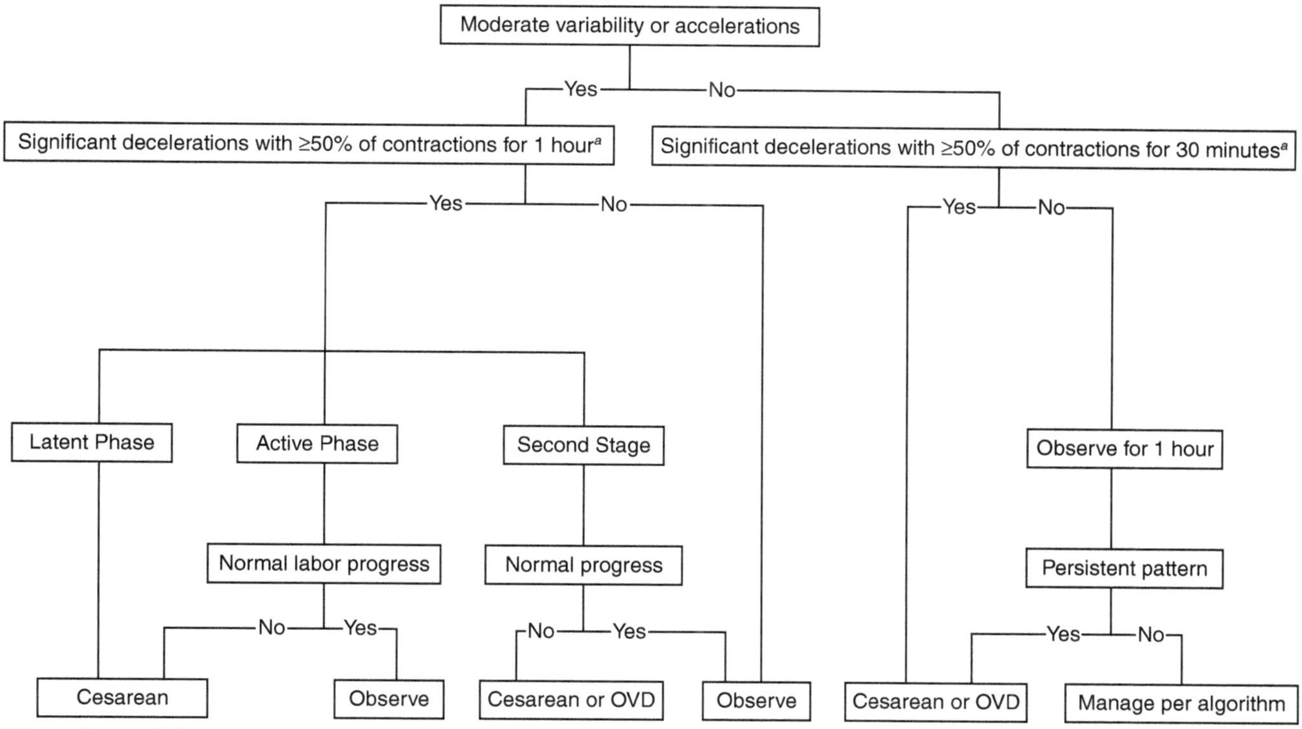

OVD, operative vaginal delivery.

[a]That have not resolved with appropriate conservative corrective measures, which may include supplemental oxygen, maternal position changes, intravenous fluid administration, correction of hypotension, reduction or discontinuation of uterine stimulation, administration of uterine relaxant, amnioinfusion, and/or changes in second stage breathing and pushing techniques.

Management of Category II Fetal Heart Rate Patterns: Clarifications for Use in Algorithm

1. Variability refers to predominant baseline FHR pattern (marked, moderate, minimal, absent) during a 30-minute evaluation period, as defined by NICHD.
2. Marked variability is considered same as moderate variability for purposes of this algorithm.
3. Significant decelerations are defined as any of the following:
   - Variable decelerations lasting longer than 60 seconds and reaching a nadir more than 60 bpm below baseline.
   - Variable decelerations lasting longer than 60 seconds and reaching a nadir less than 60 bpm regardless of the baseline.
   - Any late decelerations of any depth.
   - Any prolonged deceleration, as defined by the NICHD. Due to the broad heterogeneity inherent in this definition, identification of a prolonged deceleration should prompt discontinuation of the algorithm until the deceleration is resolved.
4. Application of algorithm may be initially delayed for up to 30 minutes while attempts are made to alleviate category II pattern with conservative therapeutic interventions (e.g. correction of hypotension, position change, amnioinfusion, tocolysis, reduction or discontinuation of oxytocin).
5. Once a category II FHR pattern is identified, FHR is evaluated and algorithm applied every 30 minutes.
6. Any significant change in FHR parameters should result in reapplication of algorithm.
7. For category II FHR patterns in which algorithm suggests delivery is indicated, such delivery should ideally be initiated within 30 minutes of decision for cesarean.

(continued)

FIGURE 5-15 (Continued)

8. If at any time tracing reverts to category I status, or deteriorates for even a short time to category III status, the algorithm no longer applies. However, algorithm should be reinstituted if category I pattern again reverts to category II.
9. In fetus with extreme prematurity, neither significance of certain FHR patterns of concern in more mature fetus (e.g., minimal variability) or ability of such fetuses to tolerate intrapartum events leading to certain types of category II patterns are well defined. This algorithm is not intended as guide to management of fetus with extreme prematurity.
10. Algorithm may be overridden at any time if, after evaluation of patient, physician believes it is in best interest of the fetus to intervene sooner.

FHR, fetal heart rate; *NICHD, Eunice Kennedy Shriver* National Institute of Child Health and Human Development

Note: Reprinted from American Journal of Obstetrics and Gynecology, 209(2), 91–92. S. L. Clark, M. P. Nagette, T. J. Garite, R. K. Freeman, D. A. Miller, K. R. Simpson, M. A. Belfort, G. A. Dildy, J. T. Parer, R. L. Berkowitz, M. D'Alton, D. J. Rouse, L. C. Gilstrap, A. M. Vintzileos, J. P. van Dorsten, F. H. Boehm, L. A. Miller, & G. D. Hankins. "Intrapartum management of category II fetal heart rate tracings: Towards standardization of care" Copyright 2013, with permission from the American College of Obstetricians and Gynecologists.

Evolution of FHR Patterns over Time

The most important factors in interpreting FHR patterns are the degree of FHR variability and the evolution of the tracing over time in the context of the entire clinical picture (Clark et al., 2013; Fox et al., 2000; Macones et al., 2008; Parer et al., 2006). In interpreting indeterminate tracings, it is also essential to take into account the estimated proximity to birth, any maternal or fetal factors presenting threats to fetal reserve, and the specific logistics of the birth setting. In the absence of catastrophic events, the gradual nature of pattern evolution and the reliability of moderate FHR variability as a predictor of adequacy of fetal oxygenation indicate that there is usually a period of time, in the range of approximately 60 minutes, when observing the evolution of many FHR patterns can be safe practice. Furthermore, close observation often may be continued when moderate variability or accelerations are present and labor is progressing normally (Clark et al., 2013). Naturally, the presence of concerning factors in a given patient may warrant more prompt intervention. During this period of ongoing close observation and reevaluation, the bedside provider can do the following:

- Arrange for consultation
- Request in-house, bedside evaluation of FHR tracings
- Initiate interventions aimed at resolution of FHR changes
- Initiate preparations for operative or surgical birth when birth rather than continued observation appears warranted
- Secure the presence of anesthesia providers and the neonatal resuscitation team (Fox et al., 2000; Lyndon, O'Brien-Abel, & Simpson, 2014).

Overall interpretation of the urgency of FHR findings will take into account the specific current FHR characteristics in combination with other factors such as maternal medical and obstetric history, gestational age, labor progress, and proximity or remoteness from birth as well as institutional factors such as availability and response time of anesthesia, surgical personnel, and pediatric support for birth should the pattern progress. Suggested general guidelines for management of selected tracings are presented in Figure 5-16, and a management algorithm for indeterminate tracings was presented in Figure 5-15.

The challenge in assessing pattern evolution is the potential for loss of situation awareness with resulting lack of recognition or appreciation of an increased threat to fetal well-being. This rarely occurs when there is an acute event such as severe maternal hypotension, cord prolapse, or uterine rupture. Acute events typically present dramatic and recognizable FHR changes that prompt a rapid response from the perinatal team. Acute events differ from close observation of FHR characteristics over time. Although intrauterine resuscitation techniques supporting

FIGURE 5-16 Fetal Monitoring Decision Tree

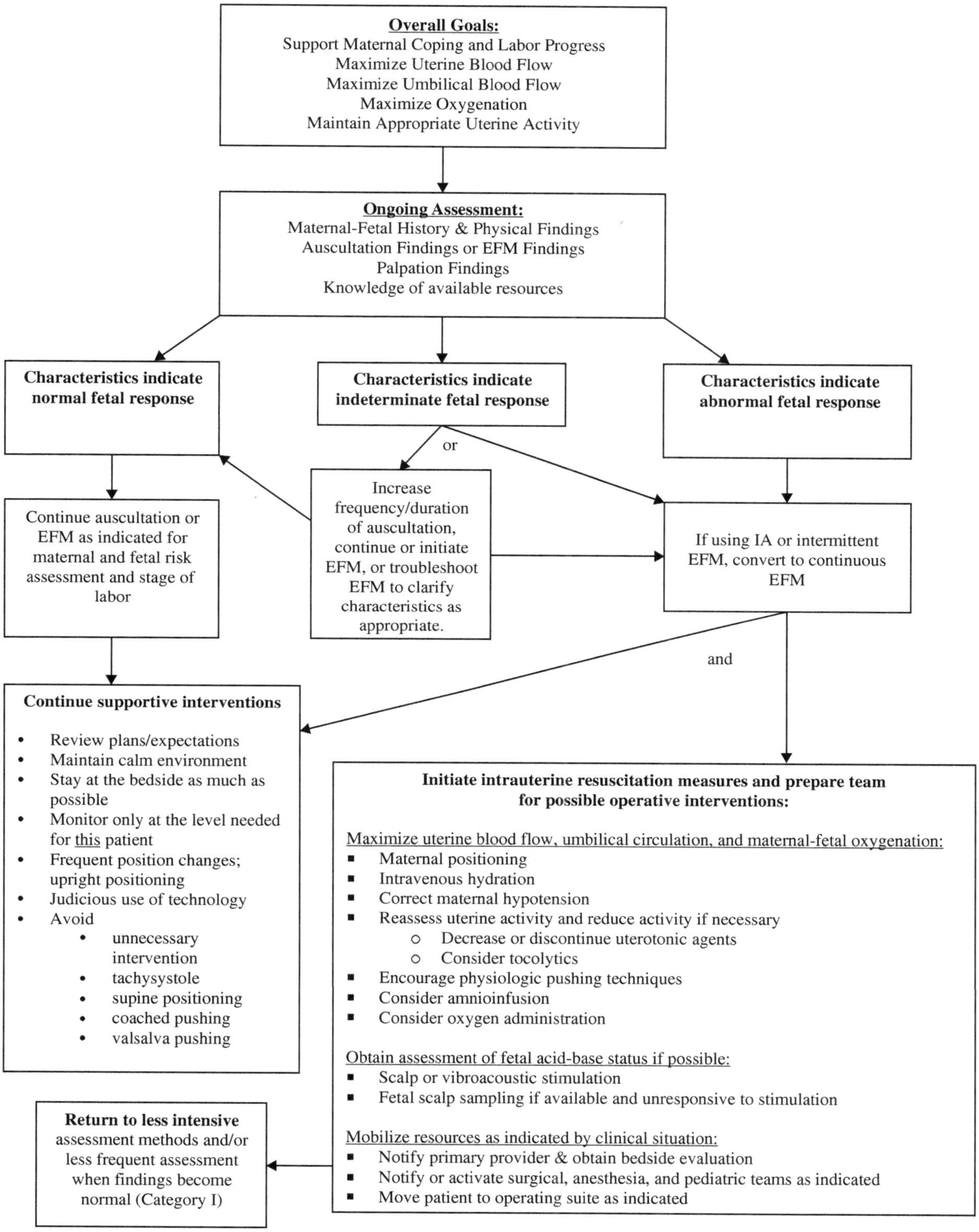

improvement of maternal-fetal exchange are often the most appropriate approach to concerning characteristics of the FHR, clinicians also need to be aware of the risk of failure to recognize more subtle signs of progressive fetal deterioration over longer periods or when they are focused on a perceived imminent endpoint such as vaginal birth "in just a few more pushes."

When the FHR evolves from a baseline within normal limits with moderate variability and accelerations to tachycardia, minimal to absent variability and recurrent late, variable, or prolonged decelerations, risk of fetal deterioration to hypoxemia and eventually acidemia is significant (Clark et al., 2013). Oxytocin-induced tachysystole can exacerbate the situation, so it is important to carefully titrate the oxytocin infusion based on contraction frequency and the fetal response (ACOG, 2010; Bakker et al., 2007). If the usual intrauterine resuscitation techniques do not result in pattern resolution, expeditious birth should be considered. A request for bedside evaluation by the primary care provider is warranted so that plans can be made and implemented for fetal rescue in a timely manner.

There is consensus on interpretation of tracings at the end of the continuum: tracings with absent FHR variability and recurrent late or variable decelerations or bradycardia are believed by most experts to be associated with a significant risk for fetal acidemia. Birth should be expedited in these cases unless evidence of fetal well-being can be ascertained without delay (Parer & Ikeda, 2007). Intrauterine resuscitation techniques are appropriate while preparing for birth, but they must not delay such preparations. It should be noted that there is no clear evidence to suggest the optimal decision-to-delivery interval in the setting of a category III tracing, as expeditious delivery must occur in a fashion that balances maternal and fetal risks and benefits (ACOG, 2010).

INTERPRETATION OF INTERMITTENT AUSCULTATION FINDINGS ACROSS THE CONTINUUM

The three-tiered EFM interpretation system also has implications for the interpretation and communication of FHR data obtained using IA. Using a common language for discussion of fetal status is a key principle for effective clinical communication and has the potential to decrease communication errors. For the purposes of interpreting auscultation findings, two categories are presented herein: Category I and Category II (Box 5-3). The definitions of these categories are consistent with the terminology used to interpret EFM patterns, but refer only to auscultation.

Category I auscultated FHR characteristics are normal (Box 5-3). Normal IA findings include all of the following characteristics: FHR baseline between 110 and 160 bpm, regular rhythm, and the absence of FHR decreases or decelerations. Normal FHR characteristics are predictive of fetal well-being at the time they are observed and may be followed with routine supportive measures.

Category II auscultated FHR characteristics include all findings that are not classified as normal (Box 5-3). Irregular rhythm, presence of decreases or decelerations from baseline, tachycardia, and bradycardia are all indeterminate IA findings. They cannot be classified as abnormal without information about FHR variability, as the patterns identified in Category III all include

BOX 5-3 Interpretation of Auscultation Findings

CATEGORY I

Category I FHR characteristics by auscultation include **all** of the following:

- Normal FHR baseline between 110 and 160 bpm
- Regular rhythm
- Presence of or absence of FHR increases or accelerations from the baseline rate
- Absence of FHR decreases or decelerations from the baseline

CATEGORY II

Category II FHR characteristics by auscultation include **any** of the following:

- Irregular rhythm
- Presence of FHR decreases or decelerations from the baseline
- Tachycardia (baseline >160 bpm > 10 minutes in duration)
- Bradycardia (baseline <110 bpm > 10 minutes in duration)

assessment of variability. Category II FHR characteristics require evaluation, ongoing surveillance, and reevaluation, consistent with the assessment of the overall clinical circumstances. This may include, but is not limited to continuous electronic fetal monitoring, use of intrauterine resuscitation techniques, ruling out maternal heart rate, and assessment of the continuation of indeterminate findings. As with EFM, auscultation findings and management needs are interpreted in the context of the overall clinical picture. Preparations to expedite birth in emergent situations (e.g., apparent significant fetal bradycardia) should be undertaken simultaneously with efforts to ameliorate, verify, and determine the precise nature of the FHR findings.

SUMMARY

Fetal heart monitoring is a complex psychomotor and interpretative skill that requires specialized education and practice. The care of childbearing women is enhanced when registered nurses, physicians, and midwives use standardized language for communicating FHR findings and engage in ongoing collaborative dialogue regarding FHR interpretation in the context of specific clinical cases. Timely identification and communication of FHR findings is essential to optimal maternal-fetal care. Systematic assessment, accurate interpretation, and effective teamwork will lead to selection of the most appropriate physiologic interventions for the condition of a given mother and fetus. These interventions and their physiologic rationales are discussed in Chapter 6.

Case Study: Mary

Age:	24 years old
Gravidity/Par:	G3 P1011
Gestational Age:	40-1/7 weeks
Medical History:	Tuberculosis at age 19—treated with INH, negative chest X-ray
Surgical History:	Unremarkable
Psychosocial History:	Migrant worker; single parent; father of baby not involved
Past Obstetric History:	Normal spontaneous vaginal birth at 39-2/7 weeks; spontaneous abortion at 9 weeks requiring dilation and curettage
Current Obstetric History:	Normal prenatal laboratory results Rh negative: received RhoGAM at 28 weeks Second trimester ultrasound consistent with last menstrual period (LMP), normal anatomy Five prenatal visits in community clinic

Mary presented to obstetric triage for decreased fetal movement for 4 days. Her membranes were intact. Vaginal examination (VE) revealed a cervix that was 2 cm dilated, 75% effaced, and a fetal vertex that was −2 station. Her vital signs were as follows: oral temperature, 97.8° F (36.5° C); blood pressure, 110/68 mmHg; pulse, 92 bpm; respiration, 20 breaths per minute. This tracing occurred within the first 15 minutes of monitor placement.

Mary: Triage Tracing Using Ultrasound and Tocodynamometer

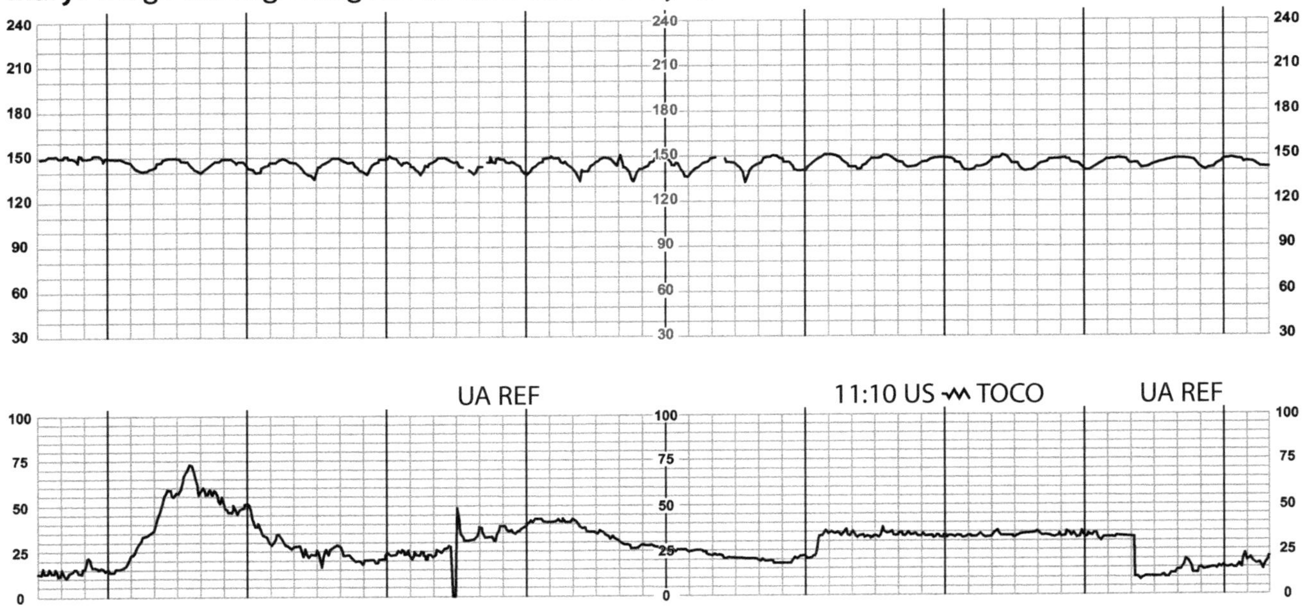

Case Study Exercise: Mary

1. Baseline FHR:	**145 bpm**	
2. Variability	Absent (undetectable)	_____
	Minimal (>0 but 5 bpm)	_____
	Moderate (6–25 bpm)	_____
	Marked (>25 bpm)	_____
	Unable to determine	**Sinusoidal**
3. Contractions	Frequency:	**Irregular**
	Duration:	**90–110 seconds**
	Intensity:	**Palpate**
	Resting tonus:	**Palpate**

4. Accelerations and decelerations. When present, circle P if periodic or E if episodic.

Accelerations	P	E
Early decelerations	P	
Variable decelerations	P	E
Late decelerations	P	
Prolonged decelerations	P	E
None present		

5. Interpretation	Category I	________
	Category II	________
	Category III	________

6. List possible underlying physiologic mechanisms or rationales for observed patterns.
- **Severe fetal anemia**
- **Rh isoimmunization**
- **Abruptio placentae**
- **Fetal–maternal hemorrhage**
- **Associated with an abnormal fetal acid-base status at present**
- **Narcotic or analgesic administration or ingestion**
- **Fetal thumbsucking**
- **Unknown etiology**

7. List in order of priority the physiologic goal(s) for observed patterns.
- **Maximize oxygenation.**
- **Maximize uteroplacental blood flow.**
- **Reduce uterine activity.**

8. List interventions to achieve the physiologic goals and actions needed (physiologic based, instrumentation based, and further assessments).
- **Administer maternal supplemental oxygen at 10 Liters/minute via a tight nonrebreather face mask.**
- **Change maternal position to maximize uterine blood flow.**
- **Hydrate with intravenous (IV) fluids.**
- **Notify provider for immediate bedside evaluation.**
- **Prepare for possible emergent birth if FHR pattern cannot be improved.**
- **Alert neonatal team for possible emergent birth.**

- **Interview the woman about fetal activity patterns prior to admission.**
- **Assess for current or previous vaginal bleeding.**
- **Assess for uterine tenderness or abdominal pain.**
- **Question woman about recent trauma, abuse (e.g., abdominal trauma), and medication use (legal and illegal substances).**
- **Review prenatal records for Rh status and RhoGAM® administration.**
- **Consider fetal surveillance techniques such as biophysical profile.**
- **Evaluate FHR responses to interventions.**
- **Consider Kleihauer-Betke test and drug screen profile.**
- **Palpate uterus to validate uterine monitoring data.**
- **Keep provider notified of FHR pattern (undulating tracing) and evaluate maternal–fetal response to interventions.**

REFERENCES

American College of Obstetricians and Gynecologists. (2003). Dystocia and augmentation of labor. Practice bulletin no. 49. *Obstetrics & Gynecologgy, 102*(6), 1445–1454.

American College of Obstetricians and Gynecologists. (2006). Umbilical cord blood gas and acid-base analysis. Committee Opinion No. 348. *Obstetrics and Gynecology, 108*(5), 1319–1322.

American College of Obstetricians and Gynecologists. (2009). Intrapartum fetal heart rate monitoring: nomenclature, interpretation, and general management principles. Practice Bulletin No. 106. *Obstetrics and Gynecology, 114*(1), 192–202. doi: 10.1097/AOG.0b013e3181aef106.

American College of Obstetricians and Gynecologists. (2010). Management of intrapartum fetal heart rate tracings. Practice Bulletin No. 116. *Obstetrics and Gynecology, 116*(5), 1232–1240. doi: 10.1097/AOG.0b013e3182004fa9

Andres, R. L., Saade, G., Gilstrap, L. C., Wilkins, I., Witlin, A., Zlatnik, F., & Hankins, G. V. (1999). Association between umbilical blood gas parameters and neonatal morbidity and death in neonates with pathologic fetal acidemia. *American Journal of Obstetrics and Gynecology, 181*(4), 867–871.

Association of Women's Health, Obstetric and Neonatal Nurses. (2009a). Fetal heart monitoring (Position statement). Washington, DC: Author.

Association of Women's Health, Obstetric and Neonatal Nurses. (2009b). The role of unlicensed assistive personnel (nursing assistive personnel) in the care of women and newborns. Position statement. *Journal of Obstetric, Gynecologic and Neonatal Nursing,* 38(6), 745–747. doi:10.1111/j.1552-6909.2009.01080.x.

Bakker, P. C., Kurver, P. H., Kuik, D. J., & Van Geijn, H. P. (2007). Elevated uterine activity increases the risk of fetal acidosis at birth. *American Journal of Obstetrics and Gynecologgy, 196*(4), 313.e1–313.e36.

Ball, R. H., & Parer, J. T. (1992). The physiologic mechanisms of variable decelerations. *American Journal of Obstetrics & Gynecology, 166*(6, Pt. 1), 1683–1688.

Beard, R. W., Filshie, G. M., Knight, C. A., & Roberts, G. M. (1971). The significance of the changes in the continuous fetal heart rate in the first stage of labour. *Journal of Obstetrics and Gynaecology of the British Commonwealth, 78*(10), 865–881.

Berkus, M. D., Langer, O., Samueloff, A., Xenakis, E. M., & Field, N. T. (1999). Electronic fetal monitoring: What's reassuring? *Acta Obstetricia et Gynecologica Scandinavica, 78*(1), 15–21.

Cahill, A. G., Roehl, K. A., Odibo, A. O., & Macones, G. A. (2012). Association of a typical decelerations with acidemia. *Obstetrics and Gynecology, 120*(6), 1387–1393. doi: http://10.1097/AOG.0b013e3182733b6e

Cibils, L. A. (1975). Clinical significance of fetal heart rate patterns during labor. II. Late decelerations. *American Journal of Obstetrics and Gynecology, 123*(5), 473–494.

Clark, S. L., Gimovsky, M. L., & Miller, F. C. (1984). The scalp stimulation test: A clinical alternative to fetal scalp blood sampling. *American Journal of Obstetrics and Gynecology, 148*(3), 274–277.

Clark, S. L., Nageotte, M. P., Garite, T. J., Freeman, R. K., Miller, D. A, Simpson, K. R., . . . Hankins, G. D. V. (2013). Intrapartum management of category II fetal heart rate tracings: Towards standardization of care. *American Journal of Obstetrics and Gynecology, 209*(2), 89–97. doi:10.1016/j.ajog.2013.04.030

Copel, J. A., Friedman, A. H., & Kleinman, C. S. (1997). Management of fetal cardiac arrhythmias. *Obstetrics and Gynecology Clinics of North America,* 24(1), 201–211.

Crane, J. M., Young, D. C., Butt, K. D., Bennett, K. A., & Hutchens, D. (2001). Excessive uterine activity accompanying induced labor. *Obstetrics and Gynecology,* 97(6), 926–931.

Dalton, K. J., Dawes, G. S., & Patrick, J. E. (1977). Diurnal, respiratory, and other rhythms of fetal heart rate in lambs. *American Journal of Obstetrics and Gynecology, 127*(4), 414–424.

Dawes, G. S., Visser, G. H., Goodman, J. D., & Levine, D. H. (1981). Numerical analysis of the human fetal heart rate: Modulation by breathing and movement. *American Journal of Obstetrics and Gynecology, 140*(5), 535–544.

Dawood, M. Y. (1995). Pharmacologic stimulation of uterine contraction. *Seminars in Perinatology, 19*(1), 73–83.

Dellinger, E. H., Boehm, F. H., & Crane, M. M. (2000). Electronic fetal heart rate monitoring: Early neonatal outcomes associated with normal rate, fetal stress, and fetal distress. *American Journal of Obstetrics & Gynecology, 182*(1, Pt. 1), 214–220.

Feinstein, N, Sprague, A., & Trepanier, M.-J. (2009). *Fetal heart rate auscultation* (2nd ed.). Washington, DC: Association of Women's Health, Obstetric and Neonatal Nurses.

Fox, M., Kilpatrick, S., King, T., & Parer, J. T. (2000). Fetal heart rate monitoring: Interpretation and collaborative management. *Journal of Midwifery and Women's Health, 45*(6), 498–507.

Freeman, R. K., Garite, T. J., Nageotte, M. P., & Miller, L. A. (2012). *Fetal heart rate monitoring* (4th ed.). Philadelphia, PA: Lippincott Williams & Wilkins.

Friedman, D. M. (1992). Fetal echocardiography in the assessment of lupus pregnancies. *American Journal of Reproductive Immunology, 28*(3-4), 164–167.

Garite, T. J., & Simpson, K. R. (2011). Intrauterine resuscitation during labor. *Clinical Obstetrics and Gynecology, 54*(1), 28–39. doi: 10.1097/GRF.0b013e31820a062b

Garite, T. J. (2012). Intrapartum fetal evaluation. In S. G. Gabbe, J. R. Neibyl, J. L. Simpson, M. B. Landon, H. L. Galan, E. R. M. Jauniaux, & D. A. Driscoll (Eds.), *Obstetrics: Normal and problem pregnancies* (6th ed., pp. 330–361). Philadelphia: Saunders.

Gull, I., Jaffa, A. J., Oren, M., Grisaru, D., Peyser, M. R., & Lessing, J. B. (1996). Acid accumulation during end-stage bradycardia in term fetuses: How long is too long? *British Journal of Obstetrics and Gynaecology, 103*(11), 1096–1101.

Hammacher, K., Huter, K. A., Bokelmann, J., & Werners, P. H. (1968). Foetal heart frequency and perinatal condition of the foetus and newborn. *Gynaecologia, 166*(4), 349–360.

Jackson, M., Holmgren, C. M., Esplin, M. S., Henry, E., & Varner, M. W. (2011). Frequency of fetal heart rate categories and short-term neonatal outcome. *Obstetrics and Gynecology, 118*(4), 803-808. doi:10.1097/AOG.0b013e31822f1b50

James, L. S., Yeh, M. N., Morishima, H. O., Daniel, S. S., Caritis, S. N., Niemann, W. H., & Indyk, L. (1976). Umbilical vein occlusion and transient acceleration of the fetal heart rate. Experimental observations in subhuman primates. *American Journal of Obstetrics and Gynecology, 126*(2), 276–283.

Kamoshita, E., Amano, K., Kanai, Y., Mochizuki, J., Ikeda, Y., Kikuchi, S., . . . Unno, N. (2010). Effect of the interval between onset of sustained fetal bradycardia and cesarean delivery on long-term neonatal neurologic prognosis. *International Journal of Gynecology and Obstetrics, 111*(1), 23–27. doi:10.1016/j.ijgo.2010.05.022

King, T. L. (2012). Fetal assessment. In S. T. Blackburn (Ed.), *Maternal, fetal, and neonatal physiology: A clinical perspective* (4th ed., pp. 163–182). Maryland Heights, MO: Saunders Elsevier.

Kleinman, C. S., & Nehgme, R. A. (2004). Cardiac arrhythmias in the human fetus. *Pediatric Cardiology, 25*(3), 234–251.

Korhonen, J., & Kariniemi, V. (1994). Emergency cesarean section: The effect of delay on umbilical arterial gas balance and Apgar scores. *Acta Obstetricia et Gynecologica Scandinavica, 73*(10), 782–786.

Krebs, H. B., Petres, R. E., & Dunn, L. J. (1981). Intrapartum fetal heart rate monitoring. V. Fetal heart rate patterns in the second stage of labor. *American Journal of Obstetrics and Gynecology, 140*(4), 435–439.

Krebs, H. B., Petres, R. E., & Dunn, L. J. (1983). Intrapartum fetal heart rate monitoring. VIII. Atypical variable decelerations. *American Journal of Obstetrics and Gynecology, 145*(3), 297–305.

Krebs, H. B., Petres, R. E., Dunn, L. J., Jordaan, H. V., & Segreti, A. (1979). Intrapartum fetal heart rate monitoring. I: Classification and prognosis of fetal heart rate patterns. *American Journal of Obstetrics and Gynecology, 133*(7), 762–772.

Lee, C. Y., Di Loreto, P. C., & O'Lane, J. M. (1975). A study of fetal heart rate acceleration patterns. *Obstetrics and Gynecology, 45*(2), 142–146.

Lee, S. T., & Hon, E. H. (1963). Fetal hemodynamic response to umbilical cord compression. *Obstetrics and Gynecology, 22,* 553–562.

Leung, A. S., Leung, E. K., & Paul, R. H. (1993). Uterine rupture after previous cesarean delivery: Maternal and fetal consequences. *American Journal of Obstetrics and Gynecology, 169*(4), 945–950.

Leveno, K. J., Quirk, J. G., Jr., Cunningham, F. G., Nelson, S. D., Santos-Ramos, R., Toofanian, A., & DePalma, R. T. (1984). Prolonged pregnancy. I: Observations concerning the causes of fetal distress. *American Journal of Obstetrics and Gynecology, 150*(5, Pt. 1), 465–473.

Low, J. A., Lindsay, B. G., & Derrick, E. J. (1997). Threshold of metabolic acidosis associated with newborn complications. *American Journal of Obstetrics and Gynecology, 177,* 1391–1394. doi: 10.1016/S0002-9378(97)70080-2

Low, J. A., Victory, R., & Derrick, E. J. (1999). Predictive value of electronic fetal monitoring for intrapartum fetal asphyxia with metabolic acidosis. *Obstetrics and Gynecology, 93*(2), 285–291.

Lyndon, A., O'Brien-Abel, N., & Simpson, K. R. (2014). Fetal assessment during labor. In K. R. Simpson & P. A. Creehan (Eds.), *Perinatal nursing* (4th ed., pp. 445–492). Philadelphia, PA: Lippincott.

MacLennan, A. (1999). A template for defining a causal relation between acute intrapartum events and cerebral palsy: International consensus statement. *British Medical Journal, 319*(7216), 1054–1059.

Macones, G. A., Hankins, G. D., Spong, C. Y., Hauth, J. D., & Moore, T. (2008). The 2008 National Institute of Child Health Human Development workshop report on electronic fetal monitoring: Update on definitions, interpretations, and research guidelines. *Obstetrics and Gynecology, 112*(3), 661–666. doi:10.1097/AOG.0b013e3181841395; and *Journal of Obstetric, Gynecologic and Neonatal Nursing, 37*(5), 510–515. doi:10.1111/j.1552-6909.2008.00284.x

Manseau, P., Vaquier, J., Chavinie, J., & Sureau, C. (1972). Le rythme cardiaque foetal "sinusoidal" aspect evocateur de souffrance fortale au cours de a grossesse. *Journal de Gynecologie, Obstetrique et Biologie de la Reproduction, 1*(4), 343–352.

Martin, C. B., Jr. (1978). Regulation of the fetal heart rate and genesis of FHR patterns. *Seminars in Perinatology, 2*(2), 131–146.

Martin, C. B., Jr. (1982). Physiology and clinical use of fetal heart rate variability. *Clinics in Perinatology, 9*(2), 339–352.

Modanlou, H. D., & Freeman, R. K. (1982). Sinusoidal fetal heart rate pattern: Its definition and clinical significance. *American Journal of Obstetrics & Gynecology, 142*(8), 1033–1038.

Modanlou, H. D., & Murata, Y. (2004). Sinusoidal heart rate pattern: Reappraisal of its definition and clinical significance. *Journal of Obstetrics and Gynaecology Research, 30*(3), 169–180.

Nageotte, M. P., & Gilstrap, L. C. (2009). Intrapartum fetal surveillance. In R. K. Creasy, R. Resnik, J. D. Iams, C. J. Lockwood, & T. R. Moore (Eds.), *Creasy & Resnik's maternal-fetal medicine: Principles and practice* (6th ed., pp. 397–417). Philadelphia, PA: Saunders.

National Institute of Child Health and Human Development Research Planning Workshop. (1997). Electronic fetal heart rate monitoring: Research guidelines for interpretation. *American Journal of Obstetrics and Gynecology, 177*(6), 1385–1390; and *Journal of Obstetric, Gynecologic, and Neonatal Nursing, 26*(6), 635–640.

O'Brien-Abel, N. E., & Benedetti, T. J. (1992). Saltatory fetal heart rate pattern. *Journal of Perinatology, 12*(1), 13–17.

Paine, L. L., Benedict, M. I., Strobino, D. M., Gregor, C. L., & Larson, E. L. (1992). A comparison of the auscultated acceleration test and the nonstress test as predictors of perinatal outcomes. *Nursing Research, 41*(2), 87–91.

Paine, L. L., Zanardi, L. R., Johnson, T. R., Rorie, J. A., & Barger, M. K. (2001). A comparison of two time intervals for the auscultated acceleration test. *Journal of Midwifery and Women's Health, 46(2),* 98–102.

Parer, J. T. (1997). *Handbook of fetal heart monitoring* (2nd ed.). Philadelphia, PA: W. B. Saunders.

Parer, J. T., Dijkstra, H. R., Vredebregt, P. P., Harris, J. L., Krueger, T. R., & Reuss, M. L. (1980). Increased fetal heart rate variability with acute hypoxia in chronically instrumented sheep. *European Journal of Obstetrics, Gynecology, and Reproductive Biology, 10*(6), 393–399.

Parer, J. T., & Ikeda, T. (2007). A framework for standardized management of intrapartum fetal heart rate patterns. *American Journal of Obstetrics & Gynecology, 197*(1), 26.e1–26.e6.

Parer, J. T., King, T., Flanders, S., Fox, M., & Kilpatrick, S. J. (2006). Fetal acidemia and electronic fetal heart rate patterns: Is there evidence of an association? *Journal of Maternal-Fetal and Neonatal Medicine, 19*(5), 289–294.

Parer, J. T., & Livingston, E. G. (1990). What is fetal distress? *American Journal of Obstetrics and Gynecology, 162*(6), 1421–1425.

Patrick, J., Campbell, K., Carmichael, L., Natale, R., & Richardson, B. (1982). Patterns of gross fetal body movements over 24-hour observation intervals during the last 10 weeks of pregnancy. *American Journal of Obstetrics and Gynecology, 142*(4), 363–371.

Paul, R. H., Suidan, A. K., Yeh, S., Schifrin, B. S., & Hon, E. H. (1975). Clinical fetal monitoring. VII: The evaluation and significance of intrapartum baseline FHR variability. *American Journal of Obstetrics and Gynecology, 123*(2), 206–210.

Phaneuf, S., Rodríguez Liñares, B., TambyRaja, R. L., MacKenzie, I. Z., & López Bernal, A. (2000). Loss of myometrial oxytocin receptors during oxytocin-induced and oxytocin-augmented labour. *Journal of Reproduction and Fertility, 120*(1), 91–97.

Porter, T. F., & Clark, S. L. (1999). Vibroacoustic and scalp stimulation. *Obstetrics and Gynecology Clinics of North America, 26*(4), 657–669.

Reddy, A., Moulden, M., & Redman, C. W. (2009). Antepartum high-frequency fetal heart rate sinusoidal rhythm: Computerized detection and fetal anemia. *American Journal of Obstetrics and Gynecology, 200*(4), 407.e1–407.e6. doi:10.1016/j.ajog.2008.10.026

Reed, K. L. (1989). Fetal arrhythmias: Etiology, diagnosis, pathophysiology, and treatment. *Seminars in Perinatology, 13*(4), 294–304.

Ridgeway, J. J., Weyrich, D. L., & Benedetti, T. J. (2004). Fetal heart rate changes associated with uterine rupture. *Obstetrics and Gynecology, 103*(3), 506–512.

Simpson, K. R. (2007). Intrauterine resuscitation during labor: Review of current methods and supportive evidence. *Journal of Midwifery and Women's Health, 52*(3), 229–237. doi:10.1016/j.jmwh.2006.12.010

Simpson, K. R. (2013). *Cervical ripening and induction and augmentation of labor* (4th ed.). Washington, DC: Association of Women's Health, Obstetric, and Neonatal Nurses.

Simpson, K. R., & James, D. C. (2008). Effects of oxytocin-induced uterine hyperstimulation during labor on fetal oxygen status and fetal heart rate patterns. *American Journal of Obstetrics and Gynecology, 199*(1), 34 e31–35. doi: 10.1016/j.ajog.2007.12.015

Sklansky, M. (2009). Fetal cardiac malformations and arrhythmias: Detection, diagnosis, management, and prognosis. In R. K. Creasy, R. Resnik, J. D. Iams, C. J. Lockwood, & T. R. Moore (Eds.), *Creasy & Resnik's maternal-fetal medicine: Principles and practice* (6th ed., pp. 305–345). Philadelphia, PA: Saunders.

Spong, C. Y., Rasul, C., Collea, J. V., Eglinton, G. S., & Ghidini, A. (1998). Characterization and prognostic significance of variable decelerations in the second stage of labor. *American Journal of Perinatology, 15*(6), 369–374. doi:10.1055/s-2007-993959

Timor-Tritsch, I. E., Dierker, L. J., Hertz, R. H., Deagan, N. C., & Rosen, M. G. (1978). Studies of antepartum behavioral state in the human fetus at term.

American Journal of Obstetrics and Gynecology, 132(5), 524–528.

Williams, K. P., & Galerneau, F. (2003). Intrapartum fetal heart rate patterns in the prediction of neonatal acidemia. *American Journal of Obstetrics and Gynecology, 188*(3), 820–823.

Wright, R. G., Shnider, S. M., Levinson, G., Rolbin, S. H., & Parer, J. T. (1981). The effect of maternal administration of ephedrine on fetal heart rate and variability. *Obstetrics and Gynecology, 57*(6), 734–738.

Zeeman, G. G., Khan-Dawood, F. S., & Dawood, M. Y. (1997). Oxytocin and its receptor in pregnancy and parturition: Current concepts and clinical implications. *Obstetrics and Gynecology, 89*(5, Pt. 2), 873–883.

CHAPTER 6

Physiologic Interventions for Fetal Heart Rate Patterns

Kathleen Rice Simpson

INTRODUCTION

The goal of fetal monitoring is ongoing assessment of fetal oxygenation to promote fetal safety. The clinician can best develop an understanding of fetal physiologic status by thoroughly assessing the maternal medical and obstetric history; current risk factors; and physical assessment findings, including fetal heart rate (FHR) characteristics and uterine activity. Selection of appropriate interventions to maximize fetal oxygenation is based on these assessment data and other relevant clinical information. This chapter reviews concepts for collaborative diagnosis and interventions based on assessment and interpretation of FHR characteristics in the context of the ongoing clinical condition of the mother and fetus (Figure 6-1). The dynamic physiologic response model is used to conceptualize fetal status as the basis for interventions (Figure 6-2). Independent and collaborative interventions are discussed, with emphasis on the goal of supporting or improving fetal oxygenation.

PROMOTING FETAL WELL-BEING

Fetal well-being requires a hemodynamically stable, well-oxygenated mother and a well-oxygenated fetus. The mother's condition is a significant determinant of fetal well-being. To promote fetal oxygenation, essential clinical criteria must be met, including adequate maternal cardiac output, blood pressure, hemoglobin levels, and oxygen saturation; adequate blood flow to the uterus and placenta; adequate placental function; normal uterine activity; and uninterrupted umbilical blood flow to the fetus (e.g., absence of umbilical cord compression). During labor, clinicians have limited ability to influence some of these criteria, such as adequacy of placental function. However, clinicians can support fetal well-being by implementing interventions based on the specific physiologic goals of supporting maternal coping and labor progress, and maintaining appropriate uterine activity. Upright positioning and frequent position changes can promote labor progress. Maintaining a calm environment; minimizing fear, anxiety, and pain; and assisting a woman to cope with labor may decrease her catecholamine production, thereby promoting adequate blood flow and fetal oxygenation. Likewise, maintaining appropriate levels of uterine activity, avoiding tachysystole, and using a physiologic approach to pushing support optimal fetal oxygenation and maternal–fetal adaptation to the labor process.

FIGURE 6-1 The Collaborative Process and Fetal Heart Monitoring

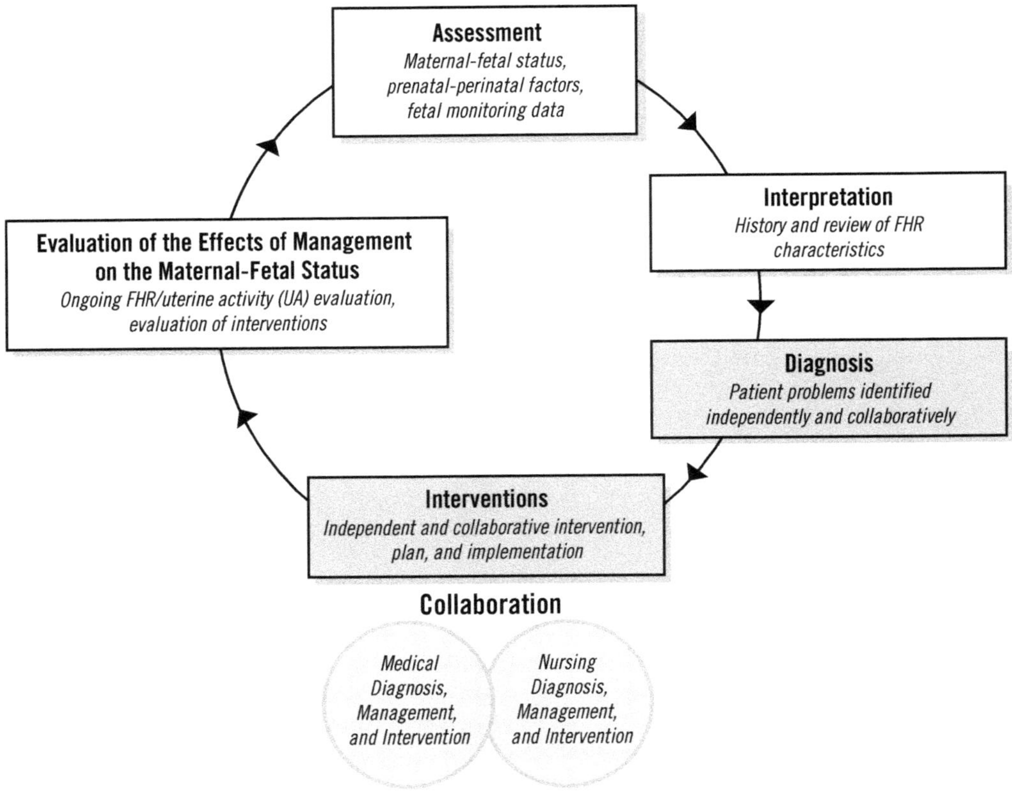

FIGURE 6-2 The Dynamic Physiologic Response Model

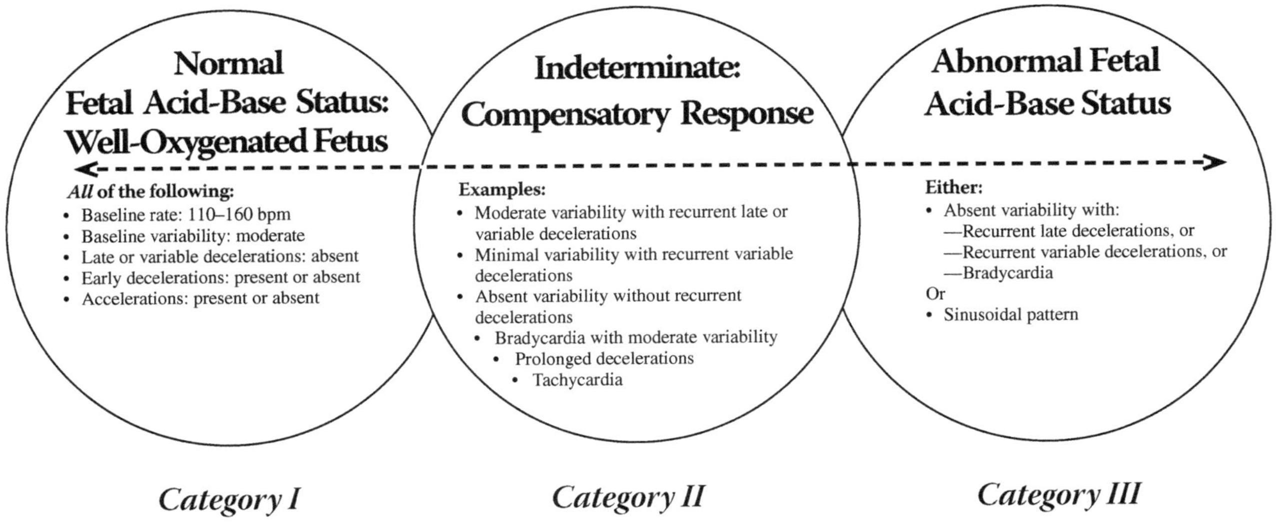

This diagram is not meant to be all inclusive. All patterns must be treated with interventions that are based on suspected underlying physiologic causes and evaluation of individual patient presentation.

CLASSIFICATION OF ELECTRONICALLY OBTAINED FETAL HEART RATE PATTERNS

The 2008 National Institute of Child Health and Human Development (NICHD) Workshop guidelines proposed a three-tiered system for classification of intrapartum EFM findings: category I (normal), category II (indeterminate), and category III (abnormal) (Macones et al., 2008). The Society of Obstetricians and Gynaecologists of Canada (SOGC; 2007) uses the terms "normal," "atypical," and "abnormal" in their *Fetal Health Surveillance: Antepartum and Intrapartum Consensus Guideline* (see Table 5-6 in Chapter 5).

A normal (category I) FHR tracing has a baseline rate of 110-160 bpm, moderate baseline FHR variability, and no late or variable decelerations. Normal tracings may or may not have accelerations or early decelerations. Experts generally agree that this type of FHR tracing confers an extremely high predictability of a normally oxygenated fetus (American College of Obstetricians and Gynecologists [AOCG], 2010; NICHD, 1997; Macones et al., 2008). Normal FHR tracings may be followed with routine measures to support labor progress, maternal coping, and fetal oxygenation. At the other end of the continuum from completely normal tracings are abnormal (category III) FHR patterns requiring prompt evaluation and attempts to expeditiously resolve the abnormal findings (ACOG, 2010). Category III FHR tracings are those with a sinusoidal pattern or absent variability *in conjunction with* bradycardia or recurrent late or variable decelerations (Macones et al., 2008).

The majority of intrapartum FHR tracings may be interpreted as indeterminate (category II) at any one time during labor (Jackson, Holmgren, Esplin, Henry, & Varner, 2011). Indeterminate (category II) includes, but is not limited to, tracings with *moderate or minimal variability* and recurrent late or variable decelerations, baseline tachycardia, marked variability, prolonged decelerations, and the absence of an acceleratory response to fetal stimulation. In a recent study of 48,444 women in term labor, normal (category 1) FHR patterns were noted 77.9% of the time, while indeterminate (category II) and abnormal (category III) FHR patterns were noted 22.1% and .004% of the time, respectively (Jackson et al., 2011). The percentage of time the FHR patterns were classified in each category changed over the course of labor. For example, as compared to the previously mentioned data representing the entire labor, during the 2 hours immediately prior to birth, 60.9% of FHR tracings were category I, 39.1% were category II, and 0.006% were category III (Jackson et al., 2011). Most patients (83.6%) had FHR patterns consistent with at least two of the three interpretive categories during their labor (Jackson et al., 2011). Indeterminate (category II) tracings require evaluation, continued surveillance, initiation of appropriate corrective measures when indicated, and reevaluation (ACOG, 2010). Supportive actions to promote maternal and fetal adaptation to labor are usually indicated and should be based on the specific characteristics of the indeterminate FHR pattern.

Parer, King, Flanders, Fox, and Kilpatrick (2006) conducted a review of 18 fetal monitoring studies to test for relationships between fetal heart characteristics, the duration of specific FHR patterns, and newborn acidemia versus newborn vigor. Fetal acidemia was defined as a cord pH of <7.15, and newborn vigor was defined as a 5-minute Apgar score ≥7. The association between acidemia and the presence of late or variable decelerations was only 23%, but this was the most consistent predictor of newborn acidemia. However, the association between moderate variability in this review with an absence of acidemia or presence of newborn vigor was 98%, whether or not decelerations or bradycardia were present. Additional findings included a progressive relationship between depth of decelerations or bradycardia and the severity of newborn acidemia, and the observation that newborn acidemia generally developed over a period of approximately an hour in the context of decreasing FHR variability in conjunction with decelerations. Acidemia only developed rapidly in the context of sudden and profound bradycardia. These findings are consistent with the results of a systematic review by the National Collaborating Centre for Women's and Children's Health (NCCWCH; 2007) on both specific and overall features of FHR patterns as they relate to neonatal outcomes. Thus, there is supportive evidence for associations between category III patterns and some category II patterns and risk for significant fetal acidemia. The predictive value of grading schemes for the depth, duration, and/or absolute nadir of decelerations requires further research (Macones et al., 2008).

Interventions aimed at improving fetal oxygenation via one or more intrauterine resuscitation techniques should be used when category II or III FHR patterns are present. Ideally, members of the perinatal team have a shared method of interpreting FHR patterns and an agreed-upon management guideline for specific FHR patterns.

SYSTEMATIC INTERPRETATION OF THE FETAL HEART RATE TRACING

Appropriate interventions require an accurate interpretation of the characteristics of both the FHR and uterine activity and their relationship with each other. Attention should be given to the overall clinical picture and to the trends in the FHR pattern over time. Although the experienced clinician may assess the individual characteristics of the FHR simultaneously, a detailed and thorough evaluation of each component may be useful when planning appropriate interventions. The method of monitoring used determines which characteristics can be assessed.

A systematic fetal monitoring assessment includes, but is not limited to, the following data:

Baseline FHR Characteristics

- Baseline rate
- Rhythm (with auscultation)
- Variability
- Sinusoidal

Baseline Changes

- Presence or absence of accelerations
- Presence or absence of decelerations
    - Early
    - Late
    - Variable
    - Prolonged

Uterine Activity

- Frequency
- Duration
- Intensity
- Resting tone

The clinician may review these physiologic data through the following process:

- What is the baseline FHR?
- Is it within normal limits for this fetus?
- If not, what clinical factors could be contributing to this baseline rate?
- Is there evidence of moderate baseline variability?
- If not, does fetal stimulation elicit an acceleration of the FHR appropriate for gestational age?
- What clinical factors could be contributing to this baseline variability?
- Are there periodic or episodic FHR patterns?
- If so, what are they and what are the appropriate interventions (if any)?
- Does the FHR pattern suggest a chronic or acute maternal-fetal condition?
- Is uterine activity normal in frequency, duration, intensity, and resting tone?
- What is the relationship between FHR and uterine activity?
- What is the relationship between FHR and maternal vital signs?
- If the FHR pattern is not normal, what types of interventions would be appropriate to maximize fetal oxygenation?
- Do these appropriate interventions resolve the situation?
- If not, are further interventions needed?
- Is the FHR pattern such that notification of the physician or midwife is warranted?
- Is the FHR pattern such that actions should be initiated for expeditious birth?
- What steps should be taken in the case of clinical disagreement between caregivers regarding FHR interpretation and/or appropriate response to the FHR patterns? (Simpson, 2006)

INTERVENTIONS FOR CATEGORY II AND III FETAL HEART RATE PATTERNS

Intrauterine Resuscitation Techniques

When an indeterminate or abnormal FHR pattern is identified, initial assessment may include a cervical exam to rule out umbilical cord prolapse, rapid cervical dilation, or rapid descent of the fetal head; review of uterine activity to rule out tachysystole; and evaluation of maternal vital signs, in particular temperature and blood pressure, to rule out maternal fever or maternal hypotension. Further information about fetal status can be obtained by an assessment of variability, and determining if accelerations (either spontaneous or stimulated) are present, since moderate variability and accelerations are highly predictive of normal fetal acid-base status at the time they are observed (ACOG, 2010). These assessment data can guide the timing and type of appropriate interventions to attempt to resolve the pattern. The physiologic goals for intrauterine resuscitation include the following:

- Support maternal coping and labor progress.
- Maximize uterine blood flow.
- Maximize umbilical circulation.
- Maximize oxygenation.
- Maintain appropriate uterine activity.

Intrauterine resuscitation refers to a series of techniques that include but may not be limited to:

- Maternal repositioning
- Reduction of uterine activity
- Intravenous (IV) fluid bolus
- Correction of maternal hypotension
- Oxygen administration
- Amnioinfusion during first-stage labor
- Modification of maternal pushing efforts during second-stage labor

The type of resuscitative technique is based on the specific characteristics of the FHR pattern. In some cases, a combination of techniques will be required to resolve the pattern. A summary of the goals and techniques for intrauterine resuscitation are presented in Table 6-1.

TABLE 6-1 Intrauterine Resuscitation

GOAL	TECHNIQUES/METHODS
Promote fetal oxygenation	Lateral positioning (either left or right)
	IV fluid bolus of at least 500 mL of lactated Ringer's solution
	Discontinuation of oxytocin/removal of dinoprostone insert (prostaglandin E_2)/withholding of next dose of misoprostol
	Pushing with every other or every third contraction or discontinuation of pushing temporarily (during second-stage labor)
	Oxygen administration at 10 L/min via nonrebreather face mask (discontinue as soon as possible based on the fetal response)
Reduce uterine activity	Discontinuation of oxytocin/removal of dinoprostone insert (prostaglandin E_2)/withholding of next dose of misoprostol
	IV fluid bolus of at least 500 mL of lactated Ringer's solution
	Lateral positioning (either left or right)
	If no response, terbutaline 0.25 mg subcutaneously may be considered
Alleviate umbilical cord compression	Repositioning
	Amnioinfusion (during first-stage labor)
	Pushing with every other or every third contraction or discontinuation of pushing temporarily (during second-stage labor)
	If prolapse umbilical cord is noted, elevation of the presenting fetal part as preparations are underway for expeditious birth may be effective
Correct maternal hypotension	Lateral positioning (either left or right)
	IV fluid bolus of at least 500 mL of lactated Ringer's solution
	If no response, ephedrine 5–10 mg IV push may be considered

Note: IV, intravenous.
Adapted from "Fetal assessment during labor." By A. Lyndon, N. O'Brien-Abel, & K. R. Simpson. (2013). In K. R. Simpson & P. A. Creehan (Eds.), *AWHONN's perinatal nursing* (4th ed., p. 461). Copyright 2013 by the Association of Women's Health, Obstetric and Neonatal Nurses.

Although intrauterine resuscitation techniques are commonly used (ACOG, 2010; ACOG & American Academy of Pediatrics [AAP], 2014; SOGC, 2007), supportive data for their effectiveness could be more robust (Garite & Simpson, 2011; Simpson, 2007). It is generally believed that these interventions improve maternal blood flow to the placental intervillous space and oxygen delivery to the fetus. There are data to suggest that these techniques can improve fetal oxygen status, but it is important to remember that there is no evidence that any of these techniques individually or collectively will reverse fetal acidemia. If the clinical characteristics of the FHR patterns are such that they represent a serious, immediate risk to the fetus (e.g., bradycardia unresponsive to other intervention), these techniques should be initiated only if doing so does not delay expeditious birth (Garite & Simpson, 2011; Simpson, 2007).

Lateral Positioning or Change in Position

Lateral positioning alters the relationship between the umbilical cord, fetal parts, and the uterine wall, and is usually performed to minimize or correct umbilical cord compression and decrease the frequency of uterine contractions. In a lateral position, the uterus does not compress the vena cava or aorta; thus, maternal cardiac return and cardiac output are maximized, and blood flow to the uterus is optimal (ACOG, 2010; Clark et al., 1991; Freeman, Garite, Nageotte, & Miller, 2012). Several studies have compared the effects of right lateral, left lateral, and supine maternal positions on fetal oxygen status; the findings of each suggest that lateral positioning on either side is more favorable for enhancing fetal oxygenation when compared with a supine position (Aldrich et al., 1995; Carbonne, Benachi, Leveque, Cabrol, & Papiernik, 1996; Simpson & James, 2005b). When compared with supine positioning, upright and lateral positions are associated with fewer "nonreassuring" FHR characteristics (Abitbol, 1985; Gupta, Hofmeyr, & Shehmar, 2012). A lateral position or a change in position can resolve or decrease the severity of late, variable, and/or prolonged decelerations (Abitbol, 1985; Freeman et al., 2012). Lateral positioning may also modify or eliminate late decelerations if the etiology is decreased uterine blood flow (usually secondary to supine positioning and inferior vena caval compression) (Abitbol, 1985; Freeman et al., 2012). The supine position should be avoided in general to prevent compression of the vena cava and supine hypotensive syndrome. When indeterminate or abnormal FHR patterns are occurring, changing maternal position to where the FHR pattern is most improved is typically an effective therapeutic strategy (Freeman et al., 2012; Garite & Simpson, 2011).

Reduction of Uterine Activity

Care should be taken to maintain appropriate intervals between contractions by avoiding tachysystole and using timely measures to reduce uterine activity when it occurs. Normal contraction frequency in the active phase of labor is every 2–3 minutes (ACOG, 2003). Assessments of maternal pain, coping, and uterine tenderness also contribute to the interpretation of uterine activity but are not required to make a determination of excessive uterine activity or tachysystole. *Hypertonus* generally refers to uterine resting tone above 20–25 mmHg.

Uterine activity is determined by the number of contractions present in a 10-minute period, averaged over 30 minutes (ACOG, 2009b, 2010; Macones et al., 2008):

- Normal: $\leq$5 contractions in 10 minutes.
- Tachysystole: $>$5 contractions in 10 minutes. Tachysystole is further qualified by the presence or absence of associated FHR decelerations.

This definition is primarily based on expert opinion, as there are only a few published studies in the literature evaluating the effects of uterine activity on fetal well-being. Although fetal assessment during labor has been the subject of numerous research studies, uterine activity assessment has received much less attention in the literature. Quantification of uterine activity as it relates to labor progress and fetal status has not been well studied. This gap in knowledge presents a challenge for determining the level of appropriate uterine activity during labor to effect normal labor progress when using pharmacologic agents to stimulate uterine contractions, as well as the limits of uterine activity to ensure ongoing fetal well-being during labor.

In the past, some clinicians have reserved the term *tachysystole* for a contraction frequency of >5 contractions in 10 minutes with evidence that the fetus is not tolerating this contraction pattern, as demonstrated by late decelerations or fetal bradycardia. Definitions of tachysystole that include evidence of category II or III FHR changes are not clinically appropriate because such definitions may delay interventions to reduce uterine activity while fetal status is threatened. Some clinicians have included the woman's perception of pain in their determination of tachysystole; however, this factor is not a reliable indicator of the potential physiologic implications of the frequency, duration, and intensity of uterine contractions (Simpson, 2013; Simpson & Miller, 2011).

Tachysystole can result in a progressive adverse effect on fetal oxygenation (Bakker, Kurver, Kuik, & Van Geijn, 2007; Simpson & James, 2008). Evidence suggests that *less than five* contractions in 10 minutes may be optimal for supporting fetal well-being (Bakker et al., 2007; Simpson & James, 2008). Uterine contractions cause an intermittent decrease in blood flow to the intervillous space where oxygen exchange occurs. If this intermittent interruption of blood flow reaches an abnormal level as a result of too-frequent contractions, the fetus is at risk for hypoxemia (ACOG & AAP, 2014). When fetal oxygenation is sufficiently impaired to produce metabolic acidosis from anaerobic glycolysis, direct myocardial depression occurs (ACOG & AAP, 2014). As fetal deterioration progresses, the fetus will likely respond with late decelerations and the FHR will lose variability and reactivity (ACOG & AAP, 2014). The more time between contractions, the more time there is to maximally perfuse the placenta and deliver oxygen to the fetus (Caldeyro-Barcia, 1992; Freeman et al., 2012).

As a contraction begins, the fetus uses the reservoir of oxygen (fetal reserve) in the intervillous space; restricted blood flow prevents complete recovery until some time after the contraction when full oxygenation has been restored (Paternoster, Micaglio, Tambuscio, Bracciante, & Chiarenza, 2001). In most healthy fetuses, the physiologic effects of intermittent contractions of normal labor are well tolerated (Paternoster et al., 2001). Earlier research concerning the effects of uterine contractions on fetal oxygen saturation ($FSpO_2$) found that $FSpO_2$ decreased during contractions, reaching the lowest level 92 seconds after the peak of the contraction, with approximately 90 seconds required for $FSpO_2$ to return to normal levels (McNamara & Johnson, 1995). When contractions are occurring every 2 minutes or more, recovery of $FSpO_2$ to previous baseline levels is incomplete (Johnson et al., 1994). The $FSpO_2$ decreases incrementally after each contraction, and the fetus becomes hypoxemic, recovering only when oxytocin is discontinued (Johnson, van Oudgaarden, Montague, & McNamara, 1994). Comparable effects of too-frequent contractions on fetal oxygen levels were noted by Peebles et al. (1994). Contraction intervals of less than 2–3 minutes are less favorable on fetal cerebral oxygen saturation when compared with longer contraction intervals. Peebles et al. (1994) concluded that contractions occurring repeatedly at intervals less than 2–3 minutes were likely to result in progressive fetal cerebral desaturation.

Bakker et al. (2007) studied uterine activity involving 1,433 labors and births and found five or more contractions in 10 minutes during the last hour of the first stage of labor was significantly associated with a higher incidence of neonatal acidemia (umbilical arterial pH $\leq$ 7.11) at birth when compared to contractions that were less frequent. Simpson and James (2008) found five or more contractions in 10 minutes over a 30-minute period during first-stage labor was associated with a 20% decrease in fetal oxygen saturation while six or more contractions in the same period was associated with a 29%

decrease. When contractions were fewer than five in 10 minutes over a 30-minute period, there was no change in fetal oxygen saturation. Significantly more "nonreassuring" fetal heart rate (FHR) changes, such as absent and minimal variability and late and recurrent decelerations were also noted when contractions were more than five in 10 minutes as compared to periods when contractions were less frequent (Simpson & James, 2008). These findings are consistent with the earlier studies suggesting contraction intervals closer than every 2–3 minutes are associated with progressive fetal oxygen desaturation. In a more recent study of 50,335 births over a 28-month period in a single hospital system, tachysystole was found in 10.65% (n = 5363) of EFM tracings (Heuser et al., 2013). The majority of patients with tachysystole had only one event of tachysystole, which lasted on average approximately 1 hour (Heuser et al., 2013). Tachysystole was associated with an increased risk of neonatal morbidity as measured by a composite neonatal outcome including sepsis, intraventricular hemorrhage, necrotizing entercolitis, pneumothorax, and 5-minute Apgar score <7 (Heuser et al., 2013).

More research from well-designed studies with adequate sample sizes are needed to guide clinical practice with regard to safe and appropriate levels of uterine activity during labor induction and augmentation. While tachysystole can be the result of endogenous maternal oxytocin and prostaglandins, most tachysystole results from administration of exogenous pharmacologic agents. Tachysystole alone and tachysystole accompanied by FHR changes are more common during cervical ripening and labor induction than during spontaneous labor (Crane, Young, Butt, Bennett, & Hutchens, 2001; Heuser et al., 2013).

Reduction of uterine activity can occur either by decreasing or discontinuing the oxytocin infusion, having the mother assume a lateral position, and/or administering an intravenous fluid bolus of lactated Ringer's solution (ACOG, 2010; Freeman et al., 2012; SOGC, 2007). Simpson and James (2008) found that simultaneous initiation of all three interventions resolved oxytocin-induced tachysystole more rapidly than when used individually, as follows:

- Oxytocin discontinuation: resolution = 14.2 minutes
- Oxytocin discontinuation + an IV fluid bolus of at least 500 mL of lactated Ringer's solution: resolution = 9.8 minutes
- Oxytocin discontinuation + an IV fluid bolus of at least 500 mL of lactated Ringer's solution + change to lateral position: resolution = 6.1 minutes

From the perspective of fetal safety, interventions for tachysystole should not be delayed until the FHR exhibits indeterminate or abnormal findings (Simpson, 2008, 2013). Late decelerations are a frequent result of excessive stimulation of contractions with oxytocin (Caldeyro-Barcia, 1992; Freeman et al., 2012; Shenker, 1973). If FHR decelerations occur with tachysystole, reduction of contraction activity will optimize fetal oxygenation (ACOG, 2010; Freeman et al., 2012). When the FHR pattern is abnormal or indeterminate with recurrent late, variable, or prolonged decelerations, oxytocin should be discontinued. The next dose of pharmacologic agents used to ripen the cervix or stimulate contractions should be delayed until uterine activity and FHR patterns return to normal (Simpson, 2013).

Although tachysystole should be identified and treated in a timely manner, its effects on the fetus based on the FHR characteristics can be used to guide the interventions chosen. A suggested clinical protocol for interventions during tachysystole with and without FHR changes is presented in Table 6-2. Each component of this suggested protocol is based on one or more of the following: the physiologic effects of oxytocin on maternal-fetal status, limited available evidence on interventions for tachysystole, promulgated professional practice guidelines, and the opinions of experts (ACOG & AAP, 2014; ACOG, 2010; Arias, 2000; Bakker et al., 2007; Bakker & van Geijn, 2008; Caldeyro-Barcia, 1992; Freeman et al., 2012; Johnson et al., 1994;

TABLE 6-2 Suggested Clinical Protocol for Oxytocin-Induced Tachysystole

OXYTOCIN-INDUCED TACHYSYSTOLE (NORMAL FHR)
• Assist the mother to a lateral position. • Give IV fluid bolus of at least 500 mL lactated Ringer's solution as indicated. • If uterine activity has not returned to normal after 10–15 minutes, decrease oxytocin rate by at least half; if uterine activity has not returned to normal after 10–15 more minutes, discontinue oxytocin until uterine activity is less than five contractions in 10 minutes. • To resume oxytocin after resolution of tachysystole: If oxytocin has been discontinued for less than 20–30 minutes, the FHR is normal, and contraction frequency, intensity, and duration are normal, resume oxytocin at no more than half the rate that caused the tachysystole and gradually increase the rate as appropriate based on unit protocol and maternal-fetal status. If the oxytocin is discontinued for more than 30–40 minutes, resume oxytocin at the initial dose ordered.
OXYTOCIN-INDUCED TACHYSYSTOLE (INDETERMINATE OR ABNORMAL FHR)
• Discontinue oxytocin. • Assist the mother to a lateral position. • Give IV fluid bolus of at least 500 mL of lactated Ringer's solution as indicated. • Consider oxygen at 10 L/min via nonrebreather face mask (discontinue as soon as possible based on the FHR pattern). • If no response, consider 0.25 mg terbutaline SQ. • To resume oxytocin after resolution of tachysystole: If oxytocin has been discontinued for less than 20–30 minutes, the FHR is normal, and contraction frequency, intensity, and duration are normal, resume oxytocin at no more than half the rate that caused the tachysystole and gradually increase the rate as appropriate based on unit protocol and maternal-fetal status. If the oxytocin is discontinued for more than 30–40 minutes, resume oxytocin at the initial dose ordered.

Note: IV, intravenous; SQ, subcutaneous.
Adapted from "Labor and birth" by K. R. Simpson & N. O'Brien-Abel. In K. R. Simpson & P. A. Creehan (Eds.), *AWHONN's perinatal nursing* (4th ed., pp. 343–444). Copyright 2013 by the Association of Women's Health, Obstetric and Neonatal Nurses.

Leduc, Biringer, Lee, & Dy, 2013; Peebles et al., 1994; Seitchik, Amico, Robinson, & Castillo, 1984; Simpson, 2008; Simpson & James, 2008). Thus, the components of the suggested protocol individually and collectively have not been rigorously evaluated in a prospective clinical trial and should be viewed as guidelines to be used in conjunction with independent professional judgment.

When tachysystole occurs or fetal status is such that oxytocin is discontinued, data are limited to guide the decision regarding the timing and dosage of subsequent IV oxytocin administration. Physiologic and pharmacologic principles may be used to determine the most appropriate dosage. If oxytocin has been discontinued for less than 20–30 minutes, the FHR is normal, and contraction frequency, intensity, and duration are normal, a suggested protocol may include restarting oxytocin at least at a lower rate of infusion than before the tachysystole occurred. In this clinical situation, many practitioners restart the infusion at half the rate that caused the tachystole and gradually increase the rate as appropriate based on unit protocol and maternal-fetal status. However, if the oxytocin is discontinued for more than 30–40 minutes, most of the exogenous oxytocin is metabolized and plasma levels are similar to that of a woman who has not received IV oxytocin (Seitchik et al., 1984). In this clinical situation, a suggested protocol may include restarting the oxytocin at or near the initial dose ordered. There are individual differences in myometrial sensitivity and the response to oxytocin during labor (Arias, 2000; Smith & Merrill, 2006; Ulmsten, 1997). It may be necessary to use a lower dose and lengthen the interval between dosage increases when there is evidence of the patient's previous sensitivity to the drug.

Administration of tocolytics is another option that is occasionally used as a temporary measure to provide intrauterine resuscitation for a prolonged deceleration, or for other indeterminate or abnormal FHR patterns resulting from tachystole, by reducing uterine activity (ACOG, 2010; Caldeyro-Barcia, 1992). It is presumed that the reduction in uterine activity as the result of tocolytic administration may improve uteroplacental blood flow, thereby improving fetal oxygenation (Pullen et al., 2007). A subcutaneous dose of terbutaline 0.25 mg is often used for this purpose; however, there are only limited supportive data regarding terbutaline or other tocolytics as an intervention for intrauterine resuscitation. Nitroglycerine is used in some institutions for intrauterine resuscitation; however, when compared with terbutaline, nitroglycerine results in a significant decrease in maternal mean arterial blood pressure and is less effective as a tocolytic in reducing uterine activity (Pullen et al., 2007). According to the latest Cochrane Review (three studies included), betamimetic therapy appears to be able to reduce the number of FHR abnormalities; however, there is not enough evidence based on clinically important outcomes to evaluate the use of these medications for suspected fetal compromise (Kulier & Hofmeyr, 2000).

One strategy to prevent tachysystole is to use a physiologic dosage regimen for oxytocin induction and augmentation (ACOG, 2009a; NCC-WCH, 2007). Beginning at 1–2 milliunits per minute and increasing by 1–2 milliunits per minute no more frequently than every 30–40 minutes will minimize risk of oxytocin side effects. A meta-analysis of low-dose versus high-dose oxytocin for labor induction by Crane and Young (1998) found that this type of protocol resulted in fewer episodes of excessive uterine activity, fewer operative vaginal births, a higher rate of spontaneous vaginal birth, and a lower rate of cesarean birth. The side effects of oxytocin are generally dose related; tachysystole and FHR tracings that are indeterminate (category II) or abnormal (category III) are the most common side effects (ACOG, 2009a). Low-dose oxytocin protocols and longer intervals between increases in the oxytocin rate are associated with less tachysystole with related FHR changes (ACOG, 2009a).

Intravenous Fluid Administration

When a pregnant woman is hypovolemic or hypotensive, blood volume is shifted away from the uterus, decreasing uteroplacental perfusion and oxygen delivery to the fetus. It is believed that administration of fluids maximizes maternal intravascular volume and is therefore protective against decreases in uteroplacental perfusion. A reduction in uterine blood flow can occur following administration of regional anesthesia because the sympathectomy causes dilation of peripheral vessels, lower peripheral resistance, and a potential drop in uteroplacental blood flow. There are data to suggest that increasing IV fluids will positively affect uterine blood flow and thus fetal oxygenation, even in women who are normotensive and well hydrated. One study found that $FSpO_2$ was significantly increased after at least a 500-mL bolus of lactated Ringer's solution over 20 minutes in normotensive women who were otherwise receiving lactated Ringer's solution at 125 mL per hour (Simpson & James, 2005b). The increase in $FSpO_2$ was greatest with a 1000-mL IV fluid bolus. The positive effects on fetal oxygen status continued for more than 30 minutes after the IV fluid bolus (Simpson & James, 2005b). Thus, an IV fluid bolus of 500–1000 mL may be useful as an intrauterine resuscitation technique. However, caution should be exercised when increasing IV fluids or giving repeated IV fluid boluses. It is important to remember that some clinical situations such as preeclampsia, preterm labor treated with magnesium sulfate, or preterm labor treated with corticosteroids and beta-sympathomimetic medications carry an increased risk for pulmonary edema that might necessitate fluid restriction. Oxytocin has an antidiuretic effect, so prolonged use can also lead to fluid overload if IV fluids are used too liberally. An extreme effect of fluid overload related to excessive use of oxytocin is water intoxication.

Some clinicians believe that IV solutions containing glucose can improve FHR variability; however, there is no supportive evidence for this practice. Intravenous fluid boluses of glucose-containing solutions should generally be avoided because there is evidence to suggest that maternal IV administration of glucose can have potentially detrimental effects on fetal status, including increased fetal lactate and decreased fetal pH

(Phillipson, Kalihan, Riha, & Pimental, 1987; Wasserstrum, 1992). If the fetus is hypoxemic (a possibility when the FHR is indeterminate or abnormal), relatively small elevations in glucose can lead to lactic acidosis (Phillipson et al., 1987; Wasserstrum, 1992). IV solutions with glucose can cause fetal hyperglycemia and subsequent reactive hypoglycemia, hyperinsulinism, acidosis, jaundice, and transient tachypnea in the newborn after birth (Carmen, 1986; Dumoulin & Foulkes, 1984; Grylack, Chu, & Scanlon, 1984; Kenepp et al., 1982; Mendiola, Grylack, & Scanlon, 1982; Romney & Gabel, 1966; Singhi, 1988; Sleutel & Golden, 1999; Sommer, Norr, & Roberts, 2000). A bolus of IV solution containing glucose also can cause marked maternal hyperglycemia (Mendiola et al., 1982; Wasserstrum, 1992). Thus, when the clinical situation is such that a bolus of IV fluids may be necessary to rapidly expand plasma volume for the woman in labor, the research indicates that these IV fluids should not contain glucose, especially if birth is imminent (American College of Nurse-Midwives [ACNM], 2008; Cerri et al., 2000; Simpson & O'Brien-Abel, 2013).

As a preventative measure, adequate hydration in labor should be maintained (Garite & Simpson, 2011). Labor can be compared to sustained exercise during which participants do not ingest adequate amounts of fluid and become clinically dehydrated (ACNM, 2008; Freeman et al., 2012). The increased insensible fluid loss associated with labor has the potential to lead to a decrease in intravascular volume if fluid replacement is inadequate, which can result in a decrease in uterine blood flow (Garite, Weeks, Peters-Phair, Pattillo, & Brewster, 2000). Although oral hydration may be appropriate for most healthy women during labor (ACNM, 2008), IV replacement fluids often are provided simultaneously. Findings from two studies suggest that the usual amount of IV fluids of 125 mL per hour may not be sufficient to support adequate labor hydration (Eslamian, Marsoosi, & Pakneeyat, 2006; Garite et al., 2000). In these randomized clinical trials, women who received 250 mL per hour of IV fluids had shorter labors and were less likely to require oxytocin augmentation than women who received 125 mL per hour.

Oxygen Administration

Maternal oxygen therapy is commonly used for intrauterine resuscitation and appears to be beneficial in improving fetal oxygen status during labor. In a classic study of the effects of maternal oxygen administration on the fetus, 100% oxygen via face mask corrected "nonreassuring" FHR patterns by decreasing the baseline FHR during fetal tachycardia and reducing or eliminating late decelerations (Althabe, Schwarcz, Pose, Escarcena, & Caldeyro-Barcia, 1967). There is evidence that fetal oxygen levels will increase as a result of maternal oxygen administration of 10 L per minute via nonrebreather face mask (Aldrich, Wyatt, Spencer, Reynolds, & Delpy, 1994; Bartnicki & Saling, 1994; Dildy, Clark, Loucks, van den Berg, & Jongsma, 1995; Haydon et al., 2006; McNamara, Johnson, & Lilford, 1993; Simpson & James, 2005b). Fetuses with lower oxygen saturation appear to achieve the greatest increase in oxygen levels with maternal oxygen administration (Haydon et al., 2006; Simpson & James, 2005b).

Although healthy women in labor have nearly 100% SpO_2 (usually between 96% and 99%), increasing inspired oxygen increases blood oxygen tension and results in more oxygen delivered to the fetus (McNamara et al., 1993). There is a more rapid increase in $FSpO_2$ when oxygen is given as compared with the decrease in $FSpO_2$ when it is discontinued, suggesting that the fetus responds to the new placental oxygen gradient by accepting oxygen more rapidly than it gives it up. In two studies, $FSpO_2$ levels higher than those preceding administration of oxygen to the mother persisted 30 minutes after the oxygen was discontinued (Dildy et al., 1995; Simpson & James, 2005b). Fetal hemoglobin has a higher affinity for oxygen than adult hemoglobin, and fetal hematocrit is higher than that of adults. These physiologic factors allow for a steeper increase in fetal oxygen concentration and $FSpO_2$ during maternal oxygen therapy.

The method that provides the highest fraction of inspired oxygen (FiO_2) should be used when oxygen is administered to the mother. The nonrebreather face mask works best because the FiO_2 at 10 L per minute is approximately 80–100%, as compared with a simple face mask (FiO_2 27%–40%) or nasal cannula (FiO_2 31%) (Simpson & James, 2005b).

There is scant evidence concerning how long maternal oxygen therapy should be continued and its effects on the mother and fetus (Simpson, 2008). Both *hypo*xia and *hyper*oxia can result in production of oxygen-free radicals, which can cause oxidative stress and subsequent adverse effects such as damage to cell membranes, cell structures, and cellular lipoproteins and DNA (Klinger, Beyene, Shah, & Perlman, 2005). These effects are more pronounced when oxygen is reintroduced after a period of hypoxia and are thought to be the genesis of reperfusion injuries in the newborn (Blackburn, 2006; Khaw & Ngan Kee, 2004; Klinger et al., 2005). The newborn's brain is particularly vulnerable to oxidative stress because neuronal membranes are rich in polyunsaturated fatty acids and have a relative deficiency of several important antioxidant enzymes (Blackburn, 2006). Antioxidants are normal physiologic defense mechanisms that delay or prevent oxidative stress and formation of free radicals or damaging by-products; however, these defenses are limited in newborns, especially preterm babies, because of lowered intracellular antioxidant enzymes and other defense systems (Blackburn, 2005, 2006).

Data regarding the potential deleterious effects of hyperoxia on newborns during resuscitation at birth and in the first few hours of life (Klinger et al., 2005; Vento et al., 2001, 2003) prompted the neonatal experts who develop guidelines for neonatal resuscitation to make changes in their recommendations for care for depressed babies at birth in 2006 and 2011 (AAP & American Heart Association [AHA], 2011). Room air (21% FiO_2) is now considered the preferred initial alternative to 100% oxygen for neonatal resuscitation in selected clinical situations and for preterm babies. Titration of FiO_2 to the resultant oxygen saturation of the baby using a pulse oximeter and blended oxygen is recommended when oxygen is administered for neonatal resuscitation. Findings from later studies have confirmed the potential adverse effects of oxygen for the extremely preterm baby and illustrated the clinical challenges of determining the most effective therapeutic dose without causing harm (SUPPORT Study Group of the Eunice Kennedy Shriver NICHD Neonatal Research Network et al., 2010). Damage to the baby from the oxidative stress produced by high levels of oxygen and associated oxygen-free radical activity and its by-products may be minimized by these techniques (AAP & AHA, 2011). However, it remains uncertain whether oxidative stress has a causal role or is merely a consequence of the physiologic sequelae associated with hypoxia and asphyxia (Blackburn, 2006; Higgins, Bancalari, Willinger, & Raju, 2007).

Although transfer of oxygen from the mother to the fetus via passive diffusion as well as placental equilibrium prevent fetal hyperoxia as a result of maternal oxygen administration (Khaw & Ngan Kee, 2004), even small increases in maternal and fetal PO_2 as a result of maternal oxygen administration can produce oxygen-free radical activity in mothers and their fetuses (Khaw, Wang, Ngan Kee, Pang, & Rogers, 2002). The potential long-term effects on the mother and fetus are unknown. Only one human study has involved measurement of by-products of oxygen-free radical activity in mothers and fetuses after mothers at term were given oxygen prior to birth (Khaw et al., 2002). In this study, 22 women were randomized to receive oxygen at 60% FiO_2 prior to cesarean birth (mean oxygen exposure, 53 minutes; range, 33–150 minutes), compared with a control group of 22 women who did not receive oxygen. Levels of by-products of oxygen-free radical activity in the mothers were noted within 10 minutes of maternal oxygen administration, peaked at 30 minutes, and continued to be detected at abnormally high ranges throughout the 60 minutes of monitoring. Levels of oxygen-free radical activity also were noted in the umbilical arterial and venous cord blood at birth of fetuses whose mothers received 60% oxygen at levels significantly higher than the control group (Khaw et al., 2002). There is evidence that some by-products of oxygen-free radical activity cross the placenta, whereas others do not (Rogers, Mongelli, Tsang, & Wang, 1999).

Conversely, fetal hypoxia and acidemia (umbilical artery pH < 7.15; base excess < -8) during labor also have been shown to cause abnormally elevated levels of by-products of oxygen-free radical activity (Rogers et al., 1997). Based on the research, withholding oxygen from mothers in labor when the FHR pattern is indeterminate or abnormal to prevent possible adverse effects of oxygen-free radicals is not recommended. The potential effects of progressive fetal hypoxemia and acidemia have been demonstrated (ACOG & AAP, 2014), so clinical interventions to avoid these conditions are warranted (Simpson, 2008). Oxygen therapy via the mother to the fetus can be beneficial in increasing fetal oxygen levels (Aldrich et al., 1994; Dildy et al., 1995; Haydon et al., 2006; McNamara et al., 1993; Simpson & James, 2005b); however, prolonged use should be discouraged until more data are available regarding the potential risks to the mother and fetus (NCCWCH, 2007). If other intrauterine resuscitation techniques have not resulted in resolution of the FHR pattern, maternal oxygen therapy has been shown to be reasonable (Dildy et al., 1995; Haydon et al., 2006; Simpson & James, 2005b). However, oxygen should be discontinued as soon as possible based on the fetal response. Much more data are needed on the effects of longer periods of maternal oxygen administration on the mother and baby (Simpson, 2008). When oxygen is chosen for intrauterine resuscitation, it is assumed that other sources of potential fetal physiologic stress have been minimized; thus, oxytocin should not be infusing concurrently with maternal oxygen administration.

Interventions for Anesthesia-Related Hypotension

Conduction anesthetics increase the risk of decreased placental blood flow secondary to maternal hypotension resulting from sympathetic blockade. If maternal repositioning and IV fluid bolus are not successful in resolving FHR changes, ephedrine may be given to increase vascular tone and thus maternal blood pressure (ACOG, 2005). Ephedrine is the usual agent and has not been found to be associated with adverse fetal outcomes, although it does cross the placenta (Freeman et al., 2012; Miller, Miller, & Tucker, 2013; Wong, 2009).

Amnioinfusion

Amnioinfusion, the transcervical instillation of fluid into the amniotic cavity, is a reasonable therapeutic option to attempt to resolve recurrent variable FHR decelerations by correcting umbilical cord compression resulting from decreased amniotic fluid or oligohydramnios (ACOG, 2006, 2010). Rupture of amniotic membranes is required. Amnioinfusion has been found to significantly resolve patterns of "moderate to severe" variable decelerations but does not affect late decelerations or patterns with absent variability (Hofmeyr & Lawrie, 2012; Mino, Puertas, Miranda, & Herruzo, 1999; Miyazaki & Nevarez, 1985). Amnioinfusion may be used in the presence of recurrent variable decelerations in first-stage labor that have been unresolved with maternal position changes.

Although amnioinfusion has been shown to dilute thick, meconium-stained amniotic fluid and decrease the incidence of meconium below the newborn's vocal cords (Klingner & Kruse, 1999; Pierce, Gaudier, & Sanchez-Ramos, 2000), in a large international study of 1,998 women in term labor, amnioinfusion did not reduce risk of moderate or severe meconium aspiration syndrome or perinatal death (Fraser et al., 2005). Based on available evidence, amnioinfusion is no longer recommended as an intervention for meconium-stained fluid (ACOG, 2006, 2010).

Amnioinfusion does not seem to affect the length of labor (Strong, 1997) and appears to be safe for women who are attempting a vaginal birth after a previous cesarean birth (Hicks, 2005; Ouzounian, Miller, & Paul, 1996). Prophylactic amnioinfusion for oligohydramnios is not necessary and has not been shown to prevent the development of variable decelerations (Hofmeyr & Lawrie, 2007). Because of its efficacy in resolving variable decelerations, risk of cesarean birth related to a "nonreassuring" FHR pattern may be decreased with amnioinfusion (Hofmeyr & Lawrie, 2007). Based on available evidence, amnioinfusion should be limited to the management of variable decelerations (ACOG, 2006). Contraindications may include vaginal bleeding, uterine anomalies, and active infection such as human immunodeficiency virus or herpes simplex virus. Careful monitoring and documentation of fluid infused is important to avoid iatrogenic polyhydramnios (Box 6-1).

BOX 6-1 Amnioinfusion

Amnioinfusion is a reasonable therapeutic option when there are recurrent variable decelerations as a result of a decrease in amniotic fluid (ACOG, 2006, 2010; Hofmeyr & Lawrie, 2012).

An institutional protocol may include the following:

- Contraindications (e.g., vaginal bleeding, uterine anomalies, active infections such as HIV or herpes, impending birth)
- Who can perform amnioinfusion
- Who can insert the intrauterine pressure catheter
- What type of fluid may be used (normal saline or lactated Ringer's solution)
- What instillation method may be used (gravity flow or infusion pump)
- What infusion techniques may be used (bolus, continuous, or a combination of both)
- When and why the procedure should be altered (e.g., loss of large amount of fluid resulting from position change or coughing, increased uterine resting tone, reappearance of variable decelerations, or no fluid return)

General guidelines for the procedure are as follows:

- The amnioinfusion procedure and the indication should be explained to the woman and her support persons prior to initiation.
- During amnioinfusion, room temperature normal saline or lactated Ringer's solution is infused into the uterus transcervically via an intrauterine pressure catheter.
- The initial bolus is usually 250–500 mL given over a 20- to 30-minute period using either an infusion pump or gravity flow. Both methods are appropriate and seem to be equally efficacious.
- Some protocols allow for a continuous infusion of 2–3 mL per minute (120–180 mL per hour) after the bolus until resolution of the variable decelerations (Miller et al., 2013). Usually the maximal amount of fluid infused is 1000 mL (Miller et al, 2013.).
- If variable decelerations have not resolved after infusion of 800-1000 mL, the infusion may be discontinued and alternative approaches used (Miller et al., 2013).
- During bolus of the infusion and maintenance rate, approximate amount of fluid returning should be noted and recorded to avoid iatrogenic polyhydramnios.
- Assessment of fluid return can be accomplished by weighing the underpads (1 mL of fluid equals ≈ 1 gram of weight) (Miller et al., 2013).
- As a general consideration, if 250 mL has infused with no return, the amnioinfusion is discontinued until the fluid has returned.
- Overdistention is more likely when the presenting part obstructs flow, thus releasing the fluid by gently elevating the presenting part may be a successful intervention.
- A dual-lumen intrauterine catheter is preferred so that estimate of uterine resting tone can be assessed during the infusion.
- Uterine resting tone may appear higher than normal during the procedure (from 25 to 40 mmHg). If there is a concern about an elevated uterine resting tone (>40 mmHg), temporarily discontinue the infusion to attempt a more accurate assessment. If the uterine resting tone exceeds 25 mmHg while the infusion is temporarily discontinued for assessment of uterine resting tone, consider discontinuing the infusion.
- Warming of the solution may not be necessary for full-term fetuses but may be appropriate for preterm or growth-restricted fetuses. Fetal bradycardia may occur if the solution is colder than room temperature and/or is infused too rapidly (Miller et al., 2013). Some providers prefer to warm the solution to body temperature. If the solution is warmed, acceptable temperatures are 93–96° F (34–37° C). The safest method to warm the solution is by use of an electronic blood/fluid warmer. Microwaves and other types of warming techniques should not be used to heat the solution.

BOX 6-1 (Continued)

- Assessment and documentation:
  - Contraction intensity and frequency should be continually assessed during the procedure.
  - In addition to assessments appropriate for the first stage of labor, additional assessments may include:
    - Fundal height and leakage of fluids
    - Amount, color, and odor of fluid leaking from vagina
    - Fetal response such as resolution of the variable decelerations
- Documentation may include the maternal and fetal response; uterine resting tone; fluid output; and type, rate, and amount of solution infused.

Note: FHR, fetal heart rate; HIV, human immunodeficiency virus.

Modification of Maternal Pushing Efforts during Second-Stage Labor

Indeterminate or abnormal FHR patterns may occur during the second stage of labor. The continuation of coached pushing in the presence of these FHR patterns can lead to iatrogenic fetal stress as evidenced by recurrent variable or prolonged decelerations, loss of normal baseline, minimal or absent variability, tachycardia, and bradycardia (Freeman et al., 2013). Although most fetuses tolerate decelerations during pushing, some fetuses enter the second stage of labor with less physiologic reserve than others. The active pushing phase of the second stage of labor is the most physiologically stressful part of labor for the fetus (Piquard, Schaefer, Hsiung, Dellenbach, & Haberey, 1989; Roberts, 2002). When compared with the passive fetal descent phase, the active pushing phase results in more FHR decelerations (Hansen, Clark, & Foster, 2002; Piquard et al., 1988; Simpson & James, 2005a) and a progressive adverse effect on fetal acid-base status (Nordstrom, Achanna, Nuka, & Arulkumaran, 2001) and $FSpO_2$ (Simpson & James, 2005a). Shortening the active pushing phase by delaying pushing until maternal urge to push can promote fetal well-being (Hansen et al., 2002; Nordstrom et al., 2001; Piquard et al., 1988; Simpson & James, 2005a). Prolonged active pushing may have a negative effect on fetal status and the condition of the baby at birth (Piquard et al., 1988).

Fetal assessment data (either from electronic fetal monitoring or intermittent auscultation) should be used to guide maternal pushing efforts and to minimize the risk of iatrogenic negative FHR changes. There is ample evidence that fetal status in the last 1–2 hours prior to birth has significant implications on neonatal well-being at birth (Heuser et al., 2013; Jackson et al., 2011). "Abnormal" FHR characteristics (variable and late decelerations and bradycardia) during second-stage labor are associated with higher rates of operative vaginal birth, Apgar scores lower than 7 at 1 minute, umbilical artery pH < 7.2, and admission to the neonatal intensive care unit (NICU) when compared with "normal" FHR patterns (Sheiner et al., 2001). "Abnormal" changes (a decrease) in FHR variability in the last hour prior to birth are associated with an increased risk of fetal acidemia (umbilical artery pH < 7.05) compared with normal variability (Siira et al., 2005). ("Abnormal" and "normal" were used by the researchers to describe FHR patterns in the Sheiner et al. [2001] and Siira et al. [2005] studies, but these descriptions may not correspond precisely with the 2008 NICHD definitions of these terms.) Variable and late decelerations occurring with every one to two contractions in the 30 minutes prior to birth are associated with lower 1-minute and 5-minute Apgar scores, more cases of umbilical artery pH < 7.2, and more admissions to the NICU when compared with decelerations occurring less frequently during this time period (Kazandi, Sendag, Akercan, Terek, & Gundem, 2003). Minimal to absent variability, bradycardia, prolonged decelerations, and late decelerations with absence of accelerations in the last hour prior to birth are associated with significant fetal acidemia (umbilical artery pH < 7.0) (Williams & Galerneau, 2002, 2003). Recurrent late or variable decelerations and minimal variability with absence of accelerations in the 2 hours prior to birth are associated with fetal acidemia (umbilical artery pH < 7.1) (Sameshima & Ikenoue, 2005). Using a five-tiered FHR classification system to evaluate 2,472 EFM tracings of fetuses >35 weeks' gestation in the last 3 hours prior to birth, Elliot, Warrick, Graham, and Hamilton (2010) reported a positive association between the duration and severity of FHR tracings, suggesting fetal compromise and an increased risk of neonatal metabolic acidosis and neurologic morbidity. Jackson et al. (2011) found there was an association between neonatal morbidity (1- and 5-minute Apgar scores <7 and admission to the NICU) and the percentage of time the FHR pattern in the last 2 hours prior to birth was indeterminate (category II). As the percentage of time extended beyond 50% and beyond 75%, there were significant increases in babies with low Apgar scores and NICU admissions (Jackson et al., 2011). When decelerations are occurring with most contractions during the second stage of labor, the fetus is at risk for metabolic acidosis at birth (Hamilton, Warrick, Knox, O'Keeffe, & Garite, 2012). The higher the ratio of decelerations with contractions, the greater the risk (Hamilton et al., 2012).

Suggestions for care during second-stage labor to promote fetal well-being are presented in Box 6-2. Temporarily discontinuing pushing to allow the fetus to recover when the FHR is indeterminate or abnormal and limiting pushing to every other or every third contraction to maintain normal FHR characteristics can be effective methods to minimize risk of progressive fetal oxygen desaturation (Simpson & James, 2005a). Sustained coached closed-glottis pushing, that is, "take a deep breath and hold it for 10 to 15 seconds," and pushing more than four times with each contraction should be avoided (Association of Women's Health, Obstetric and Neonatal Nurses [AWHONN], 2008; Barnett & Humenick, 1982; Caldyro-Barcia et al., 1981; Simpson & James, 2005a). Instead, three to four pushing efforts per contraction lasting 6–8 seconds each is more appropriate for the mother and fetus (Figure 6-3) (AWHONN, 2008; Barnett & Humenick, 1982; Caldyro-Barcia et al., 1981; Roberts, 2002; Roberts & Hanson, 2007; Simpson & James, 2005a). A baseline FHR should be identifiable between contractions. Some fetuses develop metabolic acidemia if recurrent variable or late decelerations continue over a long period, especially if accompanied by tachysystole (Bakker et al., 2007; Kazandi et al., 2003). Sustained pushing efforts in the presence of an indeterminate or abnormal FHR pattern during second-stage labor characterized by recurrent late and/or variable decelerations, a rising baseline rate, and decreasing variability increase the risk of fetal harm, such as fetal hypoxic and ischemic injuries (Hamilton et al., 2012; Shifrin & Ater, 2006), and should be avoided.

BOX 6-2 Second-Stage Labor Care to Promote Fetal Well-Being

- For women with epidural anesthesia who do not feel the urge to push when they are completely dilated, consider delaying pushing until the urge to push is felt (up to 2 hours for nulliparous women and up to 1 hour for multiparous women).
- Discourage prolonged breath-holding. Instead, instruct the woman to bear down and allow her to choose whether or not to hold her breath while pushing.
- Discourage more than three pushing efforts with each contraction and more than 6-8 seconds of each pushing effort.
- Avoid counting to 10 to promote sustained breath-holding during pushing efforts.
- Take steps to maintain a normal FHR pattern while pushing. Maternal pushing efforts may need to be modified based on the FHR pattern. Push with every other or every third contraction if necessary to avoid recurrent FHR decelerations. Reposition as necessary for FHR decelerations.
- Avoid tachysystole during the second stage of labor.

Note: FHR, fetal heart rate.
Adapted from "Nursing care and management of the second stage of labor (Evidence-Based Clinical Practice Guideline, 2nd ed.)" by the Association of Women's Health, Obstetric and Neonatal Nurses. Copyright 2008 by the Association of Women's Health, Obstetric and Neonatal Nurses.

FIGURE 6-3 Coached Closed-Glottis (Valsalva) Pushing during the Second Stage of Labor: Effect on Maternal Hemodynamics and Fetal Status

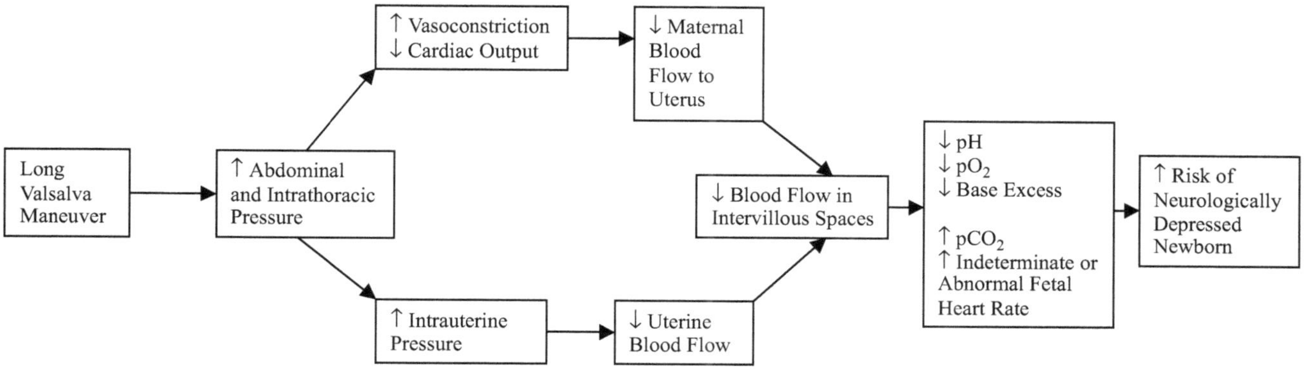

Adapted from "Infant outcome in relation to second stage labor pushing method." by M. M. Barnett and S. S. Humenick. 1982. *Birth and the Family Journal, 9*(4), p. 222. Copyright 1982 by Wiley Blackwell. Adapted with permission.

As a potential preventative measure, shortening the active pushing phase by delaying active pushing until the woman feels the urge to can mimimize fetal stress (Hansen et al., 2002; Piqard et al.,) 1989; Roberts, 2002; Simpson & James, 2008). In the absence of an urge to push, delaying pushing for up to 2 hours for nulliparous women and up to 1 hour for multiparous women is suggested with regional analgesia/anesthesia (Fraser et al., 2000; Hansen et al., 2002; Mayberry, Hammer, Kelly, True-Driver, & De, 1999; Simpson & James, 2008; Sprague et al., 2006). These guidelines are consistent with recommendations for labor management and diagnosis of failed induction and arrest disorders from the NICHD, the Society for Maternal-Fetal Medicine (SMFM), and ACOG (ACOG & SMFM, 2014; Spong, Berghella, Wenstrom, Mercer, & Saade, 2012). These guidelines suggest defining second-stage labor arrest as no progress (descent or rotation) for ≥4 hours in nulliparous women with an epidural, ≥3 hours in nulliparous women without an epidural, ≥3 hours in multiparous women with an epidural, and ≥2 hours in multiparous women without an epidural (Spong et al., 2012). Extending the expected time frame for birth to occur after the cervix is found to be 10 cm can allow adequate time for both passive fetal descent and active pushing, and promote vaginal birth given that there is evidence of fetal well-being.

Interventions to Support Coping and Labor Progress

In many modern labor and birth settings, nurses, physicians, and midwives are often pressed for time and caring for more than one woman simultaneously. It is important to maintain a caring connection with each individual woman and her family and to assess and respond to each woman's needs, desires, and potential risk factors. Asking women about their expectations, providing accurate information, maintaining open communication, and staying engaged with women and their families increases the woman's trust and sense of control, therefore supporting her coping and improving her overall perception of her birth experience. The following aspects of care during labor and birth may promote coping, labor progress, and a positive childbirth experience:

- Include the woman as a full partner in her care.
- Review plans/expectations with the woman and her partner, friends, or family members.
- Maintain a calm environment whenever possible.
- Include family members as per the desires of the woman.
- Remain at the bedside as much as possible and per the desires of the woman.
- Assess maternal and fetal status at the level appropriate for the woman.

- Encourage frequent position changes, especially to an upright position.
- Minimize use of technology as appropriate to the woman's clinical condition.
- Avoid unnecessary interventions.

SUMMARY

All members of the perinatal team should ideally have a common understanding of the physiologic and pathophysiologic characteristics of frequently occurring FHR patterns and shared expectations for how and when to intervene when FHR characteristics are indeterminate or abnormal (Fox, Kilpatrick, King, & Parer, 2000). Knowledge related to FHM is not exclusive to one discipline. Decisions regarding initial and subsequent interventions for indeterminate and abnormal FHR patterns should be individualized to each clinical situation on the basis of ongoing assessment and the maternal-fetal response. Although indeterminate or abnormal FHR patterns can develop at any time during labor despite excellent clinical care, in some cases, the need for intrauterine resuscitation may be the result of iatrogenic fetal compromise. Careful vigilance is required to avoid supine maternal positioning, hypotension, dehydration, oxytocin-induced tachysystole, elective amniotomy at high fetal station, and continued coached pushing when recurrent decelerations or abnormal FHR patterns are present. When FHR characteristics are suggestive of acute or evolving fetal compromise, members of the interdisciplinary perinatal team should remain composed and provide clear directions to the woman as well as other team members to decrease patient anxiety and promote an effective and timely team response. While explaining the situation to the woman and her support persons, a calm, factual, concise statement regarding the concerns about fetal status and the need to provide interventions to potentially resolve the condition may be beneficial. Ideally, an ongoing explanation is provided concurrent with the team efforts to improve fetal status.

A decision tree that addresses the issues of intrapartum goals, physiologic interventions, and the use of additional measures such as monitoring equipment modifications is offered in Figure 6-4. This decision tree provides a general process outline, which must be interpreted and modified as appropriate, in light of the perinatal team's clinical assessment of the mother and fetus.

FIGURE 6-4 Fetal Heart Monitoring Decision Tree

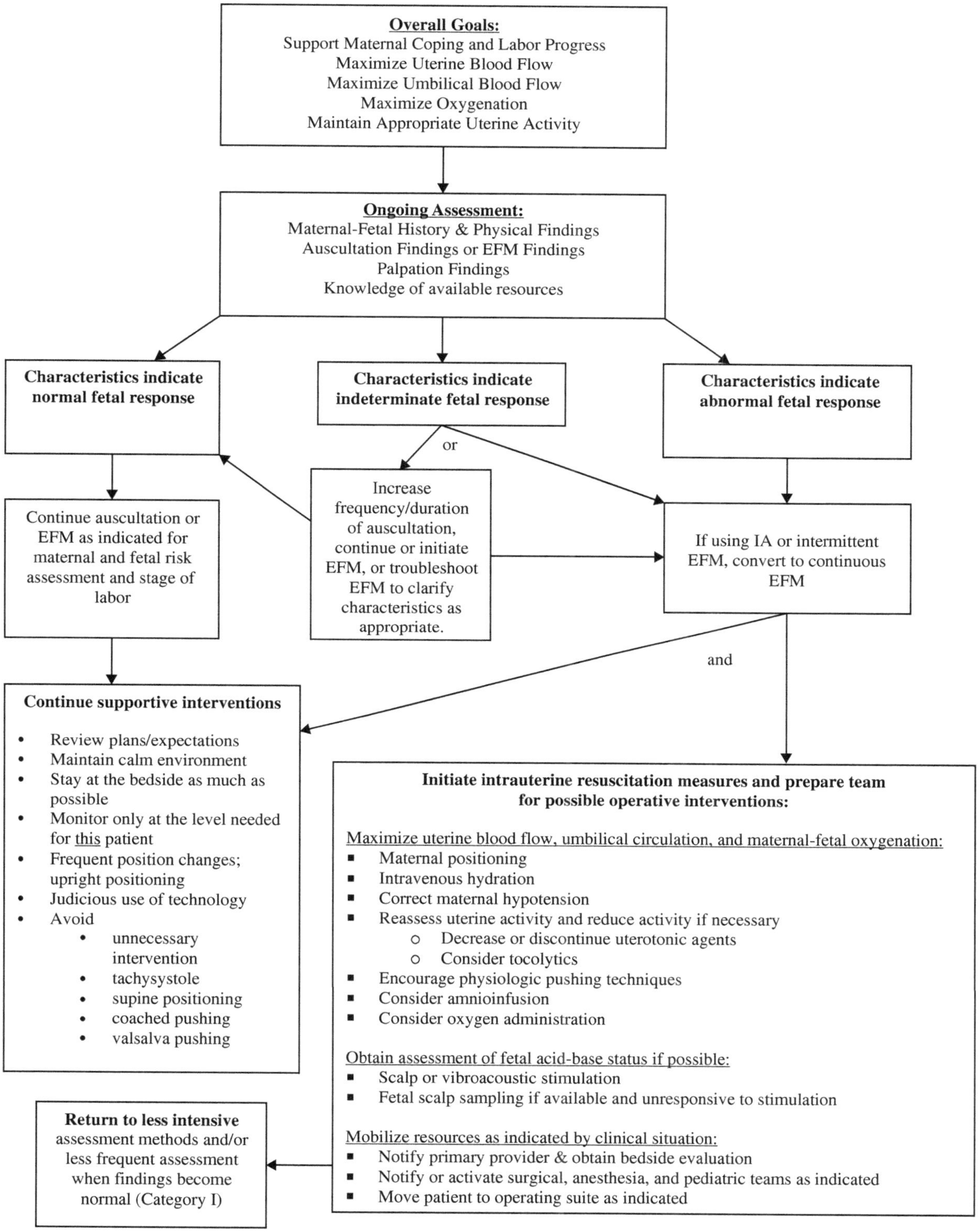

Case Study: Lori

Age:	36 years old
Gravidity/Parity:	G2P1001
Gestational Age:	41-1/7 weeks
Medical History:	Unremarkable
Surgical History:	Laparoscope for endometriosis
Psychosocial History:	Unremarkable
Past Obstetric History:	Previous cesarean birth for breech presentation
Current Obstetric History:	Advanced maternal age—normal quad screen Low-lying placenta on ultrasound

Lori presented to OB triage at 0350 for q 3- to 5-minute contractions and bloody show. This was her third visit to triage in 24 hours. She was admitted for therapeutic rest using morphine sulfate. VE on admission revealed a cervix that was 1 cm dilated, 90% effaced, and fetal vertex at −3 station. Lori progressed to 4 cm dilated, 100% effaced, and a fetal vertex at −1 station by 0645. Lori continued to contract q 3–4 minutes but her VE had not changed when she was examined at 0915. The membranes were artificially ruptured at this time for a large amount of clear fluid. Internal monitors were also placed at this time. At 1230 a vaginal examination revealed a cervix dilated 5 cm, 100% effaced and the fetal vertex at 0 station. Lori requested an epidural at this time. The initial dosing rates of the epidural caused hypotension requiring two doses of ephedrine.

Lori: Labor and Delivery EFM Tracing at 1300 Using Fetal Spiral Electrode and Intrauterine Pressure Catheter

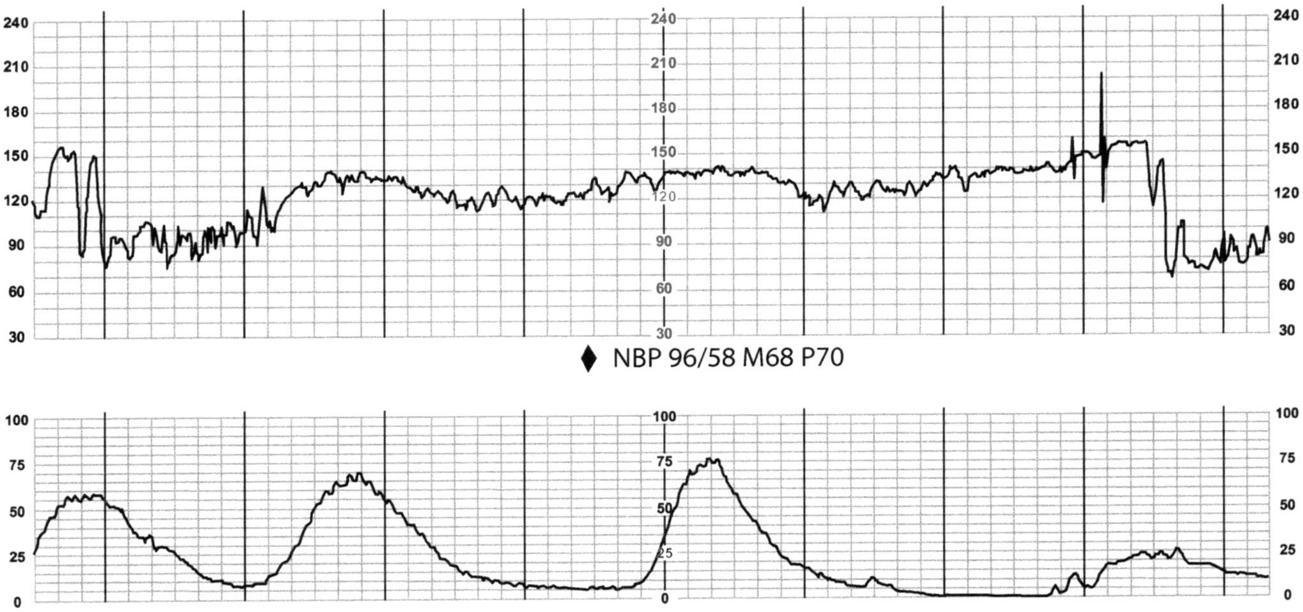

Case Study Exercise D: Lori

1. Baseline FHR: **140 bpm**

2. Variability

Absent (undetectable)	________
Minimal (>0 but ≤5 bpm)	________
Moderate (6–25 bpm)	________
Marked (>25 bpm)	________
Unable to determine	________

3. Contractions

Frequency:	**q 2–3 minutes**
Duration:	**90–100 seconds**
Intensity:	**55–75 mmHg**
Resting tone:	**5 mmHg**

4. Accelerations and decelerations. When present, circle P if periodic or E if episodic.

Accelerations	P	E
Early decelerations	P	
Variable decelerations	**P**	E
Late decelerations	**P**	
Prolonged decelerations	P	E
None present		

5. Interpretation

Category I	________
Category II	________
Category III	________

There is a mixed pattern of decelerations according to NICHD terminology. NICHD definitions emphasize the abruptness or gradualness of the onset of the deceleration. According to the definitions, the first, third, and last decelerations are variable, and the second deceleration is late. (The third deceleration reaches its nadir in less than 30 seconds). Some participants may feel strongly that these are late decelerations based on the timing and the etiology (maternal hypotension). When interpreting the FHR pattern, it is important to evaluate the baseline variability, the evolution of the pattern over time, the overall clinical picture, and the fetal response to interventions.

6. List possible underlying physiologic mechanisms or rationales for observed patterns.

- Uteroplacental insufficiency related to maternal hypotension
- Decreased uteroplacental perfusion related to postmature placenta and abnormal placentation
- Associated with an indeterminate fetal acid-base status at present
- Possible decreasing fetal reserves and hypoxia
- Fetal behavioral state change (fetal sleep cycle)
- Possible cord compression

7. List in order of priority the physiologic goal(s) for observed patterns.

- Maximize uteroplacental blood flow.
- Maximize oxygenation.
- Reduce uterine activity.

8. List actions and interventions indicated based on overall interpretation (physiologic based, instrumentation based, and further assessments).

- Change maternal position to promote uteroplacental blood flow.
- Assess maternal vital signs (blood pressure):
  - Repeat ephedrine sulfate doses as ordered/indicated.
- Give intravenous (IV) fluid bolus to increase maternal blood volume and increase placental perfusion.
- Consider oxygen at 10 liters/minute via face mask. Discontinue oxygen administration as soon as possible based on the fetal response.
- Consider tocolytic medication if hypotension resolved.
- Consider vaginal examination to evaluate labor progress.
- Continue to assess deceleration pattern and variability and monitor evolution of tracing.
- Review previous tracing segments to evaluate variability and periodic/episodic changes.
- Notify provider of FHR pattern (decelerations and variability), interventions, and patient response.
- Evaluate FHR response to interventions.
- Palpate uterus to validate uterine monitoring data.
- Continue routine assessments and interventions for labor, such as maternal comfort measures.
- Prepare for birth if FHR pattern deteriorates.
- Alert neonatal team for possible emergent birth.

REFERENCES

Abitbol, M. M. (1985). Supine position in labor and associated fetal heart rate changes. *Obstetrics and Gynecology, 65*(4), 481–486.

Aldrich, C. J., D'Antona, D., Spencer, J. A., Wyatt, J. S., Peebles, D. M., Delpy, D. T., & Reynolds, E. O. (1995). The effect of maternal posture on fetal cerebral oxygenation during labour. *British Journal of Obstetrics and Gynaecology, 102*(1), 14–19.

Aldrich, C. J., Wyatt, J. S., Spencer, J. A., Reynolds, E. O., & Delpy, D. T. (1994). The effect of maternal oxygen administration on human fetal cerebral oxygenation measured during labour by near infrared spectroscopy. *British Journal of Obstetrics and Gynaecology, 101*(6), 509–513.

Althabe, O., Jr., Schwarcz, R. L., Pose, S. V., Escarcena, L., & Caldeyro-Barcia, R. (1967). Effects on fetal heart rate and fetal pO2 of oxygen administration to the mother. *American Journal of Obstetrics and Gynecology, 98*(6), 858–870.

American Academy of Pediatrics & American Heart Association. (2011). *Textbook of neonatal resuscitation* (6th ed.). Elk Grove Village, IL: Authors.

American College of Nurse-Midwives. (2008). Providing oral nutrition to women in labor (Clinical Bulletin No. 10). *Journal of Midwifery and Women's Health, 53*(3), 276–283. doi:10.1016/j.jmwh.2008.03.006

American College of Obstetricians and Gynecologists. (2003). Dystocia and the augmentation of labor (Practice Bulletin No. 49; Reaffirmed, 2011). *Obstetrics and Gynecology, 102*(6), 1445–1454.

American College of Obstetricians and Gynecologists. (2005). Inappropriate use of the terms fetal distress and birth asphyxia (Committee Opinion No. 326). *Obstetrics and Gynecology, 106*(6), 1469–1470.

American College of Obstetricians and Gynecologists. (2006). Amnioinfusion does not prevent meconium aspiration syndrome (Committee Opinion No. 346; Reaffirmed, 2012). *Obstetrics and Gynecology, 108*(4), 1053.

American College of Obstetricians and Gynecologists. (2009a). Induction of labor (Practice Bulletin No. 107). *Obstetrics and Gynecology, 114*(2, Pt. 1), 386–397. doi:10.1097/AOG.0b013e3181b48ef5

American College of Obstetricians and Gynecologists. (2009b). Intrapartum fetal heart rate monitoring: Nomenclature, interpretation, and general management principles (Practice Bulletin No. 106). *Obstetrics and Gynecology, 114*(1), 192–202.

American College of Obstetricians and Gynecologists. (2010). Management of intrapartum fetal heart rate tracings (Practice Bulletin No. 116). *Obstetrics and Gynecology, 116*(5), 1232–1240. doi:10.1097/AOG.0b013e3182004fa9

American College of Obstetricians and Gynecologists & American Academy of Pediatrics. (2014). *Neonatal encephalopathy and neurologic outcome* (2nd ed.). Washington, DC: Authors.

American College of Obstetricians and Gynecologists & Society for Maternal-Fetal Medicine. (2014). *Safe prevention of the primary cesarean delivery* (Obstetric Care Consensus No.1). Washington, DC: Author. doi:10.1097/01.AOG.0000444441.04111.1d

Arias, F. (2000). Pharmacology of oxytocin and prostaglandins. *Clinical Obstetrics and Gynecology, 43*(3), 455–468.

Association of Women's Health, Obstetric and Neonatal Nurses. (2008). *Nursing management of the second stage of labor* (Evidence-Based Clinical Practice Guideline). Washington, DC: Author.

Bakker, P. C., Kurver, P. H., Kuik, D. J., & Van Geijn, H. P. (2007). Elevated uterine activity increases the risk of fetal acidosis at birth. *American Journal of Obstetrics* and *Gynecology, 196*(4), 313.e1313.e6. doi:10.1016/j.ajog.2006.11.035

Bakker, P. C., & van Geijn, H. P. (2008). Uterine activity: Implications for the condition of the fetus. *Journal of Perinatal Medicine, 36*(1), 30–37. doi:10.1515/JPM.2008.003

Barnett, M. M., & Humenick, S. S. (1982). Infant outcome in relation to second stage labor pushing method. *Birth and the Family Journal, 9*(4), 221–229.

Bartnicki, J., & Saling, E. (1994). The influence of maternal oxygen administration on the fetus. *International Journal of Gynaecology and Obstetrics, 45*(2), 87–95.

Blackburn, S. (2005). Free radicals in perinatal and neonatal care, Part 1: The basics. *Journal of Perinatal and Neonatal Nursing, 19*(4), 298–300.

Blackburn, S. (2006). Free radicals in perinatal and neonatal care, Part 2: Oxidative stress during the perinatal and neonatal period. *Journal of Perinatal and Neonatal Nursing, 20*(2), 125–127.

Caldeyro-Barcia, R. (1992). Intrauterine fetal reanimation in acute intrapartum fetal distress. *Early Human Development, 29*, 27–33.

Caldeyro-Barcia, R., Giussi, G., Storch, E., Poseiro, J. J., Lafaurie, N., Kettenhuber, K., & Ballejo, G. (1981). The bearing down efforts and their effects on fetal heart rate, oxygenation and acid base balance. *Journal of Perinatal Medicine, 9*(Suppl. 1), 63–67.

Carbonne, B., Benachi, A., Leveque, M. L., Cabrol, D., & Papiernik, E. (1996). Maternal position during labor: Effects on fetal oxygen saturation measured by pulse oximetry. *Obstetrics and Gynecology, 88*(5), 797–800.

Carmen, S. (1986). Neonatal hypoglycemia in response to maternal glucose infusion before delivery. *Journal of Obstetric, Gynecologic and Neonatal Nursing, 15*(4), 319–323.

Cerri, V., Tarantini, M., Zuliani, G., Schena, V., Redaelli, C., & Niconlini, U. (2000). Intravenous glucose infusion in labor does not affect maternal and fetal acid base balance. *Journal of Maternal-Fetal Medicine, 9*(4), 204–208.

Clark, S. L., Cotton, D. B., Pivarnik, J. M., Lee, W., Hankins, G. D., Benedetti, T. J., & Phelan, J. P. (1991). Position change and central hemodynamic profile during normal third trimester pregnancy and post partum. *American Journal of Obstetrics and Gynecology, 164*(3), 883–887.

Crane, J. M., & Young, D. C. (1998). Meta-analysis of low-dose versus high-dose oxytocin for labour induction. *Journal of the Society of Obstetricians and Gynaecologists of Canada, 20*, 1215–1223.

Crane, J. M., Young, D. C., Butt, K. D., Bennett, K. A., & Hutchens, D. (2001). Excessive uterine activity accompanying induced labor. *Obstetrics* and *Gynecology, 97*(6), 926–931.

Dildy, G. A., Clark, S. L., Loucks, C. A., van den Berg, P. P., & Jongsma, H. W. (1995). Effects of maternal inhalation of 40% oxygen on fetal oxygen saturation. *American Journal of Obstetrics and Gynecology, 172*(6), 1939–1943.

Dumoulin, J. G., & Foulkes, J. E. (1984). Ketonuria during labour. *British Journal of Obstetrics and Gynaecology, 91*(2), 97–98.

Elliott, C., Warrick, P. A., Graham, E., & Hamilton, E. F. (2010). Graded classification of fetal heart rate tracings: Association with neonatal metabolic acidosis and neurologic morbidity. *American Journal of Obstetrics and Gynecology, 202*(3), 258.e1-e8. doi:10.1016/j.ajog.2009.06.026

Eslamian, L., Marsoosi, V., & Pakneeyat, Y. (2006). Increased intravenous fluid intake and the course of labor in nulliparous women. *International Journal of Gynaecology and Obstetrics, 93*(2), 102–105. doi:10.1016/j.ijgo.2006.01.023

Fox, M., Kilpatrick, S., King, T., & Parer, J. T. (2000). Fetal heart rate monitoring: Interpretation and collaborative management. *Journal of Midwifery and Women's Health, 45*(6), 498–507.

Fraser, W. D., Hofmeyr, J., Lede, R., Faron, G., Alexander, S., Goffinet, F., . . . Wei, B. (2005). Amnioinfusion for the prevention of the meconium aspiration syndrome. *New England Journal of Medicine, 353*(9), 909–917. doi:10.1056/NEJMoa050223

Fraser, W. D., Marcoux, S., Krauss, I., Douglas, J., Goulet, C., & Boulvain, M. (2000). Multicenter, randomized, controlled trial of delayed pushing for nulliparous women in the second stage of labor with continuous epidural analgesia. *American Journal of Obstetrics and Gynecology, 182*(5), 1165–1172.

Freeman, R. K., Garite, T. J., Nageotte, M. P., & Miller, L. A. (2012). *Fetal heart rate monitoring* (4th ed.). Philadelphia, PA: Lippincott Williams & Wilkins.

Garite, T. J., & Simpson, K. R. (2011). Intrauterine resuscitation during labor. *Clinical Obstetrics and Gynecology, 54*(1), 28–39. doi:10.1097/GRF.0b013e31820a062b

Garite, T. J., Weeks, J., Peters-Phair, K., Pattillo, C., & Brewster, W. R. (2000). A randomized controlled trial of the effect of increased intravenous hydration on the course of labor in nulliparous women. *American Journal of Obstetrics and Gynecology, 183*(6), 1544–1548.

Grylack, L. J., Chu, S. S., & Scanlon, J. W. (1984). Use of intravenous fluids before cesarean section: Effects on perinatal glucose, insulin, and sodium homeostasis. *Obstetrics and Gynecology, 63*(5), 654–658.

Gupta, J. K., Hofmeyr, G. J., & Shehmar, M. (2012). Position in the second stage of labour for women without epidural anaesthesia. *Cochrane Database of Systematic Reviews,* Issue 5 (Article No. CD002006). doi:10.1002/14651858.CD002006.pub3

Hamilton, E., Warrick, P., Knox, E., O'Keeffe, D., & Garite, T. (2012). High uterine contraction rates in births with normal and abnormal umbilical artery gases. *Journal of Maternal–Fetal and Neonatal Medicine, 25*(11), 2302–2307. doi:10.3109/14767058.2012.691578

Hansen, S. L., Clark, S. L., & Foster, J. C. (2002). Active pushing versus passive fetal descent in the second stage of labor: A randomized controlled trial. *Obstetrics and Gynecology, 99*(1), 29–34.

Haydon, M. L., Gorenberg, D. M., Nageotte, M. P., Ghamsary, M., Rumney, P. J., Patillo, C., & Garite, T. J. (2006). The effect of maternal oxygen administration during labor on fetal pulse oximetry. *American Journal of Obstetrics and Gynecology, 195*(3), 735–738. doi:10.1016/j.ajog.2006.06.084

Heuser, C. C., Knight, S., Esplin, M. S., Eller, A. G., Holmgren, C. M., Richards, D., . . . Jackson, G. M. (2013). Tachysystole in term labor: Incidence, risk factors, outcomes, and effect on fetal heart tracings. *American Journal of Obstetrics and Gynecology, 209*, e1–e6. doi:10.1016/j.ajog.2013.04.004

Hicks, P. (2005). Systematic review of the risk of uterine rupture with the use of amnioinfusion after previous cesarean delivery. *Southern Medical Journal, 98*(4), 458–461.

Higgins, R. D., Bancalari, E., Willinger, M., & Raju, T. N. (2007). Executive summary of the workshop on oxygen in neonatal therapies: Controversies and opportunities. *Pediatrics, 119*(4), 790–796. doi:10.1542/peds.2006-2200

Hofmeyr, G. J., & Lawrie, T. A. (2012). Amnioinfusion for potential or suspected umbilical cord compression in labour. *Cochrane Database of Systematic Reviews,* Issue 2 (Article No. CD000013). doi:10.1002/14651858.CD000013.pub2

Jackson, M., Holmgren, C. M., Esplin, M. S., Henry, E., & Varner, M. W. (2011). Frequency of fetal heart rate categories and short-term neonatal outcome. *American Journal of Obstetrics & Gynecology, 118*(4), 803–808.

Johnson, N., van Oudgaarden, E., Montague, I., & McNamara, H. (1994). The effect of oxytocin-induced hyperstimulation on fetal oxygen. *British Journal of Obstetrics and Gynaecology, 101*(9), 805–807.

Kazandi, M., Sendag, F., Akercan, F., Terek, M. C., & Gundem, G. (2003). Different types of variable decelerations and their effects to neonatal outcome. *Singapore Medical Journal, 44*(5), 243–247.

Kenepp, N. B., Kumar, S., Shelley, W. C., Stanley, C. A., Gabbe, S. G., & Gutsche, B. B. (1982). Fetal and neonatal hazards of maternal hydration with 5% dextrose before caesarean section. *Lancet, 1*(8282), 1150–1152.

Khaw, K. S., & Ngan Kee, W. D. (2004). Fetal effects of maternal supplementary oxygen during caesarean section. *Current Opinion in Anaesthesiology, 17*(4), 309–313.

Khaw, K. S., Wang, C. C., Ngan Kee, W. D., Pang, C. P., & Rogers, M. S. (2002). Effects of high inspired oxygen fraction during elective caesarean under spinal anaesthesia on maternal and fetal oxygenation and lipid peroxidation. *British Journal of Anaesthesia, 88*(1), 18–23.

Klinger, G., Beyene, J., Shah, P., & Perlman, M. (2005). Do hyperoxaemia and hypocapnia add to the risk of brain damage after intrapartum asphyxia? *Archives of Disease in Childhood: Fetal and Neonatal Edition, 90*(1), F49–F52.

Klingner, M. C., & Kruse, J. (1999). Meconium aspiration syndrome: Pathophysiology and prevention. *Journal of the American Board of Family Practice, 12*(6), 450–466.

Kulier, R., & Hofmeyr, G. J. (2000). Tocolytics for suspected intrapartum fetal distress. *Cochrane Database of Systematic Reviews,* Issue 2 (Article No. CD000035).

Leduc, D., Biringer, A., Lee, L., & Dy, L. (2013). Induction of labour (SOGC Clinical Practice Guideline No. 296). *Journal of Obstetrics and Gynaecology of Canada, 35*(9), 840–860.

Lyndon, A., O'Brien-Abel, N., & Simpson, K. R. (2013). Labor and birth. In K. R. Simpson & P. A. Creehan (Eds.), *AWHONN's perinatal nursing* (4th ed., pp. 445–492). Philadelphia, PA: Lippincott Williams & Wilkins.

Macones, G. A., Hankins, G. D., Spong, C. Y., Hauth, J. D., & Moore, T. (2008). The 2008 National Institute of Child Health Human Development workshop report on electronic fetal monitoring: Update on definitions, interpretations, and research guidelines. *Obstetrics and Gynecology, 112, 661–666.* doi:10.1097/AOG.0b013e3181841395; and *Journal of Obstetric, Gynecologic and Neonatal Nursing, 37,* 510–515. doi:10.1111/j.1552-6909.2008.00284.x

Mayberry, L. J., Hammer, R., Kelly, C., True-Driver, B., & De, A. (1999). Use of delayed pushing with epidural anesthesia: Findings from a randomized controlled trial. *Journal of Perinatology, 19*(1), 26–30.

McNamara, H., & Johnson, N. (1995). The effect of uterine contractions on fetal oxygen saturation. *British Journal of Obstetrics and Gynaecology, 102*(8), 644–647.

McNamara, H., Johnson, N., & Lilford, R. (1993). The effect on fetal arteriolar oxygen saturation resulting from giving oxygen to the mother measured by pulse oximetry. *British Journal of Obstetrics and Gynaecology, 100*(5), 446–449.

Mendiola, J., Grylack, L. J., & Scanlon, J. W. (1982). Effects of intrapartum maternal glucose infusion on the normal fetus and newborn. *Anesthesia and Analgesia, 61*(1), 32–35.

Miller, L. A., Miller, D., & Tucker, S. M. (2013). *Pocket guide to fetal monitoring: A multidisciplinary approach.* St. Louis, MO: Mosby.

Miño, M., Puertas, A., Miranda, J. A., & Herruzo, A. J. (1999). Amnioinfusion in term labor with low amniotic fluid due to rupture of the membranes: A new indication. *European Journal of Obstetrics, Gynecology, and Reproductive Biology, 82*(1), 29–34.

Miyazaki, F. S., & Nevarez, F. (1985). Saline amnioinfusion for relief of repetitive variable decelerations: A prospective randomized study. *American Journal of Obstetrics and Gynecology, 153*(3), 301–306.

National Collaborating Centre for Women's and Children's Health. (2007). *Intrapartum care: Care of healthy women and their babies during childbirth.* London, UK: Royal College of Obstetricians and Gynaecologists Press.

National Institute of Child Health and Human Development Research Planning Workshop. (1997). Electronic fetal heart rate monitoring: Research guidelines for interpretation. *American Journal of Obstetrics and Gynecology 177*(6), 1385–1390, and *Journal of Obstetric Gynecology and Neonatal Nursing, 26*(6), 635–640.

Nordstrom, L., Achanna, S., Nuka, K., & Arulkumaran, S. (2001). Fetal and maternal lactate increase during active second stage labour. *British Journal of Obstetrics* and *Gynaecology, 108*(3), 263–268.

Ouzounian, J. G., Miller, D. A., & Paul, R. H. (1996). Amnioinfusion in women with previous cesarean births: A preliminary report. *American Journal of Obstetrics and Gynecology, 174*(2), 783–786.

Parer, J. T., King, T., Flanders, S., Fox, M., & Kilpatrick, S. J. (2006). Fetal acidemia and electronic fetal heart rate patterns: Is there evidence of an association? *Journal of Maternal-Fetal and Neonatal Medicine, 19*(5), 289–294. doi:10.1080/14767050500526172

Paternoster, D. M., Micaglio, M., Tambuscio, B., Bracciante, R., & Chiarenza, A. (2001). The effects of epidural analgesia and uterine contractions on fetal oxygen saturation during the first stage of labour.

International Journal of Obstetric Anesthesia, 10(2), 103–107.

Peebles, D. M., Spencer, J. A., Edwards, A. D., Wyatt, J. S., Reynolds, E. O., Cope, M., & Delpy, D. T. (1994). Relation between frequency of uterine contractions and human fetal cerebral oxygen saturation studied during labour by near infrared spectroscopy. *British Journal of Obstetrics and Gynaecology, 101*(1), 44–48.

Phillipson, E. H., Kalihan, S. C., Riha, M. M., & Pimental, R. (1987). Effects of maternal glucose infusion on fetal acid-base status in human pregnancy. *American Journal of Obstetrics and Gynecology, 157*(4, Pt. 1), 866–873.

Pierce, J., Gaudier, F. L., & Sanchez-Ramos, L. (2000). Intrapartum amnioinfusion for meconium-stained fluid: Meta-analysis of prospective clinical trials. *Obstetrics and Gynecology, 95*(6, Pt. 2), 1051–1056.

Piquard, F., Hsiung, R., Mettauer, M., Schaefer, A., Haberey, P., & Dellenbach, P. (1988). The validity of fetal heart rate monitoring during second stage of labor. *Obstetrics and Gynecology, 72*(5), 746–751.

Piquard, F., Schaefer, A., Hsiung, R., Dellenbach, P., & Haberey, P. (1989). Are there two biological parts in the second stage of labor? *Acta Obstetricia et Gynecologica Scandinavica, 68*(8), 713–718.

Pullen, K. M., Riley, E. T., Waller, S. A., Taylor, L., Caughey, A. B., Druzin, M. L., & El-Sayed, Y. Y. (2007). Randomized comparison of intravenous terbutaline vs nitroglycerine for acute intrapartum fetal resuscitation. *American Journal of Obstetrics and Gynecology, 197*(4), 414e1-414e6. doi:10.1016/j.ajog.2007.06.063

Roberts, J. E. (2002). The "push" for evidence: Management of the second stage. *Journal of Midwifery and Women's Health, 47*(1), 2–15.

Roberts, J., & Hanson, L. (2007). Best practices in second stage labor care: Maternal bearing down and positioning. *Journal of Midwifery and Women's Health, 52*(3), 238–245.

Rogers, M. S., Mongelli, M., Tsang, K. H., & Wang, C. C. (1999). Fetal and maternal levels of lipid peroxides in term pregnancies. *Acta Obstetricia et Gynecologica Scandinavica, 78*(2), 120–124.

Rogers, M. S., Wang, W., Mongelli, M., Pang, C. P., Duley, J. A., & Chang, A. M. (1997). Lipid peroxidation in cord blood at birth: A marker of fetal hypoxia during labour. *Gynecologic and Obstetric Investigation, 44*(4), 229–233.

Romney, S. L., & Gabel, P. V. (1966). Maternal glucose loading in the management of fetal distress. *American Journal of Obstetrics and Gynecology, 96*(5), 698–709.

Sameshima, H., & Ikenoue, T. (2005). Predictive value of late decelerations for fetal acidemia in unselective low-risk pregnancies. *American Journal of Perinatology, 22*(1), 19–23.

Seitchik, J., Amico, J., Robinson, A. G., & Castillo, M. (1984). Oxytocin augmentation of dysfunctional labor. IV Oxytocin pharmacokinetics. *American Journal of Obstetrics and Gynecology, 150*(3), 225–228.

Sheiner, E., Hadar, A., Hallak, M., Katz, M., Mazor, M., & Shoham-Vardi, I. (2001). Clinical significance of fetal heart rate tracings during the second stage of labor. *Obstetrics and Gynecology, 97*(5, Pt 1), 747–752.

Shenker, L. (1973). Clinical experience with fetal heart rate monitoring of one thousand patients in labor. *American Journal of Obstetrics and Gynecology, 115*(8), 1111–1116.

Shifrin, B. S., & Ater, S. (2006). Fetal hypoxic and ischemic injuries. *Current Opinion in Obstetrics and Gynecology, 18*(2), 112–122. doi:10.1097/01.gco.0000192984.15095.7c

Siira, S. M., Ojala, T. H., Vahlberg, T. J., Jalonen, J. O., Valimaki, B. A., Rosen, K. G, & Ekholm, E. M. (2005). Marked fetal acidosis and specific changes in power spectrum analysis of fetal heart rate variability recorded during the last hour of labour. *BJOG: International Journal of Obstetrics and Gynaecology, 112*(4), 418–423.

Simpson, K. R. (2006). Critical illness during pregnancy: Considerations for evaluation and treatment of the fetus as the second patient. *Critical Care Nursing Quarterly, 29*(1), 20–31.

Simpson, K. R. (2007). Intrauterine resuscitation during labor: Review of current practice and supportive evidence. *Journal of Midwifery and Women's Health, 52*(3), 229–237.

Simpson, K. R. (2008). Intrauterine resuscitation during labor: Should maternal oxygen administration be a first-line measure? *Seminars in Fetal and Neonatal Medicine, 13*(6), 362–367. doi:10.1016/j. siny.2008.04.016

Simpson, K. R. (2013). *Cervical ripening and labor induction and augmentation* (Practice Monograph). Washington, DC: Association of Women's Health, Obstetric and Neonatal Nurses.

Simpson, K. R., & James, D. C. (2005a). Effects of immediate versus delayed pushing during second stage labor on fetal well-being: A randomized clinical trial. *Nursing Research, 54*(3), 149–157.

Simpson, K. R., & James, D. C. (2005b). Efficacy of intrauterine resuscitation techniques in improving fetal oxygen status during labor. *Obstetrics and Gynecology, 105*(6), 1362–1368. doi:10.1097/01.AOG.0000164474.03350.7c

Simpson, K. R., & James, D. C. (2008). Effects of oxytocin-induced uterine hyperstimulation on fetal oxygen status and fetal heart rate patterns. *American Journal of Obstetrics and Gynecology, 199,* 34.e1-34.e5. doi:10.1016/j.ajog.2007.12.015

Simpson, K. R., & Miller, L. (2011). Assessment and optimization of uterine activity during labor. *Clinical*

Obstetrics and Gynecology, 54(1), 40–49. doi:10.1097/GRF.0b013e31820a06aa

Simpson, K. R., & O'Brien-Abel, N. (2013). Labor and birth. In K. R. Simpson & P. A. Creehan (Eds.), *AWHONN's perinatal nursing* (4th ed., pp. 343–444). Philadelphia, PA: Lippincott Williams & Wilkins.

Singhi, S. (1988). Effect of maternal intrapartum glucose therapy on neonatal blood glucose levels and neurobehavioral status of hypoglycemic term infants. *Journal of Perinatal Medicine, 16*(3), 217–224.

Sleutel, M., & Golden, S. S. (1999). Fasting in labor: Relic or requirement. *Journal of Obstetric, Gynecologic and Neonatal Nursing, 28*(5), 507–512.

Smith, J. G., & Merrill, D. C. (2006). Oxytocin for induction of labor. *Clinical Obstetrics and Gynecology, 49*(3), 594–608.

Society of Obstetricians and Gynaecologists of Canada. (2007). Fetal health surveillance in labour: Antepartum and intrapartum consensus guideline. *Journal of the Society of Obstetricians and Gynaecologists of Canada, 29*(9, Suppl. 4), S3–S56.

Sommer, P. A., Norr, K., & Roberts, J. (2000). Clinical decision-making regarding intravenous hydration in normal labor in a birth center setting. *Journal of Midwifery and Women's Health, 45*(2), 114–121.

Sprague, A. E., Oppenheimer, L., McCabe, L., Brownlee, J., Graham, I. D., & Davies, B. (2006). The Ottawa Hospital's Clinical Practice Guidelines for the second stage of labour. *Journal of Obstetrics and Gynaecology of Canada, 28*(9), 769–779.

Spong, C. Y., Berghella, V., Wenstrom, K. D., Mercer, B. M., & Saade, G. R. (2012). Preventing the first cesarean delivery: Summary of a joint Eunice Kennedy Shriver National Child Health and Human Development, Society for Maternal-Fetal Medicine, and American College of Obstetricians and Gynecologists workshop. *Obstetrics and Gynecology, 120*(5), 1181–1193. doi:http://10.1097/AOG.0b013e3182704880

SUPPORT Study Group of the Eunice Kennedy Shriver NICHD Neonatal Research Network, Carlo, W. A., Finer, N. N., Walsh, M. C., Rich, W., Gantz, M. G., . . . Higgins, R. D. (2010). Target ranges of oxygen saturation in extremely preterm infants. *New England Journal of Medicine, 362*(21), 1959–1969. doi:10.1056/NEJMoa0911781

Strong, T. H., Jr. (1997). The effect of amnioinfusion on the duration of labor. *Obstetrics and Gynecology, 89*(6), 1044–1046.

Ulmsten, U. (1997). Onset and forces of term labor. *Acta Obstetricia et Gynecologica Scandinavica, 76*(6), 499–514.

Vento, M., Asensi, M., Sastre, J., Garcia-Sala, F., Pallardo, F. V., & Vina, J. (2001). Resuscitation with room air instead of 100% oxygen prevents oxidative stress in moderately asphyxiated term neonates. *Pediatrics, 107*(4), 642–647.

Vento, M., Asensi, M., Sastre, J., Lloret, A., Garcia-Sala, F., & Vina, J. (2003). Oxidative stress in asphyxiated term infants resuscitations with 100% oxygen. *Journal of Pediatrics, 142*(3), 240–246.

Wasserstrum, N. (1992). Issues in fluid management during labor: General considerations. *Clinics in Obstetrics and Gynecology, 35*(3), 505–513.

Williams, K. P., & Galerneau, F. (2002). Fetal heart rate parameters predictive of neonatal outcome in the presence of a prolonged deceleration. *Obstetrics and Gynecology, 100*(5, Pt 1), 951–954.

Williams, K. P., & Galerneau, F. (2003). Intrapartum fetal heart rate patterns in the prediction of neonatal acidemia. *American Journal of Obstetrics and Gynecology, 188*(3), 820–823.

Wong, C. A. (2009). Epidural and spinal analgesia/anesthesia for labor and vaginal delivery. In D. H. Chestnut, L. S. Polley, L. C. Tsen, & C. A. Wong (Eds.), *Chestnut's obstetric anesthesia: Principles and practice* (4th ed., pp. 429–492). Philadelphia, PA: Elsevier.

CHAPTER 7

Assessment of Fetal Oxygenation and Acid-Base Status

Rebecca Cypher

INTRODUCTION

Antepartum and intrapartum clinical management decisions often have an impact on fetal oxygenation and perinatal outcomes, including fetal acid-base status and the metabolic condition at birth. The Apgar score, originally designed to assess the need for neonatal resuscitation, may not correlate with the fetal heart rate (FHR) tracing and acid-base status nor predict future adverse neurologic development. The primary focus of this chapter is to highlight key concepts of fetal oxygenation and acid-base status. Indirect and direct adjunct techniques used to assess fetal oxygenation are reviewed.

FETAL ACID-BASE BALANCE: KEY CONCEPTS

As discussed in Chapter 2, the placenta is a low-resistance structure that serves as the interface between the mother and the fetus. At term, 90% of total uterine blood flow is directed to the placenta as a result of maternal arterial vasodilation and placental growth (Ross, Ervin, & Novak, 2012). Several independent physiologic functions occur in the placenta including nutrient uptake for fetal growth and development, disposal of fetal waste products, secretion of hormones to sustain pregnancy, and exchange of oxygen and carbon dioxide between the mother and fetus (Rampersad, Cervar-Zivkovic, & Nelson, 2011). Blood flow to and within the placenta is approximately 500–600 mL/minute (Blackburn, 2013; Huckabee, 1962). Oxygen is transferred from the environment to the fetus via maternal-fetal blood exchange along a pathway that includes the maternal lungs, heart, vasculature, uterus, placenta, and umbilical cord (Miller & Miller, 2012). This oxygenated blood flows to the fetus through a single umbilical vein. Two umbilical arteries branch onto the chorionic plate of the placenta and into the intervillous space where nutrients, oxygen, and waste products are exchanged with maternal blood. Deoxygenated blood from the fetus then flows back through the umbilical arteries in the umbilical cord to the placenta (Blackburn, 2013). A number of factors influence the transfer of oxygen to the fetus, including environmental factors; maternal cardio-pulmonary status; and the structure and function of the uterus, placenta, and umbilical cord (Blackburn, 2013; King & Parer, 2000; Ross et al., 2012; Society of Obstetricians and Gynaecologists of Canada [SOGC], 2007; Yancy & Harlass, 1993). For example, tobacco smoke can cause an acute reduction of blood flow to the intervillous space due to various mechanisms that include vasoconstriction of peripheral and uterine blood vessels (Lehtovirta

& Forss, 1978; Zdravkovic, Genbacev, McMaster, & Fisher, 2005).

Fetal acid-base balance is determined by a number of factors: adequacy of maternal oxygenation and acid-base balance during the antepartum and intrapartum period; blood flow to and across the placenta; and the ability of the fetus to oxygenate the vital organs' tissues (Dildy, 2005; Greene, 1999; Nageotte & Gilstrap, 2009). Uterine contractions during labor create a temporary disruption in blood flow and exchange of oxygen and carbon dioxide to and from the fetus. The fetus with adequate oxygenation will adapt to this normal decrease in oxygen exchange when there are adequate rest periods between contractions. If the fetus is not adequately oxygenated or excessive uterine activity is present for a prolonged period of time, there may be a progressive accumulation of carbon dioxide (hypercapnia) and a decrease in oxygen content (hypoxemia) that may result in fetal acidemia in umbilical cord gases, specifically a lower pH value in the umbilical artery (Bakker, Kurver, Kuik, & Van Geijn, 2007; Greene, 1999; Hamilton, Warrick, Knox, O'Keefe, & Garite, 2012; Ross, 2011). The fetus responds to the oxygen disruption with a physiologic compensatory mechanism in which there is a redistribution of blood flow: increased cardiac output to preserve blood flow to the vital organs (brain, myocardium, and adrenal glands), continual maintenance of blood flow to the placenta, and decreased flow to other organs including the kidneys, gastrointestinal tract, and muscles (Martin, 2008; Perlman, 2012).

There is a finite limit to the fetus' ability to sustain the necessary physiological responses required to maintain adequate oxygenation along the disrupted oxygenation pathway (Hamilton, Warrick, Knox, et al., 2012). If sufficient oxygenation is not restored a series of sequential physiologic steps occurs: hypoxemia, hypoxia, metabolic acidosis, and finally if severe enough and of sufficient duration, metabolic acidemia. Specifically, recurrent or sustained disruption in the oxygen pathway may lead to reduced oxygen uptake by fetal hemoglobin as the pH decreases (hypoxemia). In turn, this leads to inadequate oxygenation of the tissues (hypoxia), which activates lactic acid production as the fetus converts to an anaerobic metabolic pathway. Lactic acid diffuses across the placenta but if the fetal buffering system cannot correct the excess hydrogen ion production, lactic acid accumulates in the tissue resulting in metabolic acidosis. Eventually the blood pH falls because of the buildup of pyruvic and lactic acid in the tissues leading to metabolic acidemia in the arterial cord blood and potential injury (Brouillette & Waxman, 1997; Campbell, Vintzileos, & Nochimson, 1986; Greene, 1999; King, 2013; D. A. Miller, 2011; Miller & Miller, 2012).

Acidosis may not always lead to acidemia if corrective interventions are implemented as the fetus may still possess compensatory mechanisms that maintain tissue oxygenation and reduce energy consumption. In addition to preferential circulatory streaming to the vital organs and a higher hemoglobin concentration, the fetus may suppress trunk, limb, breathing, and eye movement to reduce oxygen requirements (Brouillette & Waxman, 1997; Martin, 2008). The following sections include terminology used when describing fetal acid-base status or physiology, a description of the means by which the fetus meets its normal metabolic needs, and physiologic and pathophysiologic factors that may affect the fetal acid-base balance.

Terminology

Several terms are used to describe fetal and adult acid-base physiology and blood gas values (Culver, 2008; King & Parer, 2000; Zamudio, 2011):

- Normoxia: normal levels of oxygen
- Hypoxia: inadequate cellular and tissue oxygenation
- Hypoxemia: inadequate oxygen content in blood
- Hypercapnia: increase in carbon dioxide in blood
- Acidemia: increase in hydrogen ions in blood
- Acidosis: increase in hydrogen ions in tissue
- Metabolic acidosis: low bicarbonate (base excess) in the presence of normal pressure of carbon dioxide (PCO_2) values
- Respiratory acidosis: high PCO_2 with normal bicarbonate levels
- Asphyxia: hypoxia with metabolic acidosis

Additionally, the terms "fetal distress" and "birth asphyxia" are sometimes linked with fetal acid-base status. On occasion, "fetal distress" has been used as an antepartum or intrapartum diagnosis and "birth asphyxia" as a neonatal diagnosis. Neither term should be used in clinical practice because both are imprecise and nonspecific. There is little predictive value associated with these terms at birth as "the infant may be in good condition as determined by the Apgar score or umbilical cord blood gas analysis or both" (American College of Obstetricians and Gynecologists [ACOG], 2005). Instead, if a "category II" or "category III" FHR finding is interpreted during a bedside evaluation of the FHR tracing, a written description of the FHR characteristics and associated uterine activity is more appropriate than "fetal distress" or the FHR category. Documenting and communicating specific components of the FHR characteristics and uterine activity reflects the clinician's assessment of the FHR findings rather than relying on a summary term or category (L. Miller, 2011). This is especially true for category II tracings, which are believed to cover a wide spectrum of potential fetal states, are indeterminate, and may occur in many laboring women (Macones, Hankins, Spong, Hauth, & Moore, 2008). For example, a clinician may document "FHR: BL 175, minimal variability with recurrent late decelerations," or "FHR: BL 155 with moderate variability and intermittent variable decelerations."

There is an assumption that when there is a disruption along the oxygenation pathway—a prolapsed umbilical cord for instance—a category I finding can rapidly evolve to a category II finding. Corrective interventions, such as a maternal position change and supplemental oxygen, are initiated. If these interventions are ineffective, a category II finding can advance to a category III finding paralleling the progression of normoxia to asphyxia resulting in neurologic injury (King & Parer, 2000). However, in 2014, the American College of Obstetricians and Gynecologists (ACOG) and the American Academy of Pediatrics (AAP) published a revised consensus report defining category elements that are more likely to play a role in the development of neonatal encephalopathy from hypoxia-ischemia during the peripartum or intrapartum period. (Box 7-1).

Box 7-1 Neonatal Signs Consistent with an Acute Peripartum or Intrapartum Event

- Agpar score of less than 5 at 5 minutes and 10 minutes
- Fetal umbilical artery acidemia defined as an umbilical arterial cord blood sample of pH less than 7.0 or base deficit greater than or equal to 12 mmol/L or both
- Neuroimaging evidence of acute brain injury detected on brain magnetic resonance imaging or magnetic resonance spectroscopy consistent with hypoxia-ischemia in infants born at or greater than 35 weeks' gestation
- Presence of multisystem organ failure consistent with hypoxic-ischemic encephalopathy

Contributing Factors Consistent with an Acute Peripartum or Intrapartum Event

- Sentinel hypoxic event occurring immediately before or during labor
  - Uterine Rupture
  - Severe abruptio placentae
  - Umbilical cord prolapse
  - Amniotic fluid embolus with coincident severe and prolonged maternal hypotension and hypoxemia
  - Maternal cardiovascular collapse
  - Fetal exsanguination from vasa previa or massive fetomaternal hemorrhage
- Fetal heart rate patterns consistent with an acute peripartum or intrapartum event
- Timing and type of brain injury patterns based on imaging studies consistent with an etiology of an acute peripartum or intrapartum event
- No evidence of other proximal or distal factors that could be contributing factors
- Developmental outcome is spastic quadriplegia or dyskinetic cerebral palsy

ACOG & AAP (2014).

Physiologic and Pathophysiologic Factors Affecting Intrapartum Acid-Base Assessment

The energy-consuming process of metabolism is called *anabolism,* whereas *catabolism* refers to the energy-releasing process. There are three phases of catabolism in which proteins, lipids, and polysaccharides are broken down. In phase one, large molecules are broken down into smaller subunits: proteins into amino acids, polysaccharides into simple sugars, and fats into fatty acids and glycerol. In phase two, molecules that enter cells are broken down in the cytoplasm of the cell. Sugars are broken down into pyruvate, which then enters the mitochondria and is converted to the acetyl groups, which include adenosine triphosphate (ATP). Glycolysis, the breakdown of glucose, can occur both aerobically and anaerobically. In phase three, the acetyl group is degraded to water and carbon dioxide (King & Parer, 2000; McCance, 2009; Ross et al., 2012).

In normal cellular glucose metabolism, ATP is generated from the oxidation of glucose to water and carbon dioxide, which then provides the energy for other cellular processes (Greene, 1999; King & Parer, 2000; McCance, 2009). For aerobic cellular metabolism to occur, oxygen must be present. Two classes of acids are produced when the fetus exhibits normal metabolism: volatile acids (e.g., carbonic acid) and nonvolatile acids (e.g., lactic acid), also known as fixed acids (Armstrong & Stenson, 2007; Thorp & Rushing, 1999).

The end result of aerobic metabolism in the fetus is carbonic acid, which is formed by the hydration of carbon dioxide during oxidative metabolism. It is found in very low concentrations in the plasma. The fetus can tolerate the amount of carbonic acid normally produced from aerobic metabolism because carbonic acid dissociates into water and carbon dioxide, thus diffusing very rapidly across the placenta as long as there is adequate intervillous and umbilical blood flow (Culver, 2008; Freeman, Garite, Nageotte, & Miller, 2012; King, 2013).

The primary variable that alters fetal oxygenation during the labor course is interruption in the blood flow to the placenta that occurs when the spiral arteries are compressed during uterine contractions. Throughout pregnancy, 70–90% of uterine blood flow circulates through the intervillous space unless factors such as uterine contractions decrease the volume flowing to the spiral arteries (King, 2013). Specifically, there is a temporary decrease in oxygen exchange to the fetus and carbon dioxide away from the fetus when the spiral arteries supplying the intervillous space are constricted at intrauterine pressures exceeding approximately 30 mmHg. Characteristic hemodynamic changes show that blood flow begins to decrease within seconds after a detectable rise in intra-amniotic fluid pressure, which continues during the ascending phase of the uterine contraction. Blood flow to the intervillous space tends to stabilize after the peak intensity is reached and then returns to the precontractile baseline level when the contraction is completed (Brotanek, Hendricks, & Yoshida, 1969; Greene, 1999; Harbert, 1982). The duration of spiral artery compression depends on the duration and intensity of the contraction (Figure 7-1). The fetus usually tolerates these transitory interruptions (no more than 60 seconds with sufficient resting time of at least 2 minutes) without a major change in oxygen content (Bakker & van Geijn, 2008; Garite, 2012; Greene, 1999; King & Parer, 2000) as the fetus has several compensatory mechanisms that have been mentioned previously for managing these transient periods of hypoxia (see Chapter 2).

Additional factors, such as a chronic placental abruption or maternal hypertension, may affect uteroplacental perfusion and fetal oxygenation (Bakker & van Geijn, 2008; Simpson & James, 2008). When placental transfer of oxygen is restricted over a long period of time, fetal metabolism proceeds into anaerobic metabolism and lactic acid accumulates (Blechner, 1993; Helwig, Parer, Kilpatrick, & Laros, 1996; Miller & Miller, 2012). Fetal acid-base status depends on maternal factors as well as transplacental transfer of gases. The normoxic fetus has a pH level slightly lower than the maternal pH level and is affected by the acid-base balance of the mother. During labor, intrauterine vessels are

Figure 7-1 Uteroplacental Blood Flow and the Influence of Intramyometical Pressure

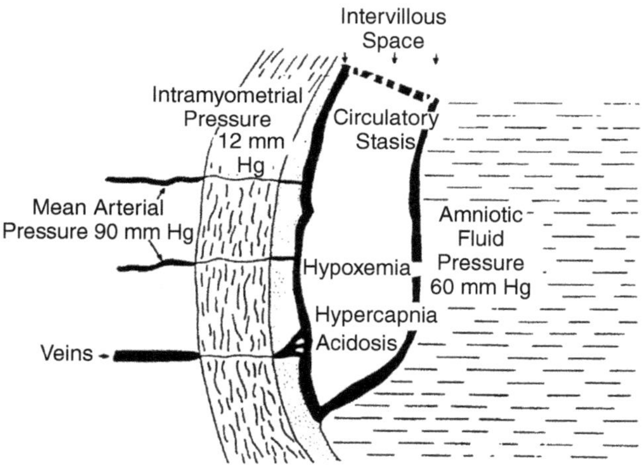

At the acme, or peak of a contraction of greater than 50 mmHg, uteroplacental blood flow ceases temporarily. This causes the fetus to be dependent upon placental reserve. There may be a brief alteration of contraction effectiveness.
Adapted from Freeman, et al., 2012; Poseiro (1969).

constricted, thereby decreasing blood flow to the intervillous space and transfer of carbon dioxide, a waste product of cellular metabolism, away from the fetus. Normally the fetus can adjust to brief episodes of oxygen pathway disruptions and continue to maintain aerobic metabolism because of the coordinated responses that include behavioral, cardiovascular, metabolic, and hormonal modifications (Greene, 1999; Ross et al., 2013). Aerobic metabolism is maintained until oxygen in the intervillous space is reduced to 50% of the normal level, at which point the fetus is unable to compensate for the progressive accumulation of carbon dioxide and hypoxemia (Bobrow & Soothill, 1999; King & Parer, 2000; Wilkening & Meschia, 1983). This process eventually results in metabolic acidosis, and finally if severe enough and of sufficient duration, metabolic academia (Effros & Swenson, 2010; Greene, 1999; King, 2012; Miller & Miller, 2012).

Anaerobic glucose metabolism occurs when oxygen is unavailable and cellular oxidation of hydrogen ions cannot take place. When placental transfer of oxygen is restricted over a long period, energy is released through the conversion of pyruvate to lactic acid. Continued hypoxia results in the accumulation of this nonvolatile acid (Blechner, 1993; D. A. Miller, 2011a). Plasma bicarbonate and hemoglobin, the two most important buffers in the blood, permit the maintenance of the pH at a relatively constant level during short periods of anaerobic metabolism (Freeman, Garite, Nageotte, & Miller, 2012).

Early in anaerobic metabolism, when oxygen stores are depleted, glucose is initially converted to pyruvic acid through a series of chemical reactions while lactic acid and carbon dioxide build up. As pyruvic and lactic acid accumulate from continued anaerobic metabolism, increasing amounts of hydrogen ion are released that lower the pH. In the absence of oxygen, lactic acid cannot be broken down and it accumulates, resulting in metabolic acidemia. Hydrogen ions are toxic to cells but are buffered by bicarbonate, hemoglobin, and plasma proteins. Buffers resist the changes in pH and are a mixture of a weak acid and its salt base. Buffers are the first line of defense in counteracting the continuous metabolic production of hydrogen ions by the tissues. They also maintain acid-base homeostasis by keeping blood pH in a normal range. Over time, as the ATP supply is exhausted, the fetus will accumulate lactic acid in the bloodstream. When these buffers are depleted, there is marked increase in hydrogen ions and a fall in pH, resulting in acidosis. This chain of events leads to cell death unless oxygenation is restored (Blechner, 1993; Greene, 1999; King, 2013). In other words, the fetus attempts to redistribute cardiac output to preserve cerebral perfusion and maintain cellular integrity but if interruption of blood flow is severe or prolonged there is increased risk for cerebral and end organ damage (Perlman, 2012).

After birth, excretion of nonvolatile acids occurs through the kidneys. However, because of the immaturity of the fetal renal system, excretion of accumulated acids must take place via the placenta. These acids must therefore cross the placenta into the maternal circulation for excretion by the maternal kidneys; however, this diffusion is much slower than carbon dioxide diffusion. Excretion may require hours rather than seconds to completely clear the buildup of nonvolatile acids, even after sufficient oxygen is restored for aerobic metabolism. When these acids accumulate, fetal metabolic acidosis occurs (Freeman et al., 2012; Thorp & Rushing, 1999). With the addition of oxygen (at the cellular level), lactic acid is converted into carbon dioxide, which enters the umbilical arteries and is transported into the maternal circulation for excretion through the maternal system. The process of reversing metabolic acidosis with adequate oxygenation can take 20–30 minutes or longer, depending on the degree of acidosis. Therefore, fetuses with metabolic acidosis *in utero* may exhibit decreasing variability, possible loss of variability, neurologic compromise, and even intrauterine death.

The fetus can develop respiratory acidemia as a result of several circumstances, including excessive uterine activity (Bakker et al., 2007), an acute onset of umbilical cord compression, recurrent variable decelerations, or decreased uteroplacental perfusion (Armstrong & Stenson, 2007; Freeman et al., 2012). If situations such as these are not corrected, respiratory acidemia may occur. For example, variable decelerations occurring during a labor complicated by oligohydramnios may be a result of recurrent episodes of umbilical cord compression because there is an inadequate amount of amniotic fluid to cushion the umbilical cord. When umbilical cord compression or occlusion occurs, carbon dioxide produced by lactic acid conversion cannot be removed from the fetal circulation. The excess carbon dioxide is hydrolyzed, and carbonic acid is formed, resulting in respiratory acidosis. However, respiratory acidosis is easily reversed once the cord occlusion abates because carbon dioxide is quickly diffused into the maternal circulation for excretion through the maternal respiratory system. Depending on the duration of the insult, the fetus will excrete carbon dioxide across the placenta if allowed sufficient time. Once umbilical circulation is restored, a healthy fetus can be resuscitated *in utero*.

During labor, a mild maternal metabolic acidemia may develop as a result of muscle activity, catecholamine release, or relative starvation. A mixture of both respiratory and metabolic acidemia also may occur. When the supply of oxygen and the removal of carbon dioxide and fixed acids by the placenta are in balance, the fetus will maintain a normal acid-base balance within a narrow range. If these processes are interrupted, the fetus may develop acidemia (Thorp & Rushing, 1999).

FETAL OXYGENATION AND ACID-BASE ASSESSMENT

A key principle in understanding fetal oxygenation in the antepartum and intrapartum period is that moderate variability with or without accelerations reliably predicts the absence of fetal metabolic acidemia at the time the FHR tracing is reviewed (Macones et al., 2008; Miller & Miller, 2011; Parer, King, Flanders, Fox, & Kilpatrick, 2006). Conversely, the opposite of this statement is not always true as the absence of accelerations or moderate variability does not reliably predict metabolic acidemia (Stout & Cahill, 2011). Consequently, clinicians may need to use adjunct methods of assessing fetal acid-base status in order to interpret category II and III FHR findings. These methods may be especially useful in evaluating the fetal condition in the setting of minimal variability with recurrent late or variable decelerations (ACOG, 2010; Low, Victory, & Derrick, 1999). The fetal condition can be evaluated when intermittent auscultation or EFM is used with other adjunct methods of evaluation, including indirect and direct approaches (Greenberg, Druzin, & Gabbe, 2012; Kim, Khandelwal, Gaughan, Agar, & Reece, 2003; King, 2013; SOGC, 2007). The direct method is one in which actual blood sampling occurs; indirect methods are those in which acid-base levels are implied on the basis of a less direct measure, the fetal response, or both. Regardless of which method is used, these are assessments that must be repeated periodically if the tracing does not respond to corrective measures (Simpson, 2012).

Indirect Methods of Acid-Base Assessment during the Intrapartum Period

Indirect methods for evaluation of oxygenation and acid-base values include fetal scalp stimulation and vibroacoustic stimulation (VAS), which are used to elicit an acceleration. This fetal response is typically associated with a nonacidotic fetus, generally with a pH of ≥ 7.19, and a normoxic central nervous system (Clark, Gimovsky, & Miller, 1982, 1984; Elimian, Figueroa, & Tejani, 1997). Elicitation of FHR accelerations following scalp stimulation or VAS is probably related to a change in the fetal behavioral state (Martin, 2008; Porter & Clark, 1999). Although an acceleration response is associated with fetal well-being, the absence of acceleration does not predict fetal compromise. Decisions to use additional direct assessments of acid-base status are based on various factors, including the maternal–fetal history, labor progress, current maternal status, and individual institutional guidelines.

Fetal Scalp Stimulation

Fetal scalp stimulation is a noninvasive procedure that may provide information about the acid-base status of the fetus in the setting of an indeterminate (category II) FHR finding in labor. Historically, scalp stimulation was performed by one of two methods: pinching the fetal scalp with an Allis clamp or applying gentle digital pressure to the scalp through a dilated cervix for 15 seconds. Fetal scalp stimulation may be used when there is minimal variability or no spontaneous accelerations. This procedure is performed during segments of baseline, not during decelerations or a bradycardia as it is not a method of intrauterine resuscitation (ACOG, 2010; Clark et al., 1984; Freeman et al., 2012). Accelerations, spontaneous or induced, of 15 bpm or more in amplitude for a duration of 15 seconds or longer typically reflect a pH of ≥ 7.19 and the absence of acidosis (Clark, Gimovsky & Miller, 1982, 1984; Garite, 2012) (Figure 7-2). The absence of an acceleratory response to stimulation is an indeterminate finding (Macones et al., 2008).

General guidelines for the procedure are as follows:

- Explain the procedure to the patient.
- Place the patient in a lateral position.
- Perform a vaginal examination.
- Apply gentle digital pressure on the fetal scalp.
- Perform stimulation when the FHR is at baseline and in between decelerations.
- Document the procedure and response per institutional policy.

Vibroacoustic Stimulation

FHR accelerations and movement induced by VAS were first reported by Sontag and Wallace in 1934. Auditory development in the fetus involves formation of ear structures in the first 20 weeks of gestation, and development of the auditory system's neurosensory parts after 20 weeks gestational age. The auditory system becomes functional at approximately 25–28 weeks' gestation (Graven & Brown, 2008; Greenburg et al., 2012). The acoustic environment of the fetus is composed of continuous cardiovascular, respiratory, and intestinal sounds of the pregnant woman. Vibrations on the external surface of the mother's abdomen can also induce sounds within the uterus. Sounds penetrate the tissues and fluid surrounding the fetal head and stimulate the inner ear though a bone conduction route. The fetus hears low-frequency sounds below 300 Hz. In fact, the fetus can likely detect vowels and rhythmic patterns of music (Gerhardt & Abrams, 2000). A commercially distributed vibroacoustic stimulator, a battery-powered artificial larynx, or both are used to deliver auditory and vibratory stimulus to the fetus. These devices may be hand-held or attached by a connector to the fetal monitor. The vibroacoustic stimulator may be placed over the fetal vertex or fetal breech. Identical FHR responses and increases in fetal movement can be observed after stimulation over either position (Eller, Robinson, & Newman, 1992).

Yao and colleagues (1990) reported that movements occurred more frequently after VAS set at 103 dB and at 109 dB. If the artificial larynx

Figure 7-2 Fetal Scalp Stimulation Elicits FHR Acceleration

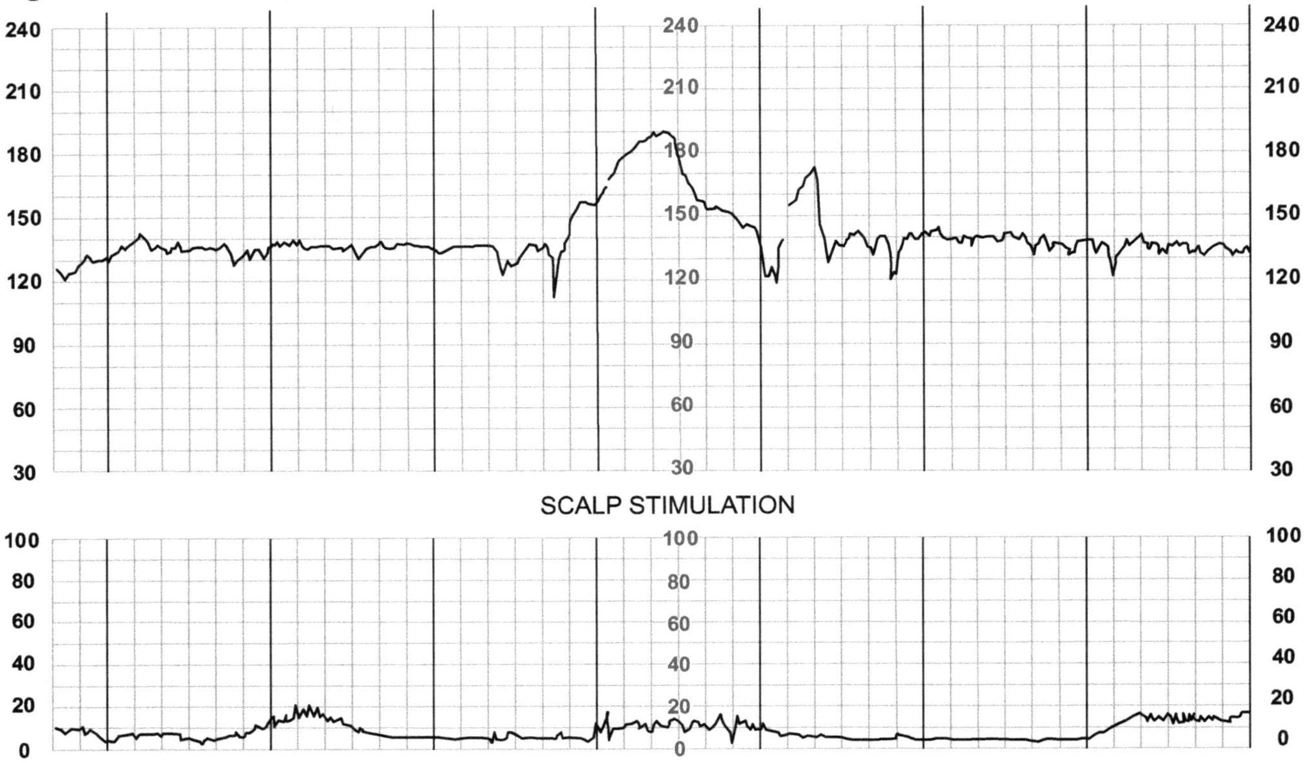

is set at 103 dB, it will usually be sufficient to elicit accelerations (Yao et al., 1990). The static and dynamic forces of the vibrator and the distance from the fetal head are also factors in the transmission of the sound (Gerhardt & Abrams, 2000). The use of VAS in antepartum testing is discussed in Chapter 10.

A reactive non-stress test (NST) after VAS appears to be as reliable as a spontaneous acceleration demonstrating that there is an intact central nervous system and no disruption in the oxygentation pathway to the fetal heart (Greenberg et al., 2012). Occasionally, a fetus will respond to VAS with a prolonged acceleration or deceleration, particularly when oligohydramnios is present (Miller, Rabello, & Paul, 1996). Some medications have been associated with altered responses to VAS. These include beta-adrenergic blocking agents, corticosteroids, and magnesium sulfate, which have been associated with decreased reactivity and a blunted response (Rotmensch, Celentano, Liberati, Sadan, & Glezerman, 1999; Sherer, 1994; Sherer & Bentolila, 1998). The effect of intrauterine growth restriction on fetal response to VAS has also been studied. It has been noted that FHR accelerations are shorter in duration and body movements are fewer in these fetuses when compared with normal-size fetuses (Porter & Clark, 1999). In fetuses between 26 and 32 weeks' gestation that are small for gestational age, researchers reported a limited response, suggesting delayed functional maturation of fetal sensory receptors (Gagnon, Hunse, & Foreman, 1989).

The benefits of VAS must be weighed against the effect on the predictive reliability of the test and the safety of the procedure. VAS produces significant increases over baseline intrauterine sound pressure levels, which average 72–88 decibels (dB) (Smith, Satt, Phelan, & Paul, 1990), to sound levels between 98 and 111 dB. Although prolonged exposure to sound levels above 110 dB has been shown to be associated with acoustic injury, several studies have shown that there is no evidence of either hearing loss or neurological damage because amniotic fluid attenuates sound vibration and intensity (Arulkumaran et al., 1991, 1992; Nyman, Barr, & Westgren, 1992).

Intrapartum Use of Vibroacoustic Stimulation

There has been discussion about extending the use of VAS during the intrapartum period for fetal assessment (Lin, Vassallo, & Mittendorf, 2001; Skupski, Rosenberg, & Eglinton, 2002). One of the earliest studies found VAS to be as reliable as fetal scalp sampling for determining acidosis during the first stage of labor (Smith, Ngueyn, Phelan, & Paul, 1986). Of those fetuses that responded to VAS with FHR accelerations ≥15 bpm ≥15 seconds duration, none were found to have an acidotic pH. The predictive value was 100% for a normal scalp pH. A prospective observational study examined the association between accelerations, spontaneous or induced by VAS, and subsequent scalp pH values in the presence of abnormal FHR tracings. FHR accelerations that were induced by VAS were associated with scalp blood pH values of 7.25 or higher (Irion et al., 1996). To date, there are no randomized controlled trials that address the safety and efficacy of VAS in the intrapartum period so clinical judgment should be utilized when using VAS intrapartum.

Fetal Pulse Oximetry

The fetal pulse oximeter was first introduced in the 1990s as an adjunct to intrapartum fetal assessment in an effort to measure fetal oxygenation and acid-base balance. The fetal pulse oximeter was based on existing technology that had already had a definitive impact on patient care in a variety of settings including critical care, anesthesia, and neonatal resuscitation (Dildy, 2011; Garite, 2013). The principle theory behind pulse oximetry is that arterial hemoglobin oxygen saturation can be estimated by how much red and infrared light is absorbed by oxygenated (oxyhemoglobin) and deoxygenated hemoglobin (deoxyhemoglobin). The percentage of oxyhemoglobin, also known as arterial oxygen saturation, is calculated by obtaining the ratio of red and infrared light absorbed into the tissue through a sensor. The fraction is displayed as a percentage and represents the mean of the measurements obtained during the previous 3–6 seconds (Fouzas, Priftis, & Anthracopoulos, 2011).

A number of randomized controlled trials concluded there was limited support for using fetal pulse oximetry in the presence of an indeterminate or abnormal fetal heart rate tracing because the technology did not reduce the overall cesarean birth rate and the device was particularly difficult to place from a technological standpoint (Dildy, 2011; Garite, 2013). The manufacturer removed the product from the market in January 2006. The product is no longer available but more important is the data that was gleaned about fetal oxygenation, the critical threshold for causing metabolic acidosis and acid-base balance.

As previously discussed, persistent fetal hypoxia may lead to acidosis, neurologic injury, tissue and organ damage, and ultimately, death (Dildy, Clark, & Loucks, 1996; King & Parer, 2000). However, the fetus often becomes hypoxemic for short periods of time and may revert to a normal acid-base balance without becoming acidotic. The critical threshold of when hypoxia would likely cause metabolic acidosis was largely unknown and the data that emerged with fetal pulse oximetry technology answered this key question. The fetus is presumed to be adequately oxygenated in a range of 30–65% saturation (Dildy, Thorp, Yeast, & Clark, 1996; Nijland, Jongsma, Nijhuis, van den Berg, & Oeseburg, 1995; Richardson, Carmichael, Homan, & Patrick, 1992). Metabolic acidosis does not develop until the saturation level falls below 30% for at least 10-15 minutes (Seelbach-Gobel, Heupel, Kuhnert, & Butterwegge, 1999). This value was also validated in a randomized controlled trial conducted concurrently in nine medical centers across the United States (Garite et al., 2000). Although it is not used clinically in the United States, the use of fetal pulse oximetry in research contributed to our understanding of the effects of common interventions on fetal oxygenation (Haydon et al., 2006; Simpson & James, 2005, 2008).

DIRECT METHODS OF ACID-BASE ASSESSMENT

Direct methods of acid-base assessment are those in which actual blood sampling occurs. Examples of methods used during the intrapartum period include fetal scalp sampling and umbilical cord blood sampling. *In utero* techniques such as percutaneous umbilical blood sampling (PUBS) allow for evaluation of fetal blood gases as well as other laboratory parameters but technical limitations and the fact that sampling only provides insight at that point in time make PUBS impractical for use during the intrapartum period (Neerhof & Thaete, 2008).

Fetal Scalp Sampling

Intrapartum fetal scalp sampling, a method of estimating capillary blood pH, was first reported in the 1960s (Saling & Schneider, 1967) and continues to be used in other countries (Garite, 2013). Today, fetal scalp sampling in the United States is not used in obstetrical practice due to significant technical, facility, and clinical limitations (Garite, 2013). In addition, two consensus-based concepts in fetal heart rate interpretation have also acknowledged that "moderate fetal heart rate variability reliably predicts the absence of fetal metabolic acidemia at the time it is observed" and "the presence of fetal heart rate accelerations (either spontaneous or stimulated) reliably predicts the absence of fetal metabolic acidemia" (Macones et. al, 2008, p. 513). Therefore, less invasive methods, such as fetal scalp stimulation, have been advocated for to reduce the need for fetal scalp sampling in acid-base assessment (Clark et al., 1984; Elimian et al., 1997; Goodwin, Milner-Masterson, & Paul, 1994). In Canada and Europe, updated clinical guidelines and references recognize fetal scalp sampling in situations of fetal compromise but acknowledge that this method should be used when technically possible and in the absence of contraindications (National Collaborating Centre for Women's and Children's Health [NCC-WCH], 2007; SOGC, 2007). The technique also is used for clinical experience and indirect research comparisons (Neilson, 2008).

Contraindications

Contraindications to fetal scalp sampling include but are not limited to (NCC-WCH, 2007; SOGC, 2007):

- Fetal coagulopathy, whether determined or suspected (hemophilia)
- Maternal infections that increase the risk of maternal–fetal transmission (e.g., human immunodeficiency virus, hepatitis, herpes simplex)
- Prematurity (< 34 weeks' gestation)

Factors and Limitations

Factors and limitations that may affect fetal scalp sampling include (Clark & Paul, 1985; SOGC, 2007; Whitworth & Bricker, 2006):

- Availability of 24-hour access to blood gas analysis equipment with rapid turnaround
- Insufficient training and/or continuing opportunity to maintain proficiency
- Ruptured membranes and accessible presenting part
- Adequate cervical dilation and effacement (which may limit feasibility of obtaining sample)
- Maternal positioning
- Maternal consent
- Time lapse for filling the capillary tube
- Misinterpretation of pH data or lack of reporting of base deficit or base excess
- Contamination of the sample with hair, caput, air from slow blood flow, and meconium (which may affect accuracy of results)
- Blood clotting in capillary tube before sample reaches the laboratory

Interpretation of Results

Results obtained from fetal scalp sampling reflect fetal acid-base status only at the time of the sampling and are interpreted in the context of the clinical situation (Clark & Paul, 1985; Whitworth & Bricker, 2006); thus, repeat testing is often necessary. The information should be evaluated in the context of the total clinical situation at the time of sampling, including FHR characteristics and patterns, uterine contraction pattern, and any maternal factors that could affect the fetal acid-base status. Repeat testing is typically performed to assess trends in values, for example, whether the pH is rising or falling. Furthermore, pH as a sole value reported is a less satisfactory measure of acidemia than a combination of pH and base deficit because of variations of acidemia that may be present at the time of blood sampling (SOGC, 2007). A study performed by Bowen, Kochenour, Rehm, and Woolley (1986) showed that 10% of samples obtained at the time of birth were found to be below the values found in the umbilical artery; this suggests that there may be factors in the fetal scalp that are responsible for the falsely low fetal scalp pH value.

Mothers with complications such as asthma, dehydration, and hyperventilation may need a simultaneous arterial blood gas sample for comparative evaluation with the fetal scalp sample. Typically, fetal scalp blood pH is approximately 0.1 unit below the maternal pH, which will guide the clinician when significant maternal acidosis or alkalosis is suspected.

Umbilical Cord Blood Sampling

Umbilical cord blood acid-base analysis can be used as an objective method of quantifying fetal acid-base balance and oxygenation at the time of cord clamping when umbilical circulation ceases (Table 7-1) (Armstrong & Stenson, 2007). The pH, PCO_2 and PO_2 of the blood can be measured; the bicarbonate concentration and percentage oxygen saturation are determined from these measurements. From the measured values and the hemoglobin level, the base excess and base deficit can be calculated. The pH and the base excess or base deficit are useful values in assessing the fetal condition at the time of collection when establishing whether an acute intrapartum event is sufficient to cause cerebral palsy (ACOG, 2006; ACOG & AAP, 2014). Uncommonly, other than acute intrapartum events, conditions such as fetal anemia in an Rh isoimmunized pregnancy or parvovirus infection may impact umbilical artery values (Bobrow & Soothill, 1999; Soothill, Nicolaides, & Rodeck, 1987; Soothill, Nicolaides, Rodeck, Clewell, & Lindridge, 1987). Box 7-2 describes the process of umbilical cord blood sampling. A finding of normal umbilical blood gas measurements precludes the presence of acidemia at or immediately before birth (Gregg & Weiner, 1993) and is a more objective measure than the Apgar score, especially in the preterm fetus (ACOG, 2006; Dickinson, Erikson, Meyer, & Parisi, 1992).

TABLE 7-1 Normal Ranges of Umbilical Cord Arterial Blood Gas Values

ARTERIAL MEASURE[a]	NORMAL MEAN VALUE RANGE[b]	RANGE (±2 STANDARD DEVIATIONS)
Ph	7.20–7.29	7.02–7.43
PCO_2 (mmHg)	49.2–56.3	21.5–78.3
Bicarbonate (mEq/L)	22.0–24.1	14.8–29.2
Base deficit (mEq/L)	2.7–8.3	2.0–16.3
PO_2 (mmHg)	15.1–23.7	2.0–37.8

Thorp and Rushing (1999).
[a]Venous values reflect maternal acid-base status and are generally higher than arterial values that reflect fetal acid-base status. Venous values may be normal despite arterial values reflecting fetal acidemia.
[b]These figures represent the range of normal mean values reported in a review of studies of umbilical arterial cord blood gases.

The specific interval and optimal timing between birth and umbilical cord clamping has not been established in the literature or formal clinical guidelines (ACOG, 2012). Recent reviews suggest that umbilical cord clamping at birth could be delayed for at least 30–60 seconds, with the infant maintained at or below the level of the placenta (Arca, Botet, Palacio, & Carbonell-Estrany, 2010; Mercer & Erickson-Owens, 2012; Rabe, Reynolds, & Diaz-Rossello, 2008). The clinical neonatal benefits include increased blood volume, reduced need for blood transfusion, up to a 50% reduction in intraventricular hemorrhage in preterm infants, and lower frequency of iron-deficiency anemia in term infants (ACOG, 2012; Eichenbaum-Pikser & Zasloff, 2009). Timing of delayed umbilical cord clamping needs to be balanced with timely resuscitation of the newborn.

When indicated, a double-clamped segment of the umbilical cord is obtained at birth.

Box 7-2 Umbilical Cord Blood Gas Sampling Procedure

General Guidelines

- Obtain two or three 1-mL heparinized syringes with a short, small-gauge needle for optimal control with minimal injury to the vessels.
- Heparin is the only acceptable anticoagulant for umbilical cord blood gases.
- Prepare labels with patient's name, medical record number, and sample site.
- Obtain a double-clamped cord segment after the delivery.
- Obtain a blood sample from the umbilical artery first because it is often more difficult to get and the umbilical vein may help support the umbilical artery.)
- Avoid air bubbles or carefully expel excess air from each syringe.
- Cap each syringe.
- Label the specimen(s) and send specimen(s) to the laboratory for analysis.
- Document that the cord blood samples were collected and sent to the laboratory for analysis; document the results when available.

ACOG (2006); Scheans (2011); Wallman (1997).

Alterations in umbilical cord blood acid-base values can occur within 5–10 seconds of neonatal breathing after birth or in situations of delayed umbilical cord clamping in which placental circulation persists allowing for changes in fluid volume and ongoing placental metabolism and gas exchange (Armstrong & Stenson, 2006; Lievaart & de Jong, 1984; Wiberg, Kallen, & Olofsson, 2008). With delayed cord clamping, small changes in umbilical cord pH can occur within 60 seconds of birth (Ulrich & Ackerman, 1972) and after 60 minutes cord umbilical arterial or venous pH can drop by more than 0.2 pH units (Armstrong & Stenson, 2006). Similar changes, while less predictable, can occur in blood that is sampled from placental surface with the pH falling at twice the rate of the cord pH (Lynn & Beeby, 2007). These changes are not detected if the cord is doubly clamped at birth (Armstrong & Stenson, 2006; Duerbeck, Chaffin, & Seeds, 1992; Hilger, Holzman, & Brown, 1981). Cord blood banking may also necessitate the need for earlier cord clamping in order to obtain a sufficient amount of umbilical cord blood for stem cell harvesting (Eichenbaum-Pikser & Zasloff, 2009).

Indications and Contraindications

There is a lack of consensus among experts and professional organizations regarding whether umbilical cord gas sampling should be performed routinely at every delivery or solely in selected high-risk situations when an adverse perinatal outcome may be suspected (ACOG, 2006; NCC-WCH, 2007; SOGC, 2007). The cord blood can be analyzed if "a serious abnormality that arose during the birth process or a problem with the neonate's condition, or if both persist at or beyond the first 5 minutes" (ACOG, 2006, p. 1321) or according to facility protocol. Analysis of the cord blood can be delayed while Apgar scores are being assigned. The umbilical cord segment may be discarded if the infant appears stable and the 5-minute Apgar score is satisfactory (ACOG, 2006). Suggested indications for umbilical cord blood sampling may include but may not be limited to the following (ACOG, 2006; Freeman et al., 2012):

- Cesarean birth for fetal compromise
- Low 5-minute Apgar score
- Severe intrauterine growth restriction
- Abnormal fetal heart rate tracing within 1 hour of birth (e.g., category II or III patterns)
  - Recurrent late decelerations
  - Fetal tachycardia
  - Absent variability
  - Recurrent variable decelerations (especially with decreasing FHR baseline variability, increasing FHR baseline, or when the deceleration meets at least two of the following criteria: drop of depth 60 bpm or less, nadir of and duration of 60 seconds or longer) (Freeman et al, 2012; Hamilton, Warrick, & O'Keeffe, 2012; Ross et al., 2013)
  - Recurrent prolonged decelerations
  - Bradycardia
- Delivery of high-risk patients (e.g., maternal thyroid disease, multifetal gestations, unexpected fetal anomaly)

- Intrapartum fever (≥ 100.4° F)
- Preterm birth < 34 weeks' gestation
- Moderate or thick meconium
- Unexplained intrapartum vaginal bleeding
- Operative vaginal birth (forceps or vacuum)
- Shoulder dystocia
- Vaginal birth of a fetus with a malpresentation (e.g., breech)

Umbilical cord blood sampling may be helpful in clarifying fetal acid-base status at birth and may also assist planning the clinical management of selected newborns such as those neonates requiring neuroprotective cooling for suspected neonatal hypoxic-ischemic encephalopathy (Shankaran et al., 2012; Thorp & Rushing, 1999). There are no known contraindications for the use of umbilical cord blood sampling, but it may preclude other uses of the cord, such as harvesting blood for stem cells.

A double-clamped segment of the umbilical cord is stable for blood gas assessment for at least 1 hour (ACOG, 2006; Armstrong & Stenson, 2006; Duerbeck et al., 1992). The cord blood sample in a heparinized syringe is stable for up to 1 hour (Duerbeck et al. 1992; Strickland, Gilstrap, Hauth, & Widmer, 1984), but not longer. Residual heparin and air should be expelled because it has been reported that the addition of heparin or air can decrease the pH, PCO_2, and bicarbonate (Kirshon & Moise, 1989). Umbilical cord segments and cord blood samples do not need to be placed on ice because they will remain relatively stable at room temperature for up to 1 hour with no significant changes in the pH value (Duerbeck et al., 1992; Hilger et al., 1981; Manor, Blickstein, Hazan, Flidel-Rimon, & Hagay, 1998). Many facilities no longer transport samples on ice because of the short amount of time required between obtaining the specimen and performing the test.

Umbilical artery samples reveal details on the blood returning to the placenta and provide fundamental information about fetal status at the time of birth, including the presence and severity of fetal acidosis. Umbilical vein samples reflect placental function and acid-base status at the time of birth and confirm the accuracy of umbilical artery samples. Both umbilical vein and artery samples should be collected and analyzed whenever possible to prevent debate over whether a true arterial specimen was obtained (ACOG, 2006b; Armstrong & Stenson, 2007; Riley & Johnson, 1993; Thorp & Rushing, 1999).

Umbilical arterial and venous samples should be collected using separate syringes and labeled immediately. The sample values can then be reviewed to verify that the samples originate from two separate vessels and are accurate (Westgate, Garibaldi, & Greene, 1994; Armstrong & Stenson, 2007). This will also assist in identifying if an intrapartum event may have caused fetal acidosis, if present (Riley & Johnson, 1993). For example, in an umbilical cord prolapse, the umbilical arterial blood value may be more acidotic compared with the normal values in the venous sample because it reflects information on the blood returning to the placenta from the fetus (Riley & Johnson, 1993). The umbilical arterial values are also an accurate assessment of fetal metabolic status at the time of birth and appear to correlate best with the Apgar score (Thorp, Dildy, Yeomans, Meyer, & Parisi, 1996; Thorp, Sampson, Parisi, & Creasy, 1989). The umbilical venous values are an important addition to umbilical cord sampling because they confirm accuracy of the values obtained from the artery and assist in determining if acidosis is metabolic or respiratory (Armstrong & Stenson, 2007; Freeman et al., 2012; Riley & Johnson, 1993).

Obtaining cord blood samples from the umbilical cord can be difficult at times. The umbilical arteries, which carry deoxygenated blood away from the fetus, have smaller lumens, thicker walls, and contain less blood than the umbilical vein. Therefore, the distended umbilical vein that carries oxygenated blood to the fetus may provide some support to the artery, making sampling easier (ACOG, 2006; Armstrong & Stenson, 2007). If the umbilical cord vessels are poorly filled, blood can be milked with the thumb and forefinger from the placenta toward the clamp. After the umbilical vessels become distended, the cord can be clamped again to isolate a segment that can be used for sampling (Riley & Johnson, 1993).

In the event umbilical cord samples are unobtainable or insufficient such as when a thin cord in the pregnancy is complicated by intrauterine growth restriction, a sample can be obtained from the umbilical vessels that traverse the chorionic (fetal) surface of the placenta. Umbilical vessels become very obvious when they can be traced back to the umbilical cord at the insertion site on the placenta (ACOG, 2006; Riley & Johnson, 1993; Thorp & Rushing, 1999). The smaller, thick-walled arteries consistently cross over the larger, thin-walled veins (Smart, 1962). Results of the sample obtained from the placental vessels will offer a close estimate but not necessarily an equivalent of all the blood gas measurements because the placenta remains metabolically active for several minutes after cord clamping (Armstrong & Stenson, 2006; Nodwell, Carmichael, Ross, & Richardson, 2005; Riley & Johnson, 1993).

Factors Affecting Sampling and Interpretation of Results

Factors that may affect umbilical cord blood sampling and interpretation include the following:

- Differences in methodology, such as duration of procedure or air bubbles in sample
- Differences in heparin concentration
  - Spurious metabolic acidosis resulting from use of too much heparin or too concentrated a solution (Thorp & Rushing, 1999)
  - Bicarbonate and partial PCO_2 values show an inverse relationship with the volume of heparin (Duerbeck et al., 1992)
- Sampling of venous and not arterial blood

Interpretation of Umbilical Cord Blood Acid-Base

Interpretation of umbilical cord blood gas results requires a basic understanding of acid-base terminology and the clinical implications associated with acidosis and acidemia. The fetus, compared to the adult, survives in a hypoxemic, normocarbic, nonacidotic environment before the onset of labor. During the course of labor, some tissue hypoxia occurs as a result of uterine contractions that may result in fetal acidosis and ultimately acidemia depending on the type and duration of the oxygen pathway disruption (Bakker et al., 2007; Brouillette & Waxman, 1997; Hamilton, Warrick, Knox, et al., 2012). Limited data implies that metabolic acidemia does not appear abruptly but evolves gradually over a period of 60 minutes (Parer et al., 2006). As previously discussed, respiratory acidosis occurs when an elevated PCO_2 level is present (i.e., the value is more than two standard deviations above the mean). Normally, carbon dioxide diffuses rapidly across the placenta. The rate of carbon dioxide diffusion is related to the rate of blood flow on both sides of the placenta. Respiratory acidosis can develop rapidly but also can be corrected rapidly.

Metabolic acidosis takes longer to develop and longer to resolve; it is present when levels of lactic acid and other acids become elevated. These acids are the end product of anaerobic metabolism. Elevation of the acids consumes fetal base buffers, exhausting the fetal capacity to regulate pH. Metabolic acidosis is more serious than respiratory acidosis because it reflects a more prolonged hypoxic insult (Wallman, 1997). A fetus may experience respiratory and metabolic acidosis simultaneously. When this occurs it is referred to as mixed acidosis (Table 7-2).

For umbilical cord blood, the normal mean arterial blood pH values ranged from 7.20 to 7.29 in a review of studies that monitored umbilical cord arterial blood gas values, with a full range of normal pH values (± 2 standard deviations) from 7.02 to 7.43 (Thorp & Rushing, 1999). Traditionally, cord blood pH values below 7.20, defined as acidemia, have been considered pathologic or clinically significant. However, published data suggest that the lower range of normal for umbilical artery pH is between 7.10 and 7.19 and that the original threshold of 7.2 may not be reasonable (Blackstone & Young, 1993; Dildy, 2005; Gilstrap, Leveno, Burris,

TABLE 7-2 Significance of Deviation from Normal Values

TYPE OF ACIDOSIS	PH	PO_2	PCO_2	HCO_3	BASE DEFICIT
Respiratory	Decreased	Variable	Increased	Normal	Normal
Metabolic	Decreased	Decreased	Normal	Decreased	Increased
Mixed	Decreased	Decreased	Increased	Decreased	Increased

Gilstrap et al. (1989); Helwig et al. (1996); Yeomans et al. (1985).

Williams, & Little, 1989; Goldaber & Gilstrap, 1993; Low, 1988; Riley & Johnson, 1993; Sykes et al., 1982; Thorp et al., 1989; Yeomans, Hauth, Gilstrap, & Strickland, 1985). Blood pH values below 7.00 have been associated with adverse neonatal outcomes and more clearly represent a threshold for significant fetal acidemia (Andres et al., 1999; Gilstrap et al., 1989; Goldaber, Gilstrap, Leveno, Dax, & McIntire, 1991).

Although normal blood values are often described in ranges, it may be helpful to identify a specific number to use a frame of reference when evaluating cord blood values (see Table 7-3). All umbilical cord blood values should be evaluated in relationship to the specific clinical findings and situation for any given infant. In addition to pH levels, the PO_2, PCO_2, bicarbonate, and base deficit or excess values are also considered.

Plasma bicarbonate is one base buffer used to raise (or normalize) pH levels. In metabolic acidosis, an excess of hydrogen ions is released. As a result, bicarbonate is depleted, so the values are decreased in metabolic acidosis (Freeman et al., 2012; Gimovsky & Caritis, 1982). Thus, a base deficit exists when fetal base buffers are below normal values. The base deficit or excess is not measured directly but is calculated for the pH, PCO_2, and bicarbonate blood values. The terms "base deficit" and "base excess" are often confusing, but they basically measure the same thing: base buffers in the blood specimen that help to determine the type of acidosis. When the base buffers are depleted, a base deficit exists and metabolic acidosis is present. Although this is expressed as a negative base excess by some laboratories instead of base deficit, the principle is the same.

TABLE 7-3 Single-Digit Value Guideline for Initial Assessment of Normal and Abnormal Umbilical Cord Blood Acid-Base Values

	NORMAL VALUES	METABOLIC ACIDEMIA	RESPIRATORY ACIDEMIA
pH	≥ 7.10	<7.10	<7.10
PO_2 (mmHg)	≥ 20	<20	Variable
PCO_2 (mmHg)	<60	<60	>60
Bicarbonate (mEq/L)	>22	<22	≥ 22
Base deficit (mEq/L)	≤ 12	>12	<12
Base excess (mEq/L)	≥ -12	<-12	>-12

Note: The values presented are suggested as a guide for evaluating acid-base status. All umbilical cord blood values should be evaluated in relation to the specific clinical findings and situation for a given patient. Note that greater absolute values of base deficit or excess are associated with acidemia.
Andres et al. (1999); Low, Lindsay, and Derrick (1997).

Remember that for numbers with negative values, the further to the left of zero they move on a number line, the lesser their value. A base excess of −12 is a lower number than −11. Numbers further from zero, whether expressed as base deficit or negative base excess, indicate inadequate base buffer reserves and increasing metabolic acidosis (the higher the number, the more severe the acidosis). Conversely, the closer to "0" the base deficit or negative base excess is, the more buffers remain in the specimen and are outside the range of metabolic acidosis.

SUMMARY

Assessment of fetal well-being is an important component of antepartum and intrapartum care. A variety of methods for direct and indirect fetal acid-base monitoring have been developed, each with potential challenges to successful clinical implementation (Dildy, 2005). Research to identify additional effective assessment strategies is needed. Health care providers are challenged to understand the circumstances that affect fetal oxygenation, select the appropriate method of acid-base assessment, and intervene in a timely manner to maximize fetal oxygenation.

Case Study: Eleanor

Age:	28
Gravidity/Parity:	G3 P1011
Gestational Age:	41-4/7 weeks
Medical History:	Unremarkable
Surgical History:	Cesarean section
Psychosocial History:	Unremarkable
Past Obstetric History:	Previous low transverse cesarean section for arrest of dilation at 6 cm; spontaneous abortion at 6 weeks
Current Obstetric History:	Normal prenatal laboratory results. Second trimester ultrasound consistent with LMP, normal anatomy

Eleanor presented to labor and delivery at 1330 with spontaneous rupture of membranes that occurred at 1100. The fluid was meconium stained. She stated her contractions started some time last evening and gradually became more frequent and regular through the night. After her membranes ruptured, the contractions became more intense, occurring every 3 minutes; she rated her pain as 6 on a 1–10 scale. The FHR was normal, with a baseline of 140, moderate variability, and spontaneous accelerations. She was having contractions every 2–3 minutes, lasting 60–90 seconds, and moderate on palpation. A VE on admission revealed a cervix that was 2 cm dilated, 50% effaced, and a fetal vertex that was –2 station. Her vital signs were as follows: oral temperature, 97.8° F (36.5° C); blood pressure, 112/58 mmHg; pulse, 86 bpm; and respirations, 22 breaths per minute. Eleanor requested an epidural shortly after admission because of the increasing intensity of contractions. A vaginal examination at 1640 revealed a cervix that was 6 cm dilated, 75% effaced, and fetal vertex at 0 station. The physician placed an IUPC to monitor contractions. At 1800, Eleanor's cervix remained 6 cm and an oxytocin infusion was started due to inadequate Montevideo units (140–180 mmHg).

The FHR gradually changed to a baseline of 135 bpm, minimal variability, and recurrent variable decelerations with an occasional late deceleration. The nurse performed intrauterine resuscitation maneuvers. The physician reviewed the FHR tracing but asked that the oxytocin infusion continue at the current rate of 9 mU/minute. The nurse voiced her concern but followed the order as directed.

At 2045, the cervix was 10 cm dilated, 100% effaced, and vertex at +1 station in the occiput posterior position. At 2100, the IUPC was dislodged, and the tocodynamometer was reapplied. The physician instructed the patient to start pushing. The nurse again expressed her concern about the FHR tracing but was told by the physician that he would find another nurse to care for the patient if she refused to push with the patient.

Eleanor: Labor and Delivery at 2205 Using Fetal Spiral Electrode and Tocodynamometer

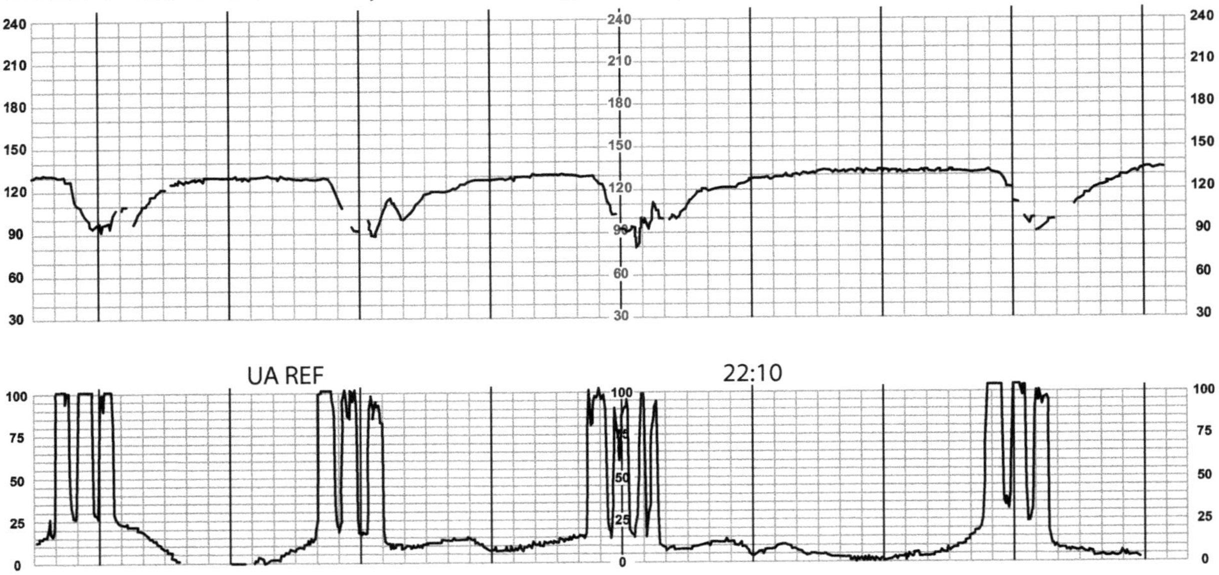

Case Study: Eleanor

1. Baseline FHR:	**130 bpm**	
2. Variability	**Absent (undetectable)**	(first 5 minutes of tracing)
	Minimal (>0 but 5 bpm)	(last 3 minutes of tracing)
	Moderate (6–25 bpm)	________
	Marked (>25 bpm)	________
3. Contractions	Frequency:	**q 2–3 minutes**
	Duration:	**50–60 seconds**
	Intensity:	**Palpate**
	Resting tone:	**Palpate**

4. Accelerations and decelerations. When present, circle P if periodic or E if episodic.

Accelerations	P	E
Early decelerations	P	
Variable decelerations	**P**	E
Late decelerations	P	
Prolonged decelerations	P	
None present		

5. Interpretation	Category I	________
	Category II	________
	Category III	________

This tracing has criteria that could be interpreted as category II or category III. It is an example of the need for clinical judgment and decision making based on the overall clinical picture: the decision to interpret as indeterminate or abnormal will depend on the preponderance of minimal versus absent variability in a larger segment of tracing.

6. List possible underlying physiologic mechanisms or rationales for observed patterns.

- **Decreased umbilical cord perfusion**
- **Umbilical cord compression**
  - **Knot in cord**
  - **Short cord**
  - **Decreased Wharton's jelly**
  - **Thin cord**
- **Associated with an indeterminate (category II) or abnormal (category III) fetal acid-base status at present**
- **Strong vagal stimulation resulting from head compression**
- **Decreasing fetal oxygen reserves related to placental changes**
- **Umbilical cord prolapse (occult)**
- **Decreased amniotic fluid (oligohydramnios)**

7. List in order of priority the physiologic goal(s) for observed patterns.

- **Maximize umbilical circulation.**
- **Maximize oxygenation.**
- **Reduce uterine activity.**
- **Maximize placental blood flow.**

8. List actions and interventions indicated based on overall interpretation (physiologic based, instrumentation based, and further assessments).
   - **Discontinue oxytocin.**
   - **Perform VE to assess fetal descent, presentation for most expeditious route of birth, and possibility of cord prolapse.**
   - **Communicate with physician and family a plan of care for most expeditious route of delivery, supporting fetal oxygenation and family desires.**
   - **If plan of care is to allow for passive descent of the fetus, continue to support physiologic goals and practice heightened surveillance of clinical situation.**
   - **If appropriate to begin active pushing, push every second or third contraction and utilize maternal positions that optimize fetal oxygenation and uterine blood flow and fetal descent.**
   - **Initiate chain of command or authority if an agreed-upon plan with physician cannot be achieved.**
   - **Continue to hydrate with IV fluids to increase maternal blood volume and maximize uterine blood flow.**
   - **Continue to administer maternal supplemental oxygen at 10 Liters/minute via a nonrebreather face mask.**
   - **Prepare for possible expedited birth.**
   - **Notify neonatal team for possible resuscitation.**
   - **Keep provider notified of FHR pattern and evaluate maternal–fetal response to interventions.**
   - **Consider fetal scalp stimulation when FHR is at baseline.**
   - **Validate uterine monitoring data.**
   - **Continue assessments and interventions based on clinical findings and facility protocols.**
   - **Keep family informed of clinical situation and involved in clinical decisions.**

REFERENCES

American College of Obstetricians and Gynecologists. (2005). Inappropriate use of the terms fetal distress and birth asphyxia (Committee Opinion No. 326). *Obstetrics and Gynecology, 106*(6), 1469–1470.

American College of Obstetricians and Gynecologists. (2006). Umbilical cord blood gas and acid-base analysis: Committee Opinion No. 348. *Obstetrics and Gynecology, 108*(5), 1319–1322.

American College of Obstetricians and Gynecologists. (2010). Management of intrapartum fetal heart rate tracings (Practice Bulletin No. 116). *Obstetrics and Gynecology, 116*(5), 1232–1240. doi:10.1097/AOG.0b013e3182004fa9

American College of Obstetricians and Gynecologists. (2012). Timing of umbilical cord clamping after birth: Committee Opinion No. 543. *Obstetrics and Gynecology, 120*(6), 1522–1526. doi:10.1097/01.AOG.0000423817.47165.48

American College of Obstetricians and Gynecologists & American Academy of Pediatrics. (2014). *Neonatal encephalopathy and neurologic outcome (2nd ed.).* Washington, DC: Author.

Andres, R. L., Saade, G., Gilstrap, L. C., Wilkins, I., Witlin, A., Zlatnik, F., & Hankins, G. V. (1999). Association between umbilical blood gas parameters and neonatal morbidity and death in neonates with pathologic fetal acidemia. *American Journal of Obstetrics and Gynecology, 181*(4), 867–871.

Arca, G., Botet, F., Palacio, M., & Carbonell-Estrany, X. (2010). Timing of umbilical cord clamping: New thoughts on an old discussion. *Journal of Maternal-Fetal and Neonatal Medicine, 23*(11), 1274–1285. doi:10.3109/14767050903551475

Armstrong, L., & Stenson, B. (2006). Effect of delayed sampling on umbilical cord arterial and venous lactate and blood gases in clamped and unclamped vessels. *Archives of Disease in Childhood: Fetal & Neonatal Edition, 91*(5), F342–F345.

Armstrong, L., & Stenson, B. (2007). Use of umbilical cord blood gas analysis in the assessment of the newborn. *Archives of Disease in Childhood: Fetal and Neonatal Edition, 92*(6), F430–F434.

Arulkumaran, S., Skurr, B., Tong, H., Kek, L. P., Yeoh, K. H., & Ratnam, S. S. (1991). No evidence of hearing loss due to fetal acoustic stimulation test. *Obstetrics and Gynecology, 78*(2), 283–285.

Arulkumaran, S., Talbert, D., Hsu, T. S., Chua, S., Anandakumar, C., & Ratnam, S. S. (1992). In-utero sound levels when vibroacoustic stimulation is applied to the maternal abdomen: An assessment of the possibility of cochlea damage in the fetus. *British Journal of Obstetrics and Gynaecology, 99*(1), 43–45.

Bakker, P. C., Kurver, P. H., Kuik, D. J., & Van Geijn, H. P. (2007). Elevated uterine activity increases the risk of fetal acidosis at birth. *American Journal of Obstetrics and Gynecology, 196*(4), 313.e1–313.e6.

Bakker, P. C., & van Geijn, H. P. (2008). Uterine activity: Implications for the condition of the fetus. *Journal of Perinatal Medicine, 36*(1), 30–37. doi:10.1515/JPM.2008.003

Blackburn, S. T. (2013). The prenatal period and placental physiology. In S. T. Blackburn (Ed.), *Maternal, fetal, and neonatal physiology: A clinical perspective* (4th ed., pp. 61–114). St. Louis, MO: Saunders.

Blackstone, J., & Young, B. K. (1993). Umbilical cord blood acid-base values and other descriptors of fetal condition. *Clinical Obstetrics and Gynecology, 36*(1), 33–46.

Blechner, J. N. (1993). Maternal-fetal acid-base physiology. *Clinical Obstetrics and Gynecology, 36*(1), 3–12.

Bobrow, C. S., & Soothill, P. W. (1999). Causes and consequences of fetal acidosis. *Archives of Disease in Childhood Fetal and Neonatal Edition, 80*(3), F246–F249.

Bowen, L. W., Kochenour, N. K., Rehm, N. E., & Woolley, F. R. (1986). Maternal–fetal pH difference and fetal scalp pH as predictors of neonatal outcome. *Obstetrics and Gynecology, 67*(4), 487–495.

Brotanek, V., Hendricks, C. H., & Yoshida, T. (1969). Changes in uterine blood flow during uterine contractions. *American Journal of Obstetrics and Gynecology, 103*(8), 1108–1116.

Brouillette, R. T., & Waxman, D. H. (1997). Evaluation of the newborn's blood gas status. National Academy of Clinical Biochemistry. *Clinical Chemistry, 43*(1), 215–221.

Campbell, W. A., Vintzileos, A., & Nochimson, D. J. (1986). Intrauterine versus extrauterine management/resuscitation of the fetus/neonate. *Clinical Obstetrics and Gynecology, 29*(1), 33–42.

Clark, S. L., Gimovsky, M. L., & Miller, F. C. (1982). Fetal heart rate response to scalp blood sampling. *American Journal of Obstetrics and Gynecology, 144*(6), 706–708.

Clark, S. L., Gimovsky, M. L., & Miller, F. C. (1984). The scalp stimulation test: A clinical alternative to fetal scalp blood sampling. *American Journal of Obstetrics and Gynecology, 148*(3), 274–277.

Clark, S. L., & Paul, R. H. (1985). Intrapartum fetal surveillance: The role of fetal scalp blood sampling. *American Journal of Obstetrics and Gynecology, 153*(7), 717–720.

Culver, B. H. (2008). Acid-base balance and control of ventilation. In R. K. Albert, S. G. Spiro, & J. R. Jett (Eds.), *Clinical respiratory medicine* (3rd ed., pp. 125–133). Philadelphia, PA: Mosby.

Dickinson, J. E., Eriksen, N. L., Meyer, B. A., & Parisi, V. M. (1992). The effect of preterm birth on umbilical cord blood gases. *Obstetrics and Gynecology, 79*(4), 575–578.

Dildy, G. A. (2005). Intrapartum assessment of the fetus: Historical and evidence-based practice. *Obstetrics and Gynecology Clinics of North America, 32*(2), 255–271, ix.

Dildy, G. A. (2011). Fetal pulse oximetry. *Clinical Obstetrics and Gynecology, 54*(1), 66–73. doi:10.1097/GRF.0b013e31820a0f71

Dildy, G. A., Clark, S. L., & Loucks, C. A. (1996). Intrapartum fetal pulse oximetry: Past, present, and future. *American Journal of Obstetrics and Gynecology, 175*(1), 1–9.

Dildy, G. A., Thorp, J. A., Yeast, J. D., & Clark, S. L. (1996). The relationship between oxygen saturation and pH in umbilical blood: Implications for intrapartum fetal oxygen saturation monitoring. *American Journal of Obstetrics and Gynecology, 175*(3, Pt. 1), 682–687.

Duerbeck, N. B., Chaffin, D. G., & Seeds, J. W. (1992). A practical approach to umbilical artery pH and blood gas determinations. *Obstetrics and Gynecology, 79*(6), 959–962.

Effros, R. M., & Swenson, E. R. (2010). Acid-base balance. In R. J. Mason, V. C. Broaddus, T. R. Martin, T. E. King, Jr., D. E. Schraufnagel, J. F. Murray, & J. A. Nadel (Eds.), *Murray & Nadel's textbook of respiratory medicine* (5th ed., pp. 134–158). Philadelphia, PA: Saunders.

Eichenbaum-Pikser, G., & Zasloff, J. S. (2009). Delayed clamping of the umbilical cord: A review with implications for practice. *Journal of Midwifery and Women's Health, 54*(4), 321–326. doi:10.1016/j.jmwh.2008.12.012

Elimian, A., Figueroa, R., & Tejani, N. (1997). Intrapartum assessment of fetal well-being: A comparison of scalp stimulation with scalp blood pH sampling. *Obstetrics and Gynecology, 89*(3), 373–376.

Eller, D. P., Robinson, L. J., & Newman, R. B. (1992). Position of the vibroacoustic stimulator does not affect fetal response. *American Journal of Obstetrics & Gynecology, 167*(4 Pt. 1), 1137–1139.

Fouzas, S., Priftis, K. N., & Anthracopoulos, M. B. (2011). Pulse oximetry in pediatric practice. *Pediatrics, 128*(4), 740–752. doi:10.1542/peds.2011–0271

Freeman, R. K., Garite, T., J., Nageotte, M. P., & Miller, L. A. (2012). Umbilical cord blood gases to assess fetal condition at birth. In R. K. Freeman, T. J. Garite, M. P. Nageotte, & L. A. Miller (Eds.), *Fetal heart rate monitoring* (4th ed., pp. 112–118). Philadelphia, PA: Lippincott Williams & Wilkins.

Gagnon, R., Hunse, C., & Foreman, J. (1989). Human fetal behavioral states after vibratory stimulation. *American*

Journal of Obstetrics and Gynecology, 161(6, Pt. 1), 1470–1476.

Garite, T. J. (2012). Intrapartum fetal evaluation. In S. G. Gabbe, J. R. Niebyl, J. L. Simpson, M. B. Landon, H. L. Galan, E. R. M. Jauniaux, & D. A. Driscoll (Eds.), *Obstetrics: Normal and problem pregnancies* (6th ed., pp. 330–361). Philadelphia, PA: Churchill Livingstone.

Garite, T. J. (2013). The search for an adequate back-up test for intrapartum fetal heart rate monitoring. *American Journal of Obstetrics and Gynecology, 208*(3), 163–164. doi:10.1016/j.ajog.2012.12.001

Garite, T. J., Dildy, G. A., McNamara, H., Nageotte, M. P., Boehm, F. H., Dellinger, E. H., . . . Swedlow, D. B. (2000). A multicenter controlled trial of fetal pulse oximetry in the intrapartum management of nonreassuring fetal heart rate patterns. *American Journal of Obstetrics and Gynecology, 183*(5), 1049–1058.

Gerhardt, K. J., & Abrams, R. M. (2000). Fetal exposures to sound and vibroacoustic stimulation. *Journal of Perinatology, 20*(8, Pt. 2), S21–S30.

Gilstrap, L. C., Leveno, K. J., Burris, J., Williams, M. L., & Little, B. B. (1989). Diagnosis of birth asphyxia on the basis of fetal pH, Apgar score, and newborn cerebral dysfunction. *American Journal of Obstetrics and Gynecology, 161*(3), 825–830.

Gimovsky, M. L., & Caritis, S. N. (1982). Diagnosis and management of hypoxic fetal heart rate patterns. *Clinical Perinatology, 9*(2), 313–324.

Goldaber, K. G., & Gilstrap, L. C., III. (1993). Correlations between obstetric clinical events and umbilical cord blood acid-base and blood gas values. *Clinical Obstetrics and Gynecology, 36*(1), 47–59.

Goldaber, K. G., Gilstrap, L. C., Leveno, K. J., Dax, J. S., & McIntire, D. D. (1991). Pathologic fetal acidemia. *Obstetrics and Gynecology, 78*(6), 1103–1107.

Goodwin, T. M., Milner-Masterson, L., & Paul, R. H. (1994). Elimination of fetal scalp blood sampling on a large clinical service. *Obstetrics and Gynecology, 83*(6), 971–974.

Graven, S. N., & Browne, J. V. (2008). Auditory development in the fetus and infant. *Newborn and Infant Nursing Reviews, 8*(4), 187–193. doi:10.1053/j.nainr.2008.10.010

Greenberg, M. B., Druzin, M. L., & Gabbe, S. G. (2012). Antepartum fetal evaluation. In S. G. Gabbe, J. R. Niebyl, J. L. Simpson, M. B. Landon, H. L. Galan, E. R. M. Jauniaux, & D. A. Driscoll (Eds.), *Obstetrics: Normal and problem pregnancies* (6th ed., pp. 237–263). Philadelphia, PA: Churchill Livingstone.

Greene, K. R. (1999). Scalp blood gas analysis. *Obstetrics and Gynecology Clinics of North America,* 26(4), 641–656, vii.

Gregg, A. R., & Weiner, C. P. (1993). Normal umbilical arterial and venous acid-base and blood gas values. *Clinical Obstetrics and Gynecology, 36*(1), 24–32.

Hamilton, E., Warrick, P., Knox, E., O'Keeffe, D., & Garite, T. (2012). High uterine contraction rates in births with normal and abnormal umbilical artery gases. *Journal of Maternal-Fetal and Neonatal Medicine, 25*(11), 2302–2307. doi:10.3109/14767058.2012.691578

Hamilton, E., Warrick, P., & O'Keeffe, D. (2012). Variable decelerations: Do size and shape matter? *Journal of Maternal-Fetal and Neonatal Medicine, 25*(6), 648–653. doi:10.3109/14767058.2011.594118

Harbert, G. M., Jr. (1982). Uterine contractions. *Clinical Obstetrics and Gynecology, 25*(1), 177–187.

Haydon, M. L., Gorenberg, D. M., Nageotte, M. P., Ghamsary, M., Rumney, P. J., Patillo, C., & Garite, T. J. (2006). The effect of maternal oxygen administration on fetal pulse oximetry during labor in fetuses with nonreassuring fetal heart rate patterns. *American Journal of Obstetrics & Gynecology, 195*(3), 735–738.

Helwig, J. T., Parer, J. T., Kilpatrick, S. J., & Laros, R. K., Jr. (1996). Umbilical cord blood acid-base state: What is normal? *American Journal of Obstetrics & Gynecology, 174*(6), 1807–1812.

Hilger, J. S., Holzman, I. R., & Brown, D. R. (1981). Sequential changes in placental blood gases and pH during the hour following delivery. *Journal of Reproductive Medicine, 26*(6), 305–307.

Huckabee, W. E. (1962). Uterine blood flow. *American Journal of Obstetrics and Gynecology, 84*, 1623–1633.

Irion, O., Stuckelberger, P., Moutquin, J. M., Morabia, A., Extermann, P., & Beguin, F. (1996). Is intrapartum vibratory acoustic stimulation a valid alternative to fetal scalp pH determination? *British Journal of Obstetrics and Gynaecology, 103*(7), 642–647.

Kim, S. Y., Khandelwal, M., Gaughan, J. P., Agar, M. H., & Reece, E. A. (2003). Is the intrapartum biophysical profile useful? *Obstetrics and Gynecology, 102*(3), 471–476.

King, T. L. (2013). Fetal assessment. In S. T. Blackburn (Ed.), *Maternal, fetal, and neonatal physiology: A clinical perspective* (4th ed., pp. 163–182). St. Louis, MO: Saunders.

King, T., & Parer, J. (2000). The physiology of fetal heart rate patterns and perinatal asphyxia. *Journal of Perinatal and Neonatal Nursing, 14*(3), 19–39.

Kirshon, B., & Moise, K. J., Jr. (1989). Effect of heparin on umbilical arterial blood gases. *Journal of Reproductive Medicine, 34*(4), 267–269.

Lehtovirta, P., & Forss, M. (1978). The acute effect of smoking on intervillous blood flow of the placenta. *British Journal of Obstetrics and Gynecology, 85*(10), 729–731.

Lievaart, M., & de Jong, P. A. (1984). Acid-base equilibrium in umbilical cord blood and time of cord clamping. *Obstetrics and Gynecology, 63*(1), 44–47.

Lin, C. C., Vassallo, B., & Mittendorf, R. (2001). Is intrapartum vibroacoustic stimulation an effective predictor of fetal acidosis? *Journal of Perinatal Medicine, 29*(6), 506–512.

Low, J. A. (1988). The role of blood gas and acid-base assessment in the diagnosis of intrapartum fetal asphyxia. *American Journal of Obstetrics and Gynecology, 159*(5), 1235–1240.

Low, J. A., Lindsay, B. G., & Derrick, E. J. (1997). Threshold of metabolic acidosis associated with newborn complications. *American Journal of Obstetrics and Gynecology, 177*(6), 1391–1394.

Low, J. A., Victory, R., & Derrick, E. J. (1999). Predictive value of electronic fetal monitoring for intrapartum fetal asphyxia with metabolic acidosis. *Obstetrics and Gynecology, 93*(2), 285–291.

Lynn, A., & Beeby, P. (2007). Cord and placenta arterial gas analysis: The accuracy of delayed sampling. *Archives of Disease in Children: Fetal and Neonatal Edition, 92*(4), F281–F285.

Macones, G. A., Hankins, G. D., Spong, C. Y., Hauth, J. D., & Moore, T. (2008). The 2008 National Institute of Child Health Human Development workshop report on electronic fetal monitoring: Update on definitions, interpretations, and research guidelines. *Obstetrics and Gynecology, 112*(3), 661–666, doi:10.1097/AOG.0b013e3181841395; and *Journal of Obstetric, Gynecologic and Neonatal Nursing, 37*(5), 510–515. doi:10.1111/j.1552-6909.2008.00284.x

Manor, M., Blickstein, I., Hazan, Y., Flidel-Rimon, O., & Hagay, Z. J. (1998). Postpartum determination of umbilical artery blood gases: Effect of time and temperature. *Clinical Chemistry, 44*(3), 681–683.

Martin, C. B., Jr. (2008). Normal fetal physiology and behavior, and adaptive responses with hypoxemia. *Seminars in Perinatology, 32*(4), 239–242. doi:10.1053/j.semperi.2008.04.003

McCance, K. L. (2009). Cellular biology. In K. L. McCance & S. E. Huether (Eds.), *Pathophysiology: The biologic basis for disease in adults and children* (6th ed., pp.1–45). St. Louis, MO: Mosby.

Mercer, J. S., & Erickson-Owens, D. A. (2012). Rethinking placental transfusion and cord clamping issues. *Journal of Perinatal and Neonatal Nursing, 26*(3), 202–217. doi:10.1097/JPN.0b013e31825d2d9a

Miller, D. A. (2011). Intrapartum fetal heart rate definitions and interpretation: Evolving consensus. *Clinical Obstetrics and Gynecology, 54*(1), 16–21. doi:10.1097/GRF.0b013e31820a04e5

Miller, D. A., & Miller, L. A. (2012). Electronic fetal heart rate monitoring: Applying principles of patient safety. *American Journal of Obstetrics and Gynecology, 206*(4), 278–283. doi:10.1016/j.ajog.2011.08.016

Miller, D. A., Rabello, Y. A., & Paul, R. H. (1996). The modified biophysical profile: Antepartum testing in the 1990s. *American Journal of Obstetrics and Gynecology, 174*(3), 812–817.

Miller, L. (2011). Intrapartum fetal monitoring: Liability and documentation. *Clinical Obstetrics and Gynecology, 54*(1), 50–55. doi: 10.1097/GRF.0b013e31820a0e27

Nageotte, M., & Gilstrap, L. (2009). Intrapartum fetal surveillance. In R. K. Creasy, R. Resnik, J. D. Iams, C. J. Lockwood, & T. R. Moore (Eds.), *Creasy & Resnik's maternal–fetal medicine: Principles and practice* (6th ed., pp. 397–417). Philadelphia, PA: W. B. Saunders.

National Collaborating Centre for Women's and Children's Health. (2007). Intrapartum care: Care of healthy women and their babies during childbirth. NICE Clinical Guideline 55. London, UK: RCOG Press. Retrieved from http://www.nice.org.uk/nicemedia/pdf/IPCNICEGuidance.pdf

Neerhof, M. G., & Thaete, L. G. (2008). The fetal response to chronic placental insufficiency. *Seminars in Perinatology, 32*(3), 201–205. doi: 10.1053/j.semperi.2007.11.002

Neilson, J. P. (2008). Fetal scalp sampling in labour. *British Medical Journal, 336*(7656), 1257–1258. doi:10.1136/bmj.39567.480972.80

Nijland, R., Jongsma, H. W., Nijhuis, J. G., van den Berg, P. P., & Oeseburg, B. (1995). Arterial oxygen saturation in relation to metabolic acidosis in fetal lambs. *American Journal of Obstetrics and Gynecology, 172*(3), 810–819.

Nodwell, A., Carmichael, L., Ross, M., & Richardson, B. (2005). Placental compared with umbilical cord blood to assess fetal blood gas and acid-base status. *Obstetrics and Gynecology, 105*(1), 129–138.

Nyman, M., Barr, M., & Westgren, M. (1992). A four-year follow-up of hearing and development in children exposed in utero to vibro-acoustic stimulation. *British Journal of Obstetrics and Gynaecology, 99*(8), 685–688.

Parer, J. T., King, T., Flanders, S., Fox, M., & Kilpatrick, S. J. (2006). Fetal acidemia and electronic fetal heart rate patterns: Is there evidence of an association? *Journal of Maternal-Fetal and Neonatal Medicine, 19*(5), 289–294.

Perlman, J. M. (2012). Cellular biology of end organ injury and strategies for prevention of injury. *Clinics in Perinatology, 39*(4), 785–802. doi:10.1016/j.clp.2012.09.002

Porter, T. F., & Clark, S. L. (1999). Vibroacoustic and scalp stimulation. *Obstetrics & Gynecology Clinics of North America, 26*(4), 657–669.

Poseiro, J. J., Mendez-Bauer, C., Pose, S. V., & Caldeyro-Barcia, R. (1969). Effect of uterine contractions on maternal blood flow through the placenta. *Perinatal Factors Affecting Human Development,* 161–171.

Rabe, H., Reynolds, G., & Diaz-Rossello J. (2008). A systematic review and meta-analysis of a brief delay in clamping the umbilical cord of preterm infants. *Neonatology, 93*(2), 138–144.

Rampersad, R., Cervar-Zivkovic, M., & Nelson, D. M. (2011). Development and anatomy of the human placenta. In H. H. Kay, D. M. Nelson, & Y. Wang (Eds.), *The placenta: From development to disease* (pp. 19–26). Oxford, UK: Blackwell.

Richardson, B. S., Carmichael, L., Homan, J., & Patrick, J. E. (1992). Electrocortical activity, electroocular activity, and breathing movements in fetal sheep with prolonged and graded hypoxemia. *American Journal of Obstetrics and Gynecology, 167*(2), 553–558.

Riley, R. J., & Johnson, J. W. (1993). Collecting and analyzing cord blood gases. *Clinical Obstetrics and Gynecology, 36*(1), 13–23.

Ross, M. G. (2011). Labor and fetal heart rate decelerations: Relation to fetal metabolic acidosis. *Clinical Obstetrics and Gynecology, 54*(1), 74–82. doi:10.1097/GRF.0b013e31820a106d

Ross, M. G., Ervin, M. G., & Novak, D. (2012). Placental and fetal physiology. In S. G. Gabbe, J. R. Niebyl, J. L. Simpson, H. L. Galan, E. R. M. Jauniaux, & D. A. Driscoll (Eds.), *Obstetrics: Normal and problem pregnancies* (6th ed., pp. 23–41). Philadelphia, PA: Churchill Livingstone.

Ross, M. G., Jessie, M., Amaya, K., Matushewski, B., Durosier, L. D., Frasch, M. G., & Richardson, B. S. (2013). Correlation of arterial fetal base deficit and lactate changes with severity of variable heart rate decelerations in the near-term ovine fetus. *American Journal of Obstetrics and Gynecology, 208*(4), 285.e1–285.e6. doi:10.1016/j.ajog.2012.10.883

Rotmensch, S., Celentano, C., Liberati, M., Sadan, O., & Glezerman, M. (1999). The effect of antenatal steroid administration on the fetal response to vibroacoustic stimulation. *Acta Obstetricia et Gynecologica Scandinavica, 78*(10), 847–51.

Saling, E., & Schneider, D. (1967). Biochemical supervision of the foetus during labour. *Journal of Obstetrics and Gynaecology of the British Commonwealth, 74*(6), 799–811.

Scheans, P. (2011). Umbilical cord blood gases: New clinical relevance for an age-old practice. *Neonatal Network, 30*(2), 123–126.

Seelbach-Gobel, B., Heupel, M., Kuhnert, M., & Butterwegge, M. (1999). The prediction of fetal acidosis by means of intrapartum fetal pulse oximetry. *American Journal of Obstetrics and Gynecology, 180*(1 Pt. 1), 73–81.

Shankaran, S., Pappas, A., McDonald, S. A., Vohr, B. R., Hintz, S. R., Yolton, K., . . . Eunice Kennedy Shriver NICHD Neonatal Research Network. (2012). Childhood outcomes after hypothermia for neonatal encephalopathy. *New England Journal of Medicine,* 366(22), 2085–2092. doi:10.1056/NEJMoa1112066

Sherer, D. M. (1994). Blunted fetal response to vibroacoustic stimulation associated with maternal intravenous magnesium sulfate therapy. *American Journal of Perinatology, 11*(6), 401–403.

Sherer, D. M., & Bentolila, E. (1998). Blunted fetal response to vibroacoustic stimulation following chronic exposure to propranolol. *American Journal of Perinatology, 15*(8), 495–498.

Simpson, L. L. (2012). When is primary cesarean appropriate: Fetal indications. *Seminars in Perinatology, 36*(5), 328–335. doi:10.1053/j.semperi.2012.04.015

Simpson, K. R., & James, D. C. (2005). Efficacy of intrauterine resuscitation techniques in improving fetal oxygen status during labor. *Obstetrics and Gynecology, 105*(6), 1362–1368.

Simpson, K. R., & James, D. C. (2008). Effects of oxytocin-induced uterine hyperstimulation during labor on fetal oxygen status and fetal heart rate patterns. *American Journal of Obstetrics and Gynecology, 199*(1), 34.e1–34.35. doi:10.1016/j.ajog.2007.12.015

Skupski, D. W., Rosenberg, C. R., & Eglinton, G. S. (2002). Intrapartum fetal stimulation tests: A meta-analysis. *Obstetrics and Gynecology, 99*(1), 129–134.

Smart, P. J. (1962). Some observations on the vascular morphology of the foetal side of the human placenta. *British Journal of Obstetrics and Gynecology, 69*, 929–933.

Smith, C. V., Nguyen, H. N., Phelan, J. P., & Paul, R. H. (1986). Intrapartum assessment of fetal well-being: A comparison of fetal acoustic stimulation with acid-base determinations. *American Journal of Obstetrics and Gynecology, 155*(4), 726–728.

Smith, C. V., Satt, B., Phelan, J. P., & Paul, R. H. (1990). Intrauterine sound levels: Intrapartum assessment with an intrauterine microphone. *American Journal of Perinatology, 7*(4), 312–315.

Society of Obstetricians and Gynaecologists of Canada & British Columbia Perinatal Health Program. (2007). Fetal health surveillance: Antepartum and intrapartum consensus guideline. *Journal of Obstetrics and Gynaecology Canada, 29*(9, Suppl. 4), S3–S56.

Sontag, L. W., & Wallace, R. F. (1934). Preliminary report of the Fels fund: Study of fetal activity. *Archives of Pediatric and Adolescent Medicine, 48*(5), 1050–1057. doi:10.1001/archpedi.1934.01960180104006

Soothill, P. W., Nicolaides, K. H., & Rodeck, C. H. (1987). Effect on anaemia on fetal acid-base status. *British Journal of Obstetrics and Gynecology, 94*(9), 880–883.

Soothill, P. W., Nicolaides, K. H., Rodeck, C. H., Clewell, W. H., & Lindridge, J. (1987). Relationship of fetal hemoglobin and oxygen content to lactate concentration in Rh isoimmunized pregnancies. *Obstetrics and Gynecology, 69*(2), 268–271.

Stout, M. J., & Cahill, A. G. (2011). Electronic fetal monitoring: Past, present, and future. *Clinics in Perinatology, 38*(1), 127–142. doi:10.1016/j.clp.2010.12.002

Strickland, D. M., Gilstrap, L. C., Hauth, J. C., & Widmer, K. (1984). Umbilical cord pH and PCO2: Effect of interval from delivery to determination. *American Journal of Obstetrics and Gynecology, 148*(2), 191–194.

Sykes, G. S., Molloy, P. M., Johnson, P., Gu, W., Ashworth, F., Stirrat, G. M., & Turnbull, A. C. (1982). Do Apgar scores indicate asphyxia? *Lancet, 1*(8270), 494–496.

Thorp, J. A., Dildy, G. A., Yeomans, E. R., Meyer, B. A., & Parisi, V. M. (1996). Umbilical cord blood gas analysis at delivery. *American Journal of Obstetrics and Gynecology, 175*(3 Pt. 1), 517–522.

Thorp, J. A., & Rushing, R. S. (1999). Umbilical cord blood gas analysis. *Obstetrics and Gynecology Clinics of North America, 26*(4), 695–709.

Thorp, J. A., Sampson, J. E., Parisi, V. M., & Creasy, R. K. (1989). Routine umbilical cord blood gas determinations? *American Journal of Obstetrics and Gynecology, 161*(3), 600–605.

Ullrich, J. R., & Ackerman, B. D. (1972). Changes in umbilical artery blood gas values with the onset of respiration. *Biology of the Neonate, 20*(5), 466–474.

Wallman, C. M. (1997). Interpretation of fetal cord blood gases. *Neonatal Network, 16*(1), 72–75.

Westgate, J., Garibaldi, J. M., & Greene, K. R. (1994). Umbilical cord blood gas analysis at delivery: A time for quality data. *British Journal of Obstetrics and Gynaecology, 101*(12), 1054–1063.

Whitworth, M. K., & Bricker, L. (2006). How to perform intrapartum fetal blood sampling. *British Journal of Hospital Medicine, 67*(9), M162–M164.

Wiberg, N., Kallen, K., & Olofsson, P. (2008). Delayed umbilical cord clamping at birth has effects on arterial and venous blood gases and lactate concentrations. *British Journal of Obstetrics and Gynaecology, 115*(6), 697–703. doi:10.1111/j. 1471-0528.2008.01708.x

Wilkening, R. B., & Meschia, G. (1983). Fetal oxygen uptake, oxygenation, and acid-base balance as a function of uterine blood flow. *American Journal of Physiology, 244*(6), H749–H755.

Yancey, M. K., & Harlass, F. E. (1993). Extraneous factors and their influences on fetal acid-base status. *Clinical Obstetrics and Gynecology, 36*(1), 60–72.

Yao, Q. W., Jakobsson, J., Nyman, M., Rabaeus, H., Till, O., & Westgren, M. (1990). Fetal responses to different intensity levels of vibroacoustic stimulation. *Obstetrics and Gynecology, 75*(2), 206–209.

Yeomans, E. R., Hauth, J. C., Gilstrap, L. C., III, & Strickland, D. M. (1985). Umbilical cord pH, PCO2, and bicarbonate following uncomplicated term vaginal deliveries. *American Journal of Obstetrics and Gynecology, 151*(6), 798–800.

Zamudio, S. (2011). Hypoxia and the placenta. In H. H. Kay, D. M. Nelson, & Y. Wang (Eds.), *The placenta: From development to disease* (pp. 43–49). Oxford, UK: Blackwell.

Zdravkovic, T., Genbacev, O., McMaster, M. T., & Fisher, S. J. (2005). The adverse effects of maternal smoking on the human placenta: A review. *Placenta, 26* (Suppl. A), S81–S86.

SECTION FOUR

Application of Fetal Heart Monitoring Data

CHAPTER 8

Communication of Fetal Heart Monitoring Information

Audrey Lyndon
Marya G. Zlatnik

INTRODUCTION

Communication is an integral component of clinical care. The quality of communication can significantly influence patient safety, quality of care, and outcomes for mothers and babies. Communication that is open, direct, accurate, and concise will increase the likelihood that information regarding patient status is known and appropriately acted on by all professionals in a timely manner. Unfortunately, communication breakdowns remain a significant contributor to adverse events in perinatal care and can result in maternal and neonatal morbidity, permanent disability, and even maternal or neonatal death. Communication issues are identified as a primary contributing factor in as many as 75% of sentinel events reported to The Joint Commission, and have consistently ranked among the top three leading causes of sentinel events from 2004 until 2012 (The Joint Commission, 2004, 2013b).

This chapter covers communications regarding fetal status, including discussions among professional colleagues and discussions with the woman and her family and support person(s). Strategies to promote respectful, collaborative communication among colleagues and with women and their families are included. Perspectives on risk management, root-cause analysis, conflict management, and the chain of resolution (also known as chain of authority or chain of command) as they relate to fetal assessment are presented as suggestions to promote safe, high-quality care for mothers and babies and to decrease professional liability exposure. Written and electronic communication specific to medical record documentation are discussed in Chapter 9.

COMMUNICATION AMONG PROFESSIONAL COLLEAGUES

Perinatal services in each institution are provided by teams of professional colleagues. Teamwork is a key factor in achieving excellence in clinical practice. In any situation requiring a real-time combination of multiple skills, experiences, and judgment, teams—not individuals—create superior performance (Gordon, Mendenhall, & O'Connor, 2013; Risser et al., 1999). Ideally, a perinatal team consists of health care professionals working collectively and in a nonhierarchical fashion toward a mutually agreed-upon and common goal: the best possible outcomes for mothers and babies (Lawrence et al., 2012; Simpson, James, & Knox, 2006). Each member contributes and is valued for his or her talents, education, experience, background, and perspective. Individual member contributions are evaluated by merit without regard for the member's status in a traditional health care hierarchy. For example, the input of a staff nurse has as much value as that of an attending physician, and the input from a resident physician is considered just as important as that of an advanced-practice nurse. The value of individual contributions is defined by existing data or merit rather than presumed organizational position (Clark, Simpson, Knox, & Garite, 2009; Sherwood, Thomas, Bennett, & Lewis, 2002). The hallmark of successful teamwork is effective communication.

Clinical interactions and communication in antepartum and intrapartum care commonly occur in a hierarchical model (based on tradition and education) even though hierarchy can be hazardous and create conditions that decrease patient safety (Knox & Simpson, 2003; Leonard & Frankel, 2011; Lyndon, 2008). Hierarchical communication regarding fetal status can be hazardous because it does not always promote trust and full exchange of information. Trust, open communication, and effective interdisciplinary teamwork are integral to promoting safe patient care. Communication implies a transfer of information. Ideally that information is accurate, timely, and conveyed with mutual respect. Teamwork is a complementary relationship of interdependence (Sherwood et al., 2002). Nurses, physicians, and midwives must rely on each other, each contributing a unique aspect of care needed for optimal outcomes. Effective teamwork improves outcomes for patients (Mazzocco et al., 2008; Neily et al., 2010).

Effective teamwork requires ongoing, consistent communication, full participation, working in synchrony, effective conflict management, continuous learning, ongoing feedback, knowledge of team goals, and acknowledgment of each other's roles and responsibilities to achieve those goals (Leonard & Frankel, 2011). Achieving an environment in which communication is reliably effective and perinatal teamwork is a reality can be a challenge because universal and institution-specific barriers may exist. Those barriers are complex and involve many interrelated factors (Box 8-1). Although some factors can be changed or overcome, others represent challenges embedded in the structure of our current health care system (Brown, 2005; Leape et al., 2012a, 2012b; Simpson & Knox, 2001). Hierarchical relationships in particular can contribute to poor communication in perinatal care (Jacobson, Zlatnik, Kennedy, & Lyndon, 2013; Lyndon et al., 2012; Simpson et al., 2006; Simpson & Lyndon, 2009), but each factor listed influences how well nurses, midwives, and physicians communicate.

An important issue that may remain an unrecognized contributor to ineffective communications in many settings is differences between clinicians in the underlying assessment of risks and benefits of common intrapartum interventions, as well as differences in philosophies about birth (Jacobson et al., 2013; Lyndon et al., 2012; Lyndon, Zlatnik, & Wachter, 2011). Both differences in risk assessment and differences in philosophy can contribute to communication breakdowns when they result in a team of clinicians who are attempting

BOX 8-1 Factors That Impede Teamwork in Perinatal Care

- Historical roles of women in society
- Traditional roles of physicians and nurses
- Institutional territory and politics
- Licensure and professional accountability
- Type and quantity of education
- Different styles of learning and information exchange
- Socialization of each group
- Philosophies about birth
- Assessment of risk/benefit ratio for common procedures
- Power of social and professional position
- Collaboration—an impediment because it assumes separation of groups
- Unresolved conflict, setting the stage for the expectation of future discord
- Availability of resources, including staffing levels, obstetric hospitalists, and consultation arrangements
- Methods and amounts of compensation
- Inability to establish common incentives

Source: Adapted from Simpson and Knox (2001).

to achieve the same goals but do not realize that they are operating from perspectives that differ. In such situations unrecognized differences in perspective do not get discussed, the active conversation does not result in a shared mental model of the situation, and the risk of communication failure or unresolvable conflict is high (Lyndon et al., 2012; Lyndon et al., 2014).

For example, many obstetricians have been trained to view "Active Management of Labor" as practiced at the Dublin Maternity Hospital as a safe and successful route to uncomplicated vaginal delivery. As practiced in many U.S hospitals, "active management" involves such elements of care as liberal use of oxytocin augmentation, early amniotomy, and higher doses of oxytocin. Many obstetricians associate these practices with low cesarean rates and a reduced risk of chorioamnionitis, but may not be aware that another critical element of the Dublin protocol was continuous one-to-one nursing or midwifery presence. A nurse who has been trained in a tradition of labor and birth as a natural process, and who is aware of the hazards of the cascade of interventions sometimes seen in the United States (including labor induction or augmentation leading to pain, epidural anesthesia leading to fetal heart rate decelerations, internal fetal and uterine monitoring leading to intra-amniotic infection, and the resultant cesarean delivery), may perceive the obstetrician's request for "pushing the pit" to be contrary to the patient's best interest (Jacobson et al., 2013; Simpson et al., 2006). As long as the underlying beliefs and mindsets are not made explicit, the stage remains set for miscommunication and frustration.

Although teamwork is a key component of safe and effective perinatal care, nurses, midwives, and physicians are accountable for their individual actions and contributions to the health care team. Professional clinicians have a body of knowledge and skills that contains an ethos of good practice. That ethos includes practice based on valid, current science; appropriate use of technology; a fiduciary relationship to the woman and her family; and responsible behavior in relation to other health care providers to uphold patient safety standards (Benner et al., 2002). Health care professionals are responsible for accurate and timely assessments, clinical interventions, and follow-up. The collaborative fetal monitoring process (Figure 8-1) is a scientific problem-solving model. Effective communication with women, families, and professional colleagues is an essential component embedded in all stages of the process.

Strategies for Improving Communications between Health Care Providers

Effective clinical communication is clear, direct, and explicit. Effective communicators avoid assuming that the other party shares their assessment of events or maternal–fetal condition. Therefore, effective communicators identify the level of urgency in the situation, concisely summarize their assessments, clearly state their recommendations for action, and seek confirmation of agreement (Gordon et al., 2013; Leonard & Frankel, 2011; Leonard, Graham, & Bonacum, 2004). Effective communicators avoid indirect strategies historically used by nurses and others such as "hinting and hoping" and avoid engaging the "doctor-nurse game" where the objective is "getting them to think it was their idea" (Gordon et al., 2013; Stein, 1968).

Complete communication between clinicians about fetal monitoring data includes a clear picture of the current assessment of maternal–fetal status and clinical needs. Specifically for fetal heart monitoring (FHM) data this will include status/stage of labor, interpretation of maternal vital signs; fetal heart rate (FHR) and uterine activity; any changes in maternal or fetal status; interventions taken; maternal–fetal responses to interventions; specific requests for actions, medical orders, or clinical assistance; and time frame in which such actions are needed.

Data concerning the FHR pattern should be conveyed using the agreed-upon definitions provided in the proceedings of the National Institute of Child Health and Human Development 2008 guidelines for EFM definitions, interpretation, and research (Macones, Hankins, Spong, Hauth, & Moore, 2008). When a clinician is concerned about indeterminate (category II) or

Figure 8-1 The Collaborative Process and Fetal Heart Monitoring

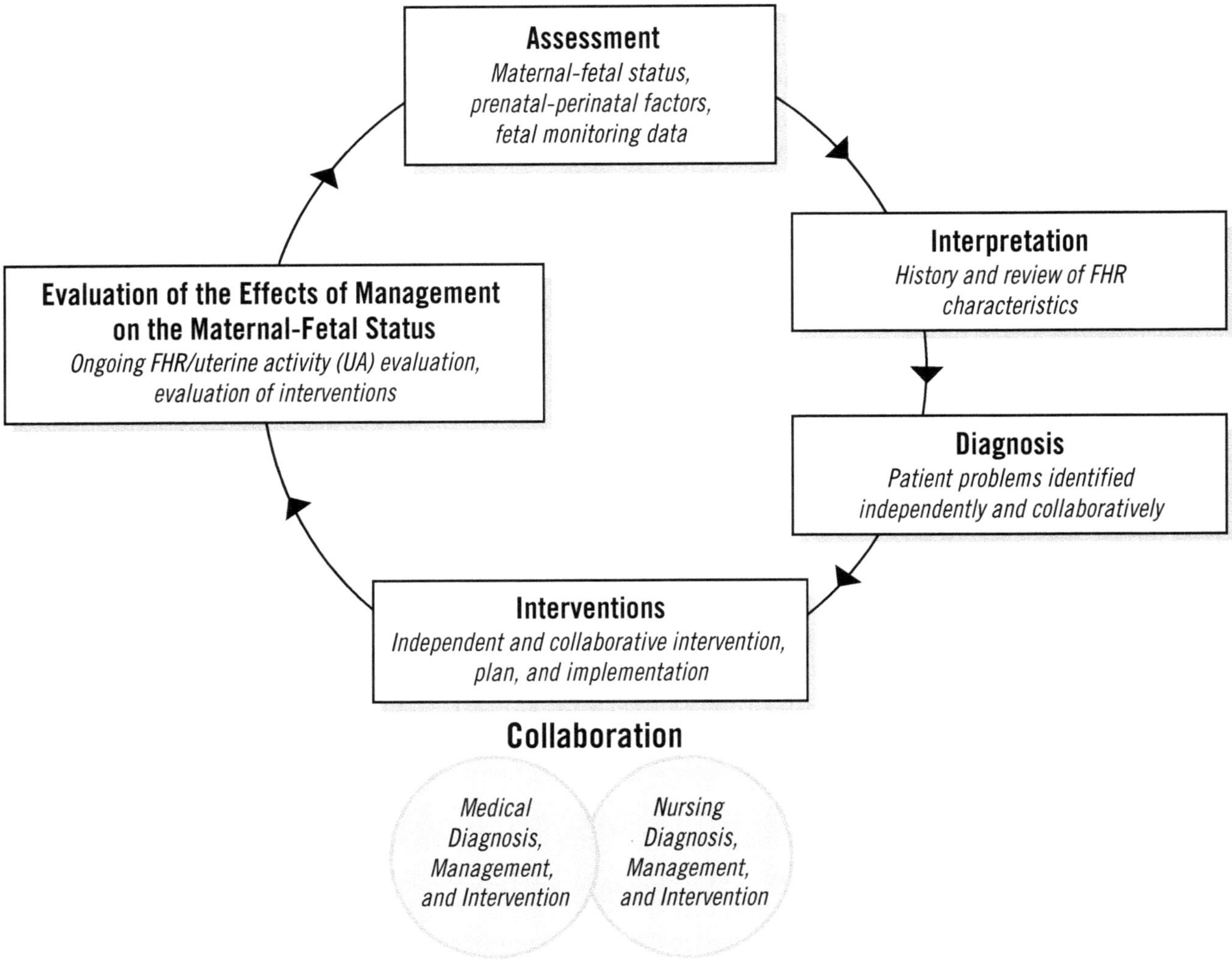

abnormal (category III) patterns, the data that should be communicated includes but is not limited to the following:

- Baseline FHR
- Variability (absent, minimal, moderate, or marked)
- Presence or absence of accelerations (appropriate for gestational age)
- Presence or absence of decelerations:
  - If decelerations are noted, type of decelerations (early, late, variable, prolonged), and whether the decelerations are recurrent
  - Clinical context (e.g., tachysystole, vaginal bleeding, recent epidural dose, rupture of membranes)
- Time frame of indeterminate or abnormal FHR changes (e.g., How long has this pattern been evolving?)
- Specific intrauterine resuscitation techniques initiated and the maternal–fetal response
- Specific, clearly stated requests for additional orders and/or direct bedside evaluation by the primary health care provider (Fox, Kilpatrick, King, & Parer, 2000)
- The time frame in which the agreed-upon plan will be accomplished and reevaluated (Brady et al., 2013)

Structuring Communication

Ideally, every clinician would speak up with confidence about their clinical concerns and would feel supported in inquiring about concerning situations. However, we know that clinicians at all levels of intrapartum care—including nurses, midwives, resident physicians, fellows, and even attending physicians—at times suppress or struggle to express their concerns for fear of the consequences that may result from questioning other team members (Jacobson et al., 2013; Lyndon et al., 2012; Maxfield, Lyndon, Kennedy, O'Keeffe, & Zlatnik, 2013; Simpson & Lyndon, 2009). While no specific individual communication strategies have been shown to be the most clinically effective, most experts agree that structured communication formats such as SBAR ("Situation, Background, Assessment, Recommendation") can be very helpful in improving communication effectiveness (Kaplan & Ballard, 2012; Leonard & Frankel, 2011).

The purpose of SBAR is to provide a consistent framework for the components of effective clinical communication described previously: urgency, assessment, and recommendations for action. To use SBAR as designed, the clinician quickly identifies him- or herself and states the nature of the immediate situation they are communicating about (**S: Situation**). The clinician then provides a summary of pertinent background information about the patient (e.g., gravidity, parity, reason for admission, any medical or obstetric risk factors, current vital signs, physical examination, and laboratory findings) (**B: Background**). Next, the clinician makes a clear statement of his or her assessment of the situation, meaning that the clinician communicates what they think is going on (**A: Assessment**). Finally, the clinician makes a direct recommendation for action or a direct request for something he or she needs for the patient (**R: Recommendation**) (Leonard, 2013). The SBAR framework is considered useful for bridging differences in communication styles between disciplines such as nursing and medicine. However, SBAR itself does not explicitly address additional essential teamwork skills of clinical assertion and closed-loop communication. Moreover, the usefulness of structuring communications is limited by the capacity of the receiving team members to listen and respond to the information conveyed in a manner that promotes psychological safety (Edmondson, 1999). Therefore, we recommend two enhancements to SBAR to address these factors: $SBAR^3$ and SBAR for Listening.

$SBAR^3$ or SBAR-R-R (Table 8-1) is a simple expansion of the SBAR format to incorporate assertion and closed-loop communication (Lyndon, Walsh, & Edwards-Silva, 2013). With **Reasoning**, the expectation is that the clinician begins the conversation prepared to articulate the reasoning for his or her request in the event that there is not mutual agreement about the recommendation. This prepares the requesting clinician to be assertive about the request, and increases the likelihood of being able to do so due to advance planning and increased self-confidence regarding the recommendation. While reasoning may only need to be used in cases where there is not initial agreement, **Ratification** should occur for all SBARs. Ratification is an explicit summary of the agreement and time frame so that all parties to the conversation are clear on the plan they are making together (Brady et al., 2013).

SBAR for Listening addresses the receiver side of clinical communication by providing a pneumonic in the SBAR-R-R framework highlighting the principles of active listening and response (Table 8-2). The first principle of effective listening is to let go of assumptions we may have about the person presenting the information or let go of assumptions about the situation, or both (**S: Set aside assumptions**). While it is normal to have and make assumptions about people and patient care situations, these assumptions get in the way of listening and can have a negative effect on communication (Purdy & Borisoff, 1997; Stone, Patton, & Heen, 2010). The second principle is to give the other person full attention (**B: Be attentive**). It is important to either stop other activities to give attention to the speaker, or ask the person who needs to discuss something to wait until you are able to give full attention to the matter (Purdy & Borisoff, 1997). After giving full attention to the speaker, it is generally useful to ask questions to clarify anything that was ambiguous and/or fill in any needed information (**A: Ask questions**), and to reflect on the information provided by the other clinician (**R: Reflect**). Intentional reflection on the information conveyed creates the space for understanding the reporting clinician's perspective,

TABLE 8-1 SBAR-R-R Communication Technique Applied to Fetal Heart Monitoring

Prepare for an SBAR-R-R by: 1. Assessing the patient 2. Reviewing recent notes and laboratory results 3. Having the medical record available during the conversation **Situation:** Always identify yourself, where you are calling from, and the name of the woman you are calling about and quickly state the main reason and the level of urgency for the call. **Background:** Give brief pertinent background information—medical history, complaints, vital signs, and interventions that have already occurred **Assessment:** Say what you think is going on **Recommendation:** Say what you think should happen or ask for specific orders **Reasoning:** If the response is not what you expect and requested, state why what you think should happen is important. What could happen if we don't do this? **Ratification:** Close the loop by confirming actions to be taken. Assure mutual agreement on the plan.
Situation I am calling about Ms. _________, who was admitted this morning for induction of labor due to worsening hypertension. I am concerned about the FHR pattern: • Baseline FHR is _________. • Variability is _________ (absent, minimal, moderate, marked) • There are recurrent _________ (variable, late, prolonged) decelerations • She needs a bedside evaluation
Background – include the following: • GPTAL @ _________ weeks • Significant OB and medical history • Cervical dilatation • Labor progress • Vital signs • Recent changes in FHR tracing baseline, variability, accelerations, decelerations • Uterine activity • Interventions already completed
Assessment • The FHR tracing is indeterminate and the decelerations do not resolve with position change. • I'm concerned the fetus is at risk for acidemia
Recommendation • I need you to come and evaluate her now. • When can I expect you?
Reasoning • The variability was moderate previously but now it is minimal and the decelerations are worsening. The fetus is stressed and may be running out of reserve. It is important that she be evaluated now to ensure fetal well-being. • If you are not able to come now, who should I call to evaluate the patient?
Ratification • Ok, I'll do_________, and you'll be here to evaluate her in_________.

Source: Adapted from Leonard (2004).

TABLE 8-2 SBAR for Listening

	SENDER	RECEIVER
S	Situation	Set aside assumptions
B	Background	Be attentive
A	Assessment	Ask questions
R	Recommendation	Reflect
R	Reasoning	Respond
R	Ratification	Ratify

and for synthesizing the information conveyed (Purdy & Borisoff, 1997). Understanding and synthesis are needed for developing an accurate grasp of the clinical situation.

The response to an SBAR should be a concise statement that summarizes understanding of the situation and a plan to address the problem or request noted in the SBAR (**R: Respond**). Ideally, the response will include the expected outcomes for the plan of care and the time frame within which these outcomes should be achieved, as stating or discussing these parameters will promote team situation awareness (Brady et al., 2013). Finally, the discussion is complete when there is a clear ratification of agreement between the two (or more) clinicians (**R: Ratify**). Developing a routine expectation that communications about patient care will include ratification provides a structure for ensuring closed-loop communication. The purpose of closed-loop communication is to verify and validate that the intent of the communication has been understood (Agency for Healthcare Research and Quality [AHRQ], n.d.).

SBAR-style structured communication strategies lie at the interface of clinician- and team-level communication processes: they require both individual and team accountability for ensuring correct and consistent use. One hallmark of team behavior is clear language, agreed-upon and understood by all members (Knox & Simpson, 2003; Leonard & Frankel, 2011). Clear language is particularly important when communication does not occur face to face. Telephone communication between clinicians should be direct and to the point. For example:

- "Based on my initial assessment, this patient is having recurrent deep variable decelerations. May I have an order for an amnioinfusion, and can you please come in to see this patient as soon as possible?"
- "I am uncomfortable with your order to start oxytocin because of the fetal heart rate pattern. I am going to wait until you are able to come in and see this patient and we can review the tracing together. When can I expect to see you?"
- "I wanted to let you know that I discontinued the oxytocin infusion because of tachysystole. I also gave an IV fluid bolus of 500 mL of lactated Ringer's solution and assisted the patient to a lateral position to improve uterine blood flow and decrease uterine activity. The FHR baseline is 150 with moderate variability and there are no decelerations. As soon as the uterine activity has returned to less than five contractions in 10 minutes, I'll restart the oxytocin. I will call you if these interventions do not reduce the number of contractions; otherwise, I will call you in an hour with a status report.
- "You ordered intermittent auscultation of the fetal heart rate, but what I am hearing during auscultation suggests decelerations. I'm calling to let you know that I am going to use continuous monitoring until I have a normal fetal heart rate tracing. I'll call you back after I assess the patient and review the tracing to let you know what is happening with the baby."
- "Your patient is fully dilated, but she doesn't feel the urge to push. I'm going to delay pushing until she feels pressure. If she doesn't have an urge to push in an hour, I will contact you regarding allowing additional time for laboring down or if patient-directed pushing techniques will need to be instituted. I'll let you know when I need you to come."
- "I'm calling for my chief resident. She just checked Ms. Jones in room 2 during a prolonged deceleration and noted a prolapsed cord. We are transferring Ms. Jones to the surgical suite and need you to come now. Anesthesia and the neonatal team have been

paged. We'll start the cesarean, but we need you to come to the unit now." (intern calling attending physician)
- "Fetal status is deteriorating quickly, and I need you here now."

Another important form of clear language that is specifically designed to support clinicians in assertion and problem resolution is referred to as "critical language." Critical language is an institution- or unit-specific word or phrase that signals the team to stop and assess the situation for safety (Leonard & Frankel, 2011). Examples from different organizations include "In the interest of patient safety," and Allina Hospitals' phrase, "I need a little clarity." Ideally, the critical language word or phrase is a neutral term, is standardized, does not trigger a defensive response from clinicians, and can be used with ease in front of women and their families (Leonard & Frankel, 2011).

Additional critical language stems from an aviation strategy known as "CUS Words" (Barker, 2009). CUS stands for *concerned, uncomfortable*, and *safety*. "I am concerned," is a critical language cue used to get other team members' attention and indicate a significant concern. "I am uncomfortable" conveys "perhaps you missed my expression of concern." "Uncomfortable" indicates an increased level of concern and a potentially unsafe situation. "This is a safety issue" is the phrase used to indicate the team needs to stop what they are doing right now to assess the situation. When used consistently and in a standardized manner, CUS words become strong cues and delineate clear communication of the clinician's perceived level of risk (Barker, 2009).

Handoff Communications

The "handoff" or transfer of patient care from one care provider to another or from one phase of care, type of unit, or type of facility to another occurs multiple times each day in the health care setting, yet it is prone to errors and omissions that have the potential to negatively affect outcomes (Abraham, Kannampallil, & Patel, 2012; Abraham, Nguyen, Almoosa, Patel, & Patel, 2011; Graham et al., 2013; Ong & Coiera, 2011). During labor, nursing, medical, or midwifery care is often transferred from one nurse, physician, or midwife to another. These transfers can be temporary or permanent and may be the result of change of shift, completion of call, duty hour limitations, covering for nursing breaks, changes in patient acuity, or a transfer of care to another team, unit, or facility.

Although the handoff process is meant to promote continuity and efficiency, there are inherent vulnerabilities because of the human factors involved in the relay of critical information (Simpson, 2005b). Other industries such as aviation, nuclear power, and emergency dispatch have developed strategies to increase the likelihood that accurate and comprehensive information is transferred and that information is received and fully understood (Patterson, Roth, Woods, Chow, & Gomes, 2004). Some of these strategies are listed in Box 8-2 and others have been added and adapted to perinatal care (ACOG, 2012; Simpson, 2005b).

While there is limited evidence to support the effectiveness of specific handoff practices in health care, there is increasing consensus that standardization of handoff practices has the potential to reduce communication breakdowns and improve patient safety (Ong & Coiera, 2011; Riesenberg, Leitzsch, & Cunningham, 2010; Riesenberg, Leitzsch, & Little, 2009; Riesenberg, Leitzsch, Massucci, et al., 2009). Some settings have demonstrated improvements in perceptions of handoff completeness and/or patient outcomes through quality improvement initiatives (Block et al., 2010; Freitag & Carroll, 2011; Graham et al., 2013; Tapia, Fallon, Brandt, Scott, & Suliburk, 2013). One technique that has been studied to improve the content of handoffs is called I-PASS (illness severity, patient summary, action list, situation awareness and contingency planning, and synthesis by receiver) (Starmer et al., 2012). I-PASS has been most studied in the context of physician-to-physician handoffs, but can be used by any two clinicians (Figure 8-2).

BOX 8-2 Strategies for Promoting Safe Handoffs

These strategies for handing off patient care to another clinician can be used both individually and collectively. They are useful for all team members and across all disciplines.

- Use face-to-face communication whenever possible with interactive questioning encouraged.
- Use confirmation summaries for verifying communication content.
- Limit interruptions during updates and handoffs.
- Develop protocols for what type and amount of information must be included in a handoff for each clinical situation (i.e., admission, labor, birth, discharge).
- Solicit outgoing team's opinions about ongoing patient status and contingency plans for various potential variations in clinical condition.
- Assess patient status together (incoming and outgoing clinicians at the bedside).
- Provide a written summary of critical information.
- Ensure incoming clinicians have knowledge of and access to the most up-to-date information.
- Ensure an unambiguous transfer of responsibility for key tasks that are left undone.
- Delay transfer of care responsibility when there is concern about status of the process or the ability of the incoming clinician to safely handle the situation.
- During emergencies, remain involved until there is assurance and evidence that each piece of critical information has been accurately transferred and received by all members of the accepting team.
- Use role playing to teach new team members how to effectively communicate during handoffs.
- Regularly observe handoffs in progress to evaluate the process and develop ideas for improvement.
- Use handoffs that are ideal and less than ideal as learning opportunities.

Source: Adapted from Simpson (2005).

FIGURE 8-2 I-PASS Tool

I-PASS
BETTER HANDOFFS. SAFER CARE.

I	Illness Severity	• Stable, "watcher," unstable
P	Patient Summary	• Summary statement • Events leading up to admission • Hospital course • Ongoing assessment • Plan
A	Action List	• To do list • Time line and ownership
S	Situation Awareness and Contingency Planning	• Know what's going on • Plan for what might happen
S	Synthesis by Receiver	• Receiver summarizes what was heard • Asks questions • Restates key action/to do items

Note: Reproduced with permission from *Pediatrics, 129*, p. 203. Copyright 2012 by the AAP.

I-PASS contains elements of SBAR, with the intent that the relevant information can be passed off quickly (e.g., when physicians hand off patient coverage at night or during emergency coverage of another nurse's patients). I-PASS handoffs begin with a statement of **illness severity**, which is usually "stable," "watcher," or "unstable." This allows the listener to prioritize the acuity of the newly acquired patients. Next, a **patient summary** includes a summary of the events of labor or situation leading to admission, labor or hospital course, ongoing assessment, and plan. **Action list** includes a "to-do" list and timeline. **Situation awareness** and contingency planning communicates the knowledge of what is going on and a plan for what might happen. Lastly, the handoff ends with a synthesis by the **receiver**, wherein the receiver summarizes what was heard, asks questions, and confirms any action plans.

An example of this communication might include: "**I** (**illness severity**), Ms. Smith in room 2 has the most worrisome tracing tonight. **P** (**patient summary**) Ms. Smith is a 16-year-old primip who presented in active labor at 9:00 A.M. this morning. Her blood pressures are elevated and she has been diagnosed with preeclampsia. Her labor has progressed spontaneously to complete dilatation, and she has been pushing for an hour with a category II tracing. Variable decelerations are seen with most contractions, variability is moderate, and the baseline is slowly rising and her temp is now 99.5°. Dr. Jones is considering an operative vaginal birth if she has not delivered in another hour. **A** (**Action list**) She's due for her next temperature and dose of GBS prophylaxis in 30 minutes. **S** (**Situation awareness**) and contingency planning: If her temp is greater than 100.4°, Dr. Jones wants her started on amp and gent." The **receiver** (**S, Summary**) replies," So I need to keep the closest eye on Ms. Smith in room 2, the patient with preeclampsia who is pushing with variables and may be getting chorio. I need to recheck her temp, dose her with antibiotics for chorio or GBS, and page Dr. Jones for birth."

There is presently limited data to support any one form of structured handoff, and very little research has been conducted in perinatal settings. One model for intrapartum handoff structure that has been published (Block et al., 2010) is displayed in Figure 8-3. Human factors research suggests that standardization with cognitive supports such as the tangible handoff card or other information summaries will support improved handoffs, but only if the information collected is clinically meaningful to the end-users (Staggers, Clark, Blaz, & Kapsandoy, 2011) in the context of an overall organizational commitment to making effective handoffs an organizational priority (Joint Commission Center for Transforming Health Care, 2013). More rigorous research is needed to determine what the specific standardization needs are for perinatal care. In the meantime, organizations should carefully assess their current handoff practices, environment, and associated clinical workload to determine the most appropriate structured format(s) to meet their needs, covering the clinical elements outlined below and following the principles outlined in Box 8-2.

Communication among clinicians during change of shift or change of responsibility for patient care should be comprehensive, although at times an acute event necessitates that one clinician cover another clinician's patient without the benefit of a comprehensive verbal report. If the medical record documentation is up-to-date, a review of the electronic fetal monitoring (EFM) tracing and labor flow record should be adequate for the clinician to assume care and ensure patient safety in acute circumstances. A comprehensive handoff report from one clinician to another about a woman in labor should include the following:

- Important maternal–fetal admission data, including pertinent laboratory tests and results
- Current assessment, including how well the mother and fetus are tolerating labor
- Characteristics of the FHR pattern and uterine activity
- Any intrauterine resuscitation measures that have been initiated, indications for the measures, and the maternal–fetal response
- Other interventions or procedures planned or completed

Figure 8-3 Tangible Handoff Tool

Labor & Delivery Tangible Handoff

Patient identification Label

Room:______ **Gravida**_____ **Para**_____ **Obstetrician:**________
Blood Type:______ **Gestational Age:**______ **Pediatrician:**________

S – Situation
Reason for admit: Spontaneous Labor; Induction; Indication:______; Cesarean Section; Pre term labor; Antepartum observe
Contact Information: Covering Obstetrician:______; Contact Number:______
Comments: Date & Time Admitted:______; Date & Time Delivered:______; LMC LFC Type of delivery:______

B – Background
Age:______ Height:______
Body Mass Iindex_____ Weight:______
Medical History:______
Surgical History:______
Current Medicationss:______
Allergies:______

A – Assessment
Adm. Vitals:Heart rate:____ Blood Pressure:____
Respiratory rate:____ Temperature:____
Oxygen saturation____
Vaginal Exam_____ **Time done**:______
Membranes:______ rupture time:______
Spontaneous: Assisted Clear
Fetal heart rate: ______BPM. Meconium
Variability:______ FHR:___ Ctx:Q___Min
Epidural Yes No Pain Level:______

R – Recommendation
Plan:

Concerns during shift

Not a permanent part of patient record

Labor & Delivery Tangible Handoff

Admission Lab Data	Ind/Aug Meds	Tocolysis:
CBC Type & screen HIV 3rd Tri	Dinoprostone: ______ Misoprostil: ______	**Magnesium:**_____Gm/Hr **Nifedipine** Due:____ **Terbutaline** Due:____ **Indomethacin** Due:____
Prenatal Labs: HIV Initial HBSAg GBS + -	Oxytocin: ______ Milliunits/ min ______	PIH Magnesium:_____Gm/Hr Antibiotics: Ampicillin Due:____ Clindamycin Due:____ Gentamicin Due:____ PenG Due:____ Other:____
Fetal Screening: U/S Pathology F/U Yes No Rhogam Yes No Date:	Fetal Echo ☐ F/U Yes ☐ No ☐ Consents: #1 #2	Lung Maturity Steroids given: 1st 2nd
Did you: **Notify Charge RN?** Prior to cross coverage **Face-to-face handoff?** **Address safety concerns**		Comments

SC = Shift Change; CC = Cross Coverage

Note: From "The tangible handoff: a team approach for advancing structured communication in labor and delivery." by M. Block, J. F. Ehrenworth, V. N. Cuce, N. Ng'ang'a, J. Weinbach, S. B. Saber, . . . M. D. Schlesinger. *Joint Commission Journal on Quality & Patient Safety, 36*, 282–7, 241. Copyright 2010 by The Joint Commission. Reprinted with permission.

- Progress of labor
- Maternal vital signs
- Current and previous dosages of pharmacologic agents that were used to ripen the cervix or induce or augment labor, if applicable, including the maternal–fetal response
- Pain status, including current and previous pain relief and comfort measures that have been used
- The woman's desires for labor and birth
- Pertinent psychosocial issues
- Anticipated clinical trajectory

When possible, clinicians should review the medical record and fetal monitor tracing together before the clinician who is giving the report leaves the unit. Doing so will ensure that all data are covered and give the clinician who is leaving an opportunity to answer questions and address concerns that the relief or oncoming clinician may have (Joint Commission Center for Transforming Health Care, 2013). Ideally, a report between nurses either occurs at the bedside where the woman can participate, and her condition can be mutually assessed and any intravenous medications mutually reviewed; or the report is followed by a visit to the patient's room for the same purpose, and the reporting nurse introduces the relief nurse to the patient and support persons in attendance.

Teamwork Practices that Enhance Communication

In addition to the strategies described above, several team-based mechanisms enhance communication, including briefings, huddles, multidisciplinary rounds, debriefings, and multidisciplinary fetal heart monitoring education that includes multidisciplinary case and fetal heart tracing reviews.

Team briefings are an important and underutilized way of communicating among team members. While SBAR and I-PASS are situational briefings that are typically oriented toward a specific patient, team briefings are short meetings that orient the entire team to the operational context of the day, shift, or procedure. For example, the preoperative checklist is designed to provide the structure for team briefing at the procedural level. An effective briefing helps the team develop a shared mental model of the situation and identify potential challenges or threats that may arise (Gordon et al., 2013; Leonard & Frankel, 2011). Multiple organizations have developed models for structuring the form and content of team briefings. Bozeman (2011) describes a systematic approach that involves twice-daily group discussion of all patients in the intrapartum unit on a service with 3,800 annual births. These 15-minute multidisciplinary rounds follow discipline-specific handoffs, are led by clinical leaders on the nursing staff, and include all disciplines (including anesthesia and pediatrics) and support staff (e.g., surgical technicians). All cases are summarized at these rounds with priority given to any urgent or potentially evolving safety concerns. Everyone in attendance is expected to reflect on questions that can help identify emerging risk (Table 8-3).

The Cleveland Clinic developed a briefing and escalation program to reduce situation awareness failures and related adverse events in a pediatric hospital (Brady et al., 2013). Similar to other programs, this model has five structured prompts that generate a huddle between the staff nurse, charge nurse, and chief resident. These prompts identify patients who are "watchers" ("gut feeling" that they are at risk for clinical deterioration); on high-risk medications; for whom the nurse has a communication concern that could impact safety; for whom the family has a concern that could impact safety; or who have a high early warning score. When any one of these prompts is positive, a huddle is triggered between the intern, staff nurse, charge nurse, and senior resident to discuss the case and develop a "robust plan" for resolving the concern. Robust planning includes a deadline and parameters for resolution or escalation (Table 8-3).

Unit- or Department-Level Strategies

Settings that have implemented comprehensive perinatal safety programs have demonstrated improvement in perinatal outcomes (Pettker et al., 2009; Simpson, Knox, Martin, George, & Watson, 2011; Simpson, Kortz, & Knox, 2009; Thanh, Jacobs, Wanke, Hense, & Sauve, 2010). Several aspects of these programs are geared toward or have communication components: team training, including practicing for emergency situations; standardization of expectations; and interprofessional case review and FHM education. Team training teaches a common set of teamwork skills, including communication formats and cross-monitoring (AHRQ, n.d.). Simulation, especially when used with effective debriefing, can improve communication by giving team members a chance to practice the necessary skills in a safe learning environment with immediate opportunity for reflection, feedback, and discussion. This type of shared learning experience can build both individual and team communication skills that may help teams achieve a shared mental model of clinical situations more quickly and effectively. Moreover, *in situ* simulation can assist the team in uncovering systems problems that may need to be resolved to promote effective communication and response (Hansen & Arafeh, 2012). Zigmont, Kappus, and Sudikoff (2011) present a detailed discussion of the principles of effective debriefing in their "3D Model of Debriefing." The stages, purpose, and example strategies for this debriefing model are presented in Table 8-4.

Common Expectations and Standardized Definitions of Fetal Heart Rate Patterns

Each institution should have a bundle of practices guiding the use of fetal monitoring (Minkoff & Berkowitz, 2009). Such a bundle would include policies related to FHR pattern interpretation, expected interventions if there is concern for maternal or fetal status and standards for communication developed by an interdisciplinary

TABLE 8-3 Approaches Used in Two Models for Team Briefing

MULTIDISCIPLINARY OBSTETRIC PATIENT SUMMARIES (BOZEMAN, 2011)	PROACTIVE IDENTIFICATION OF RISK AND ROBUST PLANNING (BRADY ET AL., 2013)
Entire team meets twice every 24 hours and reviews all intrapartum cases. All care providers participate in identifying potential risks by considering the following questions: • What potential risks exist for this patient? (Is there risk of stroke, hemorrhage, sepsis, fetal injury, etc.?) • Are there trends that indicate concern (e.g., vital signs trends, lab trends, vaginal birth after cesarean concerns, etc.)? • Is there any information or task that I don't understand or don't know how to perform? • What is the plan of care based on the given information? • Do I feel comfortable or am I concerned about the plan of care? • Do I feel qualified, or have I ever cared for a patient like this? • Are there concerns I would like to have addressed?	**All cases are screened at least every 4 hours for concerns. Identification of a concern triggers a huddle with bedside nurse, charge nurse, intern, senior resident. A robust plan is developed. If all team members do not agree with the plan, the plan is escalated to the safety officer.** **Concern:** • High warning score • Communication concern • Watcher • Family concern • High-risk medication/therapy **Planning:** • Safety manager notified **Plan:** **Team members notified:** **Expected Outcome:** (describe the yes/no criteria that will be met if the plan is successful) **Outcome deadline:** (If more than 1 hour, state why) **Escalation plan if outcomes not met:** **Notes:**

perinatal team (Fox et al., 2000; Simpson & Knox, 2005). These mutually agreed-upon practices can then be routinely used by all providers to enhance both interdisciplinary communication and patient safety. The potential for miscommunication among care providers, especially during telephone conversations regarding fetal status, are decreased when everyone is using the same terminology to describe EFM data. Thus, appropriate and timely intervention for indeterminate or abnormal FHR patterns is more likely. The major professional associations supporting clinicians who provide intrapartum care have all endorsed the NICHD terminology as the standard for describing, interpreting, and communicating fetal heart monitoring data (ACOG, 2005, 2009, 2010; American College of Nurse-Midwives, 2010b; Association of Women's Health, Obstetric and Neonatal Nurses [AWHONN], 2005, 2010).

Joint Nurse-Midwife-Physician Education Regarding Fetal Assessment

Nurses, midwives, and physicians jointly assess and manage maternal–fetal status during labor. Therefore, interdisciplinary continuing education programs provide one way to promote effective communication among providers and contribute to improving perinatal outcomes (Pettker et al., 2009; Simpson, 2005a; Simpson et al., 2009). One way to explicitly demonstrate that knowledge of fetal monitoring is not discipline-specific is to engage all disciplines in ongoing collaborative FHR monitoring education through interdisciplinary case reviews and joint FHM continuing education or certification activities. Educational collaboration among nurses, midwives, and physicians who are jointly responsible for FHR pattern interpretation and clinical interventions can enhance collaboration in everyday clinical interactions and thus

TABLE 8-4 3D Model of Debriefing

KOLB'S EXPERIMENTAL LEARNING CYCLE	3D MODEL COMPONENTS	LEARNING OUTCOMES MODEL
Concrete experience	Creating a safe environment • Introductions • Ground rules and expectations • Confidentiality • Orientation to simulation environment	Individual • . . . feels "safe" • . . . knows what to expect • . . . is prepared to complete the task
	Simulation exercise • Define objectives • Enhance realism: care-team, environment, progression • Challenging to invoke emotional response	Experience • . . . creates a change in body state for individual • . . . is realistic to evoke emotion for individual • . . . is relevant practical, and useful to individual
	Prebriefing • Ground rules • Set expectations • Explain Format	Individual • . . . knows what to expect
Reflective observation	Defusing • Discuss emotions • Recap events • Conduct needs assessment	Environment (micro) • . . . is safe for learning Individual • . . . distresses to set stage for learning • . . . engages in student-centered learning
Abstract conceptualization	Discovering • Prompt reflection through objective observation and video review • Discover mental models guiding behavior • Discuss target mental models • Cue analogical reasoning	Individual on Experience • . . . analyzes behaviors and intended outcomes Individual • . . . uses "analogical reasoning" to compare existing mental model to target mental outcomes
Active experimentation	Deepening • Prompt individual to apply new information to practice	Individual within macro-environment • . . . mentally connects target mental model to practice use within larger clinical environment
	Summary • Restate learning objectives discussed and lessons learned.	Individual • . . . leaves with practical and useful information.
	Simulation Exercise 2 • Allow individual to apply new information	Individual within microenvironment • . . . actively connects target

The 3D Model of Debriefing is based on Kolb's Experimental Learning Cycle. Adult Learning Theory, and the Learning Outcomes Model. It incorporates well-established debriefing phases and addresses the adult learner, key experiences, and the learning environment(s).

Note: From *Seminars in Perinatology, 35*(2), J. J. Zigmont, L. J. Kappus, & S. N. Sudikoff. "The 3D model of debriefing: Defusing, discovering, and deepening." pp. 52–58. Copyright 2011, Reprinted with permission from Elsevier.

promote patient safety. These interdisciplinary educational programs concerning electronic fetal monitoring can potentially accomplish the following:

- Decrease the frequency of clinical disagreement among physicians, midwives, and nurses regarding the description and interpretation of FHR patterns
- Increase the opportunity for interaction and role-modeling professional communication techniques
- Increase understanding of fellow clinicians' roles and perspectives on clinical care, FHR patterns, and approach to interventions
- Promote collaborative problem solving in the clinical setting

EFM tracing reviews work well as a form of interdisciplinary education because the presentation and discussion are associated with specific clinical cases and graphic display of FHR patterns. An interdisciplinary group of clinical leaders can identify situations that are known to produce differences of opinion in their facility, and develop case studies around these situations. Groups of nurses, physicians, and midwives can then work through the cases together to review expected responses, appropriate interpretations, and related interventions. Team discussions can lead to an increased knowledge of EFM principles for everyone involved and improve understanding of each other's roles. Developing case studies containing clinical ambiguity can be an ideal way to clarify ongoing clinical issues and expose differing levels of individual clinician tolerance of risk when interpretation and expectations of provider groups may not always be the same (Jacobson et al., 2013; Lyndon et al., 2011, 2012; Simpson, 2008). For example, physicians may expect a series of nursing interventions for a specific FHR pattern that are not the routine of nurses on the unit. In another example, there may be clinical disagreement about what to do when tachysystole is the result of oxytocin administration but the FHR pattern remains normal. Opinions may vary among nurses and primary care providers concerning when and under what circumstances oxytocin dosages should be increased or decreased, and thus may be a source of frustration (Lyndon et al., 2014; Simpson et al., 2006; Sleutel, Schultz, & Wyble, 2007). An open and proactive discussion of physiologic principles related to oxytocin administration and rationale for a course of action can result in standardization of policies and enhanced communication among providers (Lyndon et al., 2011; Simpson et al., 2006).

EFFECTIVE CONFLICT MANAGEMENT

There are many challenges to achieving teamwork in the perinatal setting, and many potential sources of conflict. Interpretation of maternal–fetal data and subsequent communication regarding those data among professional colleagues may sometimes result in conflict. Although individual expectations may differ, it is helpful to focus on clinicians' mutual commitment to childbearing women and mutual desire to achieve optimal outcomes for women and their families. Professionalism requires extending mutual respect and trust to all team members as well as the ability to respectfully resolve disagreements or differences of opinion (Knox & Simpson, 2003; Leonard & Frankel, 2011; Simpson, 2014). Strategies for improving communication in relation to multiple potential sources of conflict are listed in Table 8-5.

People often prefer to avoid situations of potential conflict or "confrontation" over differences of opinion. Moreover, nurses have often been informally trained by their peers in strategies for side-stepping potentially confrontational communication episodes. It is essential to recognize that engaging difficult conversations can actually build a stronger sense of teamwork and collegiality whereas avoiding confrontation often builds negative feelings and resentment (Stone, Patton, & Heen, 2010) in addition to potentially delaying or otherwise interfering with needed care (Lyndon et al., 2011). The principles of effective conflict resolution include those described previously for effective listening (Stone et al., 2010):

- Either avoid making, or set aside assumptions about, the other party's motivation or intentions (assume good intentions).
- Take the time to listen to the other person's understanding of events (understand his or her story).
- Recognize that perspectives often differ on both what is "risky" and what is the "right" thing to do (Lyndon et al., 2011, 2012, 2014).

Furthermore, it is essential to be aware of cultural and professional differences that may be influencing interpretation and response to the events in question.

In many situations there will be time to have a conversation with the other clinician when there is a difference of opinion or disagreement about the best course of action. In such situations it is important to consider the timing and context that

TABLE 8-5 Strategies for Improving Communication in Relation to Sources of Potential Conflict

SOURCES OF CONFLICT	APPROACH
Differing expectations for information needs, communication content and style	Team Training Structured communication tools (e.g., SBAR[a]; structured handoffs) Board rounds Huddles Attentive listening
Failure to communicate rationale	Routinely ask for plan and reasoning
Inattention to concern	Persistently restate concerns until resolved
Concerns remain unresolved	Consider instituting laborist[b] in-house if provider fatigue frequent concern or service is large with many primary providers Ensure adequate staffing and break relief Ratify plan before concluding conversation
Differing "world views", e.g., "Oxytocin Wars"[c]	Standardize oxytocin protocol Standardize fetal monitoring language and application
Fetal monitoring methods, interpretation, and management of complex tracings	Provide regular interprofessional case reviews to discuss management; role model expression of concern and positive resolution of differences Standardize expectations for notification of complications Articulate and plan for potential problems early in care Individuals take responsibility for collaboratively discussing differing views Avoid professional stereotyping as an explanation for behavior Consider instituting laborist in-house (especially at night)
Disruptive Behavior	"Good Citizen" policy consistently enforced Individuals and peers stand up to unprofessional behaviors Administrative commitment to addressing any chronic issues Availability of anonymous incident reporting system

[a]SBAR: Situation, Background, Assessment, Recommendation
[b]Laborist: An obstetric hospitalist
[c]"Oxytocin Wars": Tug of war between physicians and nurses over management of oxytocin
Note: From "Effective physician-nurse communication: A patient safety essential for labor and delivery." by A. Lyndon, M. G. Zlatnik, & R. M. Wachter, 2011. *American Journal of Obstetrics & Gynecology, 205*, p. 94. Copyright 2011 by Elsevier. Reprinted with permission.

will best support a productive dialogue (Stone et al., 2010). Finding an appropriate location for the discussion outside the patient's room or away from the central workstation may be necessary. Attention to body language and verbal cues is also important to avoid contributing to making the other party feel defensive. Asking for the other party to explain his or her point of view first is often very useful, as is attentive listening, avoiding interrupting, and asking clarifying questions to ensure your understanding. Phrases such as "I understand your concern, and I see your point. My remaining concerns are. . ." can be helpful, as is summarizing your understanding of what the other person has communicated. In acute patient care situations, there may be a perceived or actual lack of time to deal with concerns about patient care. Disagreement should always be addressed in real time if there is a concern for patient safety; in other situations the conversation can be deferred until the acute patient problem is resolved.

Unfortunately, despite professional and regulatory efforts to enforce professional behavioral standards (ACOG, 2011; The Joint Commission, 2008, 2012), disruptive behavior (e.g., rudeness; yelling; throwing things; refusal to answer questions, pages, or requests for evaluation;

demeaning body language or actions; intimidation) continues to occur in health care settings (Leape et al., 2012a, 2012b). When confronted with disrespectful or otherwise disruptive behavior it is helpful to remain calm and state that the behavior is unacceptable. "I am happy to discuss this when our conversation can be respectful," or even "We can discuss this further when you stop yelling at me," may help the other person stop what he or she is doing and reorient him- or herself to having a professional interaction. It is important to put a stop to disrespectful behavior rather than allow it to continue. Refusal to be treated with disrespect is a surprisingly powerful action that can often change the dynamic of the situation.

Chain of Resolution

Some issues of conflict in the clinical setting cannot be resolved between the caregivers immediately involved and yet need to be resolved quickly. Clinicians must initiate an appropriate course of action when their assessment of the situation indicates the issue presents a concern for patient safety, could negatively affect maternal or fetal well-being, or there is potential for the clinical situation to deteriorate rapidly (e.g., when a primary care provider does not respond to a deteriorating maternal or fetal condition). Decisive, timely nursing intervention may be necessary to avoid a potentially adverse outcome. Clinical knowledge and the use of the chain of resolution or authority are ways to attempt to resolve differences of opinion in clinical practice settings. An example of chain of resolution is presented in Figure 8-4. Steps or levels in the chain are determined by the positions and availability of personnel in each individual institution. Generally, larger institutions and academic medical centers have more steps in the chain of resolution than community and rural hospitals. If discussions with the physician or midwife do not result in appropriate care for the clinical situation, the nurse has the responsibility to use the institutional chain of resolution to ensure appropriate and timely intervention and patient safety (Simpson, 2014).

FIGURE 8-4 Example of Problem Resolution Relying on Chain-of-Resolution or Chain-of-Authority

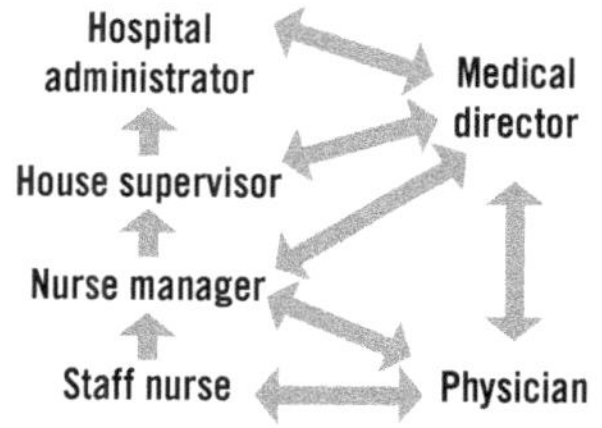

The physician or midwife should first be notified that the nurse is going to institute the chain of resolution. Sometimes this statement alone is enough to generate an appropriate clinical action or compromise. Next, the staff nurse notifies the appropriately available immediate supervisory nurse as outlined in his or her institution's chain of resolution (i.e., charge nurse, nurse manager, or nursing supervisor) to provide assistance and to review the conflict situation and possible actions and then documents in the medical record or variance report that this action has been taken as outlined in the institutional policies and protocols. In selected instances, it may be necessary to go further up the chain if the situation cannot be resolved. Due to the dynamic, rapidly evolving nature of labor birth there may not be time to use the chain of resolution in its entirety in all situations. Furthermore, the charge nurse or other supervisory personnel may need to take over the chain of resolution communications so that the primary nurse can stay at the bedside with the laboring woman. Physicians and midwives may also find themselves in situations where they need to invoke the chain of resolution in the interests of patient safety or well-being. Every clinician should know the institutional chain of resolution to facilitate rapid problem resolution when necessary.

Invoking the chain of resolution should not be a primary way of resolving clinical disagreements (Simpson, 2014). Frequent use of the chain of resolution may point to deeper underlying issues with professionalism, problematic interpersonal relationships, or other systems issues within the perinatal unit. Use of the chain of resolution should be monitored to learn from situations that lead to its invocation. A senior but neutral party should facilitate a review of each case with the parties involved, and assist the clinical team to develop plans for resolving the underlying conflict so that similar situations can be avoided (Simpson, 2014).

A key factor in perinatal clinicians' decisions about their communication strategies and other actions in conflict situations appears to be the level of administrative support they believe they will receive (Lyndon et al., 2014; Simpson & Lyndon, 2009). While strong administrative support does not guarantee that clinicians will speak up about their concerns and persist with the chain of resolution when indicated, lack of administrative support for assertive communication is cited by clinicians as a barrier to effective resolution of clinical problems. When nurses, physicians, and midwives feel that "nothing gets done" in response to concerns, or fear the repercussions of acting on their concerns, they often become resigned to not being heard (Lyndon, 2008; Lyndon et al., 2014; Simpson & Lyndon, 2009). Clinicians who are resigned in this way may either stop raising their concerns or acquiesce quickly when others do not agree with them. This compromises patient safety, as safety is enhanced when everyone takes responsibility for identifying and acting on potential hazards (Lyndon & Kennedy, 2010). Therefore, it is critical for organizations to support nurses and other clinicians who invoke the chain of resolution, whether or not they are ultimately deemed to be "correct" in their assessment of the situation (Maxfield et al., 2013; Simpson & Lyndon, 2009). A healthy work environment and strong safety culture will support effective conflict resolution and use of the chain of resolution when indicated.

COMMUNICATION WITH PREGNANT WOMEN AND THEIR FAMILIES OR SUPPORT PERSONS

Communication with women and their families during labor and birth should reflect the respect of the clinician for the dignity of the woman and her family. This includes maintaining cultural sensitivity and supporting women's autonomy. Women's involvement in decision making during birth influences her positive experience of herself and her newborn(s). On the other hand, traumatic birth experiences, which are sometimes created by the way providers interact with women, can result in psychological difficulty (Jacobson et al., 2013). Thus, the support and respect that a woman receives during birth can influence her sense of control, and may ultimately have a powerful influence on her birth experience and long-term health.

In a recent joint statement from multiple professional associations, shared decision making was highlighted as one of four key elements for achieving optimal maternal health outcomes (Lawrence et al., 2012). Shared decision making is a process in which health care providers serve as partners with women to facilitate women's fully informed participation in choosing care that is compatible with their values and preferences and aligned with the best available evidence. This implies that women should participate in choosing the method of fetal heart monitoring. In a recent nationally representative survey, a majority of women did not want nonmedically indicated intervention in the birth process, and wanted to know the risks and benefits of proposed treatments and to discuss options for treatment with their care provider (Declercq, Sakala, Corry, Applebaum, & Herrlich, 2013b). In the postpartum arm of this study, 89% of women who labored reported receiving EFM as the method of fetal surveillance some or all of the time during labor. Sixty percent of women who received EFM reported receiving it continuously, whereas 23% of women who had EFM also received some combination of monitoring methods including hand-held Doppler or stethoscope. Twelve percent of women who received EFM reported receiving intermittent monitoring (Declercq, Sakala, Corry, Applebaum, & Herrlich, 2013a). This study did not investigate whether or not women felt they were offered a choice about monitoring or if they had a choice whether it was informed. However, traditionally women have not necessarily been offered choices about methods of monitoring as continuous monitoring has been considered the routine (Declercq, Sakala, Corry, & Applebaum, 2007; Wood, 2003). The percentage of women monitored continuously is out of proportion to national rates of labor induction or prevalence of high risk conditions, suggesting that convenience and custom continue to play a role in selection of monitoring methods.

For shared decision making to occur, it is important to assess women's knowledge and preferences regarding fetal surveillance in labor. Women's preferences and the risks and benefits of methods of fetal heart monitoring are ideally discussed prior to labor. When women present in labor, the methods of monitoring that are appropriate to their clinical condition should be described and their preferences used to guide decision making. Rather than assuming that continuous EFM is the norm, it is important to keep in mind that other evidence-based options such as intermittent auscultation are frequently appropriate for laboring women (ACNM, 2010a; American Academy of Pediatrics & American College of Obstetricians and Gynecologists, 2012; AWHONN, 2008) and are recommended as the primary method of fetal surveillance for low-risk women by some organizations (ACNM, 2010a; SOGC, 2007).

Use of Translators

Caring for laboring women who are not fluent in English can be a challenge in the hospital setting. Although The Joint Commission mandates the use of interpreters in the hospital setting, many hospitals cannot provide the continuous coverage of a bilingual individual, let alone a professional, trained health care interpreter, over the length of a labor that may take days. A health care interpreter is defined by the National Council on Interpreting in Health Care as "an individual with appropriate training and experience who is able to interpret with consistency and accuracy and who adheres to a code of professional ethics" (Wilson-Stronks, Lee, Cordero, Kopp, & Galvez, 2008, p. 18). Interpreting services can also be provided via telephone or video, although this may present technological challenges during the dynamic birth process (e.g., if a laboring woman is moved quickly to the surgical suite for complications, the connection with a telephone interpreter may be lost). Furthermore, in an urgent fetal monitoring situation, the added time for translation may slow down the response to the fetal status. For this reason, a bedside nurse who is bilingual, *and who has qualified* as a hospital interpreter, is the ideal person to care for a non-English-speaking woman and her family. Although a spouse or support person who speaks English may seem like a good option, the use of family members as interpreters is unwise, as the family member may not understand completely or may edit what is said. All aspects of the labor and birth process require close attention to cultural considerations.

The concept of cultural humility refers to the ability of health care providers to engage in ongoing learning and self-reflection to understand and respond effectively to the cultural and language needs brought by the patient to the health care encounter, and to recognize and keep in check the power imbalances created by the health care encounter (Tervalon & Murray-Garcia, 1998). Cultural humility requires clinicians to value diversity, assess themselves for their own biases, acquire cultural knowledge (especially for local populations), avoid stereotyping by recognizing that each person integrates cultural values and traditions in their own way, and adapt to diversity and the cultural contexts of individuals and communities served (Tervalon & Murray-Garcia, 1998; Wilson-Stronks et al., 2008). Included in the concept of cultural humility is sensitivity to the possibility that persons from any cultural background may have low literacy and/or low health literacy. Cultural humility includes the ability to understand and respond effectively to patients with low health literacy. This means that clinicians and staff must avoid assuming that patients have read or understand forms and information sheets. In perinatal settings, clinicians must be sensitive to the laboring woman's fears and concerns, which may have cultural differences in content or expression. Furthermore, immigrant women or women from nondominant cultures may have different expectations of the birth process (Redshaw & Heikkila, 2011).

RISK MANAGEMENT AND COMMUNICATION OF FETAL HEART MONITORING INFORMATION

Along with emergency departments and perioperative services, perinatal units account for most of the claims of patient injuries and death (CRICO Strategies, 2010; Knox, Simpson, & Garite, 1999). Some of these patient injuries are related to human error and are preventable. Fetal and neonatal injuries are more common than maternal injuries. Several common recurring clinical situations account for the majority of fetal and neonatal injuries (Knox, Simpson, & Townsend, 2003; Simpson & Knox, 2005):

- Inability to recognize and/or appropriately respond to both antepartum and intrapartum fetal compromise
- Inappropriate use of oxytocin or misoprostol leading to tachysystole, uterine rupture, and fetal compromise and/or death
- Inappropriate continued coached second-stage pushing despite an indeterminate FHR pattern with decelerations or an abnormal FHR pattern
- Inability to effect a timely cesarean birth when indicated by fetal or maternal condition
- Inability to appropriately resuscitate a depressed newborn
- Inappropriate use of forceps/vacuum/fundal pressure leading to fetal trauma and/or preventable shoulder dystocia
- Inability to resolve clinical conflicts related to interpretation of and interventions for deteriorating maternal or fetal status

It is important to note that these same clinical situations have been the source of the majority of legal claims related to fetal/neonatal injuries for more than 20 years, when these data first began to be collected (Knox et al., 2003). Communication inadequacies and omissions can be associated with these recurring clinical situations. Failure to resolve a clinical conflict in a timely manner may contribute to patient injuries. In an analysis of 800 closed claims, communication breakdowns contributed to a substantial number of events, particularly in the management of second-stage labor. This problem was more acute in community hospital settings (56% of cases) than in academic medical centers (30% of cases) (CRICO Strategies, 2010).

Perinatal units should encourage the reporting of near-misses and all adverse events to enhance safety learning (Boothman & Blackwell, 2010). Routine monitoring of quality structure and processes and reporting of near misses and "incidents" allows the collection of data that provides the opportunity for problems to be solved before adverse outcomes happen (Clark, Meyers, Frye, McManus, & Perlin, 2012; Janakiraman & Ecker, 2010; Simpson, 2005a). Furthermore, these data may provide a "big picture" that elucidates recurrent problems or "accidents waiting to happen."

A sentinel event is an unexpected occurrence involving death or serious physical or psychological injury (loss of limb or function), or the risk thereof (The Joint Commission, n.d.). The phrase "or the risk thereof" includes any process variation for which a recurrence would carry a significant chance of a serious adverse outcome. In perinatal settings, these events would include maternal or term neonatal deaths or hypoxic ischemic encephalopathy. The Joint Commission mandates that these events be timely reviewed at the hospital level, including a thorough and credible root-cause analysis and developing an action plan designed to implement improvements to reduce risk. Additionally, the hospital is charged with implementing the improvements and monitoring the effectiveness of those improvements.

Types of sentinel events that are reviewable under The Joint Commission's policy include any patient death, paralysis, coma, or other major permanent loss of function associated with a medication error, patient suicide, hospital performing the wrong invasive procedure or operating on the wrong side of the patient's body, on the wrong site on the patient's body, or on the wrong patient, *any intrapartum maternal death, any perinatal death (unrelated to a congenital condition in an infant having a birth weight greater than 2,500 grams)*, patient abduction, assault, or homicide (resulting in patient death or major permanent loss of function), a patient fall that results in death or major permanent loss of function as a direct result of the injuries sustained in the fall, *hemolytic transfusion reaction involving major blood group incompatibilities,* and a *foreign body*, such as a sponge or forceps, that was left in a patient after surgery (The Joint Commission, 2013a).

Historically, adverse events related to medical errors were blamed on the clinicians involved and mistakes they may have made. This mindset assumed that errors would not occur if busy clinicians just worked harder or paid more attention. More modern thinking acknowledges that humans make errors, and we need to design our systems of care to both decrease the likelihood of errors being made and increase the potential for errors to be caught prior to adverse outcomes (Kohn, Corrigan, & Donaldson, 2000). When adverse events occur, a quality improvement technique known as root-cause analysis (RCA) can be used to explore what happened, with hopes of correcting systems problems that contributed to the error and preventing similar errors in the future. RCA is defined as an analysis of "the basic and causal factor(s) that underlie variation in performance," which in practical terms often means a multidisciplinary team reviewing an adverse event, interviewing the involved parties, and then, using a predefined protocol, attempting to analyze the sequence of events leading to the error. The analysis asks the questions: "What happened?", "Why did it happen?", and "What can be done to prevent it from happening again?" (Table 8-6) to understand the human and structural factors that led to the event (AHRQ Patient Safety Network, 2012). The RCA process, documentation, and dissemination of the results should be carefully reviewed with legal counsel, so that it is sound.

TABLE 8-6 A Framework for a Root-Cause Analysis and Action Plan in Response to a Sentinel Event (the Steps of RCA)

Overview	The Joint Commission Root-Cause Analysis and Action Plan tool has 24 analysis questions. The following framework is intended to provide a template for answering the analysis questions and aid organizing the steps in a root-cause analysis. All possibilities and questions should be fully considered in seeking "root cause(s)" and opportunities for risk reduction. For each finding continue to ask "Why?" and drill down further to uncover why parts of the process occurred or didn't occur when they should have.
Event description	Date, time, and day of the week. Detailed description of event, including a timeline. The patient's diagnoses, medications, past history. Results of autopsy or other relevant studies.
Analysis questions	For each analysis question, the root-cause analysis findings should be listed, as well as the root cause(s) and a plan of action.
Typical questions	What was the intended process flow? Were there any steps in the process that did not occur as intended? What human factors were relevant? How did equipment performance affect the outcome? Was staffing sufficient both in qualifications and number? Were there problems with communication (including verbal, written, and electronic)? What emergency and failure-mode responses have been planned and tested?
Action plan	For each of the findings identified in the analysis as needing an action, indicate the planned action expected, implementation date, and associated measure of effectiveness. In addition to the plan of action risk reduction strategies themselves, important details include the position/title of the responsible party and the method (including policy, education, audit, observation, and implementation).

AHRQ Patient Safety Network (2012); The Joint Commission (2013a).

A well-conducted RCA will generate multiple opportunities for improvement. Communication skills are very important to a successful RCA, as it is important not to close off analysis too early. The facilitator needs to ensure a safe space for all parties to state what they see in the situation. Clinicians, especially staff nurses, who may be intimidated by the process but who also may have critical ground-level observations of how things go wrong, need to keep raising what they see, so that it becomes part of the analysis (Wu, Lipshutz, & Pronovost, 2008).

SUMMARY

Communication regarding fetal status is a critical aspect of perinatal care. Verbal and written communication should be accurate, timely, and concise. A collaborative attitude and mutual respect are the foundations of a healthy interpersonal interaction. Over time, with patience and a joint commitment to the best possible outcomes for mothers and babies, respectful nonhierarchical communication styles among professional colleagues and with women and their families can be promoted and enhanced.

Perinatal care providers should develop common strategies as a team for intervening when the FHR pattern is suggestive of fetal compromise. Patient safety related to FHR assessment is dependent on competent care providers, adequate and accurate monitoring of maternal–fetal status, and timely implementation of appropriate clinical interventions. Nurses, midwives, and physicians benefit from learning about FHM in joint continuing education classes. Such classes enhance consistent communication of FHM data among professionals and provide opportunities to discuss clinical controversies and propose potential resolutions. Effective communication involves management of conflict that is often part of work among professionals with differing views and perspectives. Policies for use of the chain of resolution are helpful when conflict resolution efforts are not successful.

To ensure the robustness of patient safety systems, the perinatal team should develop and continually reevaluate effective communication and coordination strategies (Leonard & Frankel, 2011). This is particularly important in emergent situations such as a sudden, profound fetal bradycardia when the stress is high (Simpson, 2005b). The fresh perspective of the oncoming team should be valued and open interaction regarding prior, ongoing, and anticipated maternal–fetal status should be routinely expected. The effective perinatal team embraces an approach of 360-degree accountability: clinicians hold themselves accountable for effective performance and communication; clinicians and other staff hold each other accountable for effective performance and communication; and the administration holds itself accountable for providing the necessary resources and safety culture for effective communication and problem solving to be the norm for clinical care.

Case Study: Nancy

Age:	32 years old
Gravidity/Parity:	G3 P2002
Gestational Age:	38-5/7 weeks
Medical History:	Unremarkable
Surgical History:	Unremarkable
Psychosocial History:	Single; father of baby involved
Past Obstetric History:	Normal spontaneous vaginal birth at 39-6/7 weeks Normal spontaneous vaginal birth at 38-1/7 weeks
Current Obstetric History:	Normal prenatal laboratory results • Rh negative • Group B streptococcus (GBS) positive; second trimester ultrasound consistent with LMP, normal anatomy

Nancy presented to obstetric triage at 0400 with complaint of leaking small amounts of clear fluid since 0115. She also had increasing frequency and intensity of contractions prior to admission. She denied headache, blurred vision, or epigastric pain. A VE at admission showed a cervix that was 2 cm dilated, 50% effaced, and a fetal vertex that was +1 station. Her vital signs were as follows: oral temperature, 97.8° F (36.5° C); blood pressure, 126/74 mmHg; pulse, 98 bpm; and respirations, 24 breaths per minute. The patient received 2 mg Stadol for pain relief at 0845. The patient received relief, rating her pain 2–3 out of 10.

A seizure was witnessed at 1040 and the patient became unresponsive. The patient was hypotensive with a palpable pulse. An anesthesiologist was called to the bedside to assist with airway and fluid management. The charge nurse called the primary care provider to the bedside stat. Eclampsia was the presumptive diagnosis, and the patient received a loading dose of magnesium sulfate. The subsequent diagnosis, after delivery, was anaphylactoid syndrome of pregnancy, commonly referred to as an amniotic fluid embolism.

Nancy: Labor and Delivery Tracing Using Fetal Spiral Electrode and Tocodynamometer at 1050

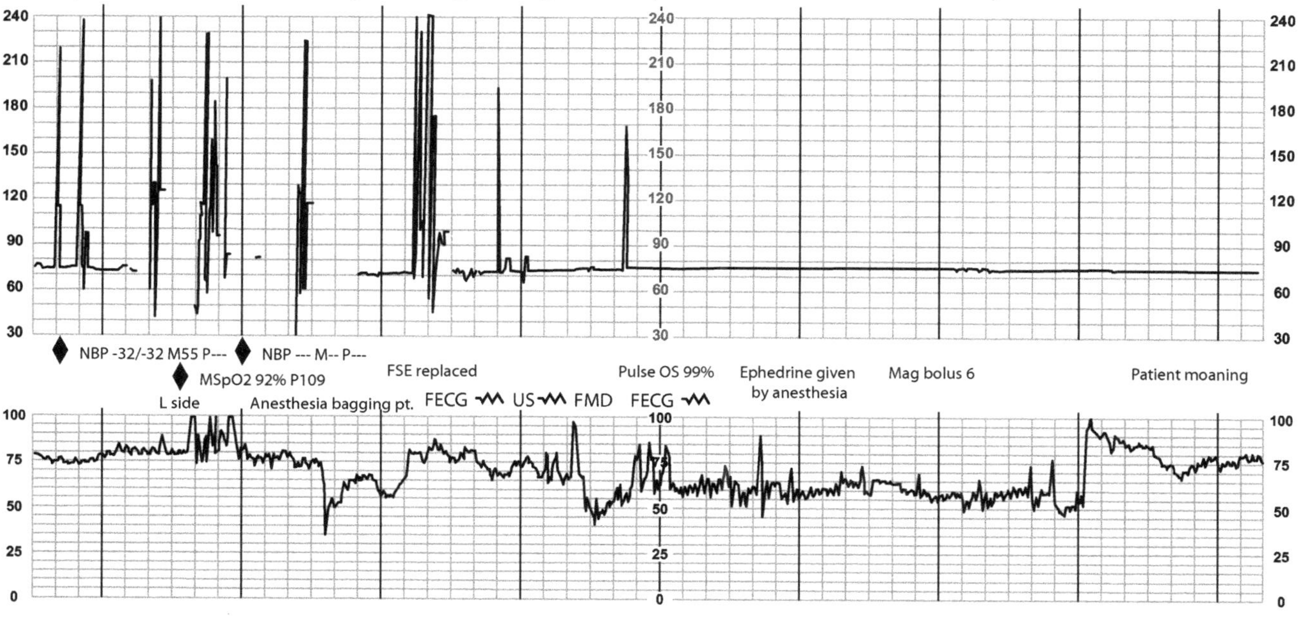

Case Study: Nancy

1. Baseline FHR: **75 bpm**

2. Variability

Absent (undetectable)	________
Minimal (>0 but 5 bpm)	________
Moderate (6–25 bpm)	________
Marked (>25 bpm)	________
Unable to determine	________

3. Contractions

Frequency:	**Unable to assess**
Duration:	**Unable to assess**
Intensity:	**Unable to assess**
Resting tone:	**Need to palpate**

4. Accelerations and decelerations. When present, circle P if periodic or E if episodic.

Accelerations	P	E
Early decelerations	P	
Variable decelerations	P	E
Late decelerations	P	
Prolonged decelerations	P (Presumed bradycardia)	E
None present		

5. Interpretation

Category I	________
Category II	________
Category III	________

6. List possible underlying physiologic mechanisms or rationales for observed patterns.
   - **Decreased uteroplacental perfusion related to maternal hypotension**
   - **Decreased maternal oxygen content and oxygen delivery to fetus related to maternal seizure**
   - **Associated with an abnormal fetal acid-base status at present**

7. List in order of priority the physiologic goal(s) for observed patterns.
   - **Maximize oxygenation.**
   - **Maximize placental blood flow.**

8. List actions and interventions indicated based on overall interpretation (physiologic based, instrumentation based, and further assessments).
   - **Maintain maternal airway and resuscitate.**
   - **Assess maternal vital signs.**
   - **Mobilize team to assist with maternal–fetal assessment and interventions.**
   - **Change maternal position with lateral tilt to maximize uterine blood flow.**
   - **Differentiate FHR from maternal pulse by manual palpation of maternal pulse, auscultation of FHR, or ultrasound of FHR.**
   - **Begin CPR as appropriate.**
   - **Prepare for perimortem cesarean if unable to resuscitate mother within 5 minutes.**
   - **Assess for alternative causes of FHR bradycardia (i.e., uterine rupture).**
   - **Maintain IV access for fluid administration to increase maternal blood volume and maximize uterine blood flow.**
   - **Prepare and administer magnesium sulfate bolus for seizure prophylaxis as ordered by provider.**

- **Prepare for emergent birth after Nancy is stabilized.**
- **Alert neonatal team to prepare for emergent birth and resuscitation.**
- **Have ephedrine 5–10 mg IV push ready to treat hypotension, if necessary.**
- **Use pulse oximeter to verify maternal oxygenation during ventilation.**
- **Evaluate FHR responses to interventions.**
- **Palpate uterus to validate uterine monitoring data.**
- **Continue assessments and interventions based on clinical findings and facility protocols.**
- **Keep family informed of clinical situation.**

REFERENCES

Abraham, J., Kannampallil, T. G., & Patel, V. L. (2012). Bridging gaps in handoffs: A continuity of care based approach. *Journal of Biomedical Informatics, 45*(2), 240–254. doi:10.1016/j.jbi.2011.10.011

Abraham, J., Nguyen, V., Almoosa, K. F., Patel, B., & Patel, V. L. (2011). Falling through the cracks: Information breakdowns in critical care handoff communication. *AMIA Annual Symposium Proceedings, 2011*, 28–37.

Agency for Healthcare Research and Quality. (n.d.). TeamSTEPPS®: Strategies and tools to enhance performance and patient safety. Retrieved from http://www.ahrq.gov/professionals/education/curriculum-tools/teamstepps/

Agency for Healthcare Research and Quality Patient Safety Network. (2012). Patient safety primers: Root cause analysis. Retrieved from http://www.psnet.ahrq.gov/primer.aspx?primerID=10

American Academy of Pediatrics & American College of Obstetricians and Gynecologists. (2012). *Guidelines for perinatal care* (7th ed.). Elk Grove Village, IL: Authors.

American College of Nurse-Midwives. (2010a). Intermittent auscultation for intrapartum fetal heart rate surveillance (replaces ACNM Clinical Bulletin #9, March 2007). *Journal of Midwifery and Women's Health, 55*(4), 397–403. doi:10.1016/j.jmwh.2010.05.007

American College of Nurse-Midwives. (2010b). Standardized nomenclature for electronic fetal monitoring (Position Statement). Silver Spring, MD: Author.

American College of Obstetricians and Gynecologists. (2005). Practice Bulletin No. 62: Intrapartum fetal heart rate monitoring. *Obstetrics and Gynecology, 105* (5, Pt. 1), 1161–1169.

American College of Obstetricians and Gynecologists. (2009). Practice Bulletin No. 106: Intrapartum fetal heart rate monitoring: Nomenclature, interpretation, and general management principles. *Obstetrics & Gynecology, 114*(1), 192–202.

American College of Obstetricians and Gynecologists. (2010). Practice Bulletin No. 116: Management of intrapartum fetal heart rate tracings. *Obstetrics and Gynecology, 116*(5), 1232–1240. doi:10.1097/AOG.0b013e3182004fa9

American College of Obstetricians and Gynecologists. (2011). ACOG Committee Opinion No. 508. Disruptive behavior. *Obstetrics and Gynecology, 118*(4), 970–972. doi:10.1097/AOG.0b013e3182358acc

American College of Obstetricians and Gynecologists. (2012). Committee Opinion No. 517. Communication strategies for patient handoffs. *Obstetrics and Gynecology, 119* (2, Pt. 1), 408–411. doi:10.1097/AOG.0b013e318249ff4f

Association of Women's Health, Obstetric and Neonatal Nurses. (2005). *NICHD transitional teaching guide.* Washington, DC: Author.

Association of Women's Health, Obstetric and Neonatal Nurses. (2008). *Fetal heart monitoring* (Position Statement). Available at www.awhonn.org

Association of Women's Health, Obstetric and Neonatal Nurses. (2010). *AWHONN intermediate fetal heart monitoring course.* Washington, DC: Kendall Hunt.

Barker, J. (2009). Improving your safety culture: Learning a lesson from the aviation industry. *Mach One Leadership, 2*(2). Retrieved from http://m1leadership.com/wp-content/uploads/2010/01/m11-newsletter-may-2009.pdf

Benner, P., Sheets, V., Uris, P., Malloch, K., Schwed, K., & Jamison, D. (2002). Individual, practice, and system causes of errors in nursing: A taxonomy. *Journal of Nursing Administration, 32*(10), 509–523.

Block, M., Ehrenworth, J. F., Cuce, V. M., Ng'ang'a, N., Weinbach, J., Saber, S. B., . . . Schlesinger, M. D. (2010). The tangible handoff: A team approach for advancing structured communication in labor and delivery. *The Joint Commission Journal on Quality and Patient Safety, 36*(6), 282–287.

Boothman, R. C., & Blackwell, A. C. (2010). Integrating risk management activities into a patient safety program. *Clinical Obstetrics and Gynecology, 53*(3), 576–585. doi:10.1097/GRF.0b013e3181eeaf42

Bozeman, L. (2011). Nurse-led multidisciplinary obstetric patient summaries: Improving collaboration, collegiality and patient safety. *Nursing for Women's Health, 15*(5), 382–391. doi:10.1111/j.1751-486X.2011.01662.x

Brady, P. W., Muething, S., Kotagal, U., Ashby, M., Gallagher, R., Hall, D., . . . Wheeler, D. S. (2013). Improving situation awareness to reduce unrecognized clinical deterioration and serious safety events. *Pediatrics, 131*(1), e298–e308. doi:10.1542/peds.2012-1364

Brown, J. P. (2005). Key themes in healthcare safety dilemmas. In M. S. Patankar, J. P. Brown, & M. D. Treadwell (Eds.), *Safety ethics* (pp. 83–126). Burlington, VT: Ashgate.

Clark, S. L., Meyers, J. A., Frye, D. R., McManus, K., & Perlin, J. B. (2012). A systematic approach to the identification and classification of near-miss events on labor and delivery in a large, national health care system. *American Journal of Obstetrics and Gynecology, 207*(6), 441–445. doi:10.1016/j.ajog.2012.09.011

Clark, S. L., Simpson, K. R., Knox, G. E., & Garite, T. J. (2009). Oxytocin: New perspectives on an old drug. *American Journal of Obstetrics and Gynecology, 200*(1), 35.e1–35.e6. doi:10.1016/j.ajog.2008.06.010

CRICO Strategies. (2010). *2010 Annual benchmarking report: Malpractice risks in obstetrics.* Retrieved from https://www.rmf.harvard.edu/Strategies/Home/Products-and-Services/Comparative-Data/Annual-Benchmark-Reports#OB

Declercq, E. R., Sakala, C., Corry, M. P., & Applebaum, S. (2007). Listening to Mothers II: Report of the Second National U. S. Survey of Women's Childbearing Experiences *Journal of Perinatal Education, 16*(4), 9–14. doi:10.1624/105812407X244769

Declercq, E. R., Sakala, C., Corry, M. P., Applebaum, S., & Herrlich, A. (2013a). *Listening to Mothers III: New mothers speak out.* Retrieved from http://transform.childbirthconnection.org/wp-content/uploads/2013/06/LTM-III_NMSO.pdf

Declercq, E. R., Sakala, C., Corry, M. P., Applebaum, S., & Herrlich, A. (2013b). *Listening to Mothers III: Pregnancy and birth.* Retrieved from http://transform.childbirthconnection.org/wp-content/uploads/2013/06/LTM-III Pregnancy-and-Birth.pdf

Edmondson, A. C. (1999). Psychological safety and learning behavior in work teams. *Administrative Science Quarterly, 44*(2), 350–383.

Fox, M., Kilpatrick, S., King, T., & Parer, J. T. (2000). Fetal heart rate monitoring: Interpretation and collaborative management. *Journal of Midwifery and Women's Health, 45*(6), 498–507.

Freitag, M., & Carroll, V. S. (2011). Handoff communication: Using failure modes and effects analysis to improve the transition in care process. *Quality Management in Health Care, 20*(2), 103–109. doi:10.1097/QMH.0b013e3182136f58

Gordon, S., Mendenhall, P., & O'Connor, B. B. (2013). *Beyond the checklist: What else healthcare can learn from aviation teamwork and safety.* Ithaca, NY: Cornell University Press.

Graham, K. L., Marcantonio, E. R., Huang, G. C., Yang, J., Davis, R. B., & Smith, C. C. (2013). Effect of a systems intervention on the quality and safety of patient handoffs in an internal medicine residency program. *Journal of General Internal Medicine, 28*(8), 986–993. doi:10.1007/s11606-013-2391-7

Hansen, S. S., & Arafeh, J. (2012). Implementing and sustaining in situ drills to improve multidisciplinary health care training. *Journal of Obstetric, Gynecologic and Neonatal Nursing, 41*(4), 559–570. doi:10.1111/j.1552-6909.2012.01376.x

Jacobson, C. H., Zlatnik, M. G., Kennedy, H. P., & Lyndon, A. (2013). Nurses' perspectives on the intersection of safety and informed decision making in maternity care. *Journal of Obstetric, Gynecologic and Neonatal Nursing, 42*(5), 577–587. doi:10.1111/1552-6909.12232

Janakiraman, V., & Ecker, J. (2010). Quality in obstetric care: Measuring what matters. *Obstetrics and Gynecology, 116*(3), 728–732. doi:10.1097/AOG.0b013e3181ea4d4f

Kaplan, H. C., & Ballard, J. (2012). Changing practice to improve patient safety and quality of care in perinatal medicine. *American Journal of Perinatology, 29*(1), 35–42. doi:10.1055/s-0031-1285826

Knox, G. E., & Simpson, K. R. (2003). Teamwork: The fundamental building block of high-reliability organizations and patient safety. In B. J. Youngberg & M. J. Hatlie (Eds.), *The patient safety handbook* (pp. 379–415). Sudbury, MA: Jones & Bartlett.

Knox, G. E., Simpson, K. R., & Garite, T. J. (1999). High reliability perinatal units: An approach to the prevention of patient injury and medical malpractice claims. *Journal of Healthcare Risk Management, 19*(2), 24–32. doi:10.1002/jhrm.5600190205

Knox, G. E., Simpson, K. R., & Townsend, K. E. (2003). High reliability perinatal units: Further observations and a suggested plan for action. *Journal of Healthcare Risk Management, 23*(4), 17–21. doi:10.1002/jhrm.5600230405

Kohn, L. T., Corrigan, J. M., & Donaldson, M. S. (Eds.). (2000). *To err is human: Building a safer health system.* Washington, DC: National Academies Press.

Lawrence, H. C., III, Copel, J. A., O'Keeffe, D. F., Bradford, W. C., Scarrow, P. K., Kennedy, H. P., . . . Olden, C. R. (2012). Quality patient care in labor and delivery: A call to action. *American Journal of Obstetrics and Gynecology, 207*(3), 147–148. doi:10.1016/j.ajog.2012.07.018

Leape, L. L., Shore, M. F., Dienstag, J. L., Mayer, R. J., Edgman-Levitan, S., Meyer, G. S., & Healy, G. B. (2012a). Perspective: A culture of respect, part 1: The nature and causes of disrespectful behavior by physicians. *Academic Medicine, 87*(7), 845–852. doi:10.1097/ACM.0b013e318258338d

Leape, L. L., Shore, M. F., Dienstag, J. L., Mayer, R. J., Edgman-Levitan, S., Meyer, G. S., & Healy, G. B. (2012b). Perspective: A culture of respect, part 2: Creating a culture of respect. *Academic Medicine, 87*(7), 853–858. doi:10.1097/ACM.0b013e3182583536

Leonard, M. W. (2004). SBAR technique for communication: A situational briefing model. *Tools.* Institute for Healthcare Improvement. Retrieved from http://www.ihi.org/knowledge/Pages/Tools/SBARTechniqueforCommunicationASituationalBriefingModel.aspx

Leonard, M. W. (2013). *SBAR technique for communication: A situational briefing model.* Retrieved from http://www.ihi.org/knowledge/Pages/Tools/SBARTechniqueforCommunicationASituationalBriefingModel.aspx

Leonard, M. W., & Frankel, A. S. (2011). Role of effective teamwork and communication in delivering safe, high-quality care. *Mount Sinai Journal of Medicine, 78*(6), 820–826. doi:10.1002/msj.20295

Leonard, M. W., Graham, S., & Bonacum, D. (2004). The human factor: The critical importance of effective teamwork and communication in providing safe care. *Quality and Safety in Health Care, 13*(Suppl. 1), i85–i90. doi:10.1136/qshc.2004.010033

Lyndon, A. (2008). Social and environmental conditions creating fluctuating agency for safety in two urban academic birth centers. *Journal of Obstetric, Gynecologic and Neonatal Nursing, 37*(1), 13–23. doi:10.1111/j.1552-6909.2007.00204.x

Lyndon, A., & Kennedy, H. P. (2010). Perinatal safety: From concept to nursing practice. *Journal of Perinatal and Neonatal Nursing, 24*(1), 22–31. doi:10.1097/JPN.0b013e3181cb9351

Lyndon, A., Sexton, J. B., Simpson, K. R., Rosenstein, A., Lee, K. A., & Wachter, R. M. (2012). Predictors of likelihood of speaking up about safety concerns in labour and delivery. *BMJ Quality and Safety, 21*(9), 791–799. doi:10.1136/bmjqs-2010-050211

Lyndon, A., Walsh, L., & Edwards-Silva, R. (2013). Teamwork and communication. In M. L. Druzin, L. E. Shields, N. L. Peterson, & V. Cape (Eds.), Preeclampsia toolkit: Improving health care response to preeclampsia (California Maternal Quality Care Collaborative Toolkit to Transform Maternity Care). Developed under contract #11-10006 with the California Department of Public Health, Maternal, Child and Adolescent Health Division. Palo Alto: California Maternal Quality Care Collaborative.

Lyndon, A., Zlatnik, M. G., Maxfield, D. G., Lewis, A., McMillan, C., & Kennedy, H. P. (2014). Contributions of clinical disconnections and unresolved conflict to failures in intrapartum safety. *Journal of Obstetric, Gynecologic and Neonatal Nursing, 43*(1), 2–12. doi: 10.1111/1552-6909.12266

Lyndon, A., Zlatnik, M. G., & Wachter, R. M. (2011). Effective physician-nurse communication: A patient safety essential for labor and delivery. *American Journal of Obstetrics and Gynecology, 205*(2), 91–96. doi:10.1016/j.ajog.2011.04.021

Macones, G. A., Hankins, G. D., Spong, C. Y., Hauth, J., & Moore, T. (2008a). The 2008 National Institute of Child Health and Human Development workshop report on electronic fetal monitoring: Update on definitions, interpretation, and research guidelines. *Journal of Obstetric, Gynecologic and Neonatal Nursing, 37*(5), 510–515. doi:10.1111/j.1552-6909.2008.00284.x and *Obstetrics and Gynecology, 112*(3), 661–666. doi: 10.1097/AOG.0b013e3181841395

Maxfield, D. G., Lyndon, A., Kennedy, H. P., O'Keeffe, D. F., & Zlatnik, M. G. (2013). Confronting safety gaps across labor and delivery teams. *American Journal of Obstetrics & Gynecology, 209*(5), 402–408.e3. doi:10.1016/j.ajog.2013.07.013

Mazzocco, K., Petitti, D. B., Fong, K. T., Bonacum, D., Brookey, J., Graham, S., . . . Thomas, E. J. (2009). Surgical team behaviors and patient outcomes. *American Journal of Surgery,197*(5), 678–685. doi:10.1016/j.amjsurg.2008.03.002

Minkoff, H., Berkowitz, R., & Greater New York Hospital Association's Perinatal Safety Committee. (2009). Fetal monitoring bundle. *Obstetrics and Gynecology, 114*(6), 1332–1335. doi:10.1097/AOG.0b013e3181bfb2bd

Neily, J., Mills, P. D., Young-Xu, Y., Carney, B. T., West, P., Berger, D. H., . . . Bagian, J. P. (2010). Association between implementation of a medical team training program and surgical mortality. *Journal of the American Medical Association, 304*(15), 1693–1700. doi:10.1001/jama.2010.1506

Ong, M. S., & Coiera, E. (2011). A systematic review of failures in handoff communication during intrahospital transfers. *Joint Commission Journal on Quality and Patient Safety, 37*(6), 274–284.

Patterson, E. S., Roth, E. M., Woods, D. D., Chow, R., & Gomes, J. O. (2004). Handoff strategies in settings with high consequences for failure: Lessons for health care operations. *International Journal for Quality in Health Care, 16*(2), 125–132. doi: 10.1093/intqhc/mzh026

Pettker, C. M., Thung, S. F., Norwitz, E. R., Buhimschi, C. S., Raab, C. A., Copel, J. A., . . . Funai, E. F. (2009). Impact of a comprehensive patient safety strategy on obstetric adverse events. *American Journal of Obstetrics and Gynecology, 200*(5), 492.e1–492.e8. doi:10.1016/j.ajog.2009.01.022

Purdy, M., & Borisoff, D. (Eds.). (1997). *Listening in everyday life: A personal and professional approach* (2nd ed.). Lanham, MD: University Press of America.

Redshaw, M., & Heikkila, K. (2011). Ethnic differences in women's worries about labour and birth. *Ethnicity and Health, 16*(3), 213–223. doi:10.1080/13557858.2011.561302

Riesenberg, L. A., Leitzsch, J., & Cunningham, J. M. (2010). Nursing handoffs: A systematic review of the literature. *American Journal of Nursing, 110*(4), 24–34. doi:10.1097/01.naj.0000370154.79857.09

Riesenberg, L. A., Leitzsch, J., & Little, B. W. (2009). Systematic review of handoff mnemonics literature.

American Journal of Medical Quality, 24(3), 196–204. doi:10.1177/1062860609332512

Riesenberg, L. A., Leitzsch, J., Massucci, J. L., Jaeger, J., Rosenfeld, J. C., Patow, C., . . . Karpovich, K. P. (2009). Residents' and attending physicians' handoffs: A systematic review of the literature. *Academic Medicine, 84*(12), 1775–1787. doi:10.1097/ACM.0b013e3181bf51a6

Risser, D. T., Rice, M. M., Salisbury, M. L., Simon, R., Jay, G. D., & Berns, S. D. (1999). The potential for improved teamwork to reduce medical errors in the emergency department. The MedTeams Research Consortium. *Annals of Emergency Medicine, 34*(3), 373–383.

Sherwood, G., Thomas, E., Bennett, D. S., & Lewis, P. (2002). A teamwork model to promote patient safety in critical care. *Critical Care Nursing Clinics of North America, 14*(4), 333–340.

Simpson, K. R. (2005a). Failure to rescue: Implications for evaluating quality of care during labor and birth. *Journal of Perinatal and Neonatal Nursing, 19*(1), 24–34.

Simpson, K. R. (2005b). Handling handoffs safely. *MCN: The American Journal of Maternal/Child Nursing, 30*(2), 152.

Simpson, K. R. (2008). Electronic fetal monitoring competence validation. In C. A. Menihan & E. Kopel (Eds.), *Electronic fetal monitoring: Concepts and applications* (2nd ed., pp. 243–252). Phildelphia, PA: Lippincott Williams & Wilkins.

Simpson, K. R. (2014). Perinatal patient safety and professional liability issues. In K. R. Simpson & P. A. Creehan (Eds.), *Perinatal nursing* (4th ed., pp. 1–40). Phildelphia, PA: Lippincott Williams & Wilkins.

Simpson, K. R., James, D. C., & Knox, G. E. (2006). Nurse-physician communication during labor and birth: Implications for patient safety. *Journal of Obstetric, Gynecologic and Neonatal Nursing, 35*(4), 547–556.

Simpson, K. R., & Knox, G. E. (2001). Perinatal teamwork: Turning rhetoric into reality. In K. R. Simpson & P. A. Creehan (Eds.), *AWHONN's Perinatal nursing* (2nd ed., pp. 53–67). Philadelphia, PA: Lippincott Williams & Wilkins.

Simpson, K. R., & Knox, G. E. (2005). Essential criteria to promote safe care during labor and birth. *AWHONN Lifelines, 9*(6), 478–483.

Simpson, K. R., Knox, G. E., Martin, M., George, C., & Watson, S. R. (2011). Michigan Health & Hospital Association Keystone Obstetrics: A statewide collaborative for perinatal patient safety in Michigan. *Joint Commisson Journal on Quality and Patient Safety, 37*(12), 544–552.

Simpson, K. R., Kortz, C. C., & Knox, G. E. (2009). A comprehensive perinatal patient safety program to reduce preventable adverse outcomes and costs of liability claims. *Joint Commission Journal on Quality and Patient Safety, 35*(11), 565–574.

Simpson, K. R., & Lyndon, A. (2009). Clinical disagreements during labor and birth: How does real life compare to best practice? *MCN: The American Journal of Maternal/Child Nursing, 34*(1), 31–39. doi:10.1097/01.NMC.0000343863.72237.2b

Sleutel, M., Schultz, S., & Wyble, K. (2007). Nurses' views of factors that help and hinder their intrapartum care. *Journal of Obstetric, Gynecologic and Neonatal Nursing,* 36(3), 203–211. doi:10.1111/j.1552-6909.2007.00146.x

Staggers, N., Clark, L., Blaz, J. W., & Kapsandoy, S. (2011). Why patient summaries in electronic health records do not provide the cognitive support necessary for nurses' handoffs on medical and surgical units: Insights from interviews and observations. *Health Informatics Journal, 17*(3), 209–223. doi:10.1177/1460458211405809

Starmer, A. J., Spector, N. D., Srivastava, R., Allen, A. D., Landrigan, C. P., Sectish, T. C., & I-PASS Study Group. (2012). I-PASS, a mnemonic to standardize verbal handoffs. *Pediatrics, 129*(2), 201–204. doi:10.1542/peds.2011-2966

Stein, L. I. (1968). The doctor-nurse game. *American Journal of Nursing, 68*(1), 101–105.

Stone, D., Patton, B., & Heen, S. (2010). *Difficult conversations: How to discuss what matters most.* New York, NY: Penguin Books.

Tapia, N. M., Fallon, S. C., Brandt, M. L., Scott, B. G., & Suliburk, J. W. (2013). Assessment and standardization of resident handoff practices: PACT project. *Journal of Surgical Research, 184*(1), 71–77. doi:10.1016/j.jss.2013.04.063

Tervalon, M., & Murray-Garcia, J. (1998). Cultural humility versus cultural competence: A critical distinction in defining physician training outcomes in multicultural education. *Journal of Health Care for the Poor and Underserved, 9*(2), 117–125.

Thanh, N. X., Jacobs, P., Wanke, M. I., Hense, A., & Sauve, R. (2010). Outcomes of the introduction of the MOREOB continuing education program in Alberta. *Journal of Obstetrics and Gynaecology Canada, 32*(8), 749–755.

The Joint Commission. (2004). Preventing infant death and injury during delivery (Sentinel Event Alert No. 30). Retrieved from http://www.jointcommission.org/Sentinel_Event_Alert__Issue_30_Preventing_infant_death_and_injury_during_delivery_Additional_Resources/

The Joint Commission. (2008). Behaviors that undermine a culture of safety. *Sentinel Event Alert,* (40), 1–3. Retrieved from http://www.jointcommission.org/sentinel_event_alert_issue_40_behaviors_that_undermine_a_culture_of_safety/

The Joint Commission. (2012). *2013 Comprehensive accreditation manual for hospitals.* Oakbrook Terrace, IL: Author.

The Joint Commission. (2013a). Sentinel event. In *Comprehensive accreditation manual for hospitals update* (pp. SE1-SE18). Retrieved from http://www.jointcommission.org/assets/1/6/CAMH_2012_Update2_24_SE.pdf

The Joint Commission. (2013b). *Sentinel event data: Root causes by event type* (2004–2012). Retrieved from http://www.jointcommission.org/assets/1/18/Root_Causes_Event_Type_04_4Q2012.pdf

The Joint Commission. (n.d.). Sentinel event. *Joint Commission Topic Library.* Retrieved from http://www.jointcommission.org/sentinel_event.aspx

The Joint Commission Center for Transforming Healthcare. (2013). *Improving transitions in care: Hand-off communications.* Retrieved from http://www.centerfortransforminghealthcare.org/assets/4/6/HOC_TST_Implementation_Guide.pdf

Wilson-Stronks, A., Lee, K. K., Cordero, C. L., Kopp, A. L., & Galvez, E. (2008). *One size does not fit all: Meeting the health care needs of diverse populations.* Retrieved from http://www.jointcommission.org/assets/1/6/HLCOneSizeFinal.pdf

Wood, S. H. (2003). Should women be given a choice about fetal assessment in labor? *MCN: The American Journal of Maternal/Child Nursing, 28*(5), 292–298.

Wu, A. W., Lipshutz, A. K., & Pronovost, P. J. (2008). Effectiveness and efficiency of root cause analysis in medicine. *Journal of the American Medical Association, 299*(6), 685–687. doi:10.1001/jama.299.6.685

Zigmont, J. J., Kappus, L. J., & Sudikoff, S. N. (2011). The 3D model of debriefing: Defusing, discovering, and deepening. *Seminars in Perinatology, 35*(2), 52–58. doi:10.1053/j.semperi.2011.01.003

CHAPTER 9

Documentation of Fetal Heart Monitoring Information

Kirsten Wisner

Linda Ali

INTRODUCTION

The main purpose of documentation is communication. Medical record documentation serves to convey information about the patient's condition and care provided to other clinicians and caregivers within the healthcare team or system. The medical record also documents services provided by clinicians for other professionals or groups such as payors, accrediting bodies, government agencies, researchers, and, in certain cases, the legal system (American Nurses Association [ANA], 2010). As such, the completeness and quality of clinical documentation not only impacts patient-care quality and the organization's ability to evaluate performance outcomes, but can have ramifications related to reimbursement, liability, risk management, and accreditation.

Achieving quality documentation of fetal heart monitoring (FHM) information depends on many factors. These include the usability, efficiency, and interoperability of the institution's information technology, fetal monitoring, and documentation systems; evidence- and standards-based documentation policies that promote the efficient capture and flow of information while allowing nurses and other clinicians to prioritize direct care; nurse staffing ratios that reasonably account for the complexity of perinatal nursing and maternal–fetal acuity; and finally, clinicians who maintain currency and fluency in the standards and guidelines governing perinatal care and maternal–fetal assessment.

This chapter aims to serve as a resource for clinicians seeking information about standards-based assessment and documentation of FHM information, as well as to assist leaders, clinical nurse specialists, educators, and others in institutional policy development. A review and summary of professional guidelines governing documentation of FHM according to monitoring method, stage of labor, and clinical scenario are presented. Current trends surrounding the transition to an electronic health record, factors contributing to the complexity of documentation in perinatal care, and documentation as it relates to liability and risk management are discussed.

OVERVIEW OF MEDICAL RECORD DOCUMENTATION

A woman's medical record may consist of several different types of documentation compiled from one or more systems whether in paper or electronic format. The medical record may be a combination of paper documentation forms, electronic or computerized entries, results from laboratories, radiological images and reports, and other recordings. The terms *medical record*, *health record*, and *medical chart* are often used interchangeably when describing one's medical history and care rendered. Documentation guidelines are governed by regulatory agencies, institutional policy, regulations such as the Health Insurance and Portability Accountability Act (HIPAA), conditions for participation for Medicare and Medicaid, eligibility for payment from third-party payers, and by guidelines and standards from specialty and professional organizations (Campos, 2009).

Data archiving is an essential component of both paper and electronic medical records systems. Each institution should have policies and procedures regarding data maintenance, storage, archiving, and retrieval of all components of the woman's medical record including fetal monitor tracing data. These policies should include system backup procedures and emergency disaster planning (Association of Women's Health, Obstetric and Neonatal Nurses [AWHONN], 2011a). Contingency plans should be developed for unexpected system failures, routine "downtime" maintenance, and software or hardware upgrades.

TYPES OF DOCUMENTATION

Electronic Documentation

The terms *electronic medical record (EMR)* or *electronic health record (EHR)* are often used interchangeably when referring to computerized medical records, electronic medical records, or other clinical information systems. They are also sometimes used imprecisely in the literature, although there is a distinction between the two terms. The EMR includes the electronic clinical records, clinical decision support systems, and computerized (physician or provider) order entry (CPOE) with order sets that link pharmacy, radiology, laboratory, and other clinical departments. The EMR provides the documentation of care provided in a specific healthcare organization. The EMR is part of the EHR which connects care delivery systems and providers (Pomerleau, 2008; Thompson, Johnston, & Spurr, 2009). The term *EMR* will be used for simplicity throughout this discussion to refer to electronic medical records and documentation systems.

In 2009, the U. S. Congress passed the Health Information Technology for Economic and Clinical Health Act (HITECH) in conjunction with the American Recovery and Investment Act (Gee & Newman, 2013). The goal of the HITECH Act is to improve health and patient care via investment in health information technology. The Act provides $27 billion in incentives through the Medicare and Medicaid reimbursement systems to assist providers and organizations in the adoption of electronic health records (HealthIT.gov, 2013). One of the objectives of the HITECH Act is to demonstrate "meaningful use" of electronic health records to show significant improvements in patient care. Meaningful use is a set of standards defined by the Centers for Medicare and Medicaid Services (CMS) that allows hospitals and healthcare providers to earn financial incentives by meeting specific criteria (Blumenthal & Tavenner, 2010; Centers for Medicare and Medicaid Services, 2012). To receive financial incentives, hospitals and healthcare providers must report clinical quality measures and other required data collected from the EMR (Gee & Newman, 2013). Hospitals and physician practices that do not achieve meaningful use by 2015 face financial penalties (Kern et al., 2013). Health care organizations in the United States are at varying stages in the process of selecting or implementing clinical information systems (Thompson et al., 2009) in response to this legislation; however, by the end of 2011, only 35% of hospitals had implemented an EMR (Tillett, 2012).

Advantages of the Electronic Medical Record

Computerization has made medical records more accessible and legible. Benefits of EMRs may include instant access, improved accuracy, improved quality, better decision making, improved documentation of meaningful use criteria, and support for coding and billing processes (Bernat, 2013). Other potential benefits include improvement in clinical efficiencies, patient outcomes, documentation of care, and decreases in medical error, duplication of testing, and need for paper chart record filing and retention (Cohen & O'Keeffe, 2008; Laramee, Bosek, Shaner-McRae, & Powers-Phaneuf, 2012).

Computerized EMRs can improve uniformity, accuracy, and retrievability of data for audits, billing, or research, and they can enhance communication and patient safety.

Certain advantages are offered by EMRs that are not possible with the paper medical record. Remote access is immediately available from the provider's office or home. Access to tools and resources can be made available to users, such as those contained in clinical decision support systems. Decision support software embedded in electronic medical record systems may contain algorithms that provide warnings about drug interactions, monitor data trending, suggest supportive care reminders, and may contain specific order sets (McGreevey, 2013). Decision support systems may also provide assistance with diagnostic interpretation, treatment planning, and medical therapy recommendations. Alerts can be programmed, and serve to remind nurses and providers to take actions to prevent complications associated with specific disorders and/or treatments (Cohen & O'Keeffe, 2008; Zusman & Vinokur, 2012). Many EMRs have templates that are designed to capture, organize, and present clinical data specific to the user's or institution's workflow design. Templates can often be customized by the system vendor to meet the specific needs of the hospital or physician's office practice. Utilization of templates is similar to documentation on specific hospital forms or checklists/flowsheets, and reduces the need for narrative notes.

In perinatal settings, such systems may interpret patient data and trigger alerts when findings deviate from preset parameters (e.g., FHR patterns or blood pressure parameters); allow access to clinical resources such as National Institute of Child Health and Human Development (NICHD) terminology definitions; assist with calculations such as estimating gestational age or a woman's Bishop Score; guide the user toward standards-based documentation; and bring references to the point-of-care (e.g., FHM policies). Decision support reduces reliance on memory and opportunities for error, and is seen as a tool to improve efficiency and patient-care safety and quality (McCartney & Barnes, 2012).

Challenges Related to EMR Implementation and Functionality

Implementation of an EMR is a considerable investment for any hospital, averaging many millions of U. S. dollars (Poissant, Pereira, Tamblyn, & Kawasumi, 2005). Projects may be delayed by competing projects, funding, or by software and hardware malfunctions and anomalies (Tillet, 2012). Other factors affecting implementation of new systems include routine system maintenance, hardware and software upgrades, interfacing with other systems within an organization as well as with external sources such as physician practices, and costs incurred for education and training. Costs associated with staff training and ongoing education may be twice that of software and hardware expenses (Cohen & O'Keeffe, 2008).

Most studies that have evaluated the impacts of EMR use have focused on physicians or primary care providers, and have been conducted in outpatient settings. Studies conducted in outpatient or perinatal network settings with physician groups suggest that EMR use can improve compliance with standards-based prenatal screening and documentation completeness. Two studies found that reminders or prompts within EMRs improved compliance with recommended first- and second-trimester laboratory and other screening tests, and the documentation of such results in prenatal records (Metz, Son, Winter, & Chae, 2011; Riley, Galang, & Green, 2011). Another study found that EMR use within a prenatal network improved communication of, and access to, prenatal screening results (Bernstein, Farinelli, & Merkatz, 2005). Systems that utilize decision support prompts may improve documentation compliance (Hasley, 2011; Riley et al., 2011).

The expectation that EMR implementation would reduce time spent on documentation by clinicians has not been realized (McCartney, 2013). While a perfectly conceived and implemented EMR and all of its associated technologies may result in time savings and improved workflow for clinicians (Thompson et al., 2009), unintended consequences may occur. The individual and cumulative effects of task complexity; system usability and hardware issues; increased volume of data entry and duplicate data entry; and the clinician's computer literacy have been examined in other high-acuity settings such as emergency and intensive care departments and found to be problematic (Callen et al., 2013; Claret et al., 2012; Kossman, 2006). A literature search by Stevenson, Nilsson, Petersson, and Johansson (2010) included five research studies between the years 2000 and 2009 that suggested nurses working in acute or inpatient settings perceived the actual systems used as slow, unreliable, complicated, and cumbersome, making it difficult to navigate within the system or obtain a comprehensive picture of how the patient was doing.

In perinatal settings, challenges exist related to electronic documentation. Some perinatal documentation systems function as stand-alone systems that do not interface with other clinical units or ancillary hospital departments. The systems used for monitoring and archiving electronic fetal monitoring data may not communicate with the EMR, requiring users to toggle between two systems when completing assessments and documentation of maternal–fetal status. This fragmentation can lead to miscommunication, omissions, and errors in care as well as potential duplication of orders or procedures resulting in increased costs. Frequently, when new technology or new systems are implemented, duplicate charting is required by nurses because of compatibility issues between new and existing systems (Ivory, 2008).

There is limited research specific to perinatal settings and how the complexity and physical arrangement of electronic systems may affect nursing workflow. In one study looking at nurses' perceptions of factors affecting staffing needs in perinatal settings, nurses reported an increase in documentation requirements overall, and more time spent documenting when using an EMR, leaving less time for direct care (Simpson, Lyndon, Wilson, & Ruhl, 2012). Poor physical layout, interruptions caused by system or hardware issues, interface problems with documentation and monitoring systems, and time spent by nurses assisting other providers with data entry or technology-related tasks are a few examples of the challenges nurses manage while also triaging and prioritizing critical decisions regarding maternal–fetal care. The collective effect of multiple system or workflow inefficiencies combined with the demanding and high-acuity nature of intrapartum settings should be considered when designing, implementing, maintaining, and evaluating technology and documentation systems. They should also be the focus of ongoing research and performance improvement initiatives in an effort to learn more about these factors as they relate to perinatal care.

The Health Insurance and Portability Accountability Act (HIPAA) requires that electronic medical records contain safeguards to protect the security of patient data. State laws also may regulate health records, data security, access, and remedies for breach. Each EMR contains an audit trail function that tracks the date and time of individual user access, data entry, any additions/deletions, or edits of information. Data cannot be entered or altered without detection (McCartney, 2009). In perinatal settings, nurses often provide uninterrupted care, completing the required documentation after care was provided. Since all documentation entries are tracked by the audit trail functionality, nurses should complete their documentation as close as possible to the time it occurred. Nurses should follow hospital policy regarding adding a late entry or an addendum in the EMR (McCartney, 2009). Documentation in paper records may be necessary during times when the electronic systems are unavailable, such as during power outages, software updates, or emergencies that interrupt access to the EMR. In these cases, hospital policy should clarify documentation details such as which forms are to be used, acceptable ink color, and how downtime information will be added to the EMR.

Flowsheets and Narrative Notes

The use of flowsheets, whether electronic or paper, can facilitate documentation of assessments and interventions. They are often designed to prompt the user to enter notations consistent with unit-specific guidelines in the perinatal setting (Simpson & Knox, 2009). Flowsheets within the EMR can be designed or customized to mimic documentation found in paper flowsheets. See Figures 9-1 to 9-5 for examples of

Figure 9-1 Sample EFM Documentation: Normal Tracing

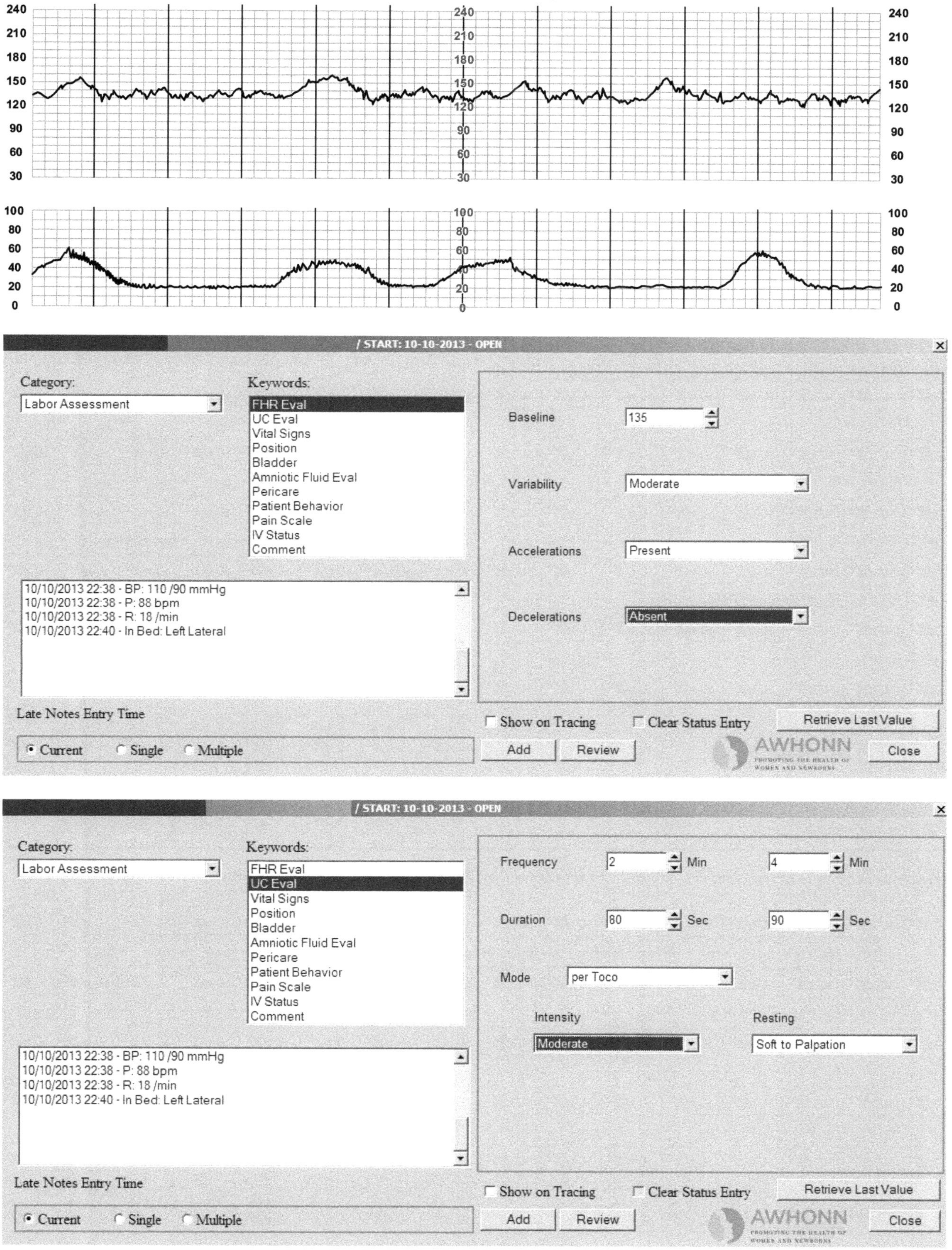

Screen shots created by and used with permission from OBIX® Perinatal Data Systems.

Figure 9-2 Sample EFM Documentation: Early Decelerations

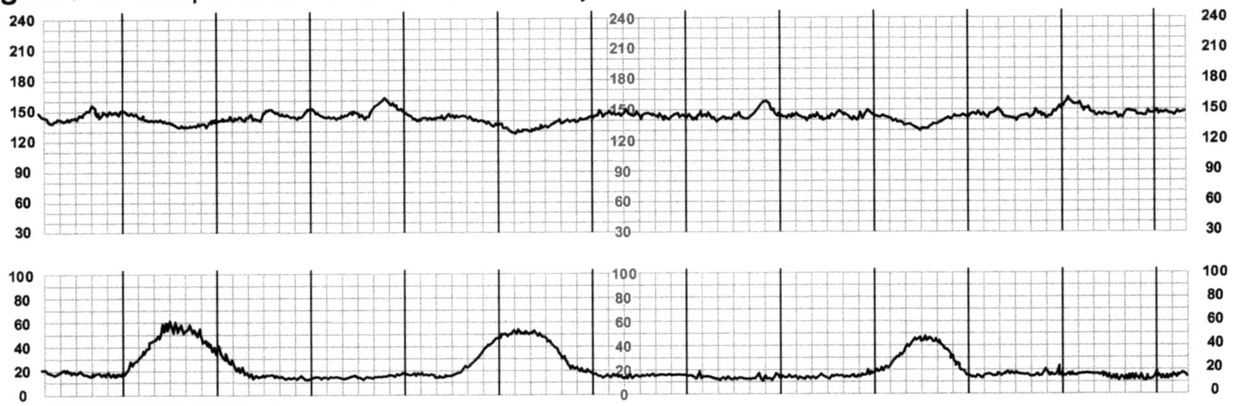

EFM Documentation Card with Dropdowns

EFM Type	continuous
Contraction Frequency	3 per 10 min
Contraction Regularity	regular
Contraction Intensity (Palpation)	strong
Contraction Duration on EFM	70 secs
Resting Phase Duration	120 secs
IUPC/Ext Toco	external
FSE/Ext FHR	external
Baseline FHR	145 bpm

☐ Baseline FHR currently indeterminate. Baseline FHR value based on previous 10 minute window.

Baseline FHR Variability	moderate (6-25 bpm)	
Sinusoidal Pattern		○ yes
FHR Accelerations	○ no	● yes
Prolonged Acceleration	○ no	○ yes

FHR Decelerations	○ no	● yes
FHR Evaluation	category I (normal)	
FHR Intervention Note		

Definitions

FHR Acceleration: Onset to peak is equal to or less than 30 seconds and duration is equal to or more than 15 seconds and less than 2 minutes from onset to return to baseline. Pregnancy less than 32 weeks - FHR acceleration is defined as an increase of 10 beats per minute or more above baseline which lasts 10 seconds or more.

Prolonged Acceleration: Acceleration is classified as prolonged if the duration is 2 minutes or more but less than 10 minutes. Accelerations that are 10 minutes or more are considered a baseline change.

Progress Notes – displayed from entry in documentation card

14:30 On electronic fetal/contractions monitoring during continuous monitoring: generally category I (normal), external tocography: regular contractions (3 per 10 min, 70 seconds each), resting phase duration: 120 seconds, contraction intensity (palpation): strong, external FHR monitor: FHR = 145 bpm, baseline FHR variability: moderate (6-25 bpm), accelerations (duration: 15 sec, peak: 163 bpm, duration: 15 sec, peak: 161 bpm), decelerations, early decelerations (duration: 45 sec, nadir: 130 bpm, recurrent). Nurse, Nurse, RN

Flowsheet View

LDR Flowsheet

Time: **MINUTE** / Select	11/26/2013 14:00	11/26/2013 14:30
Fetal Assessment		
FSE/Ext FHR	external	external
Baseline FHR	145	145
Baseline FHR Variability	moderate (6-25 bpm)	moderate (6-25 bpm)
Accelerations	yes	yes
Decelerations	yes	yes
Variable Decelerations		
Early Decelerations	yes	yes
Late Decelerations		
Prolonged Decelerations (2-10 minutes)		
Tracing Reviewed		
Fetal Movements		
Contractions		
IUPC/Ext Toco	external	external
Frequency per 10 min	3	3
Duration (sec)	70	70
Resting Phase Duration (sec)	120	120
Max Contraction Intensity (mmHg)		
Contraction Intensity (Montevideo)		

EFM Spreadsheet

EFM - Fetus 1 | Pelvic Exam Spreadsheet | ROM | Vital Signs

Time: **MINUTE**	Ctx. Freq.	Ctx. Dur.	FHR Evaluation	FHR	Variability	Reactivity	Accel's	Decel's	Tracing Reviewed	Drug
11/26/13 14:00	3	70	category I (normal)	145	moderate (6-25 bpm)		yes	yes		
11/26/13 14:30	3	70	category I (normal)	145	moderate (6-25 bpm)		yes	yes		
+										

Screen shot created by and used with permission from Perigen® PeriCALM®.

Figure 9-3 Sample EFM Documentation: Variable Decelerations

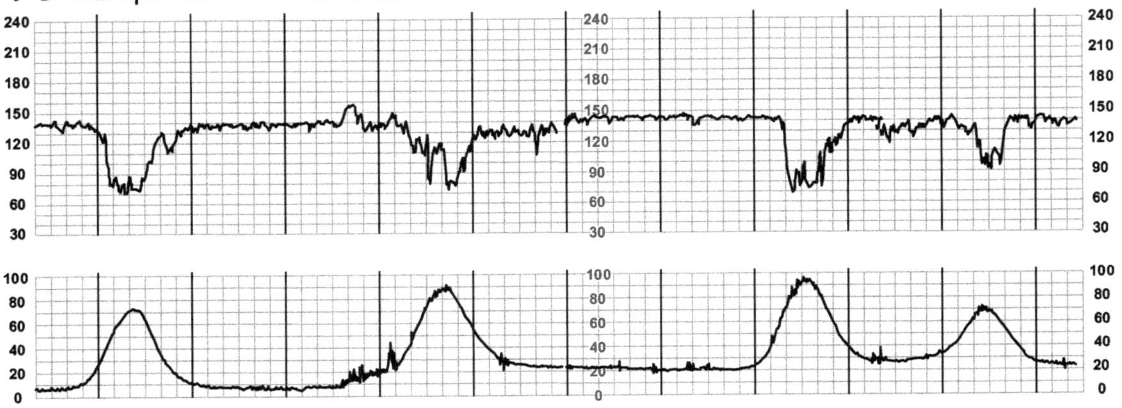

Intrapartum															
Assessment															
Date/Time		**Vital Signs**				**Fetal Heart Rate Evaluation**					**Uterine Contractions Evaluation**				
Date	**Time**	**B/P**	**T**	**P**	**R**	**Mode**	**Baseline**	**Variability**	**Accels**	**Decels**	**Mode**	**Frequency**	**Duration**	**Intensity**	**Tonus**
11/19/2013	05:30 - 05:31	120/70 mmHg	98.6 F	75 bpm	16/m	FHR Mode: FECG Placed	140 bpm	Moderate	Present	Variable	mmHg per IUPC	2-4 Min	60 - 90 Sec	70-95	
											mmHg per IUPC				8-28
											IUPC Adjusted				

EMR documentation also may be displayed as a complete notes log. Note that a log includes the time of the event and the time the event was documented.

Complete Notes Log

Note Date/Time	Entered Date/Time	Entered By	Deleted Date/Time	Deleted By	Note
11/19/2013 05:30	11/19/2013 11:00	NURSE			Cervical Exam: Dilatation: 9.0 cm /Effacement: 100 % /Station: 2 #
11/19/2013 05:30	11/19/2013 11:01	NURSE			FHR Eval: Baseline 140 bpm /Variability Moderate /Accelerations Present /Decelerations Variable
11/19/2013 05:30	11/19/2013 11:01	NURSE			FHR Mode: FECG / Placed
11/19/2013 05:30	11/19/2013 11:03	NURSE			UC Eval: Frequency: 2-4 Min
11/19/2013 05:30	11/19/2013 11:03	NURSE			UC Eval: Duration: 60-90 Sec
11/19/2013 05:30	11/19/2013 11:04	NURSE			IUPC Assess: Resting: 8-28 mmHg
11/19/2013 05:30	11/19/2013 11:04	NURSE			UC Eval: Intensity: 70-95 mmHg
11/19/2013 05:30	11/19/2013 11:04	NURSE			UC Mode: IUPC / Adjusted
11/19/2013 05:30	11/19/2013 11:04	NURSE			Pain Scale: 1
11/19/2013 05:30	11/19/2013 11:06	NURSE			Pain Management Patient Response: Coping
11/19/2013 05:30	11/19/2013 11:06	NURSE			Pain Management Patient Response: Working Well with Contractions
11/19/2013 05:30	11/19/2013 11:06	NURSE			Pain Management Intervention: Support Person Present
11/19/2013 05:30	11/19/2013 11:06	NURSE			In Bed: Right Lateral
11/19/2013 05:30	11/19/2013 11:08	NURSE			Comment: Position change for variable decelerations. Dr. Jones notified of FHR findings as above, and rapid labor progress. On his way to hospital.

****End of Notes Log****
14 Notes Printed
Transaction Notes not included in printout

Screen shot created by and used with permission from OBIX® Perinatal Data Systems.

Figure 9-4 EFM Documentation: Twin FHR Tracing

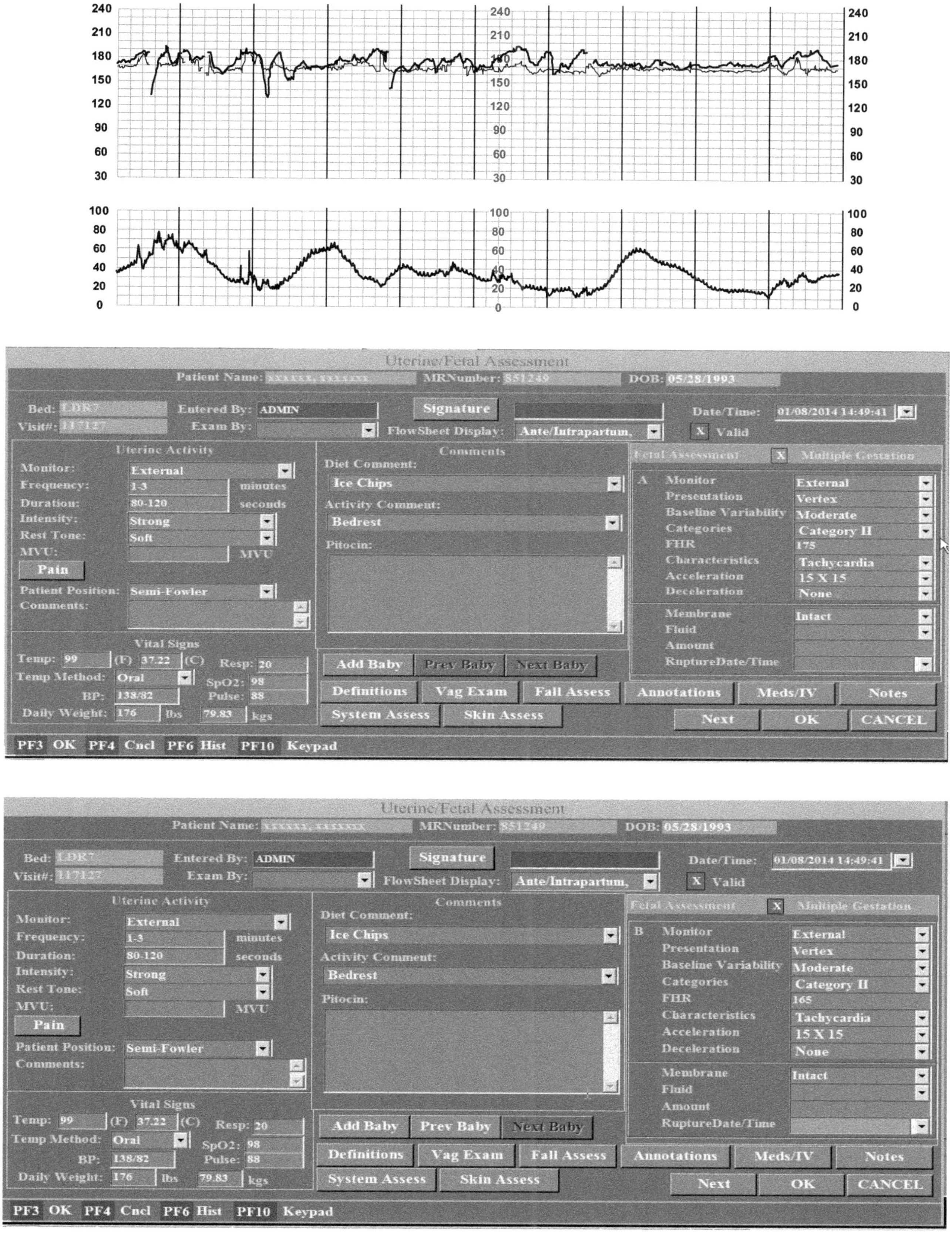

Screen shots created by and used with permission from Hill-Rom®, NaviCare® Watchchild®.

Figure 9-5 Sample Documentation for Intermittent Ausculation

...16:00 Vital Signs: Temperature: 98.7 F°. Pulse 74. Respiratory rate: 18. O2 saturation: 99%. BP 112/74 mmHg (measurement position – on left side). Mean arterial pressure : 86 mmHg. FHR Doppler/Ausculatation) : 130. Palpated:Moderate contractions q 3-4 min, duration 60-70 seconds, resting tone relaxed. Tolerating contractions well. Pain scale 3.

Nurse, Nurse, RN

✓16:30 Perform Auscultation of FHR done
...16:30 Vital signs: Temperature: 98.0 °F. Pulse:75. Respiratory rate: 18.02 saturation: 99%. BP:120/74 mmHg (measurement position - on left side). Mean arterial pressure: 89 mmHg, Pain Scale: 0, FHR (Doppler/Auscultation): 130 bpm. Palpated: Moderate contractions q3-4 min, 60-70 seconds, resting tone relaxed. Tolerating contractions well.

Nurse, Nurse, RN

Vital Signs 16:00

Temperature	98.7	°F 37.1 °C
Pulse Rate	74	bpm
Respiratory Rate	18	per min
O2 Saturation (Oximeter)	99	%
Systolic Blood Pressure	112	mmHg
Diastolic Blood Pressure	74	mmHg
Mean Arterial Pressure	86	mmHg
BP Measurement Position	on left side	
Pain Scale	0	
Orthostatic Hypotension	no	
FHR (Doppler/Auscultation)	130	bpm
Spreadsheets		
Graphs		

EFM/Contractions 16:30 | **Vital Signs 16:30** | Vitals+EFM/CTX History

Temperature	98.0	°F 36.7 °C
Pulse Rate	75	bpm
Respiratory Rate	18	per min
O2 Saturation (Oximeter)	99	%
Systolic Blood Pressure	120	mmHg
Diastolic Blood Pressure	74	mmHg
Mean Arterial Pressure	89	mmHg
BP Measurement Position	on left side	
Pain Scale	3	
Orthostatic Hypotension		
FHR (Doppler/Auscultation)	130	bpm
Spreadsheets		
Graphs		

Screen shots created by and used with permission from Perigen® PeriCALM®.

documentation using EMR. Abbreviations are commonly used to facilitate ease in documentation. Flowsheets containing abbreviations and specific guidelines for documentation should contain a "key" detailing these elements.

Narrative notes have been a traditional part of a medical record. Most documentation systems allow the use of limited narrative entries. Narrative notes can be used to document care not captured in standardized flowsheets and to summarize trends that occur over time, emergency situations, untoward events/outcomes, and communication that occurs among caregivers. Entries in narrative notes should occur in chronological order. Nursing care should be documented as close to the time it was provided whenever possible. The use of flowsheets or forms with preprinted times and limited space for notations is not recommended (Simpson & Knox, 2009).

GUIDELINES FOR DOCUMENTATION

Interpretation and Synthesis of Professional Guidelines

The following section presents a review of the major professional organization guidelines for documenting FHM information in a variety of clinical scenarios. In the United States, most women (85.4–89%) are monitored via EFM during labor (Declercq, Sakala, Corry, Applebaum, & Herrlich, 2013; Martin et al., 2005), and 60% report being monitored continuously (Declercq et al., 2013). In Canada, the use of continuous EFM is estimated to be much lower, at 37.9% (Chalmers, Kaczorowski, O'Brien, & Royle, 2012). As discussed in Chapter 8, EFM use in the United States is disproportionate to the prevalence of high-risk pregnancies or labor induction rates. All guidelines reviewed in this chapter support the use of intermittent auscultation (IA) in low-risk pregnancy, and some support the use of IA in high-risk pregnancy provided specific assessment protocols are followed. Throughout this section, terms and abbreviations such as *fetal heart monitoring (FHM)*, *electronic fetal heart monitoring (EFM)*, *fetal heart rate (FHR)*, and *fetal heart tone(s) (FHT)* and descriptors such as *continuous*, *close*, and *careful* are deliberately chosen. Distinguishing the difference between terms can be important when developing institutional policies for FHM, since such policies can have significant implications for clinical outcomes for laboring women, and workflow and perinatal quality outcomes for nursing.

For example, studies have demonstrated that mobility and upright positioning in labor facilitate labor progress and are associated with a reduction in assisted delivery, episiotomy, and abnormal FHR patterns (Gupta, Hofmeyr, & Shehmar, 2012; Lawrence, Lewis, Hofmeyr, Dowswell, & Styles, 2009). Unless continuous EFM is specifically called for, guideline language should be interpreted to support fetal surveillance using IA in order to promote maternal mobility in labor and encourage 1:1 continuous nursing support. AWHONN has undertaken a multi-year process of developing, refining, and testing a set of women's health and perinatal nursing care quality measures. The refined and tested quality measures will be submitted to the National Quality Forum (NQF) for possible endorsement. Of the 11 refined measures, two relate specifically to labor support: Measure 10a: Continuous Labor Support; 10b Some Labor Support; and Measure 11: Freedom of Movement during Labor (AWHONN, 2014). Success in achieving these perinatal nursing measures will depend on institutional policies for FHM during labor, cervical ripening and induction or augmentation of labor that promote freedom of movement for laboring women, and nursing documentation policies that reduce redundancies and allow charting at intervals that support nurses in providing continuous, uninterrupted labor support.

Recommendations for Implementation of Fetal Heart Monitoring

Guidance for fetal heart monitoring assessment and documentation may be sought from professional organizations such as the American

Academy of Pediatrics (AAP & ACOG, 2012), the American College of Obstetricians and Gynecologists (ACOG, 2009b, 2010; AAP & ACOG, 2012), the Association of Women's Health, Obstetric and Neonatal Nurses (AWHONN, 2008a); the American College of Nurse Midwives (ACNM, 2010a); the Society of Obstetricians and Gynaecologists of Canada (SOGC, 2007); and the Royal College of Obstetricians and Gynaecologists (RCOG) (National Institute for Health and Care Excellence [NICE], 2014). These recommendations are summarized according to phase or stage of labor, risk factors, clinical scenario and special circumstances throughout this section and in Tables 9-1 to 9-7. Tables 9-1 and 9-2 provide a quick summary of recommendations for assessment intervals using EFM and IA according to maternal–fetal risk status; Table 9-3, by stage of labor.

Overview

Both IA and EFM are acceptable methods for assessment of fetal status and uterine activity during labor (AAP & ACOG, 2012). Unit policies should clearly define the procedures and documentation principles associated with each method, and delineate when and how each may be used according to gestational age, diagnosis, stage of labor, and maternal or fetal risk factors

TABLE 9-1 Frequency of Fetal Heart Monitoring Assessment Using Intermittent Auscultation

ORGANIZATION	LATENT PHASE OF FIRST STAGE	ACTIVE PHASE OF FIRST STAGE		PASSIVE SECOND STAGE	ACTIVE SECOND STAGE	
		LOW RISK[a]	HIGH RISK[a]		LOW RISK	HIGH RISK
AAP & ACOG (2012)		Every 30 min	Every 15 min[b]		Every 15 min	Every 5 min[b]
ACOG (2009b)		Every 15 min[c]	EFM recommended		Every 5 min[c]	EFM recommended
ACNM (2010a)		Every 15–30 min	EFM recommended[d]	Every 15 min	Every 5 min	EFM recommended[d]
AWHONN (2008a, 2008b)	Use clinical judgment	Within the range of every 15-30 min[e]		Every 15–30 min[f]	Within the range of every 5–15 min[e]	
RCOG (NICE, 2014)		Every 15 min[g, h]	EFM recommended		Every 5 min[g, i]	EFM recommended
SOGC (2007)	On admit, then hourly	Every 15–30 min	EFM recommended[j]	Every 15 min	Every 5 min	EFM recommended

Note: AAP, American Academy of Pediatrics; ACNM, American College of Nurse-Midwives; ACOG, American College of Obstetricians and Gynecologists; AWHONN, Association of Women's Health, Obstetric and Neonatal Nurses; EFM, electronic fetal monitoring; FHM, fetal heart monitoring; IA, intermittent auscultation; NICE, National Institute for Health and Care Excellence; RCOG, Royal College of Obstetricians and Gynaecologists; SOGC, Society of Obstetricians and Gynaecologists of Canada

[a]Specific definitions of low and high risk are lacking in some guidelines. See Table 9-4 for further information.

[b]AAP and ACOG state that in the presence of risk factors, there is no difference in perinatal outcome between IA and continuous EFM if this protocol is used. The evaluation of FHR should occur before, during, and after a contraction.

[c]This frequency is suggested as a method for evaluating FHR using IA given that there are no comparative data indicating the optimal frequency for IA in the absence of risk factors.

[d]Continuous EFM is recommended for women with maternal or fetal risk factors for adverse outcomes or acidemia.

[e]Due to variation in original research protocols, factors influencing frequency of assessment should include maternal–fetal condition and risk factors and maternal response to labor.

[f]AWHONN (2008b) recommends continuing assessments at the same intervals as first stage since the intrauterine environment during passive descent is physiologically similar to first stage.

[g]The RCOG recommends uterine contraction assessments every 30 minutes throughout labor.

[h]If fetal heart rate is not within normal limits, palpate the maternal pulse to differentiate between the two heart rates.

[i]Every 15 minutes palpate the mother's pulse to differentiate between the two heart rates.

[j]During the first stage of labor, if EFM is used, even in the presence of risk factors or oxytocin administration, it is reasonable to interrupt monitoring for up to 30 minutes to allow for bathing, ambulating, or position change provided maternal–fetal assessments are stable, and if receiving oxytocin, the dose is unchanged (SOGC, 2007).

(AAP & ACOG, 2012). Women should be given information on the benefits, limitations, indications, and risks associated with IA and EFM, and participate in the decision-making process regarding the monitoring method used throughout labor (ACNM, 2010a; SOGC, 2007). For more information on the indications, benefits, and limitations of each monitoring method, see Chapter 4.

DOCUMENTATION PRINCIPLES

Documentation of Assessments and Interventions

Documentation of FHM components reflects the systematic assessment of the fetal heart rate and uterine activity. For the perinatal nurse, considerations regarding documentation of FHM assessments include accurate and timely documentation of specific components of FHM assessments, describing interventions and communications aimed at promoting or maintaining maternal–fetal stability during labor, and appropriate use of standardized language and terminology to communicate and describe findings. Nomenclature proposed by the NICHD workshop report (Macones, Hankins, Spong, Hauth, & Moore, 2008) has been adopted by professional organizations in the United States and is recommended for use when communicating FHM information (AAP & ACOG, 2012; ACNM, 2010b; ACOG, 2009b; AWHONN, 2010).

Documentation should contain succinct, factual, and objective information. In addition to a systematic admission assessment, documentation of maternal and fetal clinical information should be ongoing throughout labor and reflect continuing assessments of the woman and fetus. Since FHM assessments reveal aspects of the maternal–fetal response to labor, documentation of FHM findings should also include related interventions, communications, and maternal–fetal response. These include interventions provided with subsequent evaluation of responses; communication with providers and other team members; communication with women and their family or support persons; and communication within the chain of resolution/authority when it occurs (AWHONN, 2008a). Documentation of interventions should include efforts to support maternal coping and labor progress; maximize uterine blood flow, umbilical circulation, and oxygenation; and normalize uterine activity (AWHONN, 2010). Documentation should also capture ongoing evaluation of the maternal–fetal response to interventions and identify when/if stability has been achieved. Documentation occurs throughout all steps of clinical care and reflects how clinicians are synthesizing and responding to information obtained during the care process. See Figure 9-6.

DOCUMENTATION

Interval and Summary Documentation

Documentation intervals can, and in certain cases should, differ from assessment intervals. Institutional policies should support the ability of nurses to provide uninterrupted, continuous labor support while adhering to such policies. Periodic summary documentation may occur at less frequent intervals than recommended assessment intervals, especially when using continuous EFM (AWHONN, 2008a) since a permanent archived record of the FHR tracing is expected to be retrievable. In the case of assessments at 5-minute intervals during the active, second stage of labor when using EFM, summary documentation can occur every 30 minutes provided the nurse is continuously evaluating the EFM tracing, remains at the bedside, and there is some notation in the record that this bedside evaluation is ongoing (AWHONN, 2008a).

There is limited guidance regarding summary documentation when using IA. In general, the expectation is that IA findings are documented at each assessment interval since these entries comprise the archived record. However, given the intensity of activity required to monitor maternal–fetal status using IA while providing one-to-one (1:1) continuous labor support during active pushing, it may be reasonable to summarize findings every 15–30 minutes if the nurse is continually in attendance, FHM assessments are performed at intervals consistent with

Figure 9-6 The Collaborative Process and Fetal Heart Monitoring

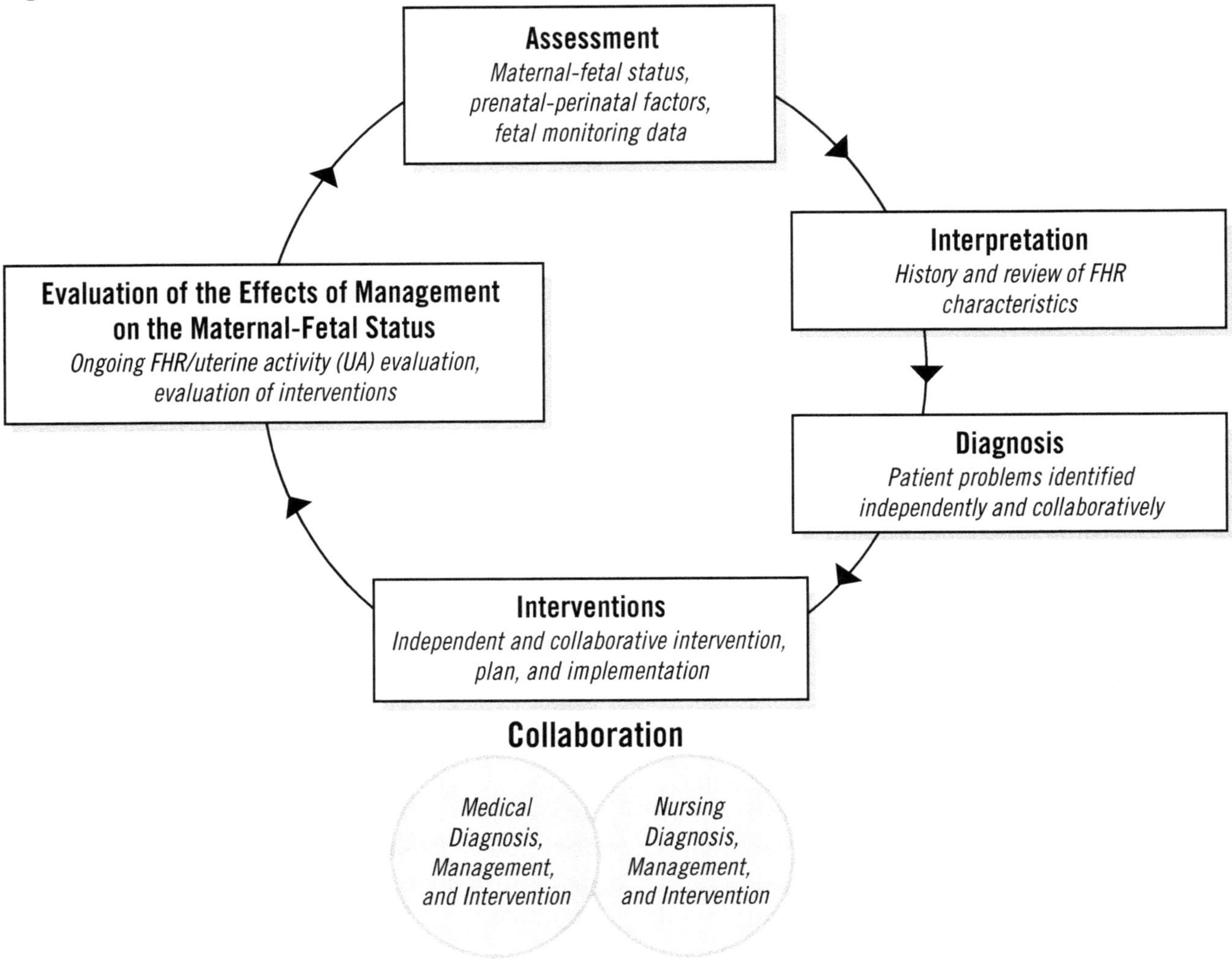

maternal–fetal condition, and there is some notation in the record that this 1:1 bedside evaluation is ongoing. Institutional policy should clearly define expectations regarding documentation intervals when using IA. If summary documentation is used during second-stage labor, the importance of ongoing assessments at 5-minute intervals should be emphasized.

SUMMARY OF DOCUMENTATION GUIDELINES

General Guidelines by Stage of Labor and Maternal–fetal Risk Status

The most recent publications by professional organizations governing obstetric practice in the U.S. and Canada containing guidance on FHM intervals by stage of labor and risk status (AAP & ACOG, 2012; ACNM, 2010a; ACOG, 2009b; AWHONN, 2008a; SOGC, 2007) all predate recent changes to the definitions of latent and active labor (ACOG, 2014; ACOG & SMFM, 2014). The consensus statement by ACOG and SMFM (2014) aimed at safely preventing primary cesarean delivery defines active labor as a dilation of ≥ 6 centimeters rather than the historical standard of 4 centimeters. This consensus statement was concerned primarily with redefining arrest of labor based on contemporary data that indicate the most accelerated phase of dilation in labor occurs at ≥ 6 centimeters in both nulliparous and multiparous women. The ACOG has also redefined active labor as beginning at ≥ 6 centimeters (ACOG, 2014). Professional organizations have not yet addressed the FHM implications for women who present in labor between 4–5 centimeters and whether they should be monitored according to guideline recommendations for latent labor. As such, the discussion that follows, and Tables 9-1, 9-2 and 9-3 which summarize FHM recommendations by stage of labor and risk status will contain some inherent ambiguity in the area of how women presenting in labor at 4–5 centimeters should be monitored.

With regard to the latent phase of labor, there have not been clinical trials examining fetal surveillance methods during this phase of labor, perhaps because many women are not in a hospital or birth center setting during this time. Formal recommendations regarding frequency of assessment during the latent phase have not been made by most professional organizations. For women who are receiving fetal surveillance during the latent phase, healthcare providers should use their clinical judgment, taking into consideration their institution's policies and procedures and the specific maternal–fetal risk factors when deciding the method and frequency of fetal surveillance during this stage of labor (AWHONN, 2008; Feinstein et al., 2008).

When using intermittent auscultation during active, first-stage labor, the FHR should be determined, evaluated, and recorded every 30 minutes if no risk factors are present, and every 15 minutes in the presence of risk factors (AAP & ACOG, 2012). When using EFM, the FHR should be evaluated at 30-minute intervals during active, first-stage labor and at 15-minute intervals during active, second-stage labor when no risk factors are present. The FHR should be evaluated at 15- and 5-minute intervals during active, first-, and second-stage labor, respectively, in the presence of risk factors (AAP & ACOG, 2012). The recording of such evaluations may occur periodically (ACOG, 2010) and be summarized at less frequent intervals than the recommended assessment intervals when using continuous EFM (AHWONN, 2008a).

The SOGC (2007) recommends IA for fetal assessment in low-risk women, with assessments every 15–30 minutes during active, first-stage labor and every 5 minutes during pushing when using IA or EFM. When EFM is used, even in the presence of risk factors or oxytocin administration, the tracing may be interrupted for up to 30 minutes to allow for ambulation, bathing, or position changes as long as the tracing has been normal, maternal–fetal assessments are stable, and the oxytocin dose is unchanged (SOGC, 2007). The RCOG (NICE, 2014) recommends FHR assessment via IA for at least 1 minute following a contraction, at 15- and 5-minute intervals during active first- and second-stage labor, respectively, and assessment of contractions every 30 minutes during these same time periods. See Tables 9-1, 9-2, and 9-3 for a summary of recommendations by stage of labor and maternal–fetal risk status.

Latent Labor, Passive Second Stage, and Admission Assessment

While there is general agreement in the professional guidelines regarding assessment during active first-stage and active second-stage labor, guidance regarding assessment and documentation during the latent phase of the first stage of labor and during passive, second-stage labor is limited. Also, guidance regarding monitoring method during triage or the admission assessment is not addressed in all guidelines. Each facility develops a policy and procedure addressing assessment intervals during each stage of labor, generally based on recommendations from professional associations in their respective countries. Clinicians in the facility should be cognizant of and practice within the policy and procedure. The SOGC (2007) recommends FHR auscultation initially, then approximately every hour thereafter for latent, first-stage labor. The ACNM, AWHONN, and SOGC distinguish passive, second-stage labor from active pushing. The ACNM and SOGC recommend assessments at 15-minute intervals during passive descent and assessments every 5 minutes during active pushing (ACNM, 2010a; SOGC, 2007). AWHONN (2008b) recommends continuing assessments at the same intervals as

TABLE 9-2 Frequency of Fetal Heart Monitoring Assessment Using Continuous Electronic Fetal Monitoring

ORGANIZATION	LATENT PHASE, FIRST STAGE	ACTIVE PHASE, FIRST STAGE		PASSIVE SECOND STAGE	ACTIVE SECOND STAGE	
		LOW RISK[a]	HIGH RISK[a]		LOW RISK	HIGH RISK
AAP & ACOG (2012); ACOG (2009b)		Every 30 min	Every 15 min		Every 15 min	Every 5 min
AWHONN (2008a, 2008b)	Use clinical judgment	Within the range of every 15–30 min[b]		Every 15–30 min[c]	Within the range of every 5–15 min[b]	
RCOG (NICE, 2014)		IA recommended	Every 15 min[d]		IA recommended	Every 5 min[e]
SOGC (2007)	On admit, then hourly	IA recommended	Every 15–30 min[f]	Every 15 min	IA recommended	Every 5 min

Note: AAP = American Academy of Pediatrics; ACNM = American College of Nurse-Midwives; ACOG = American College of Obstetricians and Gynecologists; AWHONN = Association of Women's Health, Obstetric and Neonatal Nurses; EFM = electronic fetal monitoring; FHM = fetal heart monitoring; IA = intermittent auscultation; NICE = National Institute for Health and Care Excellence; RCOG = Royal College of Obstetricians and Gynaecologists; SOOG = Society of Obstetricians and Gynaecologists of Canada

[a]Specific definitions of low and high risk are lacking in some guidelines. See Table 9-4 for further information.

[b]Due to variation in original research protocols, factors influencing frequency of assessment should include maternal–fetal condition and risk factors and maternal response to labor.

[c]AWHONN (2008b) recommends continuing assessments at the same intervals as first stage since the intrauterine environment during passive descent is physiologically similar to first stage.

[d]If fetal heart rate is not within normal limits, palpate the maternal pulse to differentiate between the two heart rates.

[e]Every 15 minutes palpate the mother's pulse to differentiate between the two heart rates.

[f]During the first stage of labor, if EFM is used, even in the presence of risk factors or oxytocin administration, it is reasonable to interrupt monitoring for up to 30 minutes to allow for bathing, ambulating, or position change provided maternal–fetal assessments are stable, and if receiving oxytocin, the dose is unchanged (SOGC, 2007).

first stage since the intrauterine environment during passive descent is physiologically similar to first stage.

The SOGC, RCOG, and AWHONN recommend IA for all low-risk, laboring women, including as first-line assessment during admission, citing a lack of evidence to support routine use of admission EFM for low-risk women (Feinstein, Sprague, & Trepanier, 2008; NICE, 2014; SOGC, 2007). The SOGC (2007) and RCOG (NICE, 2014) recommend admission fetal heart tracings for women at risk of adverse outcome. Maternal–fetal risk factors are summarized in Table 9-4. Guidance from AAP and ACOG does not specifically address admission EFM; however, both IA and EFM are considered acceptable methods of fetal surveillance in labor (AAP & ACOG, 2012), and EFM is recommended for pregnancies considered high-risk (ACOG, 2009b).

USE OF NICHD NOMENCLATURE AND CATEGORIES IN DOCUMENTATION

Historically, ambiguity of fetal monitoring terms contributed to difficulties for clinicians attempting to interpret, communicate, and manage EFM patterns. In 2008, the 1997 NICHD publication was updated. It includes standardized definitions and terminology to describe EFM characteristics and defines categories for EFM patterns. The primary purpose of developing these definitions was not necessarily for inclusion in documentation; rather, it was to facilitate more precise pattern interpretation and evidence-based management of labor (Spong, 2008).

Institutional policy should clarify expectations regarding components of FHM documentation and the use of NICHD nomenclature and categories in documentation, and consider the clinical value and/or limitations of certain

TABLE 9-3 Summary of Fetal Heart Monitoring Recommendations by Stage of Labor

Stage of Labor/ Clinical Context	Summary Recommendations
Admission Assessment OB Triage	Either EFM or IA is an acceptable/effective method of fetal surveillance in labor (AAP & ACOG, 2012). For low-risk women presenting at triage for labor admission, IA is an acceptable method of initial fetal assessment (Feinstein et al., 2008). Admission EFM is not recommended for healthy women with low-risk pregnancy. As part of the initial assessment, the FHR should be assessed by IA, and should include auscultation for one minute after a contraction (NICE, 2014). For women with high-risk pregnancy, or with risk factors for adverse perinatal outcome, admission EFM is advised (NICE, 2014; SOGC, 2007). EFM should not be used to determine or rule out if a woman is in labor (NICE, 2014; SOGC, 2007).
Latent Labor	There are no clinical trials to support a recommendation for FHM during the latent, first stage of labor. Clinicians should use clinical judgment when deciding method and frequency (AWHONN, 2008a). The SOGC (2007) recommends IA at the time of assessment/admission, and hourly thereafter.
Active Labor	For low-risk women monitored with IA, evaluate and record the FHR and UCs every 30 minutes, and every 15 minutes for women with risk factors. Assessments should preferably be performed before, during, and after a contraction. When using EFM in women without risk factors, evaluate every 30 minutes and periodically document. If risk factors are present, evaluate every 15 minutes and periodically document (AAP & ACOG, 2012; ACOG, 2009b). FHM assessments should occur within the range of every 15–30 minutes when using IA or EFM. When using continuous EFM, summary documentation may occur less frequently than assessment intervals (AWHONN, 2008a). FHM assessments should occur every 15–30 minutes using IA. EFM should be reserved for pregnancies at risk for adverse outcome. When using IA, document additional FHM assessments before and after vaginal exams, membrane rupture, medication administration, and ambulation (ACNM, 2010a). The SOGC (2007) recommends FHM assessments every 15–30 minutes. If EFM is used and the tracing is normal, it is reasonable to interrupt monitoring for up to 30 minutes to allow for bathing, ambulating, or position change provided maternal–fetal assessments are stable, and if receiving oxytocin, the dose is unchanged (SOGC, 2007). The RCOG (NICE, 2014) recommends FHR assessments every 15 minutes and UC assessments every 30 minutes for all women. When using IA, the FHR should be auscultated for 1 minute after a UC. If fetal heart rate is not within normal limits, palpate the maternal pulse to differentiate between the two heart rates. When using EFM, FHM components should be evaluated as with IA, the mother's pulse should be palpated every 15 minutes to differentiate between the two heart rates and a systematic FHM assessment documented hourly (NICE, 2014).
Second Stage, Passive Descent	AWHONN (2008b) recommends continuing assessments at the same intervals as first stage since the intrauterine environment during passive descent is physiologically similar to first stage. The SOGC recommends FHM assessments every 15 minutes (SOGC, 2007). The ACNM[a] (2010a) recommends FHR and UC assessments every 15 minutes using IA.
Second Stage, Pushing	For high-risk women monitored with IA, evaluate and record FHR and UCs every 15 minutes, and every 5 minutes for women with risk factors. Assessments should preferably be performed before, during, and after a contraction. When using EFM in women without risk factors, evaluate every 15 minutes and periodically document. If risk factors are present, evaluate every 5 minutes and periodically document (AAP & ACOG, 2012; ACOG, 2009b). FHM assessments should occur within the range of every 5–15 minutes when using IA or EFM. When using continuous EFM, summary documentation may occur less frequently than assessment intervals (AWHONN, 2008a). During 1:1 continuous labor support, summary documentation may occur every 30 minutes (AWHONN, 2008a). The ACNM (2010a) and SOGC (2007) recommend IA at 5-minute intervals when pushing. The RCOG (NICE, 2014) recommends FHR assessments every 5 minutes, after a contraction when using IA, with UC assessments every 30 minutes. Every 15 minutes palpate the mother's pulse to differentiate between the two heart rates. When using EFM, evaluation of FHR and UCs should occur at these intervals, with a systematic assessment of FHM components documented hourly (NICE, 2014).

Note: AAP = American Academy of Pediatrics; ACNM = American College of Nurse-Midwives; ACOG = American College of Obstetricians and Gynecologists; AWHONN = Association of Women's Health, Obstetric and Neonatal Nurses; EFM = electronic fetal monitoring; FHM = fetal heart monitoring; FHR = fetal heart rate; IA = intermittent auscultation; NICE = National Institute for Health and Care Excellence; RCOG = Royal College of Obstetricians and Gynaecologists; SOOG = Society of Obstetricians and Gynaecologists of Canada; UC = uterine contraction.

[a]The ACNM guideline only addresses IA.

TABLE 9-4 RCOG (NICE, 2014) and SOGC (2007): Definition of Maternal–fetal High-Risk Factors

ANTEPARTUM FACTORS: MATERNAL	INTRAPARTUM FACTORS: MATERNAL
Hypertensive disorders of pregnancy	Vaginal bleeding in labor
DM or GDM	Intrauterine infection/chorioamnionitis
Antepartum hemorrhage	Previous CS
Maternal medical disease	Membrane rupture > 24 hours at term
• Cardiac disease, anemia, hyperthyroidism, vascular or renal disease	Induced or augmented labor
Maternal MVA/trauma	Hypertonic uterus
Morbid obesity	Maternal pyrexia
Previous poor obstetrical outcome	Preterm labor
	Post-term pregnancy (> 42 weeks)
	Labor dystocia
	Abnormal VS
ANTEPARTUM FACTORS: FETAL	**INTRAPARTUM FACTORS: FETAL**
Fetal growth restriction	Meconium-stained fluid
Prematurity	Abnormal FHR on auscultation (<110 or >160 bpm baseline; any decelerations after a contraction)
Oligohydramnios	Decreased fetal activity
Abnormal umbilical artery	
Doppler velocimetry	
Isoimmunization	
Multiple pregnancy	
Breech presentation	

Note: CS, cesarean section; DM, diabetes mellitus; FHR, fetal heart rate; GDM, gestational diabetes mellitus; MVA, motor vehicle accident; VS, vital signs.

aspects of NICHD-based language. While the professional organizations have agreed upon using the NICHD nomenclature to describe and interpret EFM findings, the use of the NICHD *categories* in documentation is less well defined. ACOG (2010) recommends including a description of the FHR category and overall EFM pattern with each summary documentation interval. However, some experts have cautioned against the use of categories as a summary mechanism in documentation because of redundancy, but also since specific components of the EFM tracing (e.g., minimal vs. moderate variability) cannot be identified by the classification alone for the broadest range of EFM findings (category II tracings) (Miller, 2011). At this time, consensus has not been reached in the professional guidelines about how often and under what circumstances categories should be documented.

While certain terminology may not require further description, it may be helpful to quantify various aspects of FHM findings in some situations. For example, since early decelerations are considered clinically benign, further quantification is unnecessary. Similarly, while evaluation of length, depth, and frequency of variable or late decelerations may have clinical significance (Cahill, Roehl, Odibo, & Macones, 2012; Clark et al., 2013; Parer, King, Flanders, Fox, & Kilpatrick, 2006), quantification of late decelerations in documentation may be unnecessary since late decelerations are thought to signify transient or chronic placental insufficiency and warrant amelioration regardless of their associated characteristics. Conversely, it may be appropriate at times to quantify prolonged and variable decelerations in documentation when their characteristics are physiologically significant and relevant to the clinical response that follows their observation (Clark et al., 2013; Miller, Miller, & Tucker, 2013). When they are recurrent, variable decelerations should be evaluated further for their depth, frequency, duration, associated FHR characteristics, and uterine contraction (UC) pattern (ACOG, 2010), since findings may dictate different management strategies (see Chapter 5).

In summary, documentation of findings should generally be limited to what is clinically relevant and guided by institutional policy. Detailed documentation of deceleration depth or duration is usually discouraged; the fetal tracing is available for additional information and analysis. However, summary documentation of pattern evolution should include changes in characteristics of decelerations or other FHM components, especially as they relate to the maternal–fetal response to interventions.

DOCUMENTATION OF FETAL HEART MONITORING COMPONENTS

Documentation of Uterine Activity When Using Intermittent Auscultation

Documentation of uterine contractions when using IA reflects the clinician's subjective palpated assessment of contraction intensity, resting tone between contractions, and frequency and duration of UCs. Contraction frequency is measured as the interval from the beginning of one contraction to the beginning of the next, documented in minutes. Duration is timed from the start of the contraction to the end of the contraction and documented in seconds. Both frequency and intensity are documented as average values for the current assessment period if the observation period spans two or more contractions. Contraction strength or intensity is determined via palpation during a contraction, and documented as mild, moderate, or strong based on the ability to indent the uterus during the peak of the contraction (see Chapter 4). Uterine resting tone is assessed between contractions and documented as soft or firm (Feinstein et al., 2008).

Since FHR assessments should be considered in relationship to contractions, it is reasonable to assess contraction pattern and characteristics with each FHR assessment. Where specified in various professional organization guidelines, summary documentation of UCs is recommended as part of each auscultated FHR assessment (ACNM, 2010a; SOGC, 2007), or at 30-minute intervals (NICE, 2014).

Documentation of Uterine Activity When Using Electronic Fetal Monitoring

Assessment of uterine activity using EFM is accomplished via tocodynamometer (TOCO) or by intrauterine pressure catheter (IUPC). Contraction frequency, duration, intensity, and resting tone should be described and documented. In addition to documenting frequency and duration of contractions, contraction strength should be qualified as mild, moderate, or strong (determined via palpation) when using a TOCO, and quantified in mmHg when using an IUPC. Resting tone is documented as soft or firm (determined via palpation) when using a TOCO. When an IUPC is in place, resting tone should be documented in mmHg and verified by palpation. While the terms *strength* and *intensity* are often used interchangeably in clinical practice, documentation of contraction strength when using an IUPC indicates the peak of the contraction in mmHg, and intensity describes the peak of the contraction minus the resting tone (Miller et al., 2013). Documentation of contraction intensity can be summarized by calculating Montevideo units or by documenting the range of contraction intensity or strength in mmHg when an IUPC is in place. Institutional policy should define expectations for recording assessments of contractions, and the method for evaluation should be standardized within each institution.

Uterine activity is described as normal when there are $\leq$ 5 contractions in 10 minutes, and as tachysystole when there are $>$ 5 contractions in 10 minutes, averaged over 30 minutes. The term *tachysystole* is used whether contractions are spontaneous or induced; however, the clinical response may vary. Refer to Chapter 6 for a discussion of interventions for tachysystole. Assessment and documentation of the absence or presence of FHR decelerations should occur when tachysystole is noted (Macones et al., 2008).

Documentation of Fetal Heart Rate Components When Using Intermittent Auscultation

When using IA, baseline rate and rhythm can be assessed and documented. Since variability is visually assessed, it is not part of IA assessments. Baseline rate is determined between palpated contractions and documented as a single number if documentation is occurring at each assessment interval, or as a range if the observation period spans several assessments or summary documentation is being used. Rhythm is documented as regular or irregular. Blood flow through the umbilical cord or placenta may be heard with auscultation devices; therefore the maternal pulse should be checked to delineate maternal heart rate from FHR (ACNM, 2010a; Feinstein et al., 2008). Since baseline rate is defined as the FHR over a minimum of a 10-minute interval, more frequent auscultation would be indicated if an abnormal rate is detected in order to differentiate a bradycardic ($<$ 110 bpm) or tachycardic ($>$ 160 bpm) rate from a temporary change in FHR. Similarly, when a change in baseline is suspected via IA, the FHR should be assessed and documented again following the next contraction to further investigate the change rather than waiting until the next scheduled auscultation interval (Feinstein et al., 2008).

The terms *increases* and *decreases* (Feinstein et al., 2008) and *accelerations* and *decelerations* (ACNM, 2010a) are used to describe FHR changes from baseline when using IA. The presence or absence of increases (accelerations) and decreases (decelerations), and whether they are abrupt or gradual, should be documented with each assessment interval. If decreases (decelerations) are detected, they should be investigated further and evaluated in the context of the overall clinical picture. Since classifying types of decelerations requires visual interpretation, they should not be categorized as early, late, or variable as with EFM. Additional documentation should include whether decreases (decelerations) are intermittent or recurrent, the nadir rate, and any interventions initiated in response to them (ACNM, 2010a). Interpretation of auscultation findings may be further classified as category I or II if the documentation policy in use calls for the use of auscultation categories in the medical record. See Chapter 5 for a discussion of FHM categories when using IA.

When decreases are detected, the auscultation frequency should be increased to clarify FHR characteristics, and the clinical scenario evaluated to determine the potential cause. Interventions directed toward correcting the problem should be implemented. If the pattern persists, interventions should continue and EFM may be initiated to evaluate and classify the FHR pattern and baseline variability. All interventions, assessments, maternal–fetal responses, associated events (e.g., rupture of membranes, maternal coping), and communication with provider or other team members should be documented (Feinstein et al., 2008).

Documentation of Fetal Heart Rate Components When Using Electronic Fetal Monitoring

When using EFM, documentation of baseline FHR is determined by recording the mean FHR rounded to increments of 5 bpm, excluding decelerations, accelerations, and periods of marked FHR variability. Baseline rate is averaged during a 10-minute window, using at least 2 minutes of identifiable baseline segments (not necessarily continuous). If unable to identify baseline using these criteria, the baseline is considered indeterminate, and the clinician may refer to the previous 10-minute window for baseline determination (Macones et al., 2008). Documentation of baseline rate should always be as a single number, rounded to the nearest 5-bpm increment (140) rather than a range (140–145) when using EFM (Macones et al., 2008).

Baseline FHR variability is determined in a 10-minute window, excluding accelerations and decelerations. It is defined as fluctuations in the baseline FHR that are irregular in amplitude and frequency. The fluctuations are visually quantified as the amplitude of the peak-to-trough in bpm, and classified as *absent*, *minimal*, *moderate*, or *marked* variability based on the amplitude range in bpm.

The presence or absence of accelerations and decelerations should be documented with each assessment or summary. Decelerations are described and documented as late, early, variable, or prolonged based on specific characteristics. Additional documentation should include whether decelerations are intermittent or recurrent (Macones et al., 2008). See Chapter 5 for a review of definitions and interpretation of FHR characteristics.

CERVICAL RIPENING AND INDUCTION AND AUGMENTATION OF LABOR

Some differences are found in professional guidelines from ACOG, SOGC, and the RCOG regarding maternal–fetal assessments for women undergoing induction of labor, particularly in the case of cervical ripening with prostaglandins (PGE^1, PGE^2). In Canada and the United Kingdom, PGE^2 may be administered in outpatient settings, with less stringent monitoring protocols than in the United States. When oxytocin is used for induction or augmentation, fetal surveillance according to high-risk protocols is recommended by all professional organizations, but may not necessarily include EFM (AAP & ACOG, 2012). ACOG (2009a) recommends that FHR and uterine contractions be monitored "closely" during oxytocin for labor induction and augmentation. Table 9-5 summarizes professional organization recommendations for assessment and documentation of FHM information for women undergoing cervical ripening or induction or augmentation of labor.

DOCUMENTATION IN SPECIAL CIRCUMSTANCES

Cesarean Birth

In low-risk women admitted for scheduled primary or repeat cesarean birth, the presence of fetal heart tones (FHTs) should be confirmed and documented before surgery. There is insufficient evidence to support more frequent fetal surveillance prior to planned, scheduled cesarean in low-risk women, and decisions regarding fetal surveillance prior to surgery should be individualized (AAP & ACOG, 2012; ACOG, 2007). For unscheduled cesarean birth, fetal surveillance should continue until the abdominal prep has been initiated. When internal monitoring is in use, the FSE should remain in place until the abdominal prep is complete (AAP & ACOG, 2012).

The overarching decision regarding monitoring method, frequency, and subsequent documentation should be guided by acuity and risk factors in the case of unplanned or emergent cesarean birth. For example, in arrest of labor in a low-risk woman at 7 centimeters, IA or EFM could be used with assessments documented every 30 minutes while preparations are made for surgery. Conversely, unplanned cesarean for a deteriorating category II EFM tracing or category III tracing would warrant continuous EFM with assessments every 15 minutes for active labor or every 5 minutes for second-stage labor (AAP & ACOG, 2012).

TABLE 9-5 Fetal Heart Monitoring during Cervical Ripening or Induction and Augmentation of Labor

MEDICATION	RECOMMENDATIONS
Prostaglandin E_1(PGE$_1$) Misoprostol	Monitoring FHR and UCs is recommended for any high-risk patient in active labor. Institutional policy should address methods for maternal–fetal assessment before and during administration of prostaglandins (AAP & ACOG, 2012). Prostaglandins should be administered where continuous EFM can be implemented for an initial observation period. Further monitoring can be governed by individual indications for induction and fetal status. The patient should remain recumbent for at least 30 minutes after administration (ACOG, 2009a). In the United Kingdom, PGE$_1$ is only used for induction in cases of fetal demise (NCC-WCH, 2008). In Canada, PGE$_1$ can be administered for labor induction on an inpatient basis. Fetal well-being is assessed before administration followed by 30 minutes of EFM after administration. If any tachystystole occurs, EFM is performed for 60 minutes. (SOGC, 2013).
Prostaglandin E_2(PGE$_2$) Dinoprostone	Monitoring FHR and UCs is recommended for any high-risk patient in active labor. Institutional policy should address methods for maternal–fetal assessment before and during administration of prostaglandins (AAP & ACOG, 2012). Prostaglandins should be administered where continuous EFM can be implemented for an initial observation period. Further monitoring can be governed by individual indications for induction and fetal status. The patient should remain recumbent for at least 30 minutes after administration (ACOG, 2009a). ACOG (2009a) recommends continuous EFM for 30 minutes to 2 hours following administration of PGE$_2$ gel. Continue to monitor if regular UCs are present. The manufacturer of Cervidil® recommends careful (not continuous) monitoring of uterine activity, fetal status, and cervical dilation while the insert is in place, and that the woman be recumbent for 2 hours following placement. After that time, she may ambulate (Forest Pharmaceuticals, 2012). PGE$_2$ may be administered on an outpatient basis in Canada, with EFM for 1-2 hours after placement. Women are advised to return to the hospital with the onset of regular UCs. Once inpatient, IA is used in low-risk women (SOGC, 2007, 2013). The RCOG (NCC-WCH, 2008) recommends EFM to confirm a normal FHR tracing prior to cervical ripening; however, they cite insufficient evidence to support a recommendation regarding monitoring during induction with prostaglandins. If sent home after administration of a PGE$_2$ tablet or gel, women are advised to return at onset of UCs, or if no contractions are present 6 hours following placement. Continuous EFM is recommended for fetal assessment once contractions begin, and IA is resumed if a normal tracing is confirmed unless risk factors are present or develop (NCC-WCH, 2008). Once labor has begun following PGE$_2$, FHM is recommended per the aforementioned guideline (NCC-WCH, 2008).
Oxytocin	Close monitoring of FHR and UCs is recommended as for any high-risk patient in active labor (AAP & ACOG, 2012; ACOG, 2009a). Institutional policy should address methods for maternal–fetal assessment before and during administration of these agents (AAP & ACOG, 2012). During oxytocin induction or augmentation, FHR should be determined and evaluated every 15 minutes during the active, first stage of labor and every 5 minutes during active pushing, as well as before each dose increase (AWHONN, 2008a). Administer in labor and birth suite, where uterine activity and FHR can be recorded continuously via EFM and evaluated at a minimum of every 15 minutes during the first stage of labor, and every 5 minutes during the second stage of labor. IA or EFM telemetry may be used during ambulation or when sitting on a birthing ball or chair. If using IA, determine and record the FHR and palpate uterine contractions at least every 15–30 minutes during the first stage of labor and every 5–15 minutes during the second stage of labor based on risk status (Simpson, 2013). The SOGC (2007) recommends continuous EFM when oxytocin is used. Once the infusion rate is stable, and if the FHR tracing is normal, EFM may be interrupted for periods of up to 30 minutes to accommodate ambulation, personal care, and hydrotherapy. The RCOG (NICE, 2014) recommends continuous EFM when oxytocin is used with FHR assessments every 15 minutes in the first stage, and 5 minutes in the second stage. Uterine activity should be assessed every 30 minutes.

Note: AAP = American Academy of Pediatrics; ACNM = American College of Nurse-Midwives; ACOG = American College of Obstetricians and Gynecologists; AWHONN = Association of Women's Health, Obstetric and Neonatal Nurses; EFM = electronic fetal monitoring; FHM = fetal heart monitoring; FHR = fetal heart rate; IA = intermittent auscultation; NCC-WCH = National Collaborating Centre for Women's and Children's Health; NICE = National Institute for Health and Care Excellence; RCOG = Royal College of Obstetricians and Gynaecologists; SOOG = Society of Obstetricians and Gynaecologists of Canada; UC = uterine contraction.

Fetal Heart Monitoring: Special Considerations

Guidelines for FHM before, during, and after neuraxial analgesia/anesthesia are summarized in Table 9-6. Considerations for FHM surrounding cesarean birth, nonobstetric surgery, trauma in pregnancy, and for preterm or postdates labor are summarized in Table 9-7. While the terms *low risk* and *high risk* are used throughout FHM professional guidelines, these terms are not clearly defined in all cases. A few examples of high risk (suspected fetal growth restriction, preeclampsia, and type 1 diabetes) are offered by ACOG (2009b). More extensive criteria are presented by the RCOG (NICE, 2014) and the SOGC (2007) and are summarized in Table 9-4.

TABLE 9-6 Fetal Heart Monitoring Before, During, and After Neuraxial Analgesia/Anesthesia

AWHONN (2011b)	ASA (2007)	SOGC (2007)	RCOG (NICE, 2014)
Insufficient evidence to support definitive recommendation for frequency of FHR assessments	FHR should be monitored before and after administration of neuraxial analgesia	If protocol is in place for frequent assessments, IA may be used	Continuous EFM for at least 30 minutes during establishment of regional analgesia and after administration of each bolus ≥ 10 ml
EFM prior to initiation of procedure, and FHM before and after each analgesia/anesthesia intervention	Continuous EFM may not be necessary in every clinical situation or may not be possible during initiation of neuraxial analgesia	Recommended assessment: Every 5 minutes for 30 minutes after epidural initiated, and following top-ups (> 0.125% bupivicaine or equivalent)	
Continuous EFM may not be necessary in every clinical situation or possible during initiation of the block		PCEA does not equal top-up. Maternal hemodynamics are stable with PCEA, so additional fetal surveillance is not required	
Continuous 1:1 nursing care for first 30 minutes			
FHR, UC, BP, P, and R assessment after initiation or rebolus of a regional block, including PCEA. Continue FHR and BP assessments every 5 minutes for 15 minutes, with additional BP assessments at 30 minutes and 1 hour following procedure			
Frequency of additional FHR and BP assessments should be based on variables such as type, route, and dose of analgesia/anesthesia; maternal–fetal condition; response to medication (e.g., hypotension); and facility protocol			

Note: ASA, American Society of Anesthesiologists; AWHONN, Association of Women's Health, Obstetric and Neonatal Nurses; BP, blood pressure; EFM, electronic fetal monitoring; FHM, fetal heart monitoring; FHR, fetal heart rate; IA, intermittent auscultation; NICE, National Institute for Health and Care Excellence; P, pulse; PCEA, Patient Controlled Epidural Analgesia; PTL, preterm labor; R, respirations; RCOG, Royal College of Obstetricians and Gynaecologists; SOGC, Society of Obstetricians and Gynaecologists of Canada; UC, uterine contraction.

TABLE 9-7 Fetal Heart Monitoring in Special Circumstances

Setting/Circumstances	Recommendations
Scheduled/Elective Cesarean Birth	For scheduled primary or repeat cesarean birth, FHTs should be confirmed and documented before surgery (AAP & ACOG, 2012; ACOG, 2007). Data are insufficient to warrant further fetal monitoring prior to scheduled cesarean in low-risk women (AAP & ACOG, 2012). There are insufficient data to determine the value of fetal monitoring, either by EFM or US, prior to scheduled cesarean delivery in patients without risk factors. The decision to monitor the fetus prior to scheduled cesarean delivery should be individualized (ACOG, 2007).
Unplanned or Emergency Cesarean Birth	For unscheduled/unplanned cesarean birth, fetal surveillance should continue until the sterile prep has begun if monitored by US, and until the prep is complete if by FSE (AAP & ACOG, 2012; ACOG, 2007).
Cesarean Related to Preterm Fetus	If a cesarean is being performed related to a preterm fetus, continuous EFM should be used. The earliest gestation that this should occur will vary based on GA, EFW, and other factors influencing the fetus's likelihood of survival and/or potential for severe morbidity (ACOG, 2009b).
Nonobstetric Surgery	Pregnant women who undergo nonobstetric surgery should be managed with communication between providers. Decisions regarding FHM should be individualized, and based on GA, type of surgery, setting, and facilities available (AAP & ACOG, 2012; ACOG, 2011; AWHONN, 2011c). Each case warrants a team approach for optimal safety of the woman and fetus. Obstetric consultation is recommended prior to nonobstetric surgery and some invasive procedures (e.g., cardiac catheterization or colonoscopy) because obstetricians are uniquely qualified to discuss aspects of maternal physiology and anatomy that may affect intraoperative maternal–fetal well-being (ACOG, 2011). For a previable fetus, Doppler FHTs should be obtained before and after the procedure. For a viable fetus, EFM is recommended before and after the procedure to assess fetal well-being and detect UCs (ACOG, 2011; AWHONN, 2011c). Intraoperative EFM may be appropriate when all the following apply (ACOG, 2011): • The fetus is viable • It is physically possible to perform intraoperative EFM, and the surgery allows for safe interruption to perform an emergency cesarean if indicated • A provider with obstetric surgery privileges is available and willing to intervene during the procedure if warranted • When possible, the woman has given informed consent for an emergency cesarean birth Fetal heart rate monitoring may assist in maternal positioning and cardiorespiratory management, and may influence a decision to deliver the fetus. In select circumstances, intraoperative fetal monitoring may be considered for previable fetuses to facilitate positioning or oxygenation interventions (ACOG, 2011).
Trauma	The primary goal is maternal stabilization. If attention is focused on the fetus before the woman is stable, maternal injuries may be overlooked and circumstances capable of causing fetal compromise (maternal hypoxemia, hypovolemia, supine hypotension) may be missed. Since uterine abruption usually occurs shortly after injury, and EFM may detect it, such monitoring should be initiated as soon as the woman is stable. The recommended duration of EFM is debated, but most experts recommend EFM for 2–4 hours following the event, and continued EFM and evaluation if any of the following are present: UCs, abnormal FHR pattern, bleeding, significant uterine tenderness or irritability, serious maternal injury, or ROM. According to *Guidelines for Perinatal Care*, EFM is only recommended at viability or beyond 20–24 weeks (AAP & ACOG, 2012).
Preterm Labor	EFM is recommended for labor at <36 weeks. While evidence suggests no benefit from EFM versus IA, the incidence of other pathologies is increased in PTL, as is the risk of adverse outcome (SOGC, 2007).
Postdates Labor	IA is recommended for spontaneous, low-risk labor at ≤41.3 weeks. After 41.3 weeks, IA is appropriate if the NST and AFV are normal. EFM is recommended for labor at > 42 weeks (SOGC, 2007).

Note: AAP, American Academy of Pediatrics; ACOG, American College of Obstetricians and Gynecologists; AFV, amniotic fluid volume; AWHONN, Association of Women's Health, Obstetric and Neonatal Nurses; EFM, electronic fetal monitoring; EFW, estimated fetal weight, FHM, fetal heart monitoring; FHR, fetal heart rate; FHT, fetal heart tone(s); FSE, fetal scalp electrode; GA, gestational age; IA, intermittent auscultation; NST, non-stress test; PTL, preterm labor; SOGC, Society of Obstetricians and Gynaecologists of Canada; UC, uterine contraction; US, ultrasound.

RISK MANAGEMENT AND LIABILITY EXPOSURE

A comprehensive risk management program designed to address the litigious nature of perinatal care in the United States is multidimensional and includes system- and individual-level variables. Core efforts should revolve around avoiding preventable adverse events and limiting liability exposure (Simpson & Knox, 2000). Comprehensive, timely, and standards-based documentation is a key component of successful risk management. Documentation should capture ongoing maternal–fetal status and detail maternal–fetal response to any interventions aimed at maintaining or achieving stability (Simpson, 2014). Nursing documentation should reflect communications between the nurse, physician, and other members of the health care team as care is administered, as well as pertinent exchanges between the woman, her family, and caregivers. It should also demonstrate use of the chain of resolution when the nurse encounters an unresolved difference of opinion about clinical care that may affect patient safety, a suboptimal response from a provider, or when other communication issues arise. Close attention should be paid to ensuring that documentation reflects care provided according to specialty standards, particularly in the case of high-risk or high-liability situations such as induction or augmentation of labor, management of the second stage of labor, vaginal birth after cesarean, assisted delivery, or during unanticipated events such as shoulder dystocia or neonatal resuscitation (Simpson & Knox, 2003).

EVALUATING THE QUALITY OF MEDICAL RECORD DOCUMENTATION

Institutional policies, procedures, and protocols outline the expectations for medical record documentation (Simpson & Knox, 2009). Quality of documentation is often viewed as a reflection of the quality of care rendered (Deering, Tobler, & Cypher, 2010). Auditing clinical documentation in the medical record provides a method for evaluating and improving patient care and maintaining standards of care (ANA, 2010). Periodic medical record audits are a regulatory requirement with electronic documentation (McCartney, 2009), and are recommended with any system to promote a learning environment and decrease inaccuracies and omissions in documentation (Simpson & Knox, 2009). Audits should be conducted per hospital guidelines or policy. Audits should ideally be led by a group of volunteer nursing peers. Audits can aid in evaluating individual and team competence in different aspects of peripartum care, and information gathered can form the basis for the development of strategies aimed at improving unit performance. Evaluation of documentation audit findings can contribute to the educational needs assessments for staff continuing education requirements and identifying methods for improving providers' communication and documentation. Audits may also be one source of information on whether and how nurses and others are using the institution's chain of resolution/consultation so that positive feedback can be given for use of appropriate conflict resolution strategies (Simpson, 2014). See Box 9-1 for a sample medical record audit tool.

SUMMARY

Achieving quality documentation of FHM information is a shared responsibility of individual clinicians, administrators, healthcare organizations, and professional specialty organizations. When developing, implementing, and evaluating documentation systems and policies, it is important to bear in mind the complexity and demands of the clinical environment while keeping the woman, fetus, and family at the center of all decision making. Direct-care providers should be considered partners in system design and policy development and be an integral part of the evaluation process. Finally, it is the responsibility of all clinicians providing care to laboring women to maintain currency in research and professional standards governing peripartum care.

Box 9-1 Sample Medical Record Audit Tool

Suggested Components of a Medical Record Audit

- Are the times noted on the Admission Assessment, Labor Flow Chart, and initial EFM strip consistent with each other within a reasonable time frame?
- If elective labor induction, is gestational age of at least 39 weeks confirmed?
- If elective (e.g., repeat or scheduled) cesarean birth, is gestational age of at least 39 weeks confirmed?
- Is it documented that the physician or midwife was notified of admission within the time frame outlined in the policies and procedures?
- Is fetal well-being established on admission?
- Is fetal well-being established prior to ambulation?
- Is fetal well-being established prior to medication administration?
- Does the EFM FHR baseline rate match the FHR baseline documented?
- Does the EFM FHR baseline variability match the FHR baseline variability documented?
- If there is evidence of absent or minimal FHR variability, is it documented?
- If there is evidence of absent or minimal FHR variability, are appropriate interventions documented?
- If there are FHR decelerations on the EFM strip, are they correctly documented?
- Are appropriate interventions documented during indeterminate or abnormal FHR patterns?
- Is there documentation of physician or midwife notification during indeterminate or abnormal FHR patterns?
- If FHR accelerations are documented, are they on the EFM strip?
- Are maternal assessments documented according to policy?
- If there is evidence of an indeterminate or abnormal FHR pattern, is oxytocin dosage increased?
- If there is evidence of an indeterminate or abnormal FHR pattern, is oxytocin dosage discontinued?
- If there is evidence of uterine tachysystole, are appropriate interventions documented?
- If there is evidence of adequate labor, is oxytocin dosage increased?
- If there is evidence of uterine tachysystole, is oxytocin dosage increased or decreased?
- Does the frequency of uterine contractions on the EFM strip match what is documented?
- Is the uterine activity monitor (external tocodynamometer or intrauterine pressure catheter [IUPC]) adjusted to maintain an accurate uterine activity baseline?
- Are oxytocin dosage increases charted when there is an inaccurate uterine baseline tracing or an uninterpretable FHR tracing?
- Is the physicians' and/or midwives' documentation of fetal status consistent with the nurses' documentation?
- Are automatically generated data from blood pressure devices and pulse oximeters accurate?
- Does documentation continue during the second stage of labor?
- Are patients in the second stage of labor encouraged to push before they feel the urge to push?
- Are patients in the second stage of labor encouraged to push with contractions when the FHR is indeterminate or abnormal [i.e., are there variable or late FHR decelerations occurring with each contraction)?
- When the FHR is indeterminate or abnormal during the second stage of labor, is pushing discontinued or encouraged with every other or every third contraction to maintain a stable baseline rate and minimize decelerations?
- If the FHR is indeterminate or abnormal during the second stage of labor, is oxytocin discontinued?
- Are uterine contractions continuously monitored during the second stage of labor via external tocodynamometer or IUPC?
- Does the time of birth on the medical record match the time of birth at end of the EFM strip?
- If the patient had regional analgesia/anesthesia, is a qualified anesthesia provider involved in the decision to discharge from post anesthesia care unit (PACU) care?
- If the patient had regional analgesia/anesthesia, is the discharge from PACU care scoring evaluation documented?
- Are maternal assessments documented during the immediate postpartum period every 15 minutes for at least 2 hours?
- Are newborn assessments documented during the transition to extrauterine life at least every 30 minutes until the newborn's condition has been stable for 2 hours?

Note: From *Perinatal nursing (4th ed).* K. R. Simpson, & P. Creehan (Eds.) p. 26. Copyright 2014 by the Association of Women's Health, Obstetric and Neonatal Nurses.

Case Study: Skylar

Age:	24 years old
Gravidity/Parity:	G1P0
Gestational Age:	40-5/7 weeks
Medical History:	Unremarkable
Surgical History:	Lumpectomy for benign left breast mass Appendectomy
Psychosocial History:	Married Father of baby medically retired military veteran
Past Obstetric History:	Not applicable
Current Obstetric History:	Elevated 1-hour glucose tolerance test (GTT) = 174 mg/dL Declined 3-hour GTT and use of glucometer Second trimester ultrasound consistent with last menstrual period (LMP), normal anatomy Third trimester growth ultrasounds consistent with size and dates

Skylar presented to labor and delivery at 0030 for contractions with increasing intensity for 3 hours. Vaginal examination (VE) on admission revealed a cervix that was 4 cm dilated, 90% effaced, and a fetal vertex at 0 station. Her vital signs were as follows: oral temperature, 98.2° F (36.7° C); blood pressure, 132/87 mmHg; pulse, 79 bpm; and respirations, 24 breaths per minute. At 0345, Skylar requested an epidural. VE prior to epidural placement revealed a cervix of 7 cm dilated, 100% effaced, and vertex at 0 station with an occiput posterior position.

Skylar: Labor and Delivery EFM Tracing at 0345 Using Ultrasound and Tocodynamometer

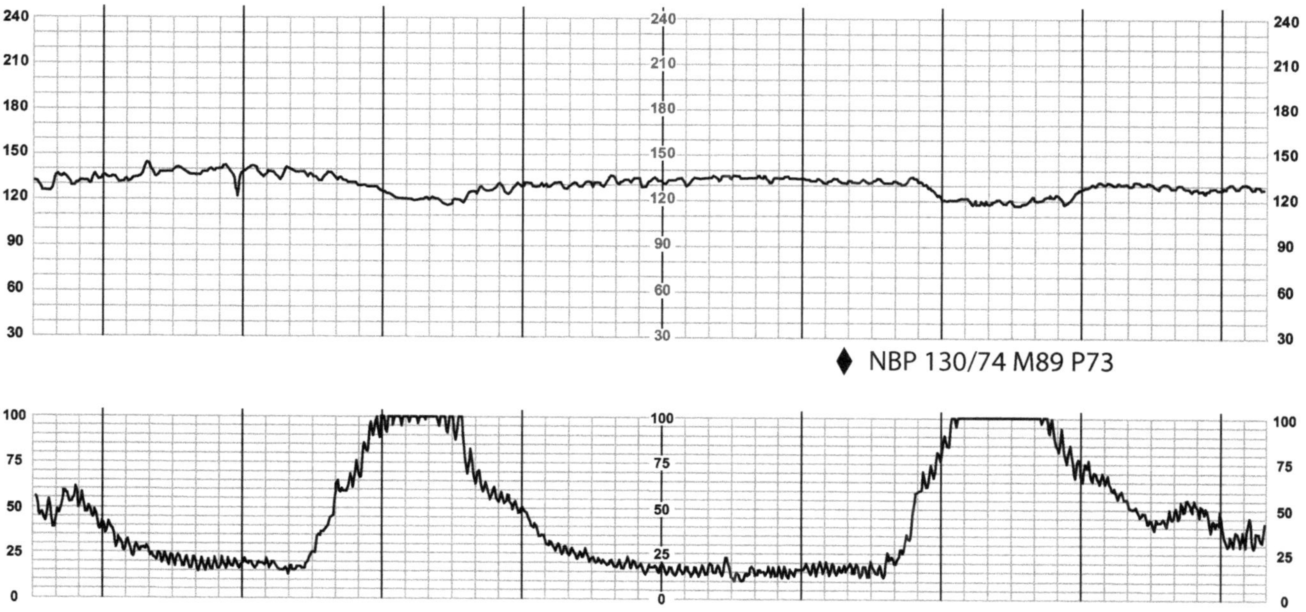

Case Study Exercise G: Skylar

1. Baseline FHR: **135 bpm**

2. Variability

Absent (undetectable)	_____
Minimal (>0 but ≤5 bpm)	**Remainder of tracing**
Moderate (6–25 bpm)	**First 2 minutes of tracing**
Marked (>25 bpm)	_____
Unable to determine	_____

3. Contractions

Frequency:	**q 4 min**
Duration:	**120–150 seconds**
Intensity:	**Palpate**
Resting tone:	**Palpate**

4. Accelerations and decelerations. When present, circle P if periodic or E if episodic.

Accelerations	P	E
Early decelerations	**P**	
Variable decelerations	P	E
Late decelerations	P	
Prolonged decelerations	P	E
None present		

5. Interpretation

Category I	First 2 minutes
Category II	Remainder of tracing
Category III	________

6. List possible underlying physiologic mechanisms or rationales for observed patterns.
   - **Primigravida in active labor**
   - **Associated with a normal to indeterminate fetal acid-base status at present**
   - **Reflex vagal response related to the following:**
     - **Head compression**
     - **Persistent occiput posterior presentation**
     - **Possible cephalopelvic disproportion**
   - **Fetal behavioral state change (fetal sleep cycle)**

7. List in order of priority the physiologic goal(s) for observed patterns.
   - **Promote maternal comfort and labor progress.**
   - **Continue to promote oxygenation.**
   - **Continue to promote uteroplacental blood flow.**
   - **Maintain appropriate levels of uterine activity.**

8. List actions and interventions indicated based on overall interpretation (physiologic based, instrumentation based, and further assessments).
   - **Review previous tracings to evaluate variability and periodic/episodic changes.**
   - **Palpate contractions to validate uterine monitoring data.**
   - **Monitor duration of uterine contractions and fetal response to contractions.**
   - **If minimal variability persists, assess FHR response to scalp stimulation, vibroacoustic stimulation, or manipulation of maternal abdomen to evaluate fetal oxygenation.**
   - **Continue to assess deceleration pattern and variability.**
   - **Change maternal position frequently to promote uteroplacental blood flow and encourage rotation of vertex to occiput anterior position.**
   - **Continue routine assessments and interventions for labor such as maternal comfort measures.**
   - **Keep provider notified of FHR pattern (decelerations and variability), interventions, and maternal–fetal response.**

Case Study: Ruth

Age:	41 years old
Gravidity/Parity:	G1 P0
Gestational Age:	39-1/7 weeks
Medical History:	Chronic hypertension controlled on methyldopa (Aldomet) twice a day
Surgical History:	None
Psychosocial History:	Married
Past Obstetric History:	Not applicable
Current Obstetric History:	*In vitro* fertilization pregnancy using donor egg and sperm Normal prenatal labs First trimester screening normal Second trimester ultrasound normal anatomy, declined amniocentesis Blood pressure ranges prenatally: 130–160s/80–90s mmHg

Ruth presented for labor induction at 0100 because of chronic hypertension. Her cervix was closed and 50% effaced on admission. A Foley bulb was placed for mechanical dilation of the cervix with a low-dose oxytocin infusion of 2 mU/minute. The Foley bulb came out spontaneously at 0720. Her cervix was 3–4 cm, 50% effaced, and the fetal vertex was at –3 station. The FHR baseline was 145 bpm with moderate variability and accelerations. Ruth progressed to 6 cm, 90% effaced, and 0 station with oxytocin. Amniotomy was performed at 1430 and a large amount of clear fluid was observed. Blood pressures during the labor were 130–150s/80s mmHg.

Ruth requested and received an epidural at 1520. Shortly after the epidural was placed, Ruth became hypotensive, with blood pressure ranges of 64–98/41–56 mmHg. The FHR baseline was 155 bpm with moderate variability. She became lightheaded and nauseated. A 5-mg dose of ephedrine was given IV push by the anesthesiologist. An increasing amount of bloody vaginal fluid was noted.

Ruth: Labor and Delivery Tracing Using Fetal Spiral Electrode and Intrauterine Pressure Catheter at 1530

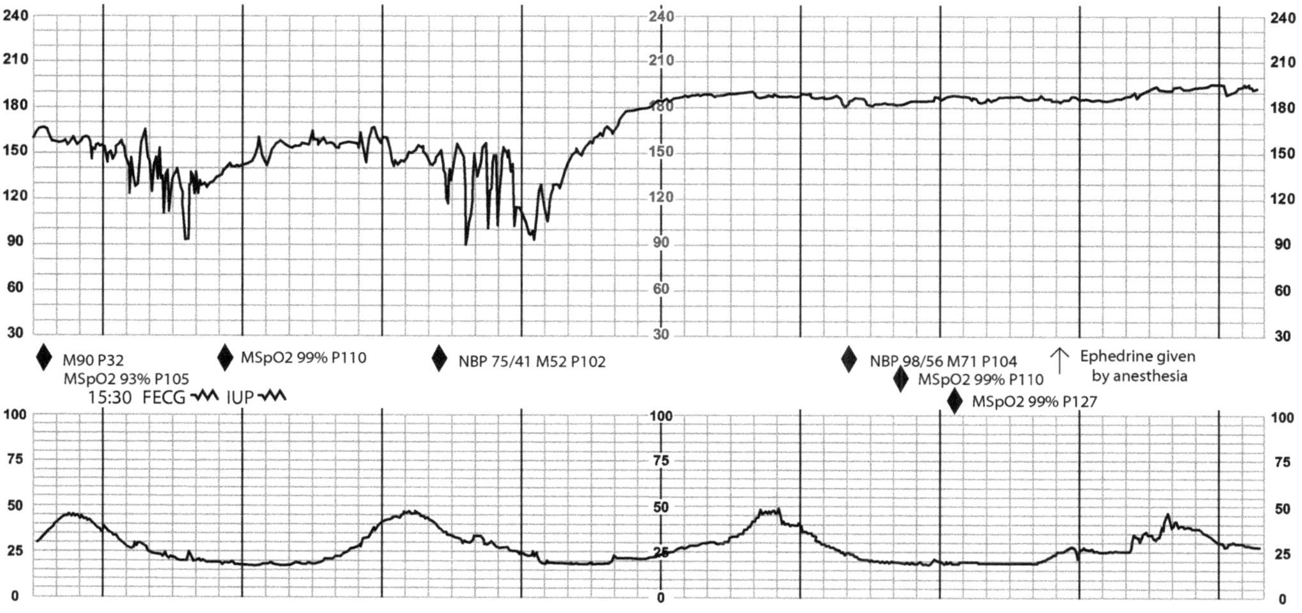

Case Study Exercise H: Ruth

1. Baseline FHR: **155 bpm initially (presumed to be stable before this segment)**
   185 bpm post decelerations

2. Variability

	Absent (undetectable)	_____
	Minimal (>0 but 5 bpm)	**In last 4 minutes**
	Moderate (6–25 bpm)	**In first 3 minutes**
	Marked (>25 bpm)	_____
	Unable to determine	_____

3. Contractions

	Frequency:	**2½–3 minutes**
	Duration:	**90–110 seconds**
	Intensity:	**45–55 mmHg**
	Resting tone:	**15–20 mmHg**

4. Accelerations and decelerations. When present, circle P if periodic or E if episodic.

Accelerations	P	E
Early decelerations	P	
Variable decelerations	P	E
Late decelerations	**P**	
Prolonged decelerations	P	E
None present		

5. Interpretation

	Category I	________
	Category II	________
	Category III	________

6. List possible underlying physiologic mechanisms or rationales for observed patterns.
   - **Decreased uteroplacental perfusion related to abrupt decrease in maternal blood pressure following epidural placement**
   - **Placental abruption related to rapid decrease in blood pressure and increasing amount of blood-tinged vaginal fluid**
   - **Fetal tachycardia as a compensatory effort following episode of suspected maternal and fetal hypoxemia**
   - **Associated with an indeterminate fetal acid-base status at present**
   - **Elevation in maternal temperature**
   - **Endogenous catecholamine response**

7. List in order of priority the physiologic goal(s) for observed patterns.
   - **Maximize placental blood flow.**
   - **Maximize oxygenation.**
   - **Reduce uterine activity.**

8. List actions and interventions indicated based on overall interpretation (physiologic based, instrumentation based, and further assessments).
   - **Change maternal position to maximize uterine blood flow and optimize oxygenation.**
   - **Hydrate with IV fluids to increase maternal blood volume and maximize uterine blood flow.**
   - **Administer maternal supplemental oxygen at 10 Liters/minute via a nonrebreather face mask.**
   - **Continue to frequently assess maternal vital signs.**

- **Evaluate fetal and maternal responses to interventions.**
- **Check maternal temperature.**
- **Notify primary care provider of changing maternal–fetal status.**
- **Provide support to decrease maternal anxiety and catecholamine response.**
- **Prepare for a possible emergent birth.**
- **Alert neonatal team for possible emergent birth.**
- **Continue assessments and interventions based on clinical findings and facility protocols.**
- **Keep family informed of clinical situation.**

Case Study Ruth: Part 2

Ruth responded to the ephedrine dose with blood pressures returning to the pre-epidural range, and her temperature was 99.0° F (37.2° C). A VE was performed because of the increased amount of bleeding and fetal tachycardia. She was 10 cm dilated, 100% effaced, and at +2 station. The IUPC was removed and a tocodynamometer applied. The patient was instructed to start pushing with every other contraction. The FHR tracing remained indeterminate, and the patient was moved to the operating room for operative vaginal delivery versus cesarean section. The fetal tracing below was recorded before Ruth was moved to the operating suite.

Ruth: Labor and Delivery Tracing Using Fetal Spiral Electrode and Tocodynamometer

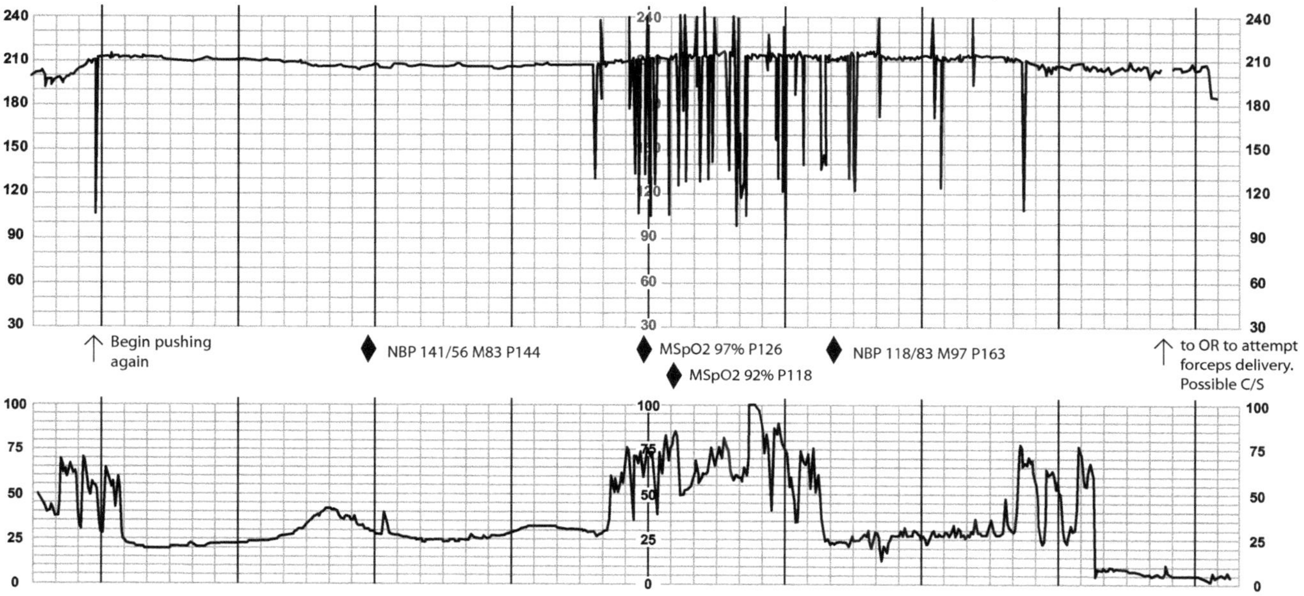

Case Study Exercise I: Ruth Part 2

1. Baseline FHR: **210 bpm**

2. Variability

Absent (undetectable)	_____
Minimal (>0 but 5 bpm)	_____
Moderate (6–25 bpm)	_____
Marked (>25 bpm)	_____
Unable to determine	_____

3. Contractions

Frequency:	**Unable to assess**
Duration:	**Unable to assess**
Intensity:	**Unable to assess**
Resting tone:	**Need to palpate**

4. Accelerations and decelerations. When present, circle P if periodic or E if episodic.

Accelerations	P	E
Early decelerations	P	
Variable decelerations	P	E
Late decelerations	P	
Prolonged decelerations		E
None present		

5. Interpretation

Category I	________
Category II	________
Category III	________

6. List possible underlying physiologic mechanisms or rationales for observed patterns.
   - **Fetal response to ephedrine**
   - **Decreased uteroplacental perfusion related to maternal hypotension**
   - **Placental abruption related to increased amount of blood-tinged vaginal fluid**
   - **Associated with an indeterminate fetal acid-base status at present**
   - **Elevation in maternal temperature**

7. List in order of priority the physiologic goal(s) for observed patterns.
   - **Maximize placental blood flow.**
   - **Maximize oxygenation.**
   - **Reduce uterine activity.**

8. List actions and interventions indicated based on overall interpretation (physiologic based, instrumentation based, and further assessments).
   - **Change maternal position to maximize uterine blood flow.**
   - **Continue IV fluid maintenance.**
   - **Continue maternal supplemental oxygen at 10 liters/minute via a nonrebreather face mask.**
   - **Palpate abdomen to evaluate uterine activity.**
   - **Adjust tocodynamometer.**
   - **Evaluate FHR responses to interventions.**
   - **Prepare to expedite birth.**
   - **Alert neonatal team about imminent birth.**
   - **Continue assessments and interventions based on clinical findings and facility protocols.**
   - **Keep family informed of clinical situation.**

REFERENCES

American Academy of Pediatrics & American College of Obstetricians and Gynecologists. (2012). *Guidelines for perinatal care* (7th ed.). Elk Grove, IL; Washington, DC: Authors.

American College of Nurse-Midwives. (2010a). Intermittent auscultation for intrapartum fetal heart rate surveillance (Clinical Bulletin). *Journal of Midwifery and Women's Health, 55*(4), 397–403. doi:10.1016/j.jmwh.2010.05.007

American College of Nurse-Midwives. (2010b). *Standardized nomenclature for electronic fetal monitoring* (Position Statement). Retrieved from http://www.midwife.org/ACNM/files/ACNMLibraryData/UPLOADFILENAME/000000000089/Standardized_Nomenclature_for_Electronic_Fetal_Monitoring_March_2010.pdf

American College of Obstetricians and Gynecologists. (2007). ACOG Committee Opinion No. 382: Fetal monitoring prior to scheduled cesarean delivery. *Obstetrics and Gynecology, 110*(4), 961–962.

American College of Obstetricians and Gynecologists. (2009a). Induction of labor (Practice Bulletin No. 107). *Obstetrics & Gynecology, 114*(2, Pt. 1), 386–397. doi:10.1097/AOG.0b013e3181b48ef5

American College of Obstetricians and Gynecologists. (2009b). Intrapartum fetal heart rate monitoring: Nomenclature, interpretation, and general management principles (Practice Bulletin No. 106). *Obstetrics andGynecology, 114*(1), 192–202. doi:10.1097/AOG.0b013e3181aef106

American College of Obstetricians and Gynecologists. (2010). Management of intrapartum fetal heart rate tracings (Practice Bulletin No. 116). *Obstetrics and Gynecology, 116*(5), 1232–1240. doi:10.1097/AOG.0b013e3182004fa9

American College of Obstetricians and Gynecologists. (2011). Nonobstetric surgery during pregnancy (ACOG Committee Opinion No. 474). *Obstetrics and Gynecology, 117*(2 Pt. 1), 420–421. doi:10.1097/AOG.0b013e31820eede9

American College of Obstetricians and Gynecologists (2014). *ReVitalize obstetric data definitions: Version 1.0.* Retrieved from http://www.acog.org/-/media/Departments/Patient-Safety-and-Quality-Improvement/2014reVITALizeObstetricDataDefinitionsV10.pdf

American College of Obstetricians and Gynecologists and Society Maternal–fetal Medicine. (2014). Safe prevention of the primary cesarean delivery (Obstetric Care Consensus Series No.1). *Obstetrics and Gynecology, 123*, 693–711. Retrieved from: http://www.acog.org/Resources-And-Publications/Obstetric-Care-Consensus-Series/Safe-Prevention-of-the-Primary-Cesarean-Delivery

American Nurses Association. (2010). *ANA's principles for nursing documentation.* Retrieved from http://www.nursesbooks.org/Main-Menu/Specialties/Staffing-Workplace/eBook-Principles-for-Nursing-Documentation.aspx

American Society of Anesthesiologists. (2007). Practice guidelines for obstetric anesthesia: An updated report by the American Society of Anesthesiologists Task Force on Obstetric Anesthesia. *Anesthesiology, 106*(4), 843–863. doi:10.1097/01.anes.0000264744.63275.10

Association of Women's Health, Obstetric and Neonatal Nurses.(2008a). *Fetal heart monitoring* (Position Statement). Washington, DC: Author.

Association of Women's Health, Obstetric and Neonatal Nurses. (2008b). *Nursing care and management of the 2nd stage of labor* (2nd ed.). Washington, DC: Author.

Association of Women's Health, Obstetric and Neonatal Nurses. (2010). *AWHONN intermediate fetal heart monitoring course instructor teaching materials.* Washington, DC: Kendall Hunt.

Association of Women's Health, Obstetric and Neonatal Nurses. (2011a). Health information technology for the perinatal setting (Position Statement). *Journal of Obstetric, Gynecologic and Neonatal Nursing, 40*(3), 383–385. doi:10.1111/j.1552-6909.2011.01246.x

Association of Women's Health, Obstetric and Neonatal Nurses. (2011b). *Nursing care of the woman receiving regional analgesia/anesthesia in labor* (2nd ed.). Washington, DC: Author.

Association of Women's Health, Obstetric and Neonatal Nurses. (2011c). *Perioperative care of the pregnant woman.* Washington, DC: Author.

Association of Women's Health, Obstetric and Neonatal Nurses. (2014). *Women's health and perinatal nursing care quality refined draft measures specifications: For testing of feasibility, validity and reliability.* Retrieved from http://www.awhonn.org/awhonn/content.do?name=02_PracticeResources/02_perinatalqualitymeasures.htm

Bernat, J. L. (2013). Ethical and quality pitfalls in electronic health records. *Neurology, 80*(11), 1057–1061. doi:10.1212/WNL.0b013e318287288c

Bernstein, P. S., Farinelli, C., & Merkatz, I. R. (2005). Using an electronic medical record to improve communication within a prenatal care network. *Obstetrics and Gynecology, 105*(3), 607–612. doi:10.1097/01.AOG.0000152344.96676.c8

Blumenthal, D., & Tavenner, M. (2010). The "meaningful use" regulation for electronic health records. *New England Journal of Medicine, 363*(6), 501–504. doi:10.1056/NEJMp1506114

Cahill, A. G., Roehl, K. A., Odibo, A. O., & Macones, G. A. (2012). Association and prediction of neonatal acidemia. *American Journal of Obstetrics and Gynecology, 207*(3), 206.e1–206.e8. doi: 10.1016/j.ajog.2012.06.046

Callen, J., Paoloni, R., Li, J., Stewart, M., Gibson, K., Georgiou, A., . . . Westbrook, J. (2013). Perceptions of the effect of information and communication technology on the quality of care delivered in emergency departments: A cross-site qualitative study. *Annals of Emergency Medicine, 61*(2), 131–144. doi:10.1016/j.annemergmed.2012.08.032

Campos, N. K. (2009). The legalities of nursing documentation. *Nursing Management, 40*(8), 16–19. doi:10.1097/01.NUMA.0000359202.59952.d2

Centers for Medicare and Medicaid Services. (2012). EHR Incentive Programs. Retrieved from http://www.cms.gov/Regulations-and-Guidance/Legislation/EHRIncentivePrograms/MeaningfulUse.html

Chalmers, B., Kaczorowski, J., O'Brien, B., & Royle, C. (2012). Rates of interventions in labor and birth across Canada: Findings of the Canadian Maternity Experiences Survey. *Birth, 39*(3), 203–210. doi:10.1111/j.1523-536X.2012.00549.x

Claret, P. G., Sebbanne, M., Bobbia, X., Bonnec, J. M., Pommet, S., Jebali, C., & de La Coussaye, J. E. (2012). First medical contact and physicians' opinion after the implementation of an electronic record system. *American Journal of Emergency Medicine, 30*(7), 1235–1240. doi:10.1016/j.ajem.2011.06.014

Clark, S. L., Nageotte, M. P., Garite, T. J., Freeman, R. K., Miller, D. A., Simpson, K. R., . . . Hankins, G. D. (2013). Intrapartum management of category II fetal heart rate tracings: Towards standardization of care. *American Journal of Obstetrics and Gynecology,* 209(2), 89–97. doi:10.1016/j.ajog.2013.04.030

Cohen, A. W., & O'Keeffe, D. F. (2008). *Implementing an electronic medical record in a perinatal practice.* Washington, DC: Society for Maternal–fetal Medicine.

Declercq, E. R., Sakala, C., Corry, M. P., Applebaum, S., & Herrlich, A. (2013). *Listening to Mothers III: New mothers speak out.* Retrieved from http://transform.childbirthconnection.org/wp-content/uploads/2013/06/LTM-III_NMSO.pdf

Deering, S. H., Tobler, K., & Cypher, R. (2010). Improvement in documentation using an electronic checklist for shoulder dystocia deliveries. *Obstetrics and Gynecology, 116*(1), 63–66. doi:10.1097/AOG.0b013e3181e42220

Feinstein, N. F., Sprague, A., & Trepanier, M.-J. (2008). *Fetal heart rate auscultation* (2nd ed.). Washington, DC: Association of Women's Health, Obstetric and Neonatal Nurses.

Forest Pharmaceuticals. (2012). Cervidil®: Brand of dinoprostone vaginal insert. St. Louis, MO: Author.

Gee, R. E., & Newman, J. (2013). Health information technology. *Obstetrics and Gynecology, 121*(6), 1161–1164. doi:10.1097/AOG.0b013e318293741e

Gupta, J. K., Hofmeyr, G. J., & Shehmar, M. (2012). Position in the second stage of labour for women without epidural anaesthesia. *Cochrane Database of Systematic Reviews,* Issue 5 (Article No. CD002006). doi:10.1002/14651858.CD002006.pub3

Hasley, S. K. (2011). Decision support and patient safety: The time has come. *American Journal of Obstetrics and Gynecology, 204*(6), 461–465. doi:10.1016/j.ajog.2010.10.901

HealthIT.gov. (2013). HITECH programs and advisory committees. Retrieved from http://www.healthit.gov/policy-researchers-implementers/hitech-programs-advisory-committees

Ivory, C. (2008). Informatics competencies for perinatal nurses: Empowering nurses to understand and use technology. *Nursing for Women's Health, 12*(1), 62–65. doi:10.1111/j.1751-486X.2007.00277.x

Kern, L. M., Malhotra, S., Barron, Y., Quaresimo, J., Dhopeshwarkar, R., Pichardo, M., . . .Kaushal, R. (2013). Accuracy of electronically reported "meaningful use" clinical quality measures: A cross-sectional study. *Annals of Internal Medicine, 158*(2), 77–83. doi:10.7326/0003-4819-158-2-201301150-00001

Kossman, S. P. (2006). Perceptions of impact of electronic health records on nurses' work. *Studies in Health Technology and Informatics, 122*, 337–341.

Laramee, A. S., Bosek, M., Shaner-McRae, H., & Powers-Phaneuf, T. (2012). A comparison of nurse attitudes before implementation and 6 and 18 months after implementation of an electronic health record. *CIN: Computers, Informatics, Nursing, 30*(10), 521–530. doi:10.1097/NXN.0b013e3182573b04

Lawrence, A., Lewis, L., Hofmeyr, G. J., Dowswell, T., & Styles, C. (2009). Maternal positions and mobility during first stage labour. *Cochrane Database of Systematic Reviews*, Issue 2 (Article No. CD003934). doi:10.1002/14651858.CD003934.pub2

Macones, G. A., Hankins, G. D., Spong, C. Y., Hauth, J., & Moore, T. (2008). The 2008 National Institute of Child Health and Human Development workshop report on electronic fetal monitoring: Update on definitions, interpretation, and research guidelines. *Obstetrics and Gynecology, 112*(3), 661–666. doi:10.1097/AOG.0b013e3181841395

Martin, J. A., Hamilton, B. E., Sutton, P. D., Ventura, S. J., Menacker, F., & Munson, M. L. (2005). Births: Final data for 2003. *National Vital Statistics Reports, 54*(2), 1–116.

McCartney, P. (2009). Audit trails and electronic record discovery. *MCN: The American Journal of Maternal/Child Nursing, 34*(1), 64. doi:10.1097/01.NMC.0000343869.79861.c7

McCartney, P. R. (2013). Evidence on electronic health record documentation time. *MCN: The American Journal of Maternal/Child Nursing, 38*(2),121. doi:10.1097/NMC.0b013e31827dbfec

McCartney, P., & Barnes, J. (2012). *Perinatal nursing informatics guide for clinical health information technology.* Washington, DC: Association of Women's Health, Obstetric and Neonatal Nurses.

McGreevey, J. D., III. (2013). Order sets in electronic health records: Principles of good practice. *Chest, 143*(1), 228–235. doi: 10.1378/chest.12-0949

Metz, J. P., Son, S. J., Winter, R. O., & Chae, S. (2011). Increasing timely and available prenatal studies by electronic health records. *Journal of the American Board of Family Medicine, 24*(4), 344–350. doi:10.3122/jabfm.2011.04.100296

Miller, L. (2011). Intrapartum fetal monitoring: Liability and documentation. *Clinical Obstetrics and Gynecology, 54*(1), 50–55. doi:10.1097/GRF.0b013e31820a0e27

Miller, L. A., Miller, D. A., & Tucker, S. M. (Eds.). (2013). Patient safety, risk management, and documentation. In *Mosby's pocket guide to fetal monitoring: A multidisciplinary approach* (7th ed., pp. 226–261). St. Louis, MO: Elsevier Mosby.

National Collaborating Centre for Women's and Children's Health. (2008). *Induction of labour* (NICE Clinical Guideline). Retrieved from http://publications.nice.org.uk/induction-of-labour-cg70

National Institute for Health and Care Excellence. (2014). Intrapartum care: Care of healthy women and their babies during childbirth (NICE Clinical Guideline 190). Retrieved from http://www.nice.org.uk/guidance/cg190

Parer, J. T., King, T., Flanders, S., Fox, M., & Kilpatrick, S. J. (2006). Fetal acidemia and electronic fetal heart rate patterns: Is there evidence of an association? *Journal of Maternal–fetal and Neonatal Medicine, 19*(5), 289–294. doi:10.1080/14767050500526172

Poissant, L., Pereira, J., Tamblyn, R., & Kawasumi, Y. (2005). The impact of electronic health records on time efficiency of physicians and nurses: A systematic review. *Journal of the American Medical Informatics Association, 12*(5), 505–516. doi:10.1197/jamia. M1700

Pomerleau, M. (2008). Electronic health record: Are you ready for the next step? *Nursing for Women's Health, 12*(2), 151–156. doi:10.1111/j.1751-486X.2008.00300.x

Riley, M., Galang, S., & Green, L. A. (2011). The impact of clinical reminders on prenatal care. *Family Medicine, 43*(8), 560–565.

Simpson, K. R. (2013). *Cervical ripening and labor induction and augmentation* (4th ed.). Washington, DC: Association of Women's Health, Obstetric and Neonatal Nurses.

Simpson, K. R. (2014). Perinatal patient safety and professional liability issues. In K. R. Simpson & P. A. Creehan (Eds.), *Perinatal nursing* (4th ed., pp. 1–40). Philadelphia, PA: Lippincott Williams & Wilkins.

Simpson, K. R., & Knox, G. E. (2000). Risk management and electronic fetal monitoring: Decreasing risk of adverse outcomes and liability exposure. *Journal of Perinatal and Neonatal Nursing, 14*(3), 40–52.

Simpson, K. R., & Knox, G. E. (2003). Common areas of litigation related to care during labor and birth: Recommendations to promote patient safety and decrease risk exposure. *Journal of Perinatal and Neonatal Nursing, 17*(2), 110–125.

Simpson, K. R., & Knox, G. E. (2009). Communication of fetal heart monitoring information. In A. Lyndon & L. U. Ali (Eds.), *Fetal heart monitoring: Principles and practices* (4th ed., pp. 177–209). Dubuque, IA: Kendall Hunt.

Simpson, K. R., Lyndon, A., Wilson, J., & Ruhl, C. (2012). Nurses' perceptions of critical issues requiring consideration in the development of guidelines for professional registered nurse staffing for perinatal units. *Journal of Obstetric, Gynecologic and Neonatal Nursing, 41*(4), 474–482. doi:10.1111/j.1552-6909.2012.01383.x

Society of Obstetricians and Gynaecologists of Canada. (2007). Fetal health surveillance: Antepartum and intrapartum consensus guideline. *Journal of Obstetrics and Gynaecology Canada, 29*(9, Suppl. 4), S3–S56.

Spong, C. Y. (2008). Electronic fetal heart rate monitoring: Another look. *Obstetrics and Gynecology, 112*(3), 506–507. doi:10.1097/AOG.0b013e318185f872

Stevenson, J. E., Nilsson, G. C., Petersson, G. I., & Johansson, P. E. (2010). Nurses' experience of using electronic patient records in everyday practice in acute/inpatient ward settings: A literature review. *Health Informatics Journal, 16*(1), 63–72. doi:10.1177/1460458209345901

Thompson, D., Johnston, P., & Spurr, C. (2009). The impact of electronic medical records on nursing efficiency. *Journal of Nursing Administration, 39*(10), 444–451. doi:10.1097/NNA.0b013e3181b9209c

Tillett, J. (2012). Implementing the electronic medical record: Building on success. *Journal of Perinatal and Neonatal Nursing, 26*(4), 284–285. doi:10.1097/JPN.0b013e318270cd3c

Zusman, E. E., & Vinokur, Y. (2012). Clinical decision support systems: Key to making EHR an improvement. *Neurosurgery, 7* (4), N12–N14.

CHAPTER 10

Antenatal Fetal Assessment and Testing

Catherine M. Treanor

INTRODUCTION

The introduction of electronic fetal monitors into obstetric care accompanied an era of expanded technology and research in fetal development and pathophysiology (Devoe, 2008). Evaluating fetal well-being was transformed as physiological markers were identified, observed, compared, and quantified and norms established (Manning, 2009; Vintzileos, 2000). Fetal effects from maternal complications such as diabetes and hypertension were defined, making it possible to differentiate fetal risk from maternal risk (Manning, 1995). Recognizing that a fetus is in danger for hypoxic injury and weighing the danger against the risk of intervening is a cornerstone of obstetric management (Manning, 2009). Many testing modalities have been implemented to identify fetuses at risk, making antepartum surveillance a fundamental component of modern prenatal care. Yet for various reasons, the ideal fetal screening test has not been developed to identify all factors that contribute to the risk for hypoxic injury or death (Manning, 1995; Signore, Freeman, & Spong, 2009). Furthermore, no single test is ideal for all high-risk fetuses (Vintzileos, 2000).

Throughout pregnancy, numerous pathophysiologic processes can place the fetus at risk for metabolic imbalance, hypoxia, or death. Early identification of those phenomena is an important first step in fetal surveillance (Vintzileos, 2000). Perinatal deaths are most often associated with (1) congenital malformations and chromosomal abnormalities, (2) prematurity and low birth weight, (3) the effects of maternal complications on the fetus/neonate, and (4) unintentional injuries (Kochanek, Kirmeyer, Martin, Strabino, & Guyer, 2012). Neurologic injury is another potential adverse fetal outcome. Insights into the origin of cerebral palsy (CP) have dispelled the commonly held belief that most cases of CP arise from intrapartum events. Neurologic injury can occur during the antepartum, intrapartum, or neonatal period (Strijbis, Oudman, van Essen, & MacLennan, 2006; Perlman, 2006). The American College of Obstetricians and Gynecologists (ACOG) and the American Academy of Pediatrics (AAP) task force on neonatal encephalopathy reported that the pathway to a diagnosis of CP progresses through a series of pathophysiologic phases, including neonatal encephalopathy, a subset of CP (ACOG & American Academy of Pediatrics [AAP], 2014. Seventy percent of neonatal encephalopathy is secondary to an antepartum event and it is important to note that depending on the type and timing of the injury, the signs and symptoms may range from mild to severe (ACOG & AAP, 2014). Approximately 4% of CP cases are attributed to intrapartum events (Perlman, 2006; Strijbis et al., 2006).

FETAL ANTEPARTUM SURVEILLANCE METHODS

Antepartum testing modalities are based on physiologic principles and are used to identify the fetus at risk for hypoxia versus the normally oxygenated fetus (Boehm & Gabbe, 2002; Perlman, 2006). The fetal response to an acute or chronic reduction in oxygen availability is a decline in activities regulated by the central nervous system (CNS), including heart rate reactivity, breathing, movement, and tone (Figure 10-1) (Manning, Harman, Menticoglou, & Morrison, 1991). Oxygenated blood is shunted to the brain, heart, and adrenal glands; if the insult is prolonged or repetitive, growth restriction and/or oligohydramnios can develop. The purpose of antepartum testing is to validate fetal well-being or identify potentially hypoxemic fetuses by the presence or absence of one or more biophysical parameters and to intervene before permanent injury or death can occur. The efficacy of antepartum surveillance to predict perinatal outcomes for different patient populations has not been clearly established, but testing is usually indicated for conditions that place the fetus at risk for uteroplacental insufficiency and fetal demise. Evaluation of factors such as the potential for fetal and neonatal survival or risk of death, the severity of maternal disease, and the risk of iatrogenic prematurity due to false-positive test results should be undertaken to help determine when to begin fetal surveillance (ACOG, 2014).

FETAL MOVEMENT DETECTION

Maternal perception of fetal movement after approximately 16 to 20 weeks of gestation is one of the oldest, simplest, least expensive, and most widely used tests of fetal well-being (Walton & Peaceman, 2012). Counting fetal movements

FIGURE 10-1 Fetal Responses to Acute and Chronic Hypoxemia and Effects on CNS-Regulated Activities

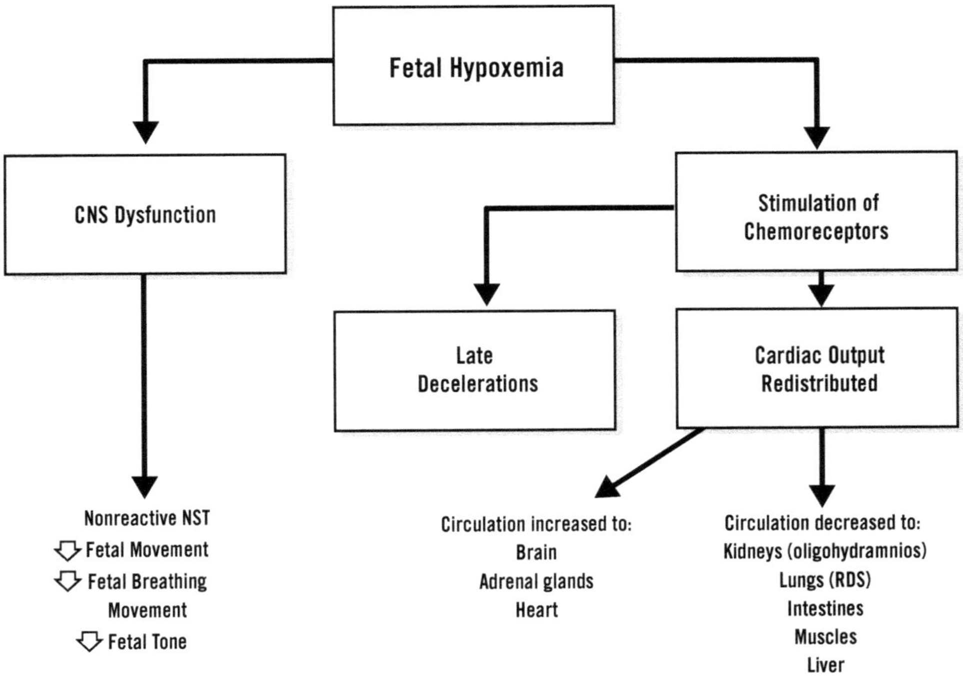

Adapted from Manning, Harmon, Menticoglou, and Morrison (1991).

during the second half of pregnancy requires no monitoring devices and is both noninvasive and cost-effective (Velazquez & Rayburn, 2002). Although a variety of fetal movement counting (FMC, or kick counting) methods are used in clinical practice, the ideal number of fetal kicks or movement or optimal duration of FMC has not been defined (AAP & ACOG, 2012; ACOG, 2014). See the "Fetal Movement Counting" section for examples of different FMC methods.

Development of Fetal Gross Body Movements

The fetus moves spontaneously by the 7th to 8th week of gestation. Maternal perception of fetal movement occurs between the 16th and 18th weeks of gestation (Blackburn, 2013). With neurologic maturation, fetal movement becomes more complex and coordinated (deVries, Visser, & Prechtl, 1982). It is well documented that fetal activity shows circadian patterns (Citro, Luisi, Mezzesimi, Cavicchioli, & Petraglia, 2005) with periods of high and low activity beginning as early as 22 weeks (Groome, Owen, Singh, Neely, & Gaudier, 1992). Total weekly movements increase, reaching a maximum between the 26th and 32nd week (Blackburn, 2013). Between the 32nd and 38th week, fetal movements decrease and then remain constant until term (Blackburn, 2013; Olesen & Svare, 2004). Intervals of quietness and activity increase with gestation, but there are no data indicating that activity is reduced toward term in normal pregnancy, although movements may be sensed differently by the mother (Heazell & Froen, 2008; Hijazi & East, 2009). Synchronization of fetal movement with fetal behavioral states (e.g., active sleep) begins early in the third trimester (Drogtrop, Ubels, & Nijhuis, 1990). Consequently, most healthy term fetuses exhibit coordinated movement patterns that correspond to specific behavioral states (Groome & Watson, 1992).

Maternal perception of fetal movement as a screening tool is based on the physiologic principle that compromised fetuses reduce activity in response to decreased oxygenation, thereby reducing oxygen requirements and conserving energy (Hijazi & East, 2009). Decreases in maternally perceived fetal movements prior to fetal death have been reported (Pearson & Weaver, 1976; Sadovsky & Yaffe, 1973). Mothers feel approximately 50% of isolated limb movements and about 80% of movements involving both the trunk and limb (de Vries & Fong, 2006). Hijazi and East's (2009) review of factors affecting maternal perception of fetal movement found that mothers perceived 33–88% of ultrasound-visualized fetal movements. A comparison of ultrasound-detected fetal movements with maternally perceived movements is presented in Table 10-1.

Fetal Movement Counting

Several different strategies for fetal movement counting (FMC) have been proposed for quantifying maternally perceived movements and for identifying potentially hypoxemic fetuses. FMC methods vary greatly according to the counting interval, number of movements considered reassuring, maternal activity during testing, and

TABLE 10-1 Comparison of Maternally Perceived and Ultrasound-Visualized Movement Patterns

MATERNAL PERCEPTION	ULTRASOUND VISUALIZED	MOTION TYPE	DURATION (SEC)	INTENSITY
Rollover, stretch	Whole fetal body	Rolling and stretching	3–30	Strong
Kick, jab, startle	Trunk and extremities	Simple or isolated	1–15	Strong
Flutter, weak kick	Lower extremities	Simple	< 1	Weak
Hiccup	Chest wall and extremities	High frequency	< 1	Weak

Source: Adapted from Rayburn (1982).

method of recording (Christensen & Rayburn, 1999), but all appear acceptable (ACOG, 2014). Typically, patients are instructed to count all fetal movements occurring in a specific time period and to contact the primary provider if a certain number of movements are not perceived during the prescribed counting interval (Rayburn, 1982). However, more valuable than any single proposed FMC guideline is the mother's perception of fetal activity in relation to previously perceived fetal movement levels (AAP & ACOG, 2012).

A suggested approach to assessing fetal well-being includes fetal movement counting starting at between the 32nd to 34th week of gestation or earlier in worrisome pregnancies (ACOG, 2014). Maternal perception of 10 distinct fetal movements within a 2-hour period is considered reassuring; once the number of movements is achieved within the time period, counts can be discontinued for that day (AAP & ACOG, 2012; ACOG, 2014). Although the presence of fetal movement within a specified protocol is usually a reliable indicator of fetal well-being, the absence of fetal movement may or may not be predictive of adverse fetal outcomes (O'Neill & Thorp, 2012). Maternal perception of fetal movement can be affected by the woman's activity as well as body habitus, fetal position, placental location, and polyhydramnios (O'Neill & Thorp, 2012; Timor-Tritsch, Dierker, Hertz, & Rosen, 1979). Therefore, an insufficient fetal movement count should be followed by a biophysical means of fetal assessment such as a nonstress test (NST), biophysical profile (BPP), or modified BPP (AAP & ACOG, 2012; ACOG, 2014).

Factors Influencing Fetal Movement

Fetal body movements and fetal movements perceived by the mother can be affected by several factors. When fetal movement is used to assess fetal well-being, one must be aware of how movement changes with gestational age and other factors. As previously mentioned, the number of movements increases between the 26th and 32nd week, decreases between the 32nd and 38th week, and then remains constant to term (Blackburn, 2013; Olesen & Svare, 2004; Rayburn, 1990). Contrary to common belief, the qualitative and quantitative measures of fetal movement do not decrease appreciably prior to labor and birth (Velazquez & Rayburn, 2002).

Fetal behavioral states (sleep-wake cycles) should also be considered when evaluating fetal movement. Fetal sleep-wake cycles vary considerably but are well established by the third trimester (Nijhuis, Prechtl, Martin, & Bots, 1982). Fetal behavioral states are presented in Table 10-2. Studies in term fetuses indicate that the mean length of the quiet state is 23 minutes and the longest period of inactivity is 75 minutes (Patrick, Campbell, Carmichael, Natale, & Richardson, 1982; Timor-Tritsch, Dierker, Hertz, Deogan, & Rosen, 1978). Fetuses spend most of their time in quiet and active sleep cycles (Pillai & James, 1990).

Fetal movement tends to decrease during periods of heavy physical activity by the mother (Manders, Sonder, Mulder, & Visser, 1997); however, low-impact exercise has only mild transitory effects, and aerobic exercise has no significant impact on movement or kick response (Hatoum, Clapp, Newman, Dajani, & Amini,1997; Szymanski & Satin, 2012). Chronic maternal anxiety and stress can also influence fetal movement. DiPietro, Costigan, and Gurewitsch (2003) discovered that

TABLE 10-2 Fetal Behavioral States

BEHAVIORAL STATE	DESCRIPTION
1F (Quiet Sleep)	• Quiet sleep • Quiescent state • Decreased FHR variability
2F (Active Sleep)	• Active sleep • Frequent whole body movements • Moderate variability • FHR accelerations
3F (Quiet Awake)	• Absent body movement • No FHR accelerations
4F (Active Awake)	• Vigorous body movement • FHR acceleration

Source: Adapted from Nijhuis et al. (1982).

when mothers were exposed to stress manipulation their fetuses demonstrated an upsurge in fetal heart rate variability and decreased motor activity, but over time stability occurred in the maternal physiological and psychological response to the stress and to a lesser but significant consistent fetal motor response as well. However, fetuses of women experiencing persistent emotional stimulation during pregnancy demonstrated increased movement, suggesting a biphasic fetal motor response (DiPietro, Hilton, Hawkins, Costigan, & Pressman, 2002). DiPietro (2012) worried that this increased fetal activity may be interpreted as an adverse effect; however, DiPietro, Kivlighan, and Costigan (2010) found that increased fetal motor activity is highly correlated with increased motor and reflex maturation at 6 months of age.

Several additional factors have been reported to affect fetal motor activity. Tobacco, sedatives, and corticosteroids decrease fetal movements (Hijazi & East, 2009) whereas caffeine intake increases fetal activity (Conde, Teves, & Figueiredo, 2011; Devoe, Murray, Youssif, & Arnaud, 1993). Fetal circadian rhythms increase fetal movement throughout the day, peaking between 2100 and 0100 hours (Hijazi & East, 2009; Patrick et al., 1982; Thaler, Goodman, & Dawes, 1980). Gross fetal body movements are unaffected by maternal glucose levels, thus dispelling a commonly held belief that juice or a meal is necessary prior to FMC (Eller, Stramm, & Newman,1992; Tan & Sabapathy, 2001; Velazquez & Rayburn, 2002).

A vigorous, active fetus is a reassuring finding while the presence of decreased fetal movement in pregnancy complications of a chronic nature correlates with a higher likelihood of subsequent fetal death (ACOG, 2014; Christensen & Rayburn, 1999). However, FMC has not been shown to prevent fetal death (ACOG, 2014; Mangesi, Hofmeyr, & Smith, 2007; Velazquez & Rayburn, 2002). Factors affecting the technique's effectiveness include varying definitions of decreased fetal movements, a lack of FMC adherence, and delayed or inadequate follow-up (Heazell & Froen, 2008; Gribbin & James, 2004). As a screening tool, FMC is appealing (Boehm & Gabbe, 2002), especially in high-risk pregnancies in which decreasing fetal movements are more often associated with chronic rather than acute compromise. FMC is of greatest value when there is long-standing placental insufficiency (Velazquez & Rayburn, 2002); however, its role in low- and high-risk pregnancies requires further investigation (O'Neill & Thorp, 2012). Research is needed to determine the ideal system for performing FMC, the optimal criteria for assessing the number of movements, the time needed for testing, the interval for repeat evaluation, gestational age at which to begin testing, and, ultimately, the efficacy of FMC to prevent fetal mortality.

Doppler-Detected Fetal Movement

The evolution of Doppler-based ultrasound technology led to advances and improvements in the processing of data between first- and second-generation electronic fetal monitors (EFMs) (Boehm, Fields, Hutchison, Bowen, & Vaughn, 1986). Today's electronic fetal monitors (also known in some European countries as cardiotocography or CTG) use a Doppler-based recording of the fetal heart rate (FHR), fetal activity, and uterine contractions to identify potentially hypoxemic fetuses (Garite, 2012; Johnson, 1994). How EFMs detect and differentiate between the fetal heart rate and fetal movement (actocardiotocography or ACTG) is an often-asked question.

Doppler transducers transmit ultra high-frequency sound waves to the moving heart valves; the sound waves are deflected back and converted into electrical signals. The raw signals are then processed by onboard algorithms that generate a baseline heart rate (Devoe, 1999). Doppler filtering systems further enable the transducer to record and distinguish low-frequency shifts from high-frequency shifts. These special band-pass filters allow for a more accurate detection of fetal movement (i.e., low-frequency shifts) from fetal cardiac activity (i.e., high-frequency shifts). Filtering systems are now incorporated into EFMs, allowing for documentation of not only FHR and variability but also fetal movement (Devoe, 1999). Several studies indicate a strong positive correlation between movements recorded with Doppler-based systems and those observed with real-time ultrasound (Pattison & McCowan, 2010). Regardless of the movement detection algorithm, Doppler-based EFM detected more than 95% of all body movements lasting more than 5 seconds and 100% of multiple movements seen during sonography (Besinger & Johnson, 1989; DiPietro, Costigan, & Pressman, 1999; Lowery et al., 1997). In addition, up to 80% of maternally perceived movements are recorded with EFM, whereas fewer than 20% of Doppler-recorded movements are detected by the mother. The large discrepancy may result from the ability of the Doppler-based device to detect small or single movements or to detect movements lasting fewer than 20 seconds (Johnson, Jordan, & Paine, 1990; Lowery et al., 1997).

The Cochrane Library (Grivell, Alfirevic, Gyte, & Devane, 2012) reviewed reports concerning the reliability of antepartum CTG in reducing perinatal morbidity and mortality as well as maternal mortality. Four randomized controlled trials (RCTs) with a combined study population of more than 1,500 women with high-risk pregnancies achieved the review criteria, but antenatal CTG had no effect on perinatal or maternal outcomes. Although in one study women with CTG experienced significantly fewer hospital admissions and shorter patient stays, the reviewers concluded there was insufficient evidence to show that the use of antenatal CTG reduced fetal mortality (Grivellet al., 2012).

NONSTRESS TEST

The nonstress test (NST) was introduced during the 1970s and has become a cornerstone of antenatal fetal surveillance. The NST evolved from early evidence that FHR accelerations were associated with fetal well-being (Lee, DiLoreto, & O'Lane, 1975) and that, conversely, the absence of FHR reactivity (acceleration) was associated with an increased risk of perinatal mortality (Rochard et al., 1976). In a subsequent investigation, contraction stress tests (CSTs) were always negative when two accelerations were recorded, and the criteria for NST reactivity (i.e., two accelerations in 20 minutes) evolved from that report (Evertson, Gauthier, Schifrin, & Paul, 1979).

The NST is technically easy to perform (Nageotte, Towers, Asrat, Freeman, & Dorchester, 1994b); lacks contraindications (Devoe & Jones, 2002); requires fewer resources than the CST and biophysical profile (Keegan & Paul, 1980); and can be used in inpatient, outpatient, and home settings (Naef et al., 1994; Reece, Hagay, Garafalo, & Hobbins, 1992). The NST is frequently the first-line fetal surveillance technique (Walton & Peaceman, 2012). Evidence supporting the NST is based on multiple time series rather than randomized controlled trials (Devoe & Jones, 2002) in view of the fact that the random allocation of pregnant women to antepartum fetal surveillance versus care that does not include fetal surveillance is unlikely in today's practice of obstetrics in the United States (ACOG, 2014). A critical review of NST testing standards and diagnostic values reveals a wide range of test sensitivity, specificity, and predictive values, suggesting the NST is better at identifying fetal well-being than fetal compromise (Devoe & Jones, 2002). A meta-analysis of four RCTs looking at gestational age, Apgar scores, NICU admissions, and seizures did not demonstrate that use of the NST reduced the incidence of perinatal death or seizures (Devoe, 2008; Grivell et al., 2012). However, O'Neill and Thorp (2012, p.725) point out that "the current practice of antenatal testing frequently involves more than one testing method and/or assessment parameter which may decrease the relevance of the efficacy of one single testing method."

Physiology of the Nonstress Test

FHR accelerations that accompany fetal movement reflect CNS alertness and activity (Freeman, Garite, Nageotte, & Miller, 2012). Rabinowitz, Persitz, and Sadovsky (1983) used simultaneous ultrasound imaging to confirm that fetal movements were virtually always present when fetal accelerations were observed. FHR reactivity reflects adequate oxygenation and normal autonomic nervous system (ANS) function (ACOG, 2014). Fetal movement and FHR accelerations are highly correlated. Typically, fetal movement increases in a linear fashion until approximately 32 weeks, when movement decreases due to the constraints of the intrauterine environment imposed by the growing fetus (Blackburn, 2013; DiPietro et al., 1999; Pillai & James, 1990). More than 95% of accelerations have a synchronous onset or begin immediately after movement (Freeman, 1975; Lee et al., 1975). The frequency and amplitude of accelerations increase with gestational age (Dawes, Houghton, Redman, & Visser, 1982; Groome, Mooney, Holland, Bentz, et al., 1997; Snijders, McLaren, & Nicolaides, 1990).

The FHR response is reflective of the nature of fetal movement. For example, a larger increase in heart rate occurs with complex movements than with isolated fetal movements (Johnson, 1994). Heart rate variation with fetal movement is an important criterion for behavior states and demonstrates normal ANS function (Dawes et al., 1982; Nijhuis et al., 1982). As FHR variability increases, so do the number of movements as well as the number and amplitude of accelerations (Dawes et al., 1982). The presence of accelerations, fetal movement, and variability usually preclude acidemia (Krebs, Petres, Dunn, & Smith, 1982; Ribbert, Snijders, Nicolaides, & Visser, 1990; Vintzileos & Knuppel, 1994; Walkinshaw, Cameron, MacPhail, & Robson, 1992). However, the absence of accelerations may be related to hypoxia, or may be due to normal fetal sleep cycles, CNS depression resulting from medications, or congenital anomalies (Freeman et al., 2012). Therefore, the absence of accelerations in the context of an NST requires further investigation. The effects of hypoxia on NST results are unclear because the sequence of the FHR changes in the transition from normal oxygenation to asphyxia is unclear. Progressive hypoxia may cause loss-of-state changes before the FHR fails to accelerate (Visser, Bekedam, & Ribbert, 1990). As fetal compromise continues, the rest cycles lengthen and eventually disappear, and FHR variability and fetal movement decrease. Subsequently, accelerations become smoother and less frequent, and they finally disappear. Before fetal death, variability has been reported to decrease to fewer than 5 beats per minute (bpm), with absent movement and FHR accelerations (Visser, Sadovsky, & Nicolaides, 1990).

Clinical Application of the Nonstress Test

A key limitation of early antenatal testing was that its use was limited primarily to inpatient settings and populations. Development of the NST, which allowed testing in the outpatient arena, quickly changed the antenatal testing experience. Formerly limited to hypertensive disorders, insulin-dependent diabetes, or other severe medical conditions, the indications for testing quickly expanded to include postdates, complaints of decreased fetal movement, and women with a history of previous fetal death (Paul & Miller, 1995).

Test Procedure and Interpretation

Assist the woman to a physiologically appropriate position, such as sidelying or semi-Fowler's with a lateral tilt. Assess fetal position with Leopold's maneuvers and apply the fetal monitor. Continuously record the FHR and uterine activity for the duration of the test. A lateral tilt position is usually recommended when performing an NST (ACOG, 2014); however, maternal semi-Fowler's position can shorten time to complete testing and has been associated with more reactive NSTs than supine positioning (Nathan, Haberman, Burgess, & Minkoff, 2000). Aortocaval compression can occur, however, when the maternal head is elevated less than 30 degrees, and maternal symptoms of supine hypotension can occur before a drop in blood pressure is recorded. Therefore, maternal position during NST should be determined by the clinical situation; supine positioning with the head lower than 30 degrees should be avoided (ACOG, 2014; Moffatt & van den Hof, 1997).

Historically, many criteria have been suggested for interpreting the NST; however, the currently accepted criteria for a reactive test is the presence of two accelerations (spontaneous or acoustically stimulated) within a 20-minute period for fetuses greater than 32 weeks' gestation (AAP & ACOG, 2012; Macones, Hankins, Spong, Hauth, & Moore, 2008). The FHR accelerations should peak at least 15 bpm above the baseline and last 15 seconds in duration from the beginning to the end of the acceleration (baseline to baseline). The peak in amplitude does not have to be sustained at 15 bpm above baseline; rather, the total duration of the increase in heart rate must be at least 15 seconds (ACOG, 2014; Macones et al., 2008). The monitoring period may be extended to 40 minutes to accommodate normal fetal sleep-wake cycles (AAP & ACOG, 2012; ACOG, 2014).

Castillo and associates (1989) recommended lower-amplitude criteria for fetuses less than 32 weeks' gestation to reduce the confounding effect of gestational age. In 1997, the National Institute of Child Health and Human Development (NICHD) workgroup on FHR monitoring concurred that a minimal threshold for acceleration should reflect gestational age norms, and this was reaffirmed in 2008. In fetuses less than 32 weeks' gestation, accelerations are defined as abrupt FHR increases peaking at least 10 bpm above the baseline, and lasting at least 10 seconds (Macones et al., 2008). Therefore a reactive NST in a fetus under 32 weeks gestation exhibits at least two 10 bpm x 10-second accelerations in a 20-minute period (ACOG, 2014).

The NST is interpreted as reactive or nonreactive (Figure 10-2a, b). A reactive NST meets the stated gestational age criteria with or without maternal perception of fetal movement. Documentation of fetal movement is not necessary (Freeman et al., 2012). A nonreactive NST is defined as fewer than two accelerations meeting the above criteria during a 40-minute period (AAP & ACOG, 2012; ACOG, 2014). A nonreactive NST typically requires additional follow-up with testing such as ultrasound or BPP (Devoe, 1999).

Variable Decelerations during a Nonstress Test

Variable decelerations occur in as many as half of NSTs (Meis et al., 1986) and are associated with umbilical cord compression (O'Leary, Andrinopoulos, & Giordano, 1980). Perinatal outcomes following NSTs with variable decelerations may vary depending on the depth, duration, and frequency of FHR changes and the overall reactivity of the NST. A reactive NST accompanied by intermittent variable decelerations lasting less than 30 seconds is not typically indicative of fetal compromise and usually requires no intervention in the absence of other conditions or cause for concern (ACOG, 2014). However "nonreassuring" intrapartum FHR patterns occurred more often following an NST with three or more variable decelerations of more than 15 seconds' duration (Glantz & D'Amico, 2001; O'Leary et al., 1980). NSTs with repetitive prolonged decelerations are associated with a greater risk of "nonreassuring" FHR patterns, cord complications (e.g., multiple nuchal or occult prolapse), and meconium staining (Jaschevatzky et al., 1998). Oligohydramnios has been reported in study groups in which NSTs revealed variable decelerations (Glantz & D'Amico; Hoskins, Frieden, & Young, 1991). The risk of cesarean birth for alterations in FHR patterns has been shown to increase progressively with the worsening severity of antepartum decelerations and decreasing amniotic fluid volume (Hoskins et al., 1991). Therefore, further evaluation is recommended when repetitive variable decelerations occur during an NST.

Efficacy of Nonstress Tests

A reactive NST with normal amniotic fluid volume is indicative of fetal well-being in 99% of pregnancies (Shalev, Zalel, & Weiner, 1993; Vintzileos et al., 1987) and has a false-negative rate (e.g., stillbirth of a nonanomalous fetus or neonate within 1 week of a reactive NST) of less than 1% (Miller, Rabello, & Paul, 1996). However, a nonreactive NST is much less reliable in predicting adverse perinatal outcomes, and false-positive rates (e.g., normal newborn after a nonreactive NST) of 50-85% or greater have been reported (Devoe, 2008; Manning, 2009). Many factors can affect the accuracy of the NST and contribute to the high rate of false-positive results; of those, a significant influence is gestational age. False-positive results occur in more

FIGURE 10-2a Reactive NST

US/ TOCO

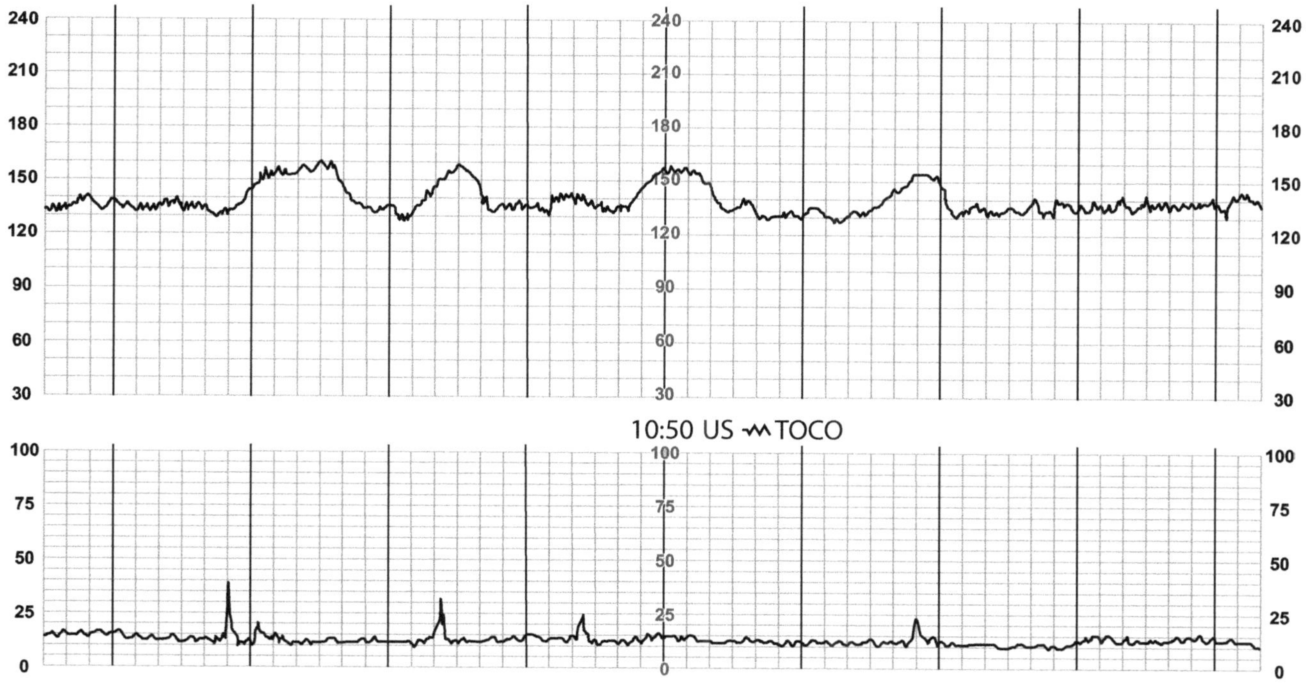

FIGURE 10-2b Nonreactive NST

US/ TOCO

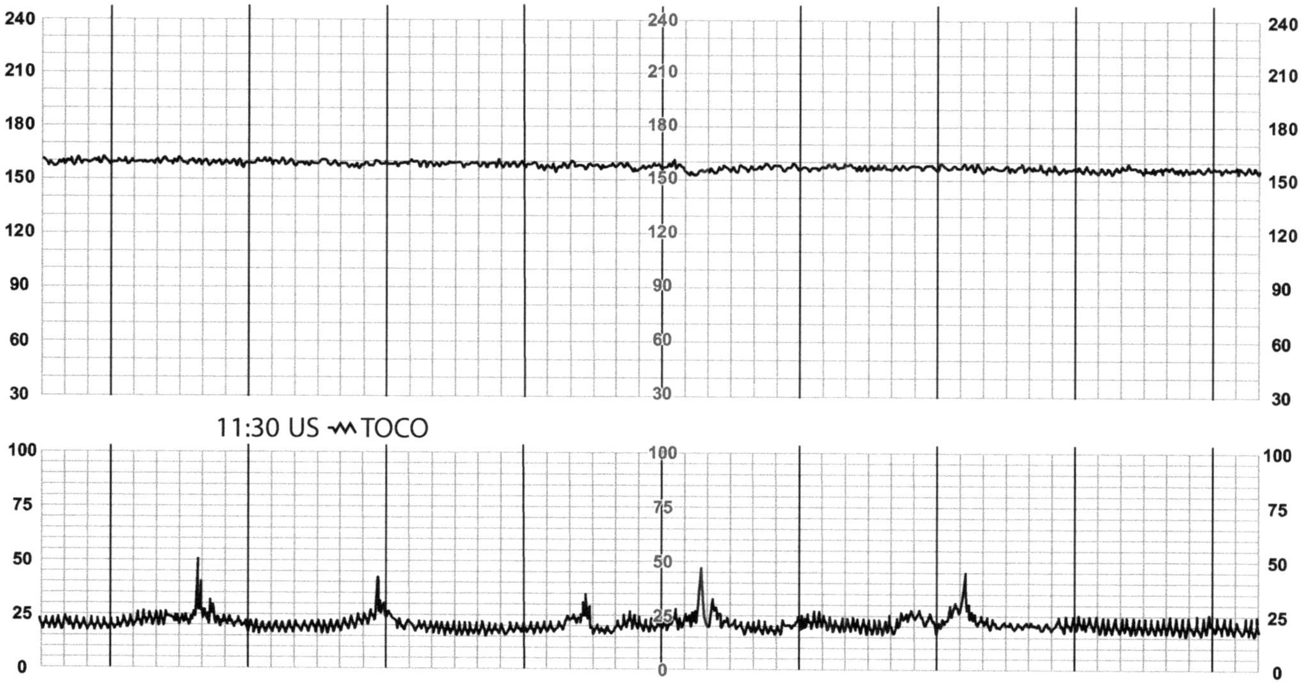

Note: From *Advanced Fetal Monitoring Course*, Association of Women's Health, Obstetric and Neonatal Nurses (AWHONN). 2005. Washington, DC: Author. Copyright 2006 by AWHONN.

than 15% of NSTs performed before 32 weeks' gestation (ACOG, 2014). The large proportion of nonreactive tests in premature fetuses is concerning because of the risk for potentially unnecessary intervention with false-positive tests.

Several conditions other than hypoxemia can reduce heart rate reactivity or interfere with fetal movement and should be considered when interpreting NSTs (Manning, 1995). During quiet sleep, the FHR tracing may have nonreactive features (e.g., diminished FHR variability, reduced fetal movement), but with a state change, the FHR can become reactive (Groome et al., 1999; Nijhuis et al., 1982). At term, the fetus is in a quiet sleep state approximately 30% of the time (Groome et al., 1999). Thus, extending the observation period until a fetus becomes more active can reduce the incidence of nonreactive NSTs (Ware & Devoe, 1994). Maternal cigarette smoking and chronic maternal stress affect the FHR, fetal movement, and NST results (Groome, Swiber, Bentz, Holland, & Atterbury, 1995; Thaler et al., 1980). Ingestion of substances such as caffeine, cocaine, morphine, sedatives, and alcohol has also been associated with false-positive NST results (Devoe et al., 1993; Kopecky et al., 2000; Rizk, Atterbury, & Groome, 1996; Vintzileos et al., 1987). In addition, poor maternal nutritional status can decrease FHR reactivity (Onyeije & Divon, 2001).

FETAL STIMULATION

Various methods of fetal stimulation have been proposed to improve the reliability of antepartum surveillance and to differentiate nonreactive NSTs caused by hypoxia from those associated with fetal sleep states or narcosis. Three methods of fetal stimulation have been reviewed by the Cochrane Collaboration, including fetal manipulation, glucose administration, and vibroacoustic stimulation (VAS). Fetal manipulation (e.g., abdominal rocking) has been used during nonreactive NSTs in two trials, with no demonstrated effect on the efficacy of antepartum testing (Tan & Sabapathy, 2010). Glucose administration increases fetal breathing, but oral (e.g., orange juice) or intravenous glucose administration did not decrease the incidence of nonreactive NSTs in two trials with fewer than 1,000 participants (Tan & Sabapathy, 2010). The reviewers concluded that there was no benefit to antepartum surveillance from either fetal manipulation or glucose administration, and further research with both methods was recommended (Tan & Sabapathy, 2010).

Vibroacoustic Stimulation

Fetal hearing begins at approximately 24–25 weeks' gestation, and auditory-provoked responses can be recorded as early as 25–26 weeks. External environmental sounds are audible to the fetus; high-frequency sounds are attenuated, but low-frequency sounds are not (Blackburn, 2013). Fetal response to sound has been studied since the 1920s.The first reported evidence of VAS-induced FHR accelerations and movement was by Sontag and Wallace (1936). Walker, Grimwade, and Wood (1971) reported a substantial increase in the number, amplitude, and duration of VAS-stimulated FHR accelerations. Subsequent VAS studies demonstrated a decrease in the number of falsely abnormal FHR pattern interpretations and shortened NST testing time without adversely affecting perinatal outcomes (Sarno & Bruner, 1990; Serafini et al., 1984; Smith, Phelan, Paul, & Broussard, 1985; Smith, Phelan, Platt, Broussard, & Paul, 1986). The expected fetal responses to VAS are FHR accelerations and increased gross body movements (Clark, Sabey, & Jolley, 1989; Sarno, Ahn, Phelan, & Paul, 1990). Although some differences in specific FHR responses have been reported (Gagnon, Hunse, & Patrick, 1988; Jensen & Flottorp, 1982), a single startle response and acceleration of the FHR in response to VAS is associated with a functional brainstem, regardless of gestational age (Groome, Mooney, Holland, Smith, & Atterbury, 1997).

The fetal response to sound has been tested using different sound intensities, frequencies, and durations. The VAS significantly increases the baseline intrauterine sound level, exposing the fetus to a sound intensity similar to the takeoff of a jet airplane (Smith, 1995). The primary device used to generate a stimulus for VAS is an artificial larynx (Clark et al., 1989; Miller-Slade et al., 1991; Sarno et al., 1990; Yao et al., 1990). The commercially available device produces 82 decibels at 1-meter air (Sarno et al., 1990). Although the long-term sequelae of VAS stimulation on hearing or cognition are not clearly understood, fetuses clinically exposed to VAS have had no reported adverse effects when the children reached 4 years of age (Nyman, Barr, & Westgren, 1992). Different stimulus durations have been used, including 1-, 2-, 3-, and 5-second durations (Clark et al, 1989; Saraçoğlu, Göl, Sahin, Türkkani, & Oztopçu, 1999; Sarno et al., 1990). A significant increase in the amplitude and duration of accelerations has been associated with 3- and 5-second stimuli durations (Pietrantoni et al., 1991).

Several investigations have explored the reliability of antepartum testing with VAS compared with other surveillance methods. Significantly more visualized or palpated fetal movements occurred after VAS than without stimulation, and evoked accelerations were associated with more than 99% of reactive NSTs (Marden, McDuffie, Allen, & Abitz, 1997) and 100% of negative CSTs (Read & Miller, 1977). Compared with standard NSTs, acoustic stimulation reduced the incidence of false-positive tests (Clark et al., 1989; Saraçoğlu et al., 1999; Serafini et al., 1984; Smith et al., 1986), and an impaired or absent response was a better predictor of perinatal outcomes than NSTs alone (Saraçoğlu et al.; Trudinger & Boylan, 1980). In addition, VAS reduced the incidence of nonreactive NSTs by as much as 50% and decreased the average test duration by 10-20 minutes (Clark et al., 1989; Miller-Slade et al., 1991; Saraçoğlu et al., 1999).

Test Procedure and Interpretation

A commercially available artificial larynx may be used to perform acoustic stimulation when indicated. The procedure includes positioning the artificial larynx on the maternal abdomen near the fetal head and applying the stimulus for 1–2 seconds (AAP & ACOG, 2012: ACOG, 2014). If the NST remains nonreactive, acoustic stimulation may be repeated up to three times, progressing to a maximum stimulation duration of 3 seconds (ACOG, 2014). A reactive NST using VAS is considered a valid indicator of fetal well-being (ACOG, 2014). However, if the NST is still nonreactive following VAS, the test should be followed with a BPP or CST (Greenberg, Druzin, & Gabbe, 2012).

No differences in perinatal outcome (e.g., meconium-stained amniotic fluid, Apgar scores < 7) have been reported following NSTs with spontaneous or stimulated accelerations (Sarno et al., 1990; Serafini et al., 1984; Smith, Phelan, Nguyen, Jacobs, & Paul, 1988). A Cochrane Collaboration review of the literature concerning fetal vibroacoustic stimulation tests revealed that VAS reduced the incidence of nonreactive antepartum NSTs and reduced the overall testing time (Tan & Smyth, 2010). The reviewers were unable to draw conclusions about the efficacy of VAS because the prevalence of perinatal morbidity and mortality in the reviewed studies was too small. In addition, the reviewers observed that there is a paucity of literature concerning fetal hearing and neurologic development after sound stimulation and that little is known about maternal anxiety and maternal satisfaction regarding testing. The reviewers concluded that VAS offered benefits by reducing the incidence of nonreactive NSTs as well as the time to complete testing, but future research was recommended to define the optimal stimulus intensity, frequency, duration, and position and to determine the efficacy, reliability, safety, and perinatal outcomes associated with VAS (Tan & Smyth, 2010).

CONTRACTION STRESS TEST AND THE OXYTOCIN CHALLENGE TEST

The CST was the first antepartum surveillance method developed following the advent of electronic FHR monitoring and quickly became a primary fetal evaluation technique, replacing technically more difficult and prognostically less accurate biochemical (estriol) analyses.

As an antepartum test, the CST evolved from animal studies in which the flow of oxygenated blood into the intervillous space ceased during uterine contractions stronger than 30 mmHg; this, in turn, resulted in transient reductions of fetal oxygen pressure (PO2) and caused late decelerations of the FHR. The mechanism for late decelerations during antepartum evaluation of a potentially chronically stressed fetus is the same as that of an acutely stressed fetus during labor (Olofsson, Thuring-Jonsson, & Marsal, 1996).

The CST is based on the principle of gradually developing uteroplacental insufficiency (Lagrew, 1995). Fetal acidemia is more likely to occur with chronic uteroplacental insufficiency and may not cause obvious changes in the fetal response during periods without uterine activity. However, in a chronically stressed fetus, the additional acute stress of even small contractions can result in hypoxemia and late decelerations (Lagrew, 1995; Paul & Miller, 1995).

Over time, the chronically stressed fetus can also develop oligohydramnios, thus reducing the normal volume of amniotic fluid that surrounds and protects the umbilical cord. Therefore, the cord may be vulnerable, and if it is compressed during uterine contractions, variable decelerations may appear on the FHR tracing (ACOG, 2014).

Clinical Application of the Contraction Stress Test

As a primary means of fetal surveillance, the CST has a low incidence of unexpected fetal death within 1 week of negative test results (AAP & ACOG, 2012). Nevertheless, Freeman et al. (2012) cite a number of concerns associated with its use as a primary surveillance technique, including:

- High false-positive rate
- Frequent equivocal test results
- Time needed to perform the test
- Cost
- Inconvenience compared with other testing techniques.

The development of the NST, BPP, modified BPP, and Doppler velocimetry has replaced the CST in many practice settings (Devoe, 2008). Relative contraindications to the CST are conditions associated with an increased risk of preterm labor and delivery, preterm rupture of membranes, previous classical uterine incision or history of extensive uterine surgery, previous uterine rupture, known placenta previa, or other uterine bleeding (AAP & ACOG, 2012; ACOG, 2014).

Uterine Contractions

Antepartum evaluation using the CST requires uterine activity that mimics the stress of early labor. The minimal number of contractions needed to adequately assess fetal health has not been clearly established, but the criteria for evaluation of the CST were extrapolated from studies performed in the 1970s (Lagrew, 1995; Paul & Miller, 1995). A primary limitation of external uterine monitoring is that only the frequency and duration of contractions—and not the intensity of contractions—can be assessed. However, the important assessment parameter for the CST is the FHR response to uterine contractions, regardless of the intensity.

Test Procedure

The CST is administered with the woman in the lateral recumbent or semi-Fowler's position, and the FHR and uterine activity are first monitored for at least 10–20 minutes with external Doppler ultrasound and tocotransducer. The presence of three or more spontaneous contractions lasting 40 seconds occurring within 10 minutes during the initial period of monitoring is sufficient to interpret the test and no stimulation is required. Contractions can be stimulated with intravenous (IV) oxytocin infusion or breast stimulation if there is no uterine activity within the first 10–20 minutes. The use of IV oxytocin for a CST, referred to as an oxytocin challenge test (OCT), is initiated at 0.5–1 milliunit per minute and increased every 15–20 minutes until at least three contractions occur in 10 minutes (AAP & ACOG, 2012). It is important to note that the oxytocin dosing regimen for a CST differs from the current recommendations for induction/augmentation of labor (Simpson & Knox, 2009). Oxytocin is designated a "high alert medication" by the Institute for Safe Medication Practices (ISMP; 2007) and increased vigilance is therefore needed during the performance of a CST to ensure safe patient care.

An alternative method for a CST is breast stimulation (ACOG, 2014). The procedure is as follows: one nipple is massaged gently through clothing for 2 minutes or until a contraction begins. If the contraction criteria are not met, the patient rests for 5 minutes and the alternate nipple is stimulated. If breast stimulation is unsuccessful (contractions have not begun), an OCT can be initiated using the technique described earlier (ACOG, 2014). Although breast stimulation has been associated with tachysystole (Schellpfeffer, Hoyle, & Johnson, 1985), similar rates of tachysystole, positive CST results, and successful tests with both IV oxytocin and breast stimulation methods have been reported in the literature (Lipitz, Barkai, Rabinovici, & Mashiach, 1987; Oki, Keegan, Freeman, & Dorchester, 1987).

Interpretation

CST interpretation is based on the presence or absence of FHR decelerations and FHR reactivity in response to uterine contractions (Figure 10-3a, b, c, d, e). ACOG (2014) categorizes CST interpretation criteria as follows:

- *Negative:* No late or significant variable decelerations are identified (Figure 10-3a). (Note: The term "significant" is not defined in ACOG [2014] or AAP/ACOG [2012] documents.)
- *Positive:* Late decelerations are identified with 50% or more of contractions, even if the contraction frequency is less than three in 10 minutes (Figure 10-3b).
- *Equivocal-Suspicious:* Intermittent late decelerations or significant variable decelerations are observed (Figure 10-3c).
- *Equivocal:* FHR decelerations that occur in the presence of contractions more frequent than every 2 minutes or lasting longer than 90 seconds (Figure 10-3d).
- *Unsatisfactory:* Fewer than three contractions occur within 10 minutes, or a tracing quality that cannot be interpreted (Figure 10-3e).

Figure 10-3a Negative CST

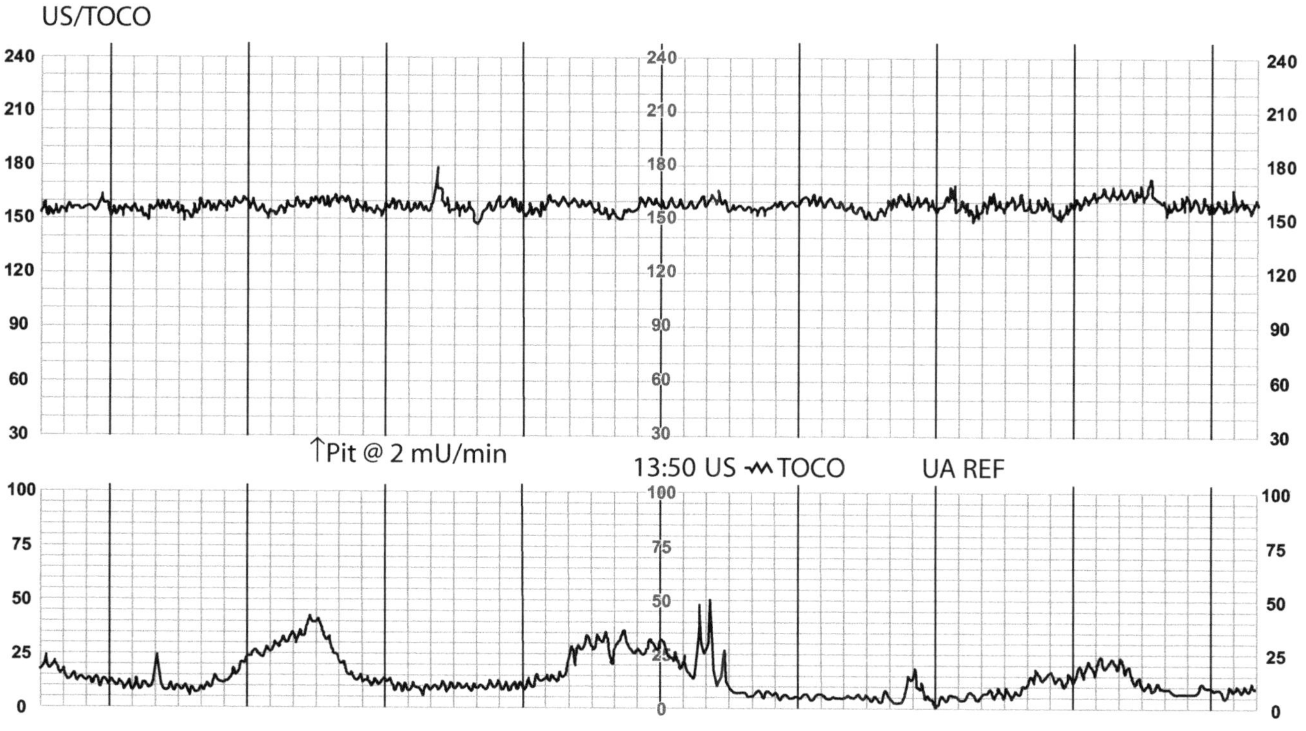

Figure 10-3b Positive CST

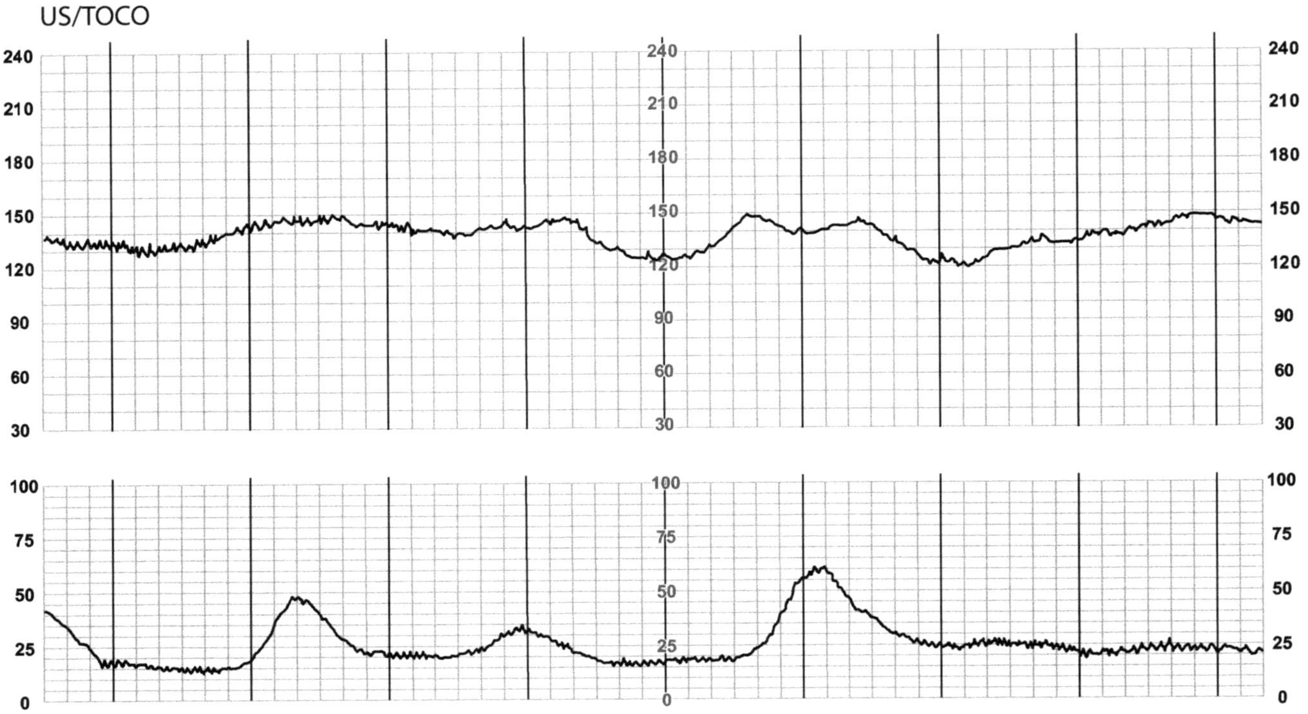

Figure 10-3c Equivocal Suspicious CST

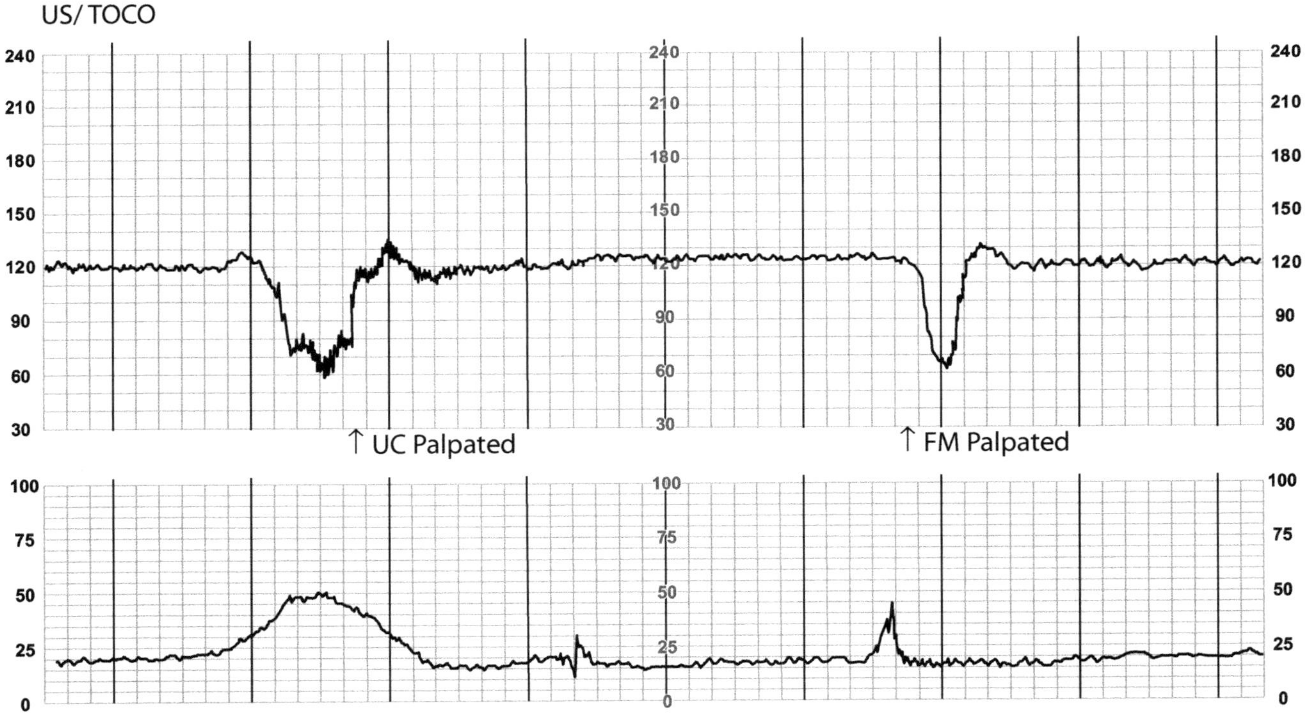

Figure 10-3d CST: Equivocal-Tachystole with FHR Decelerations

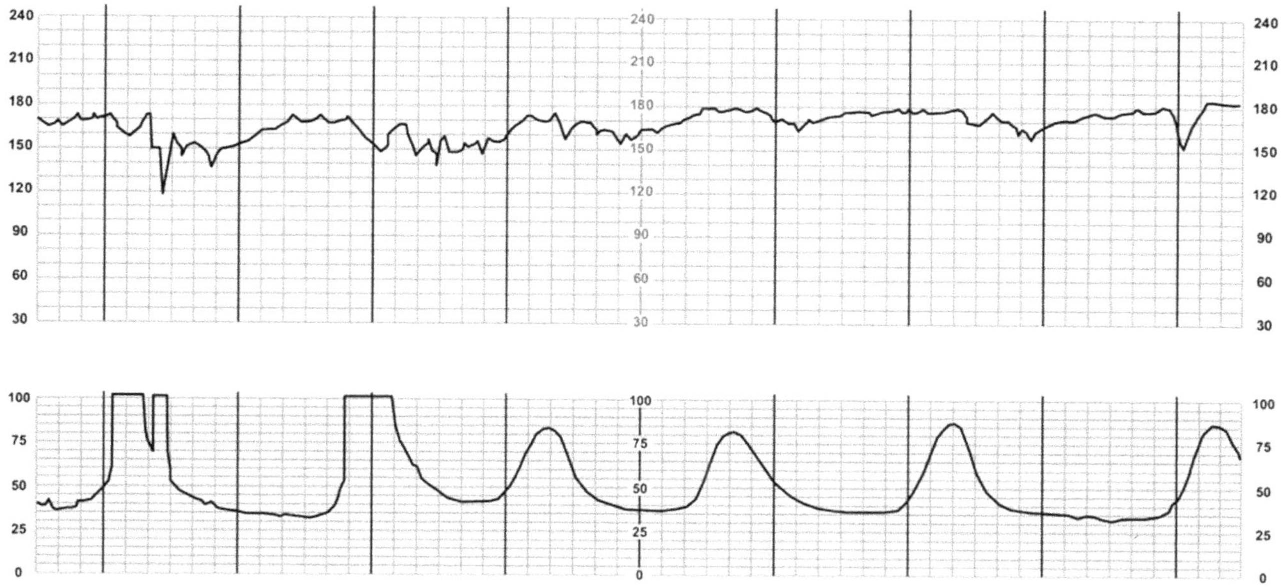

Figure 10-3e Unsatisfactory CST

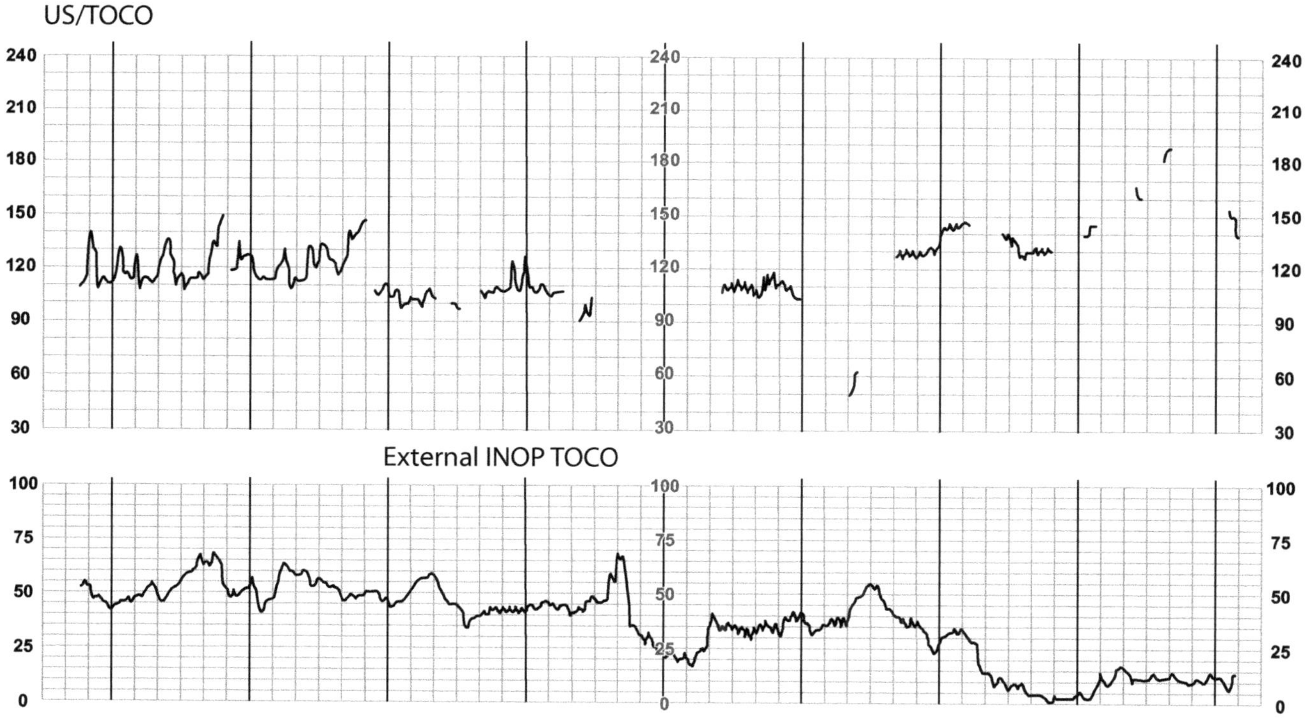

A negative CST is highly reliable and correlates with good fetal outcomes (Lagrew, 1995). In the absence of clinical deterioration, the interval between CSTs is generally 7 days, although more frequent evaluation (including NST or BPP) may be indicated for conditions such as post-term pregnancy, diabetes, intrauterine growth restriction, or hypertension (ACOG, 2014; Huddleston, 2002). Isolated or recurrent variable deceleration may occur as a result of oligohydramnios and subsequent cord compression. The appearance of variable decelerations should trigger an ultrasound evaluation of amniotic fluid volume and umbilical cord localization (Devoe, 2008). Equivocal results typically necessitate repeating the CST within 24 hours unless the woman is post term or other indications for delivery are present. Positive CSTs correlate with intrauterine growth restriction, increased incidence of late decelerations in labor, and low 5-minute Apgar scores (Lagrew, 1995). However, a significant limitation of the CST is its high false-positive rate (positive test findings in a person without disease), which can result in unnecessary intervention (Greenberg et al., 2007). False-positive rates greater than 30% have been reported following CST (Gauthier, Evertson, & Paul, 1979; Shalev et al., 1993). Therefore, management of women with positive CST results should be individualized and based on evaluation of the woman's total clinical picture (ACOG, 2014; AAP & ACOG, 2012).

FETAL BIOPHYSICAL PROFILE

In response to the high proportion of false-positive NST and CST results, Manning, Platt, and Sipos (1980) proposed an assessment of fetal well-being that combined NST results with multiple physiologic parameters observed with real-time ultrasound. The BPP was based on previous reports that fetal activities, such as breathing, decreased with hypoxia or narcosis (Manning & Platt, 1979). Furthermore, the BPP was based on the theory that acute and chronic hypoxia cause the reduction or cessation of fetal activities in a particular order, so that the absence of one or more parameters could represent the degree of fetal hypoxic stress (Manning, Morrison, Lange, & Harman, 1982).

The BPP provided improved prognostic information over other antepartum FHR tests because fetal physiologic parameters associated with both chronic (amniotic fluid volume, gross body movements, and tone) and acute (heart rate reactivity and breathing movements) hypoxia were evaluated (Manning et al., 1980). Thus, the BPP includes the assessment of the following five components: (1) fetal breathing movement, (2) gross body movement, (3) fetal tone, (4) amniotic fluid volume, and (5) FHR reactivity (NST).

The fetal activities observed during the BPP result from complex processes within the CNS and ANS, and the presence of each suggests normal neurologic function and adequate oxygenation (Vintzileos et al., 1987). Fetal activities decrease or cease as a means of reducing energy and oxygen consumption as fetal hypoxemia worsens, and it occurs in the reverse order of normal neurologic development (Table 10-3). Fetal activities that appear earliest in pregnancy (i.e., tone and movement) are usually the last to be affected; conversely, activities last to develop (i.e., breathing and FHR reactivity) are usually the first to be suppressed (Vintzileos & Knuppel, 1994). The presence of fetal activities (FHR accelerations, breathing, movement, and tone) indicates normal central oxygenation (Manning et al., 1993) depending on gestational age, whereas the clinical significance of absent activities is more difficult to determine because factors other than hypoxia can cause CNS depression

TABLE 10-3 Embryology of the CNS Centers Responsible for Fetal Activities

ACTIVITY	CNS CENTER	GESTATIONAL AGE OF DEVELOPMENT	HYPOXIA*
Tone	Cortex–subcortical	7.5–8.5 weeks	↑
Movement	Cortex–nuclei	9.0 weeks	
Breathing	Ventral Surface, 4th ventricle	20–21 weeks	
Fetal Heart rate	Posterior hypothalamus, medulla	28–32 weeks	

CNS, Central nervous system.
*The arrow indicates the order in which hypoxia affects fetal activities.
Adapted from: Manning, 1995; Vintzileos & Knuppel, 1994.

(e.g., sedatives, narcotics, anesthetics) (Manning et al., 1982; Vintzileos, Campbell, Ingardia, & Nochimson, 1983).

Clinical Application of the Biophysical Profile

Multiple studies have been undertaken worldwide to develop the scoring criteria, interpretation, and proposed management for BPP (Manning et al., 1980; Vintzileos et al., 1983). In initial descriptions, an NST was performed first, and if nonreactive after 20 minutes, the FHR was monitored for an additional 20 minutes (Vintzileos & Knuppel, 1994). An ultrasound examination followed, and a score was assigned for each parameter detected during a 30-minute observation period. The scoring criteria for BPPs are listed in Table 10-4 (Manning, 1995).

Test Procedure and Interpretation

During a real-time sonogram, the biophysical variables are monitored simultaneously until the normal criteria for each have been observed, or for a total observation period of 30 minutes. A system for BPP interpretation and management is summarized in Table 10-5. The average time to complete the BPP is 10–20 minutes when performed by an experienced sonographer (Manning, Baskett, Morrison, & Lange, 1981; Manning et al.,1982). Normal fetal gross body movement is classified by at least three rolling movements of the extremities or trunk (Vintzileos et al., 1987), and fetal tone is defined by extension of the extremities with return to flexion or by opening and closing of the fetal hand (Manning et al., 1980).

Fetal breathing is the continuous movement of the chest or abdominal walls lasting at least 30 seconds, with breath-to-breath intervals shorter than 6 seconds. Amniotic fluid volume is determined by the presence of at least one pocket of fluid measuring 2 cm or more in the vertical axis (Manning, 1995; Vintzileos & Knuppel, 1994). The NST may be performed before or after observation and assessment of the ultrasound components of the BPP (Manning, 1995; Vintzileos et al., 1987).

The usual interval between BPP examinations is 1 week (Manning et al., 1991), but more frequent testing may be used for specific high-risk conditions. In addition, the optimal gestational

TABLE 10-4 Biophysical Profile Scoring: Technique and Interpretation

BIOPHYSICAL VARIABLE	NORMAL SCORE (SCORE = 2 POINTS)	ABNORMAL (SCORE = 0 POINTS)
Fetal breathing movements	At least one episode of FBM of at least 30 seconds duration in 30 minutes	Absent FBM or no episodes >30 seconds in 30 minutes
Gross body movement	At least three discrete body/limb movements in 30 minutes (episodes of active continuous movement considered as single movement)	Two or fewer episodes of body/limb movements in 30 minutes
Fetal tone	At least one episode of active extension with return to flexion of fetal limb(s) or trunk Opening and closing of hand is considered normal tone	Either slow extension with return to partial flexion or movement of limb in full extension Absent movement
Reactive fetal heart rate (FHR)	At least two episodes of FHR accelerations of > 15 beats/min and of least 15's duration associated with fetal movement in 20 minutes	Two or greater episodes of accelerations of FHR or accelerations <15 beats/min in 20 minutes.
Qualitative amniotic fluid volume (AFV)	At least one pocket of AF that measures at least 2 cm in two perpendicular planes	Either no AF pockets or a pocket <2 cm in two perpendicular planes

Note: From "Dynamic Ultrasound-Based Fetal Assessment: The Fetal Biophysical Profile Score," by Frank Manning, 1995, *Clinical Obstetrics and Gynecology, 38*(1) p. 35. Copyright 1995 by J.B. Lippincott Company. Reprinted with permission.

TABLE 10-5 Biophysical Profile Interpretation and Suggested Management

SCORE	INTERPRETATION	PERINATAL MORTALITY WITHIN 1 WEEK WITHOUT INTERVENTION	MANAGEMENT
10/10 8 of 10 (normal fluid) 8 of 8 (NST not done)	Risk of fetal asphyxia extremely rare	1 per 1,000	• Intervention only for obstetric and maternal factors • No indication for intervention for fetal disease
8 of 10 (abnormal fluid)	Probable chronic fetal compromise	89 per 1,000	• Determine that there is functioning renal tissue and intact membranes • If so, deliver for fetal indications
6 of 10 (normal fluid)	Equivocal test, possible fetal asphyxia	Variable	• If the fetus is mature, deliver • In the immature fetus, repeat the test within 24 hours • If $< 6/10$, deliver
6 of 10 (abnormal fluid)	Probable fetal asphyxia	89 per 1,000	• Deliver for fetal indications
4 of 10	High probability of fetal asphyxia	91 per 1,000	• Deliver for fetal indications
2 of 10	Fetal asphyxia almost certain	125 per 1,000	• Deliver for fetal indications
0 of 10	Fetal asphyxia certain	600 per 1,000	• Deliver for fetal indications

Note: From "Dynamic Ultrasound-Based Fetal Assessment: The Fetal Biophysical Profile Score," by Frank Manning, 1995, *Clinical Obstetrics and Gynecology, 38*(1) p. 37. Copyright 1995 by J.B. Lippincott Company. Reprinted with permission.

age at which to initiate antepartum surveillance with the BPP has not been established with recommendations ranging from 24 to 25 weeks (Manning, 1995) to 32 weeks (ACOG, 2014; Miller et al., 1996). Gestational age must therefore be a consideration when interpreting BPP results (Oyelese & Vintzileos, 2011). As is the case with most antepartum testing methods, the interpretation of the BPP score is based on consideration of the maternal and fetal clinical situation, and a management approach based on specific pregnancy complications is also recommended (Vintzileos & Knuppel, 1994).

Efficacy of the Biophysical Profile

A BPP score of 10/10 is associated with normal fetal oxygenation and development more than 99.9% of the time (Manning, Morrison, Harmen, Lange & Menticoglau, 1987). In contrast, a significant inverse relationship exists between a worsening fetal cord pH and the absence of FHR reactivity, fetal breathing, movement, and tone—in that order (Vintzileos & Knuppel, 1994). However, there is less conformity regarding the predictive accuracy of abnormal results because of differences in study methodologies, participants, sample size, and a lack of standard criteria for BPP interpretation and divergent outcome definitions across studies. Although multiple cohort and case-controlled studies of the BPP have reported encouraging results, the BPP has been studied in only a small number of RCTs (Lalor, Fawole, Alfirevic, & Devane, 2008). Therefore, BPP scores between normal (8/10 or 10/10) and the most abnormal (0/10) require further testing and consideration when making management plans for follow-up care (Boehm & Gabbe, 2002).

Nursing Role in Biophysical Profile Testing

The BPP was developed in an antepartum testing center where the majority of ultrasound examinations were performed by nurses with special education (Manning et al., 1981). An increasing number of nurses have completed additional training to conduct a fetal assessment with real-time Doppler sonography, and the BPP interpretation by specially trained nurses has been shown to be equal to or better than that of medical subspecialists (Gegor, Paine, Costigan, & Johnson, 1994). The BPP is an ultrasound examination of limited scope that may be performed by nurses who have completed additional education and who can demonstrate competence to perform limited obstetric ultrasound (AWHONN, 2010). Nurses should verify that performing limited obstetric ultrasound is within their scope of practice as defined by state or provincial licensing bodies and is consistent with individual facility regulations (AWHONN, 2010). Nurses performing limited ultrasonography are professionally responsible for documentation of (1) specialized education including theoretical content and supervised hands-on training of initial competence; (2) ongoing competency validation via educational programs, reviews, and/or clinical update sessions; and (3) performance of ultrasound examinations in accordance with current guidelines and institutional policy (AWHONN, 2010).

Modified Biophysical Profile

Designed to simplify and decrease the time needed to complete a full BPP, the modified technique focuses on the two components most predictive of fetal outcomes, the NST and measurement of amniotic fluid volume (AAP & ACOG, 2012; ACOG, 2014). The NST as an indicator of short-term fetal well-being is the first BPP parameter impacted during an acute decline in oxygen. Amniotic fluid volume is considered a marker of long-term placental function, as decreased amniotic fluid volume can reflect a chronic decline in oxygenation status (AAP & ACOG, 2012; Devoe, 2008).

Amniotic fluid volume may reflect a normal decline near or beyond term or may be indicative of fetal hypoxia. Hypoxic fetuses demonstrate a physiologic redistribution or "shunting" of cardiac output to allow for greater oxygenation of the heart, brain, and adrenals while decreasing blood flow to other organs, such as the kidneys, gut, and skeletal system (Manning, 1995). Sustained hypoxic shunting may be followed by a decrease in renal function and then a decrease in fetal urine, which is the primary component of amniotic fluid in the third trimester. Thus, oligohydramnios can reflect long-term uteroplacental function, acute or chronic fetal asphyxia, and an increased risk for adverse perinatal outcomes (Chauhan et al., 2004). Those concepts led to the development of the modified BPP, which combines the NST and an ultrasound-obtained measure of amniotic fluid volume as a test of uteroplacental function (Nageotte, Towers, Asrat, & Freeman, 1994). Amniotic fluid volume may be assessed by either measuring the single deepest vertical cord and extremity-free pocket of fluid, or by amniotic fluid index, which represents the sum of the measurements (in centimeters) of the deepest umbilical cord-free pockets of amniotic fluid in all four abdominal quadrants (ACOG, 2014; AAP & ACOG, 2012). Oligohydramnios is commonly defined as a single 2-centimeter or less deep pocket of amniotic fluid and an AFI of 5-centimeters or less. However, randomized controlled trials (RCTs) support the use of the 2-centimeter single deepest pocket to diagnose oligohydramnios rather than the AFI (ACOG, 2014). The use of the single deepest pocket of amniotic fluid has also demonstrated a reduction in unnecessary interventions without an increase in adverse outcomes (ACOG, 2014).

A modified BPP is considered normal when the NST is reactive and if the deepest vertical pocket of amniotic fluid measures more than 2-centimeters (ACOG, 2014). The modified BPP has the advantage of requiring less time to complete, and it is associated with similar perinatal outcomes when compared with other antepartum tests (Nageotte, Towers, Asrat, Freeman, & Dorchester, 1994; Shah, Brown, Salyer, Fleischer, & Boehm, 1989).

DOPPLER ULTRASOUND VELOCIMETRY

Doppler ultra sound velocimetry is used to assess fetal blood flow primarily in the umbilical artery, middle cerebral artery, and fetal venous system (i.e., umbilical vein and ductus venosus) (Kalache & Duckelmann, 2012; Thornburg, Glantz, Giffi, & Woods, 2013). Evaluating utero-placental blood flow and fetal circulation provides important information regarding fetal adaptation and reserve, information that helps to guide fetal surveillance as well as care and management decisions (Kalache & Duckelmann, 2012; Signore et al., 2009). Doppler assessment of vascular flow, especially within the umbilical artery, is now an important adjunct in the evaluation of growth-restricted fetuses (Kalache & Duckelmann, 2012; O'Neill & Thorp, 2012; Thornburg et al., 2013). Doppler velocimetry is also enhancing the assessment and management of fetal conditions such as anemia, twin-to-twin transfusion, and cardiac function (Thornburg et al., 2013). Doppler-based studies are noninvasive, easy to perform, and have been vigorously evaluated in randomized controlled trails when compared to other fetal surveillance techniques (Boehm & Gabbe, 2002; O'Neill & Thorp, 2012).

Doppler velocimetry assesses blood flow direction, velocity, volume, and impedance or resistance to flow (O'Neill & Thorp, 2012). Doppler results obtained from the umbilical artery reflect the presence or absence of downstream resistance within the placenta. Doppler ultrasound waves are transmitted at one frequency and reflected back to the transducer at a different frequency. When directed at blood vessels, the frequency of the reflected sound is determined by the direction and velocity of the blood cells (Greenberg et al., 2012). This frequency change is called a "Doppler shift." Changes in blood flow represent systolic and diastolic shifts that occur during the cardiac cycle (Thornberget al., 2013). The Doppler test result, or S/D ratio, represents the ratio between the velocity of blood flow during systole and diastole and is a reflection of placental vascular resistance to flow (Greenberg et al., 2012). The S represents the peak systolic velocity and the D represents the velocity of flow at the end of diastole (Thornberg et al., 2013). As resistance increases, diastolic flow decreases and the S/D ratio increases (AAP & ACOG, 2012).

Umbilical artery velocimetry results correlate the best with fetal outcomes and are based on the physiologic principle that with increasing gestational age there is a decrease in placental resistance and a decrease in the systolic to diastolic ratio (Boehm & Gabbe, 2002). S/D ratios are high early in pregnancy and decrease with advancing gestational age. Doppler indices from the umbilical artery increase when 60–70% of the placental vasculature is compromised (Thompson & Trudinger, 1990). An S/D ratio greater than 3 beyond 30 weeks' gestation is considered abnormal (Greenberg et al., 2012). At the most extreme end of the spectrum, abnormal results are absent end-diastolic flow and reverse flow, respectively (Figure 10-4). When placental resistance remains elevated, there may be no

Figure 10-4 Examples of Umbilical Doppler Flow Results

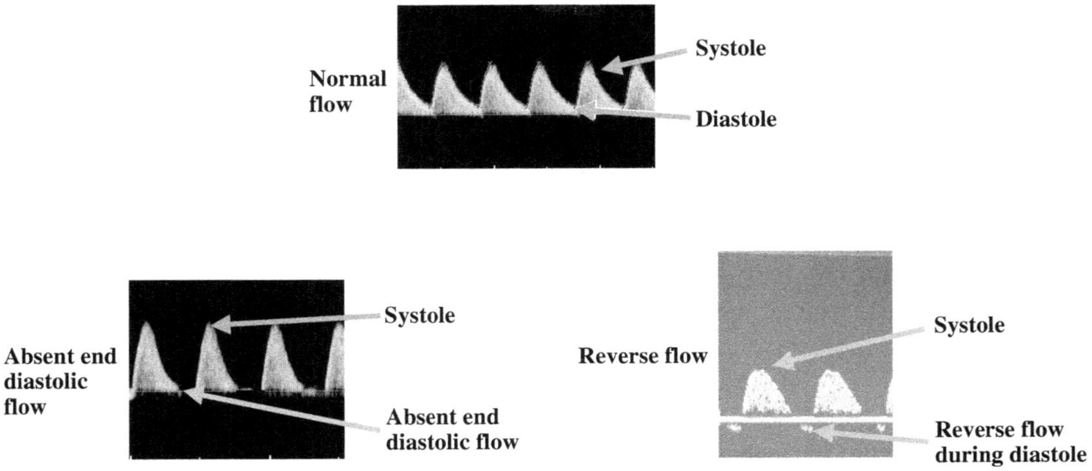

blood flow during diastole (absent end-diastolic flow); in the worst case, flow may even be reversed (reverse flow). In these cases the fetus may be severely compromised. Further testing for fetal well-being is indicated (Thornberg et al., 2013). Both absent end-diastolic flow and reverse flow are associated with an increased risk of perinatal morbidity and mortality; however, reverse flow is even more indicative of a poor outcome (Greenberg et al., 2012).

Doppler velocimetry is not recommended as a primary or independent testing modality (Greenberg et al., 2012; Signore et al., 2009), and a large number of studies have shown that blood flow investigation is of little value in low-risk pregnancies (e.g., Westergaard, Langhoff-Roos, Lingman, Marsal, & Kreiner, 2001). However, when used in high-risk pregnancies, especially in the setting of intrauterine growth restriction, the use of Doppler velocimetry significantly lowered perinatal mortality by 34% (Westergaard et al., 2001). Serial testing can be used in conjunction with other measures of fetal surveillance in growth-restricted fetuses to guide delivery timing (AAP & ACOG, 2012).

SUMMARY

A great deal remains unknown about the benefits and risks of antepartum surveillance. Adverse perinatal outcomes are infrequent and much of the existing literature suggests antenatal testing has decreased the frequency and cause of fetal death leading to good outcomes. However, in a review of the costs and benefits of fetal surveillance, Scifres and Macones (2008) stated that "in the absence of data we cannot be assured that our interventions, even if they prevent stillbirth, may not involve a tradeoff between long term neurologic dysfunction and fetal death" (p. 318). Many in the obstetric community call attention to the overwhelming limitations of reported evidence and that surveillance recommendations are based on observation and expert opinion alone (Signore et al., 2009). The majority of fetal surveillance methods do lack Level I evidence (Manning, 2009), but also face major RCT design challenges because antenatal testing is an accepted and expected component of prenatal care. Consequently designing a study comparing the outcomes of pregnancies assigned to a testing regimen versus no testing is considered unethical (Signore et al., 2009).

Numerous lists of indications for antepartum testing have been proposed and different protocols for testing recommended, but the ideal scheme has not yet been identified. Turanet al. (2007) and Kaur, Picconi, Chadha, Kruger, and Mari (2008) explored the limitations of basing management on a single testing procedure; however, the efficacy of one test to predict long-term perinatal outcomes for complicated pregnancies has not been determined. The optimal gestational age at which testing should begin continues to be the subject of research due to the confounding effects of prematurity on the predictive value of surveillance methods. Of all the surveillance techniques currently used, Doppler velocimetry-based screening is the one most rigorously evaluated in randomized trials. The inclusion of Doppler studies in high-risk pregnancies thought to be at risk for placental insufficiency is recommended. However, the optimal frequency of Doppler testing and timing of delivery based on Doppler results has not been determined (O'Neill & Thorp, 2012). Condition-specific fetal testing that takes into account the underlying pathophysiology has been proposed (Kontopoulos & Vintzileos, 2004), especially for conditions affecting uteroplacental function. Clearly the clinical value of any test is going to vary according to the underlying disease process, its rate of progression, and its propensity to cause fetal deterioration.

Research aimed at improving existing tests and technology and developing new technologies is ongoing. Nurses' responsibilities and roles are expanding in the care of high-risk pregnant women. Ongoing assessment and evaluation, patient care, education, research, and application of evidence-based interventions can improve the outcomes for both women and their newborns.

REFERENCES

American Academy of Pediatrics & American College of Obstetricians and Gynecologists. (2012). *Guidelines for perinatal care* (7th ed.). Elk Grove Village, IL: Authors.

American College of Obstetricians and Gynecologists. (2014). Antepartum fetal surveillance (Practice Bulletin No. 145). *Obstetrics and Gynecology, 124*(1), 182–192. doi:10.1097/01.AOG.0000451759.90082.7b

American College of Obstetricians and Gynecologists & American Academy of Pediatrics. (2014). *Neonatal encephalopathy and neurologic outcome* (2nd ed.). Washington, DC: Authors.

Association of Women's Health, Obstetric and Neonatal Nurses.(2006). *Advanced fetal monitoring course.* Washington DC: Author.

Association of Women's Health, Obstetric and Neonatal Nurses. (2010). *Ultrasound examinations performed by nurses in obstetrics, gynecologic, and reproductive medicine settings: Clinical competencies and education guide* (3rd ed.). Washington, DC: Author.

Besinger, R. E., & Johnson, T. R. (1989). Doppler recordings of fetal movement: Clinical correlation with real-time ultrasound. *Obstetrics and Gynecology, 74*(2), 277–280.

Blackburn, S. (2013). Neurologic, muscular, and sensory systems. In S. T. Blackburn (Ed.), *Maternal, fetal, and neonatal physiology: A clinical perspective* (4th ed., pp. 509–559). St. Louis, MO: Saunders.

Boehm, F. H., Fields, L. M., Hutchison, J. M., Bowen, A.W., & Vaughn, W. K. (1986). The indirectly obtained fetal heart rate: Comparison of first and second generation electronic fetal monitors. *American Journal of Obstetrics and Gynecology, 155*(1), 10–14.

Boehm, F. H., & Gabbe, S. G. (2002). Putting it all together. *Clinical Obstetrics, 45*(4), 1063–1068.

Castillo, R. A., Devoe, L. D., Arthur, M., Searle, N., Metheny, W. P., & Ruedrich, D. A. (1989). The preterm nonstress test: Effects of gestational age and length of study. *American Journal of Obstetrics and Gynecology, 160*(1), 172–175.

Chauhan, S. P., Doherty, D. D., Magann, E. F., Cahanding, F., Moreno, F., & Klausen, J. H. (2004). Amniotic fluid index vs. single deepest pockets technique during modified biophysical profile: A randomized clinical trial. *American Journal of Obstetrics and Gynecology, 191*(2), 661–668.

Christensen, F. C., & Rayburn, W. F. (1999). Fetal movement counts. *Obstetrics and Gynecology Clinics of North America, 26*(4), 607–621.

Citro, G., Luisi, S., Mezzesimi, A., Cavicchioli, C, & Petraglia, F. (2005). Maternal position during nonstress test and fetal heart rate patterns. *Acta Obstetricia et Gynecology Scandinavia, 84*(4), 335–338.

Clark, S. L., Sabey, P., & Jolley, K. (1989). Nonstress testing with acoustic stimulation and amniotic fluid volume assessment: 5973 tests without unexpected fetal death. *American Journal of Obstetrics and Gynecology, 160*(3), 694–697.

Conde, A., Teves, C., & Figueiredo, B. (2011). Maternal caffeine intake and associated risk factors: Effects on fetal growth and activity. *Acta Medica Portuguesa, 24*(2), 241–248.

Dawes, G. S., Houghton, C. R., Redman, C. W., & Visser, G. H. (1982). Pattern of normal fetal heart rate. *British Journal of Obstetrics and Gynaecology, 89*(4), 276–284.

Devoe, L. D. (1999). Nonstress testing and contraction stress testing. *Obstetrics and Gynecology Clinics of North America, 26*(4), 535–556.

Devoe, L. D. (2008). Antenatal fetal assessment: Contraction stress test, nonstress test, vibroacoustic stimulation, amniotic fluid volume, biophysical profile, and modified biophysical profile—an overview. *Seminars in Perinatology, 32*(4), 247–252. doi:10.1053/j.semperi.2008.04.005.

Devoe, L. D., & Jones, C. R. (2002). Nonstress test: Evidence-based use in high-risk pregnancy. *Clinical Obstetrics and Gynecology, 45*(4), 986–992.

Devoe, L. D., Murray, C., Youssif, A., & Arnaud, M. (1993). Maternal caffeine consumption and fetal behavior in normal third-trimester pregnancy. *American Journal of Obstetrics and Gynecology, 168*(4), 1105–1112.

deVries, J. I., & Fong, B. F. (2006). Normal fetal motility: An overview. *Ultrasound Obstetrics and Gynecology, 27*(6), 701–711.

deVries, J. I., Visser, G. H., & Prechtl, H. F. (1982). The emergence of fetal behavior: I. Qualitative aspects. *Early Human Development, 7*(4), 301–322.

DiPietro, J. A. (2012). Maternal stress in pregnancy: Considerations for fetal development. *Journal of Adolescent Health, 51* (2, Suppl.), S3–S8. doi:10.1016/j.jadohealth.2012.04.008

DiPietro, J. A., Costigan, K. A., & Gurewitsch, E. D (2003). Fetal response to induced maternal stress. *Early Human Development, 74*(2), 125–138.

DiPietro, J. A., Costigan, K. A., & Pressman, E. K. (1999). Fetal movement detection: Comparison of the Toitu actograph with ultrasound from 20 weeks gestation. *Journal of Maternal–Fetal Medicine, 8*(6), 237–242.

DiPietro, J. A., Hilton, S. C., Hawkins, M., Costigan, K. A., & Pressman, E. K. (2002). Maternal stress and affect influence fetal neurobehavioral development. *Developmental Psychology, 38*(5), 659–668.

DiPietro, J. A., Kivlighan, K. T., Costigan, K. A., Rubin, S. E., Shiffler, D. E., . . . Pillion, J. P. (2010). Prenatal antecedents of newborn neurological maturation. *Child Development, 81*(1), 115–130. doi:10.1111/j.1467-8624.2009.01384.x

Drogtrop, A. P., Ubels, R., & Nijhuis, J. G. (1990). The association between fetal body movements, eye movements, and heart rate patterns in pregnancies between 25 and 30 weeks of gestation. *Early Human Development, 23*(1), 67–73.

Eller, D. P., Stramm, S. L., & Newman, R. B. (1992). The effect of maternal intravenous glucose administration on fetal activity. *American Journal of Obstetrics and Gynecology, 167*(4, Pt. 1), 1071–1074.

Evertson, L. R., Gauthier, R. J., Schifrin, B. S., & Paul, R. H. (1979). Antepartum fetal heart rate testing. I. Evolution of the nonstress test. *American Journal of Obstetrics and Gynecology, 133*(1), 29–33.

Freeman, R. K. (1975). The use of the oxytocin challenge test for antepartum clinical evaluation of uteroplacental respiratory function. *American Journal of Obstetrics and Gynecology, 121*(4), 481–489.

Freeman, R. K., Garite, T. J., Nageotte, M. P., & Miller, L. A. (2012). *Fetal heart rate monitoring* (4th ed.). Philadelphia: Lippencott Williams & Wilkins.

Gagnon, R., Hunse, C., & Patrick, J. (1988). Fetal responses to vibratory acoustic stimulation: Influence of basal heart rate. *American Journal of Obstetrics and Gynecology, 159*(4), 835–839.

Garite, T. (2012). Intrapartum fetal evaluation. In S. Gabbe, J. Niebyl, J. Simpson, M. Landon, H. Galan, E. Jaunaux, & D. Driscoll (Eds.), *Obstetrics: Normal and problem pregnancies* (6th ed., pp. 330–361). Philadelphia: Churchill Livingstone.

Gauthier, R. J., Evertson, L. R., & Paul, R. H. (1979). Antepartum fetal heart rate testing. II. Intrapartum fetal heart rate observation and newborn outcome following a positive contraction stress test. *American Journal of Obstetrics and Gynecology, 133*(1), 34–39.

Gegor, C. L., Paine, L. L, Costigan, K., & Johnson, T. R. (1994). Interpretation of biophysical profiles by nurses and physicians. *Journal of Obstetric, Gynecologic, and Neonatal Nursing, 23*(5), 405–410.

Glantz, C., & D'Amico, M. L. (2001). Lack of relationship between variable decelerations during reactive nonstress tests and oligohydramnios. *American Journal of Perinatology, 18*(3), 129–135.

Greenberg, M. B., Druzin, M. L., & Gabbe, S. G. (2012). Antepartum fetal evaluation. In S. G. Gabbe, J. R. Neibyl, J. L. Simpson, M. Landon, H. Galan, E. Jaunaux, & D. Driscoll. (Eds.). *Obstetrics: Normal and problem pregnancies* (6th ed., pp. 237–263). Philadelphia: Saunders.

Gribbin, C., & James, D. (2004). Assessing fetal health. *Best Practice and Research: Clinical Obstetrics and Gynaecology, 18*(3), 411–424.

Grivell, R. M., Alfirevic, Z., Gyte, G. M., Devane, D. (2012). Antenatal cardiotocography for fetal assessment. *Cochrane Database of Systematic Reviews,* Issue 12 (Article No. CD007863). doi:10.1002/14651858.CD007863.pub3

Groome, L. J., Mooney, D. M., Holland, S. B., Bentz, L. S., Atterbury, J. L., & Dykman, R. A. (1997). The heart rate deceleratory response in low-risk human fetuses: Effect of stimulus intensity on response topography. *Developmental Psychobiology, 30*(2), 103–113.

Groome, L. J., Mooney, D. M., Holland, S. B., Smith, L. A., & Atterbury, J. L. (1997). Heart rate response in individual human fetuses to stimulation with a low-intensity sound. *Journal of Maternal–Fetal Investigation, 7*, 105–110.

Groome, L. J., Owen, J., Singh, K. P., Neely, C. L., & Gaudier, F. L. (1992). Spontaneous movement of the human fetus at 18–22 weeks of gestation: Evidence of early organization of the active rest cycle. *Journal of Maternal–Fetal Investigation, 2*, 27–32.

Groome, L. J., Swiber, M. J., Bentz, L. S., Holland, S. B., & Atterbury, J. L. (1995). Maternal anxiety during pregnancy: Effect on fetal behavior at 38 to 40 weeks of gestation. *Journal of Developmental & Behavioral Pediatrics, 16*(6), 391–396.

Groome, L. J., Swiber, M. J., Holland, S. B., Bentz, L. S., Atterbury, J. L., & Trimm, R. F., III. (1999). Spontaneous motor activity in the perinatal infant before and after birth: Stability in individual differences. *Developmental Psychobiology, 35*(1), 15–34.

Groome, L. J., & Watson, J. E. (1992). Assessment of in utero neurobehavioral development. I. Fetal behavioral states. *Journal of Maternal–Fetal Investigation, 2*, 183–194.

Hatoum, N., Clapp, J. F., III, Newman, M. R., Dajani, N., & Amini, S. B. (1997). Effects of maternal exercise on fetal activity in late gestation. *Journal of Maternal-Fetal Medicine, 6*(3), 134–139.

Heazell, A. E., & Froen, J. F. (2008). Methods of fetal movement counting and detection of fetal compromise. *Journal of Obstetrics and Gynecology, 28*(2), 147–154. doi:10.1080/01443610801912618

Hijazi, Z. R., & East, C. E. (2009). Factors affecting maternal perception of fetal movement. *Obstetrical Gynecological Survey, 64*(7), 489–497.doi:10.1097/OGX.0b013e3181a8237a

Hoskins, I. A., Frieden, F. J., & Young, B. K. (1991). Variable decelerations in reactive nonstress tests with decreased amniotic fluid index predict fetal compromise. *American Journal of Obstetrics and Gynecology, 165*(4, Pt. 1), 1094–1098.

Huddleston, J. F. (2002). Continued utility of the contraction stress test? *Clinical Obstetrics and Gynecology, 45*(4), 1005–1014.

Institute for Safe Medication Practices. (2007). *High-alert medications.* Huntingdon Valley, PA: Author. Retrieved from http://www.ismp.org/tools/highalertmedicationLists.asp

Jaschevatzky, O. E., Marom, D., Ostrovsky, P., Ellenbogen, A., Anderman, S., & Ballas, S. (1998). Significance of sporadic deceleration during antepartum testing in term pregnancies. *American Journal of Perinatology, 15*(5), 291–294.

Jensen, O. H., & Flottorp, G. (1982). A method for controlled sound stimulation of the human fetus. *Scandinavian Audiology, 11*(3), 145–150.

Johnson, T. R. (1994). Maternal perception and Doppler detection of fetal movement. *Clinics in Perinatology, 21*(4), 765–777.

Johnson, T. R., Jordan, E. T., & Paine, L. L. (1990). Doppler recordings of fetal movement. II. Comparison with maternal perception. *Obstetrics and Gynecology, 76*(1), 42–43.

Kalache, K. D., & Duckelmann, A. M. (2012). Doppler in obstetrics: Beyond the umbilical artery. *Clinical Obstetrics and Gynecology, 55*(1), 288–295. doi:10.1097/GRF.0b013e3182488156

Kaur, S., Picconi, J. L., Chadha, R., Kruger, M., & Mari, G. (2008). Biophysical profile in the treatment of intrauterine growth-restricted fetuses who weigh <1000g. *American Journal of Obstetrics and Gynecology, 199*(3), 264.e1–264.e4. doi:10.1016/j.ajog.2008.06.074

Keegan, K. A., & Paul, R. H. (1980). Antepartum fetal heart rate testing. IV. The nonstress as a primary approach. *American Journal of Obstetrics and Gynecology, 136*(1), 75–80.

Kochanek, K. D., Kirmeyer, S. E., Martin, J. A., Strabino, D. M., & Guyer, B. (2012). Annual summary of vital statistics: 2009. *Pediatrics, 129*(2), 338–348. doi:10.1542/peds.2011-3435

Kontopoulos, E. V., & Vintzileos, A. M. (2004). Condition-specific antepartum fetal testing. *American Journal of Obstetrics and Gynecology, 191*(5), 1546–1551.

Kopecky, E. A., Ryan, M. L., Barrett, J. F., Seaward, P. G., Ryan, G., Koren, G., & Amankwah, K. (2000). Fetal response to maternally administered morphine. *American Journal of Obstetrics and Gynecology, 183*(2), 424–430.

Krebs, H. B., Petres, R. E., Dunn, L. J., & Smith, P. J. (1982). Intrapartum fetal heart rate monitoring: VI. Prognostic significance of accelerations. *American Journal of Obstetrics and Gynecology, 142*(3), 297–305.

Lagrew, D. C., Jr. (1995). The contraction stress test. *Clinical Obstetrics and Gynecology, 38*(1), 11–25.

Lalor, J. G., Fawole, B., Alfirevic, Z., & Devane, D. (2008). Biophysical profile for fetal assessment in high risk pregnancies. *Cochrane Database of Systematic Reviews,* Issue 1 (Article No. CD00038). doi:10.1002/14651858.CD000038.pub.2

Lee, C. Y., DiLoreto, P. C., & O'Lane, J. M. (1975). A study of fetal heart rate acceleration patterns. *Obstetrics and Gynecology, 45*(2), 142–146.

Lipitz, S., Barkai, E., Rabinovici, J., & Mashiach, S. (1987). Breast stimulation test and oxytocin challenge test in fetal surveillance: A prospective randomized study. *American Journal of Obstetrics and Gynecology, 157*(5), 1178–1181.

Lowery, C. L., Russell, W. A., Jr., Baggot, P. J., Wilson, J. D., Walts, R. C., . . . Murphy, P. (1997). Time quantified detection of fetal movements using a new fetal movement algorithm. *American Journal of Perinatology, 14*(1), 7–12.

Macones, G. A., Hankins, G. D., Spong, C. Y., Hauth, J. D., & Moore, T. (2008). The 2008 National Institute of Child Health and Development workshop report on electronic fetal monitoring: Update on definitions, interpretation, and research guidelines. *Obstetrics and Gynecology, 112*(3), 661–666 doi:10.1097/AOG.0b013e3181841395; *Journal of Obstetric, Gynecologic and Neonatal Nursing, 37*(5), 510–515. doi:10.1111/j.1552-6909.2008.00284.x

Manders, M. A., Sonder, G. J., Mulder, E. J., & Visser, G. H. (1997). The effects of maternal exercise on fetal heart rate and movement patterns. *Early Human Development, 48*(3), 237–247.

Mangesi, L., Hofmeyr, G. J., & Smith, V. (2007). Fetal movement counting for assessment of fetal wellbeing. *Cochrane Database of Systematic Reviews,* Issue 1 (Article No.CD004909). doi: 10.1002/14651858.CD004909.pub2

Manning, F. A. (1995). Dynamic ultrasound-based fetal assessment: The fetal biophysical profile score. *Clinical Obstetrics and Gynecology, 38*(1), 26–44.

Manning, F. A. (2009). Antenatal fetal testing: A critical appraisal. *Current Opinions in Obstetrics and Gynecology, 21*(4), 348–352. doi:10.1097/GCO.0b013e32832ae0b3

Manning, F. A., Baskett, T. F., Morrison, I., & Lange, I. (1981). Fetal biophysical profile scoring: A prospective study in 1,184 high-risk patients. *American Journal of Obstetrics and Gynecology, 140*(3), 289–294.

Manning, F. A., Harman, C. R., Menticoglou, S., & Morrison, I. (1991). Assessment of fetal well-being with ultrasound. *Obstetrics and Gynecology Clinics of North America, 18*(4), 891–905.

Manning, F. A., Morrison, I., Harman, C. R., Lange, I. R., & Menticoglau, S. (1987). Fetal assessment based on fetal biophysical profile scoring: Experience in 19,221 referred high-risk pregnancies, II. An analysis of false-negative fetal deaths. *American Journal of Obstetrics and Gynecology, 157*(4 Pt. 1), 880–884.

Manning, F. A., Morrison, I., Lange, I. R., & Harman, C. (1982). Antepartum determination of fetal health: Composite biophysical profile scoring. *Clinics in Perinatology, 9*(2), 285–296.

Manning, F. A., & Platt, L. D. (1979). Maternal hypoxemia and fetal breathing movements. *Obstetrics and Gynecology, 53*(6), 758–760.

Manning, F. A., Platt, L. D., & Sipos, L. (1980). Antepartum fetal evaluation: Development of a fetal biophysical profile. *American Journal of Obstetrics and Gynecology, 136*(6), 787–795.

Manning, F. A., Snijders, R., Harman, C. R., Nicolaides, K., Menticoglou, S., & Morrison, I. (1993). Fetal biophysical profile score. VI. Correlation with antepartum umbilical venous fetal pH. *American Journal of Obstetrics and Gynecology, 169*(4), 755–763.

Marden, D., McDuffie, R. S., Jr., Allen, R., & Abitz, D. (1997). A randomized controlled trial of a new fetal acoustic stimulation test for fetal well-being. *American Journal of Obstetrics and Gynecology, 176*(6), 1386–1388.

Meis, P. J., Ureda, J. R., Swain, M., Kelly, R. T., Penry, M., & Sharp, P. (1986). Variable decelerations during nonstress tests are not a sign of fetal compromise. *American Journal of Obstetrics and Gynecology, 154*(3), 586–590.

Miller, D. A., Rabello, Y. A., & Paul, R. H. (1996). The modified biophysical profile: Antepartum testing in the 1990s. *American Journal of Obstetrics and Gynecology, 174*(3), 812–817.

Miller-Slade, D., Gloeb, D. J., Bailey, S., Bendell, A., Interlandi, E., Kline-Kaye, V., & Kroesen, J. (1991). Acoustic stimulation-induced fetal response compared to traditional nonstress testing. *Journal of Obstetric, Gynecologic, and Neonatal Nursing, 20*(2), 160–167.

Moffatt, F. W., & van den Hof, M. (1997). Semi-Fowler's positioning, lateral tilts, and their effects on nonstress tests. *Journal of Obstetric, Gynecologic and Neonatal Nursing, 26*(5), 551–557.

Naef, R. W., III, Morrison, J. C., Washburne, J. F., McLaughlin, B. N., Perry, K. G., Jr., & Roberts, W. E. (1994). Assessment of fetal well-being using the nonstress test in the home setting. *Obstetrics and Gynecology, 84*(3), 424–426.

Nageotte, M. P., Towers, C. V., Asrat, T., & Freeman, R. K. (1994). Perinatal outcome with the modified biophysical profile. *American Journal of Obstetrics and Gynecology, 170*(6), 1672–1676.

Nageotte, M. P., Towers, C. V., Asrat, T., Freeman, R. K., & Dorchester, W. (1994). The value of a negative antepartum test: Contraction stress test and modified biophysical profile. *Obstetrics and Gynecology, 84*(2), 231–234.

Nathan, E. B., Haberman, S., Burgess, T., & Minkoff, H. (2000). The relationship of maternal position to the results of brief nonstress tests: A randomized clinical trial. *American Journal of Obstetrics and Gynecology, 182*(5), 1070–1072.

National Institute of Child Health and Human Development Research Planning Workshop. (1997). Electronic fetal heart rate monitoring: Research guidelines for interpretation. *Journal of Obstetrics, Gynecology and Neonatal Nursing, 26*(6), 635–640.

Nijhuis, J. G., Prechtl, H. F., Martin, C. B., Jr., & Bots, R. S. (1982). Are there behavioral states in the human fetus? *Early Human Development, 6*(2), 177–195.

Nyman, M., Barr, M., & Westgren, M. (1992). A four-year follow-up of hearing and development in children exposed in utero to vibro-acoustic stimulation. *British Journal of Obstetrics and Gynaecology, 99*(8), 685–688.

Oki, E. Y., Keegan, K. A., Freeman, R. K., & Dorchester, W. L. (1987). The breast-stimulation contraction stress test. *Journal of Reproductive Medicine, 32*(12), 919–932.

O'Leary, J. A., Andrinopoulos, G. C., & Giordano, P. C. (1980). Variable decelerations and the nonstress test: An indication of cord compromise. *American Journal of Obstetrics and Gynecology, 137*(6), 704–706.

Olesen, A. G., & Svare, J. A. (2004). Decreased fetal movements: Background, assessment and clinical management. *Acta Obstetricia et Gynecologica Scandinavica, 83*(9), 818–826.

Olofsson, P., Thuring-Jonsson, A., & Marsal, K. (1996). Uterine and umbilical circulation during the oxytocin challenge test. *Ultrasound in Obstetrics and Gynecology, 8*(4), 247–251.

O'Neill, E., & Thorp, J. (2012). Antepartum evaluation of the fetus and fetal well being. *Clinical Obstetrics and Gynecology, 55*(3), 722–730. doi:10.1097/GRF.0b013e318253b318

Onyeije, C. I., & Divon, M. Y. (2001). The impact of maternal ketonuria on fetal test results in the setting of postterm pregnancy. *American Journal of Obstetrics and Gynecology, 184*(4), 713–718.

Oyelese, Y., & Vintzileos, A. (2011). The uses and limitations of the fetal biophysical profile. *Clinical Perinatology, 38*(1), 47–64. doi:10.1016/j.clp.2010.12.008

Patrick, J., Campbell, K., Carmichael, L., Natale, R., & Richardson, B. (1982). Patterns of gross fetal body movements over 24-hr observation intervals during the last 10 weeks of pregnancy. *American Journal of Obstetrics and Gynecology, 142*(4), 363–371.

Pattison, N., & McCowan, L. (2010). Cardiotocography for antepartum fetal assessment. *Cochrane Database of Systematic Reviews,* Issue 1 (Article No. CD001068). doi:10.1002/14651858.CD001068

Paul, R. H., & Miller, D. A. (1995). Nonstress test. *Clinical Obstetrics and Gynecology, 38*(1), 3–10.

Pearson, J. F., & Weaver, J. B. (1976). Fetal activity and fetal wellbeing: An evaluation. *British Medical Journal,* 1(6021), 1305–1307.

Perlman, J. M. (2006). Intrapartum asphyxia and cerebral palsy: Is there a link? *Clinics in Perinatology,33*(2), 335–353.

Pietrantoni, M., Angel, J. L., Parsons, M. T., McClain, L., Arango, H. A., & Spellacy, W. N. (1991). Human fetal response to vibroacoustic stimulation as a function of stimulus duration. *Obstetrics and Gynecology, 78*(5, Pt. 1), 807–811.

Pillai, M., & James, D. (1990). Are the behavioral states of the newborn comparable to those of the fetus? *Early Human Development, 22*(1), 39–49.

Rabinowitz, R., Persitz, E., & Sadovsky, E. (1983). The relation between fetal heart rate accelerations and fetal movements. *Obstetrics and Gynecology, 61*(1), 16–18.

Rayburn, W. F. (1982). Antepartum fetal assessment: Monitoring fetal activity. *Clinics in Perinatology, 9*, 1–14.

Rayburn, W. F. (1990). Fetal body movement monitoring. *Obstetrics and Gynecology Clinics of North America, 17*(1), 95–110.

Read, J. A., & Miller, F. C. (1977). Fetal heart rate acceleration in response to acoustic stimulation as a measure of fetal well-being. *American Journal of Obstetrics and Gynecology, 129*(5), 512–517.

Reddy, U. M., Abuhamad, A. Z., Levine, D., & Saad, G. R. (2014). Fetal imaging: executive summary of a Joint Eunice Kennedy Shriver Nationsl Institute of Child Health and Human Development, Society for Maternal–Fetal Medicine, American Institute of Ultrasound in Medicine, American College of Obstetricians and Gynecologists, American College of Radiology, Society for Pediatric Radiology, and Society of Radiologists in Ultrasound Fetal Imaging Workshop. *Obstetrics and Gynecology, 123,* 1070–1082.

Reece, E. A., Hagay, Z., Garafalo, J., & Hobbins, J. C. (1992). A controlled trial of self-nonstress test versus assisted nonstress test in the evaluation of fetal well-being. *American Journal of Obstetrics and Gynecology, 166*(2), 489–492.

Ribbert, L. S., Snijders, R. J., Nicolaides, K. H., & Visser, G. H. (1990). Relationship of fetal biophysical profile and blood gas values at cordocentesis in severely growth-restricted fetuses. *American Journal of Obstetrics and Gynecology, 163*(2), 569–571.

Rizk, B., Atterbury, J. L., & Groome, L. J. (1996). Reproductive risks of cocaine. *Human Reproduction Update, 2*(1), 43–55.

Rochard, F., Schifrin, B. S., Goupil, F., Legrand, H., Blottiere, J., & Sureau, C. (1976). Nonstressed fetal heart rate monitoring in the antepartum period. *American Journal of Obstetrics and Gynecology, 126*(6), 699–706.

Sadovsky, E., & Yaffe, H. (1973). Daily fetal movement recording and fetal prognosis. *Obstetrics and Gynecology, 41*(6), 845–850.

Saraçoğlu, F., Göl, K., Sahin, I., Türkkani, B., & Oztopçu, C. (1999). The predictive value of fetal acoustic stimulation. *Journal of Perinatology, 19*(2), 103–105.

Sarno, A. P., Ahn, M. O., Phelan, J. P., & Paul, R. H. (1990). Fetal acoustic stimulation in the early intrapartum period as a predictor of subsequent of fetal condition. *American Journal of Obstetrics and Gynecology, 162*(3), 762–767.

Sarno, A. P., Jr., & Bruner, J. P. (1990). Fetal acoustic stimulation as a possible adjunct to diagnostic obstetric ultrasound: A preliminary report. *Obstetrics and Gynecology, 76*(4), 668–670.

Schellpfeffer, M. A., Hoyle, D., & Johnson, J. W. (1985). Antepartal uterine hypercontractility secondary to nipple stimulation. *Obstetrics and Gynecology, 65*(4), 588–591.

Scifres, C. M., & Macones, G. A. (2008). Antenatal testing–benefits and costs. *Seminars in Perinatology, 32*(4): 318–321. doi:10.1053/j.semperi.2008.04.017

Serafini, P., Lindsay, M. B., Nagey, D. A., Pupkin, M. J., Tseng, P., & Crenshaw, C., Jr. (1984). Antepartum fetal heart rate response to sound stimulation: The acoustic stimulation test. *American Journal of Obstetrics and Gynecology, 148*(1), 41–45.

Shah, D. M., Brown, J. E., Salyer, S. L., Fleischer, A. C., & Boehm, F. H. (1989). A modified scheme for biophysical profile scoring. *American Journal of Obstetrics and Gynecology, 160*(3), 586–591.

Shalev, E., Zalel, Y., & Weiner, E. (1993). A comparison of the nonstress test, oxytocin challenge test, Doppler velocimetry, and biophysical profile in predicting umbilical vein pH in growth-retarded fetuses. *International Journal of Gynaecology and Obstetrics, 43*(1), 15–19.

Signore, C., Freeman, R., & Spong, C. (2009). Antenatal testing-a reevaluation: Executive summary of a Eunice Kennedy Shriver National Institute of Child Health and Human Development workshop. *Obstetrics and Gynecology, 113*(4), 687–701. doi:10.1097/AOG.0b013e318197bd8a

Simpson, K. R., & Knox, G. E. (2009). Oxytocin as a high-alert medication: Implications for perinatal practice. *MCN: American Journal of Maternal Child Nursing, 34*(1), 8–15. doi: 10.1097/01.NMC.0000343859.62828.ee

Smith, C. V. (1995). Vibroacoustic stimulation. *Clinical Obstetrics and Gynecology, 38*(1), 68–77.

Smith, C. V., Phelan, J. P., Nguyen, H. N., Jacobs, N., & Paul, R. H. (1988). Continuing experience with the fetal acoustic stimulation test. *Journal of Reproductive Medicine, 33*(4), 365–368.

Smith, C. V., Phelan, J. P., Paul, R. H., & Broussard, P. (1985). Fetal acoustic stimulation testing: A retrospective experience with the fetal acoustic stimulation test. *American Journal of Obstetrics and Gynecology, 153*(5), 567–569.

Smith, C. V., Phelan, J. P., Platt, L. D., Broussard, P., & Paul, R. H. (1986). Fetal acoustic stimulation testing. II. A randomized clinical comparison with the nonstress test. *American Journal of Obstetrics and Gynecology, 155*(1), 131–134.

Snijders, R. J., McLaren, R., & Nicolaides, K. H. (1990). Computer-assisted analysis of fetal heart rate patterns at 20–41 weeks' gestation. *Fetal Diagnosis and Therapy, 5*(2), 79–83.

Sontag, L. W., & Wallace, R. E. (1936). Changes in the rate of human fetal heart rate response to vibratory stimuli. *American Journal of Diseases of Children, 51*, 383.

Strijbis, E., Oudman, I., van Essen, P., & MacLennan, A. H. (2006). Cerebral palsy and the application of the international criteria for acute intrapartum hypoxia. *Obstetrics and Gynecology, 107*(6), 1357–1365.

Szymanski, L. M., & Satin, A. J. (2012). Exercise in pregnancy: Fetal response to current public health guidelines. *Obstetrics and Gynecology, 119*(3), 603–610. doi:10.1097/AOG.0b013e31824760b5

Tan, K. H., & Sabapathy, A. (2001). Fetal manipulation for facilitating tests of fetal wellbeing. *Cochrane Database of Systematic Reviews,* Issue 4 (Article No. CD003396). doi:10.1002/14651858.CD003396

Tan, K. H., & Sabapathy, A. (2010). Maternal glucose administration for facilitating tests of fetal well-being. *Cochrane Database of Systematic Reviews,* Issue 9 (Article No. CD003397). doi:10.1002/146511858.CD003397.pub2

Tan, K. H., & Smyth, R. (2010). Fetal vibroacoustic stimulation for facilitation of tests of fetal well-being. *Cochrane Database of Systematic Reviews,* Issue 1 (Article No. CD002963). doi:10.1002/14651858.CD002963

Thaler, I., Goodman, J. D., & Dawes, G. S. (1980). Effects of maternal cigarette smoking on fetal breathing and fetal movements. *American Journal of Obstetrics and Gynecology, 138*(3), 282–287.

Thompson, R. S., & Trudinger, B. J. (1990). Doppler waveform pulsatility index and resistance, pressure and flow in the umbilical placental circulation: An investigation using a mathematical model. *Ultrasound in Medical Biology, 16*(5), 449–458.

Thornburg, L. L., Glantz, J. C., Giffi, C., & Woods, J. R. (2013). Fetal assessment by Doppler velocimetry. In L. L. Thornburg, J. C. Glantz, C. Giffi, & J. R. Woods (Eds.). *Fetal heart rate monitoring: Pathophysiology and practice* (pp.143–160), Rochester, NY: University Press.

Timor-Tritsch, I. E., Dierker, L. J., Hertz, R. H., Deogan, N. C., & Rosen, M. G. (1978). Studies of antepartum behavioral state in the human fetus at term. *American Journal of Obstetrics and Gynecology, 132*(5), 524–528.

Timor-Tritsch, I. E., Dierker, L. J., Jr., Hertz, R. H., & Rosen, M. G. (1979). Fetal movement: A brief review. *Clinical Obstetrics and Gynecology, 22*(3), 583–592.

Trudinger, B. J., & Boylan, P. (1980). Antepartum fetal heart rate monitoring: Value of sound stimulation. *Obstetrics and Gynecology, 55*(2), 265–268.

Turan, S., Turan, O. M., Berg, C., Moyano, D., Bhide, A., Bower,S., . . . Baschat, A. A. (2007). Computerized fetal heart rate analysis, Doppler ultrasound and biophysical profile score in the prediction of acid-base status of growth-restricted fetuses. *Ultrasound in Obstetrics and Gynecology, 30*(5), 750–756.

Velazquez, M. D., & Rayburn, W. F. (2002). Antenatal evaluation of the fetus using fetal movement monitoring. *Clinical Obstetrics and Gynecology, 45*(4), 993–1004.

Vintzileos, A. M. (1995). Antepartum fetal surveillance. *Clinical Obstetrics and Gynecology, 38*(1), 1–2.

Vintzileos, A. M. (2000). Antenatal assessment for the detection of fetal asphyxia: An evidenced-based approach using indication-specific testing. *Annals of the New York Academy of Sciences, 900,* 137–150.

Vintzileos, A. M., Campbell, W. A., Ingardia, C. J., & Nochimson, D. J. (1983). The fetal biophysical profile and its predictive value. *Obstetrics and Gynecology, 62*(3), 271–278.

Vintzileos, A. M., Gaffney, S. E., Salinger, L. M., Kontopoulos, V. G., Campbell, W. A., & Nochimson, D. J. (1987). The relationships among the fetal biophysical profile, umbilical cord pH, and Apgar scores. *American Journal of Obstetrics and Gynecology, 157*(3), 627–631.

Vintzileos, A. M., & Knuppel, R. A. (1994). Multiple parameter biophysical testing in the prediction of fetal acid-base status. *Clinics in Perinatology, 21*(4), 823–848.

Visser, G. H., Bekedam, D. J., & Ribbert, L. S. (1990). Changes in antepartum heart rate patterns with progressive deterioration of the fetal condition. *International Journal of Biomedical Computing, 25*(4), 239–246.

Visser, G. H., Sadovsky, G., & Nicolaides, K. H. (1990). Antepartum heart rate patterns in small-for-gestational-age third-trimester fetuses: Correlations with blood gas values obtained at cordocentesis. *American Journal of Obstetrics and Gynecology, 162*(3), 698–703.

Walker, D., Grimwade, J., & Wood, C. (1971). Intrapartum noise: A component of the fetal environment. *American Journal of Obstetrics and Gynecology, 109*(1), 92–95.

Walkinshaw, S., Cameron, H., MacPhail, S., & Robson, S. (1992). The prediction of fetal compromise and acidosis by biophysical profile scoring in the small for gestational age fetus. *Journal of Perinatal Medicine, 20*(3), 227–232.

Ware, D. J., & Devoe, L. D. (1994). The nonstress test: Reassessment of the "gold standard." *Clinics in Perinatology, 21*(4), 779–796.

Walton, J. R., & Peaceman, A. M. (2012). Identification, assessment and management of fetal compromise. *Clinical Perinatology, 39*(4), 753–768. doi:10.1016/j.clp.2012.09.001

Westergaard, H. B., Langhoff-Roos, J., Lingman, G., Marsal, K., & Kreiner, S. (2001). A critical appraisal of the use of umbilical artery Doppler ultrasound in high-risk pregnancies: Use of meta-analysis in evidence-based obstetrics. *Ultrasound in Obstetrics and Gynecology, 17*(6), 466–476.

Yao, Q. W., Jakobsson, J., Nyman, M., Rabaeus, H., Till, O., & Westgren, M. (1990). Fetal responses to different intensity levels of vibroacoustic stimulation. *Obstetrics and Gynecology, 75*(2), 206–209.

CHAPTER 11

Fetal Arrhythmias

Joanne D. Barnes

INTRODUCTION

Fetal arrhythmias occur in 1–3% of pregnancies (Rasiah, Ewer, Miller, & Kilby, 2011; Strasburger, Cheulkar, & Wichman, 2007). Clinicians should be able to recognize that a rhythm disturbance may be present. Any rhythm disturbance has the potential to decrease fetal cardiac output as alterations from the normal ECG cycle are produced. When a woman is in labor, a rhythm disturbance may present an additional stressor on the fetus above and beyond the normal reductions in blood flow that occur with contractions. In some cases this can present a challenge to fetal reserve and fetal tolerance of labor. Perinatal clinicians may detect a rhythm disturbance during a routine prenatal visit, during a nonstress test (NST), or when the woman presents in labor. Clinicians caring for childbearing women should be knowledgeable about the etiology of different patterns, available treatment options, and potential outcomes and should anticipate questions that the woman and her family may ask.

The presumed mechanisms of fetal cardiac failure associated with arrhythmias include the following:

1. Decreased ventricular filling time (supraventricular tachycardia [SVT], atrial fibrillation, and atrial flutter)
2. Dissociation between atrial and ventricular depolarization causing loss of the atrial boost mechanism (supraventricular or ventricular arrhythmias)
3. Mild impairment of cardiac performance (ventricular arrhythmias)
4. Decrease in cardiac output (third-degree heart block) (Api & Carvalho, 2008; Kleinman & Nehgme, 2004; Srinivasin & Strasburger, 2008)

The most common disturbance is an irregular heart rhythm, which is usually benign (Api & Carvalho, 2008; Rasiah et al., 2011; Sharland, 2001). Irregular beats can occur secondary to isolated atrial or ventricular premature beats, producing a perceived heart rhythm irregularity or skipped beats (Kleinman & Nehgme, 2004). A premature atrial signal can also be conducted to the ventricles, resulting in ventricular contraction; if it occurs early in diastole, the signal may not be conducted at all, resulting in skipped beats (Kleinman & Nehgme, 2004).

DEFINITION

The term "arrhythmia" is described as any irregular heart rhythm (American Heart Association, 2012; Api & Carvalho, 2008). Arrhythmias fall into two broad categories:

1. *Variations in the R-R intervals.* There may be normal P waves that occur in a regular fashion preceding each QRS complex.
2. *Disordered impulse formation, impulse conduction, or a combination of both.* There will be an abnormal P-QRS relationship as evidenced by early or absent P waves; widened, bizarre-looking QRS complexes; or both.

Specific arrhythmias are typically named according to the anatomic site of aberrant impulse formation, conduction, or both and may be unassociated with uterine activity.

FETAL CARDIAC DEVELOPMENT AND FUNCTION

Three separate but related concepts are significant to any discussion of arrhythmias: (1) cardiac development, (2) differences in the adaptive mechanisms of the fetal and adult hearts, and (3) conduction physiology. An understanding of these concepts is important when discussing specific arrhythmias and the fetus' ability to withstand the changes in cardiac output that may be produced.

Cardiac Development

The fetal cardiovascular system, including the heart, blood vessels, and cells, is the first system to begin to function in the embryo and originates from the mesenchymal cells within the endoderm. By approximately the third week of development, these cells rapidly form a tube (Blackburn, 2012; Moore, Persaud, & Torchia, 2013).

During the fourth week, the tube forms a loop and begins to beat in a coordinated manner under the control of a primitive pacemaker (Blackburn, 2012; Moore et al., 2013). Soon after, differentiation of the heart regions begins, and the atrial septum begins to form from the roof of the atrium downward and the base of the atrium upward. As these continue to develop, an opening between the right and left atria, the foramen ovale, is formed. During the sixth week, the pulmonary arteries begin to form, and both the atrial and ventricular septa continue to develop. By the end of the sixth week, the valves are forming and the coronary circulation has been established. If there are alterations in any of these processes, lesions may develop and continue to evolve during the rest of gestation (Blackburn, 2012; Moore et al., 2013).

The development of the fetal cardiac conduction system also progresses over time. The sinoatrial (SA) node develops from the sinus venosus musculature during the fifth week of gestation (Blackburn, 2012; Moore et al., 2013). The SA node is then incorporated into the wall of the right atrium and will eventually lie near the entrance of the superior vena cava (Blackburn, 2012).

After the SA node is incorporated into the wall of the right atrium, cells from part of the SA node combine with cells from the atrioventricular (AV) canal to form the AV node and bundle of His. The bundle of His continues to develop into the right and left bundle branches and the Purkinje fibers, which are specialized for conduction of impulses and distributed throughout the ventricles (Blackburn, 2012; Moore, 2013). By the end of this process, there is neurogenic control of the heart, and the conduction system represents the pathway for communication of electrical impulses between the atria and the ventricles (Blackburn, 2012; Moore, 2013).

Electrical activity actually begins before the contractile apparatus of the fetal heart completely differentiates. Sympathetic innervation via the first thoracic sympathetic ganglia is usually present by day 10. The fetal cardiac muscle and the arterioles of the fetal circulation have direct sympathetic innervation. Parasympathetic innervation is present by day 80 of gestation and originates from the cardiac ganglia located on the surface and in the outflow tract of the fetal heart. Sensory innervation of the fetal heart originates from the distal ganglia of the vagus nerve, although there is little clinical evidence to show at what stage of development this begins to function (Snarr, Wessels, & McQuinn, 2011). The right and left branches of the vagus nerve innervate both the SA and the AV nodes. Early in gestation, the sympathetic nervous system has a major influence on the fetal heart rate (FHR). Parasympathetic influence on the heart increases gradually during the latter part of gestation (Pickoff, 2011).

Differences between Fetal and Adult Cardiac Functioning

The fetal heart is less able than the adult heart to alter the forces of cardiac contraction because of a number of factors, including decreased contractile mass, differences in calcium transport, differences in the pressures within the heart, and rate-dependent cardiac output. The fetal heart has approximately half the contractile mass of the adult heart because there are fewer sarcomeres, the smallest contractile units within heart muscle. Sarcomeres are arranged into myofibrils, which, in the fetus, are also fewer in number and more randomly arranged. Calcium transport into and out of the muscle cells is also limited in the fetus, resulting in cardiac muscle that is less compliant. These three factors limit the fetus' ability to alter stroke volume or the force of cardiac contractions (Blackburn, 2012).

As discussed in Chapter 2, cardiac pressures and contributions to cardiac output also differ in the fetus when compared with the adult. Right-sided pressure is higher in the fetus, and right-sided output accounts for two-thirds of the entire fetal cardiac output as a result of the shunting of blood through the patent foramen ovale and ductus arteriosus (Blackburn, 2012). The less compliant fetal myocardium and combined right and left contribution to cardiac output result in an inability of the fetus to alter its stroke volume to meet increased demand. Therefore, fetal cardiac output is rate dependent, and the fetus is dependent on maintaining a heart rate in the normal range to maintain adequate cardiac output and tissue perfusion (Blackburn, 2012).

Cardiac Physiology

When fetal arrhythmias are studied, it is important to understand normal cardiac conduction physiology and electrocardiogram (ECG) patterns. Many arrhythmias result from alterations in normal conduction patterns that are reflected as abnormal-appearing ECGs.

Cardiac cells possess unique characteristics. *Automaticity* refers to the ability of cardiac cells to contract spontaneously. *Excitability* is the readiness and ability of cardiac cells to respond to electrical stimuli. *Conductivity* is the ability to conduct an electrical stimulus between different cardiac cells. Excitability and conductivity occur through polarization and depolarization of the cellular membrane.

Cardiac cells at rest are charged. Sodium is found primarily outside the cell, whereas potassium is found inside the cell, resulting in an overall negatively charged cell, called "polarization." When stimulated by an electrical impulse, sodium rushes into the cell and potassium is forced out of the cell. This process is called "depolarization." Following depolarization is a phase known as the "refractory period," when the cell cannot respond to further electrical stimulation. After depolarization and the refractory period, the cell reverts back to its polarized, resting state (Bianchi, Crombleholme, D'Alton, & Malone, 2010). This sequence of polarization, depolarization, and refractory period is responsible for the typical ECG pattern (Figure 11-1).

Figure 11-1 Polarization/Depolarization

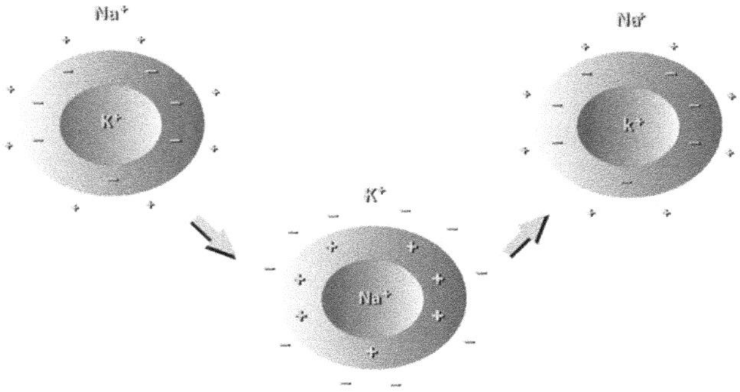

As with adult hearts, the depolarization and repolarization of the fetal cardiac muscle cells create electrical activity that can be recorded. This activity is controlled by the conduction system, composed of the SA node, AV node, the bundle of His, and Purkinje fibers. The typical cardiac impulse begins at the SA node, known as the "pacemaker of the heart." Firing of the SA node first generates an atrial contraction, which is responsible for approximately 30% of cardiac output. The impulse is then conducted down to the AV node, where it is slowed, enabling completion of atrial depolarization and contraction. As a result of atrial contraction, the ventricles fill with blood. The impulse then travels down the Bundle of His to the left and right bundle branches and through the Purkinje fibers to the ventricular muscle cells, stimulating ventricular depolarization and contraction (Table 11-1).

Each part of the conduction system has an intrinsic rate. This rate is slower when contraction impulses are generated further down the system. The SA node in a fetus has an intrinsic rate of 110–160 bpm, the normal fetal heart range. If the SA node fails and the AV node assumes the role of fetal pacemaker, the intrinsic rate falls to 50–70 bpm. If the AV node fails, the bundle of His, also called the AV junction, becomes the fetal pacemaker with an intrinsic rate of 40 bpm. This junctional rate is incompatible with continued fetal life because it is too low to maintain cardiac output.

A frequent method of monitoring cardiac conduction activity is by ECG. The typical ECG has three sections: the P wave, QRS complex, and T wave. Each section corresponds to distinct cardiac events (see Table 11-1):

1. The P wave, which is reflective of atrial depolarization and contraction (followed by a spike representing atrial repolarization, which is lost within the QRS complex).
2. The QRS complex, which is indicative of ventricular depolarization and contraction.
3. The T wave, representing ventricular repolarization and ventricular relaxation.

The ECG is a tool for assessing arrhythmias because it provides information concerning the FHR. Other evaluation modes, such as the echocardiogram, provide more detailed information about the relationships between atrial and ventricular events. It can also help identify the origin or mechanism of a variety of abnormal FHR rhythms (Api & Carvalho, 2008; Kleinman et al., 2004; Srinivasin & Strasburger, 2008) (Figure 11-2; see Table 11-1).

TABLE 11-1 Normal ECG

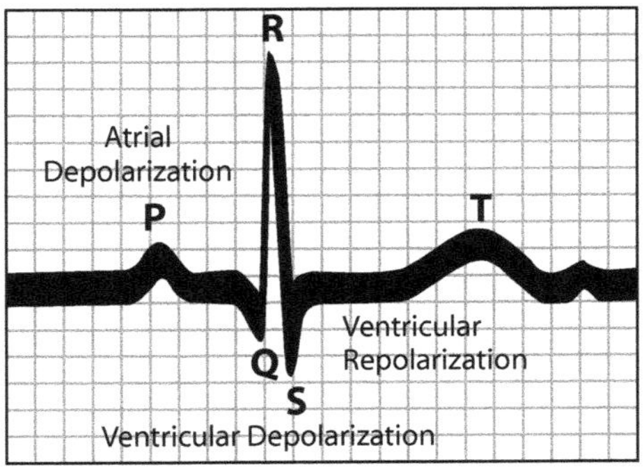

ECG COMPONENT	CARDIAC ACTIVITY
P wave	Atrial depolarization and contraction
QRS complex	Ventricular depolarization and contraction (atrial repolarization waveform lost within QRS complex)
T wave	Ventricular repolarization

Figure 11-2 Conduction System and Normal ECG of the Adult Heart

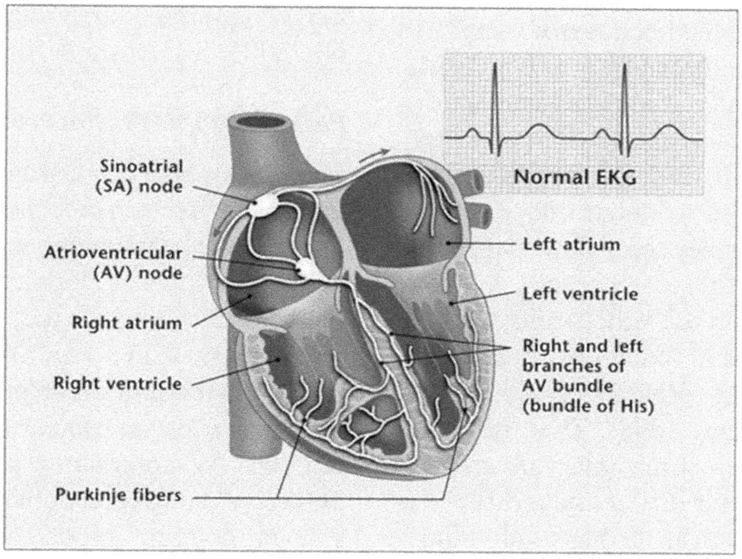

ETIOLOGIES OF FETAL RHYTHM DISTURBANCES

Fetal heart rhythm disturbances can develop in a number of ways, including conduction system defects, congenital heart defects, and infections. Conduction system defects such as AV block can develop as a result of abnormalities in development or from maternal collagen vascular diseases resulting in structural defects (Bianchi et al., 2010; Jaeggi, Laskin, Hamilton, Kingdom, & Silverman, 2010; Kleinman & Nehgme, 2004; Seferovic et al., 2006). Conduction defects can develop early in cardiac development when the cardiac tube loops to form the four-chamber heart. In the case of maternal collagen diseases such as lupus and fetal second- or third-degree AV block, maternal anti-Ro/SSA and/or anti-La/SSB antibodies cross the placenta and deposits of immunoglobulin and complement form in the atrial and ventricular myocardium. Inflammatory reaction to these deposits results in fibrosis, calcification, and, eventually, interruption of the conduction through the AV node (Jaeggi et al., 2010; Seferovic et al., 2006; Trines & Hornberger, 2004). Whether or not the fetus is affected, and, if so, the degree of resulting damage, appears to be the result of the level of maternal anti-Ro titers (Jaeggi et al., 2010).

Congenital heart defects may also result in fetal arrhythmias, although the relationship varies according to the specific defect. For example, SVT, the most frequently seen arrhythmia, is rarely associated with congenital heart defects. Atrial flutter is associated with congenital heart defects in approximately 20% of cases. However, complete heart block is associated with congenital heart defects in 50% of cases (Kleinman & Nehgme, 2004).

DIAGNOSIS OF FETAL ARRHYTHMIAS

Fetal arrhythmias may first be recognized during routine fetal assessment via fetal monitoring, either by auscultation or electronic fetal monitoring (EFM). When auscultation is used, an irregular rhythm may be heard. EFM data usually associated with fetal assessment, such as baseline, variability, and presence of accelerations or decelerations, may be obscured, depending on the frequency and type of arrhythmia. In these instances, recognition of unusual FHR characteristics should be reported promptly.

Fetal Echocardiogram

The most widely used diagnostic tool to assess fetal arrhythmias is the fetal echocardiogram. If a sustained rhythm disturbance is recognized, this diagnostic technique is recommended for direct imaging of cardiac wall motion to assess for rhythm, cardiac structure, cardiac function, and fetal well-being and to determine whether hydrops is present. Doppler color flow mapping, using pulsed Doppler, discussed below, is often used in conjunction with the echocardiogram to identify abnormal shifts in blood flow as a result of specific arrhythmias (Rasiah et al., 2011; Srinivasin & Strasburger, 2008). This tool can also be used to measure time intervals within the cardiac cycle to better differentiate different types of arrhythmias, such as further subdividing SVT as either long or short interval (Srinivasin & Strasburger, 2008). Echocardiogram is further differentiated into M-mode echocardiogram and pulsed Doppler echocardiogram.

M-Mode Echocardiogram

M-mode echocardiogram uses real-time imaging techniques to observe, time, and evaluate the sequence of electromechanical events of the fetus' cardiac activity (Kleinman & Nehgme, 2004; Srinivasin & Strasburger, 2008; Strasburger, 2005). M-mode imaging is helpful in the evaluation of contractility in abnormalities that affect heart wall motion by looking at the timing of atrial and ventricular events in the cardiac conduction cycle. The analysis of the AV contraction sequence can provide an accurate picture of the precise cardiac rhythm (Kleinman et al., 2004; Rasiah et al., 2011; Strasburger, 2005). It is also useful in determining the degree of atrial hypertrophy associated with SVT and in defining those infants with AV block who will require pacing after birth (Strasburger, 2005). Some factors may limit the data from the M-mode echocardiogram. These factors include poor resolution due to maternal obesity, oligohydramnios, and rib shadowing and difficulty obtaining a reproducible view due to fetal movement and position changes *in utero* (Comani et al., 2004). M-mode echocardiogram may be used in conjunction with other diagnostic techniques, including pulse-wave Doppler and color Doppler, when more information is required to arrive at a diagnosis (Jaeggi & Nii, 2005; Srinivasin & Strasburger, 2008).

Pulsed Doppler Echocardiogram

Pulsed Doppler echocardiogram provides information about electromechanical events as well as views of the heart chambers and the great vessels. The use of pulsed Doppler echocardiogram has been found to enhance the ability to detect cardiac malformations *in utero* (Strasburger, 2005). This technique is useful in determining atrial rate and flow reversal, ventricular rate and cardiac output, and AV contraction sequence (Strasburger, 2000). When used simultaneously with M-mode echocardiogram, blood flow velocities in the superior vena cava and ascending aorta, which can be determined with pulse Doppler echocardiogram, can provide additional information regarding atrial and ventricular events (Jaeggi & Nii, 2005; Strasburger, 2005). This additional information can provide parents with reassurance about the fetal heart, even though the incidence of structural heart defects causing arrhythmic patterns is relatively low.

These techniques are not without limitations, however. Image resolution, fetal position, and the complexity of the specific arrhythmia may limit the information obtained when these modalities are used (Carvalho et al., 2007).

Fetal Magnetocardiography

Fetal magnetocardiography (FMCG) is a noninvasive diagnostic tool used to analyze electrophysical changes of the heart as early as 20 weeks' gestation as it measures small magnetic changes that are associated with the cardiac electrical cycle (Api & Carvalho, 2008; Svirivasin & Strasburger, 2008). Compared with other common methods, FMCG provides more information that can be used to influence therapeutic decisions and thus contribute to optimal prenatal and postnatal management. FMCG can define fetal cardiac conduction and rhythm disturbances more precisely (Strasburger, 2005). It can provide information about the QRS and

QT intervals, FHR variability, and T-wave abnormalities (Api & Carvalho, 2008; Strasburger, 2005). If no arrhythmias are found after the cardiac study with FMCG, further follow-up provides no added benefit. Limitations in using this diagnostic tool include the presence of a maternal pacemaker, other devices such as clips on cerebral aneurysms, high cost, and limited accessibility (Api & Carvalho, 2008; Kumar & O'Brien, 2004; Srinivasin & Strasburger, 2008).

Tissue Doppler

Tissue Doppler velocity imaging is a rather new technique that incorporates ultrasound-based images with later computer-analyzed velocity data. Velocity curves are then produced that correlate atrial and ventricular contraction cycles. Currently, this technique is not widely used due to lack of accessibility (Api & Carvalho, 2008).

MORE COMMON CLINICALLY SIGNIFICANT FETAL ARRHYTHMIAS

Tachyarrhythmias: Sinus Tachycardia and SVT

Sinus Tachycardia

Tachycardia in the fetus is defined as a baseline rate over 160 bpm (Macones et al., 2008). Tachycardias are the second most common type of fetal arrhythmia (Kleinman & Nehgme, 2004) and may originate from within or outside of the SA node. Sinus tachycardia is considered a sinus node variant and is defined as an FHR greater than 160 bpm sustained for greater than 10 minutes (Figure 11-3). Sinus tachycardia is generally considered benign when the rate is less than 180 bpm and moderate FHR variability is present. Sinus tachycardia warrants further evaluation when the FHR is sustained at greater than 180 bpm (Jaeggi & Nii, 2005; Sharland, 2001; Strasburger, 2000). The most common causes of sinus tachycardia include the following:

1. Responses to continuous fetal activity
2. Maternal fever
3. Use of beta-sympathomimetic medications, such as terbutaline (Jaeggi & Nii, 2005)
4. Use of parasympatholytic medications, such as atropine, hydralazine, or hydroxyzine hydrochloride (Kleinman et al., 2004; Strasburger, 2000)
5. Underlying conditions, such as infections (Jaeggi & Nii, 2005; Srinivasin & Strasburger, 2008); fetal hypoxia or myocarditis (Jaeggi & Nii, 2005; Strasburger, 2000); or maternal drug ingestion of stimulants or hormones or catecholamine transfer (Pickoff, 2011; Srinivasin & Strasburger, 2008)
6. Maternal hyperthyroidism/thyrotoxicosis (Srinivasin & Strasburger, 2008; Strasburger et al., 2007).

The tachycardic fetal ECG will display normal P waves occurring in routine fashion preceding each QRS complex (see Figure 11-3). In contrast to other tachycardias, sinus tachycardia may display moderate variability within the baseline rate (Jaeggi & Nii, 2005). Sinus tachycardia generally does not exceed 200-210 bpm (Cabaniss & Ross, 2010; Jaeggi & Nii, 2005; Srinivasin & Strasburger, 2008; Strasburger, 2000). However, when it does exceed 210 bpm, the rapid rate makes it difficult to differentiate from other types of tachycardia (Strasburger, 2000).

Interventions

When sinus tachycardia is noted, the clinician should evaluate maternal hydration status and assess the woman for fever and other signs and symptoms of infection. Correction of any identifiable underlying etiology is appropriate whenever possible, as is close surveillance of the FHR tracing for maintenance of moderate variability. The primary provider should also be notified of findings.

Supraventricular Tachycardia

SVT is one of the few fetal arrhythmias with cause for concern (Figure 11–4). It is also the second most frequent cause of fetal tachycardia, after maternal infection (Api & Carvalho, 2008; Strasburger, 2005). SVT usually presents after 15 weeks' gestation; it is most commonly seen at 30-32 weeks' gestation (Menihan & Kopel, 2008; Strasburger et al., 2007). SVT is a nonsinus

Figure 11-3 Fetal Tracing: Sinus Tachycardia (Fetal Spiral Electrode and Tocodynamometer)

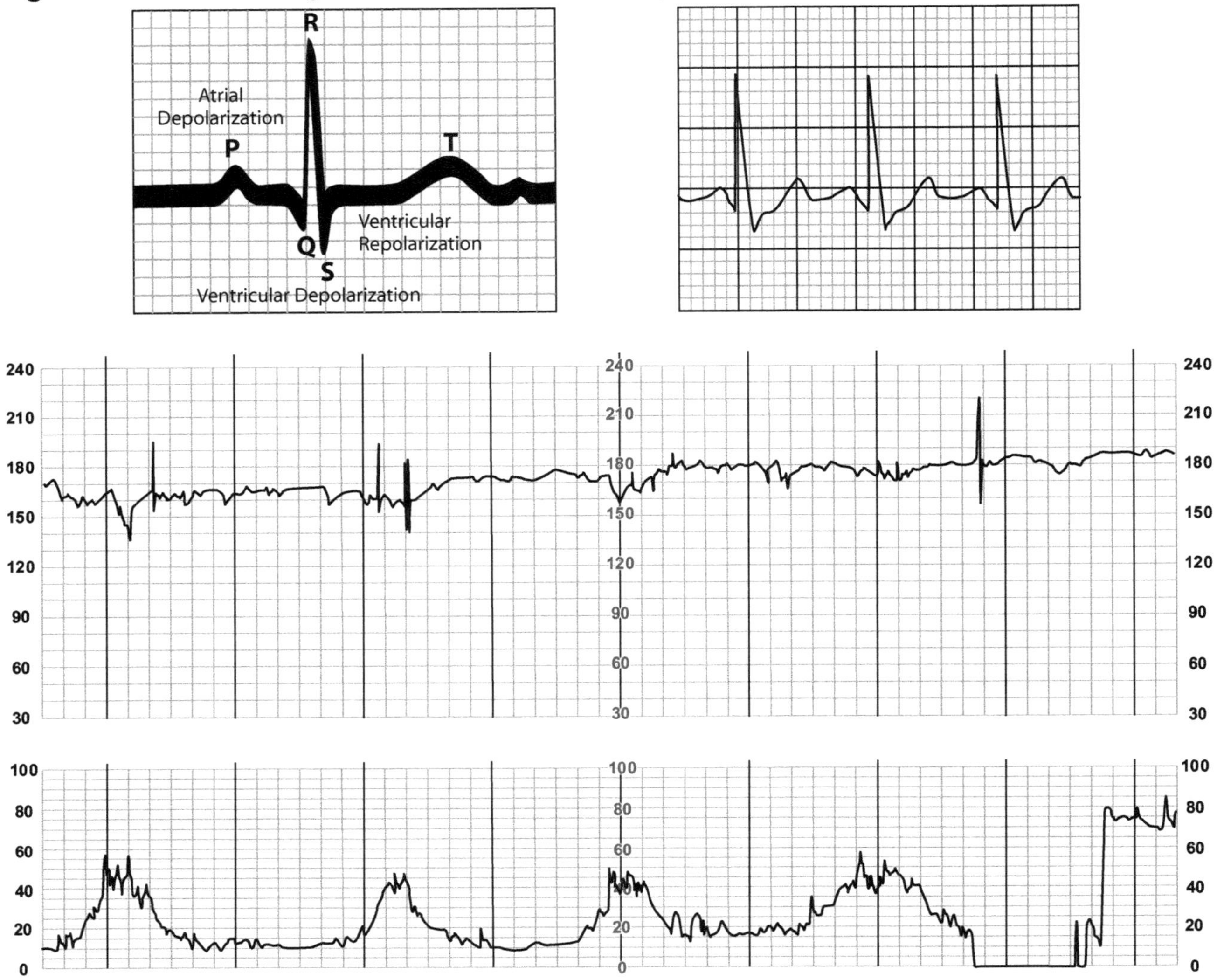

originated, sustained, rapid, regular atrial arrhythmia; it has been associated with Wolff-Parkinson-White syndrome. The rate may range from 210 to 320 bpm, but SVT rates are typically between 240 and 260 bpm (Api & Carvalho, 2008; Kleinman & Nehgme, 2004; Larmay & Strasburger, 2004; Maeno, Hirose, Kanbe, & Hori, 2009). SVT is further defined as short interval (when the following reentry mechanisms are present) or long interval (when the cycle originates in an atrial ectopic focus or as a paroxysmal junctional reciprocating tachycardia, where the electrical pathway is slower) (Maeno et al., 2009). Short-interval SVT is the most common; long-interval SVT is generally more difficult to treat (Api & Carvalho, 2008; Srinivasin & Strasburger, 2008).

Multiple electrical impulse pathways exist for the development of SVT. Reentrant or reciprocating SVT, the most common form of SVT, occurs when a circular depolarization cycle has been established between an ectopic atrial pacemaker and the AV node. An automatic SVT results from the development of an irritable ectopic focus that has assumed the role of pacemaker. Atrial flutter or fibrillation or PACs can also produce SVT (Api & Carvalho, 2008; Srinivasin & Strasburger, 2008; Strasburger et al., 2007). Most fetal SVTs are reentrant in nature (Api & Carvalho, 2008; Kleinman & Nehgme, 2004; Strasburger et al., 2007), meaning that more than one pathway conducts the impulse. The electrical impulse is carried over a secondary pathway, but the reentry of the impulse occurs over a primary pathway, creating the circular conduction pattern (Figure 11-5). On ECG, the P wave may be lost within the T wave of the previous complexes, and the QRS spike may be narrowed or widened, depending on the specific electrical pathway (see Figure 11-4). The EFM tracings may exhibit half counting of these high rates. SVT may be paroxysmal (occurring suddenly in waves or spasms) or continuous (Strasburger, 2005). In general, SVT has absent variability because of a fixed R-R interval, especially at rates greater than 240 bpm (Cabaniss & Ross, 2010; Menihan & Kopel, 2008; Strasburger, 2005).

The rapid heart rate that occurs with SVT increases the workload of the fetal heart. It also increases cardiac oxygen demand. The rapid rate results in decreased stroke volume because of decreased filling time, and cardiac output is therefore diminished. Depending on gestational age and the persistence of the SVT (sustained rates greater than 200 bpm, persisting for greater than 50% of the time), the fetus may not be able to meet its oxygen demands, resulting in the development of congestive heart failure because the heart fails as a pump. In addition, there is an increased hemolysis of red blood cells, further reducing oxygen delivery

Figure 11-4 Fetal Tracing: Supraventricular Tachycardia (Ultrasound and Tocodynamometer)

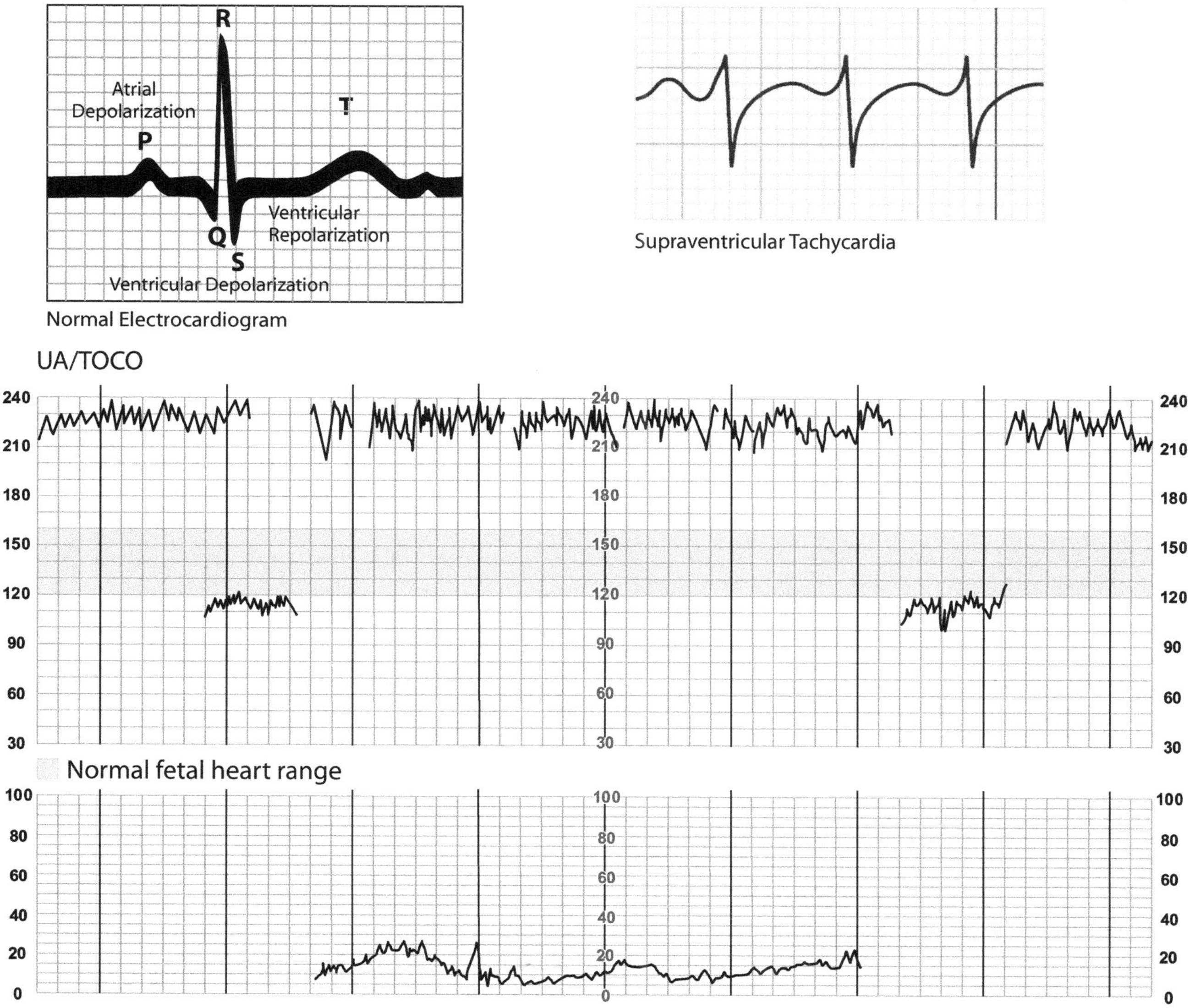

Figure 11-5 Ectopic Circular Pathway of Supraventricular Tachycardia

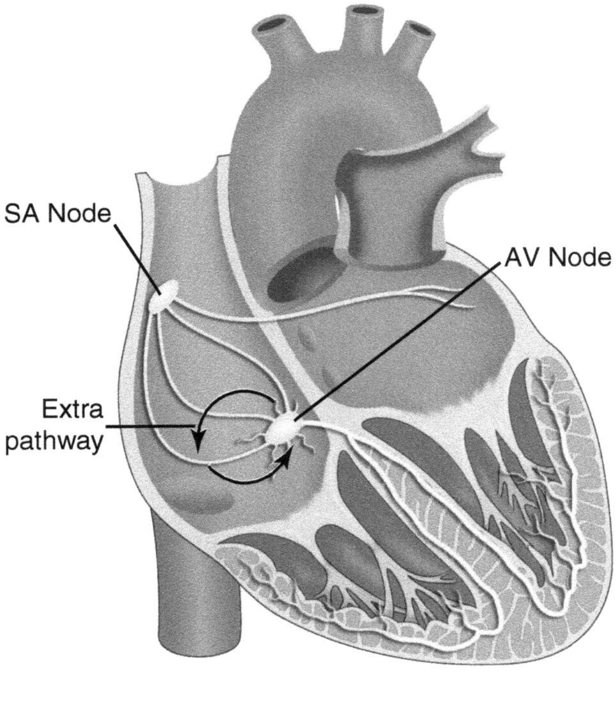

(Srinivasin & Strasburger, 2008; Strasburger, 2000, 2005; Tanel & Rhodes, 2001). Nonimmunologic hydrops fetalis—the development of generalized edema in the abdomen, scalp, liver, and spleen—and fetal death may result (Rasiah et al., 2011; Strasburger, 2000, 2005).

The rate and progression of the hydrops depend on the severity of the hemodynamic compromise, as well as gestational age (Srinivasin & Strasburger, 2008; Strasburger, 2000). The unborn, untreated fetus may develop cardiac failure and ischemic cerebral disease. Often, the fetus will demonstrate evidence of pericardial or pleural effusion, cardiomegaly, polyhydramnios, scalp edema, or ascites, all of which are suggestive of congestive heart failure (Strasburger, 2005).

Treatment

The treatment of SVT can be highly effective and improve fetal outcome. Treatment recommendations range from observation only, to prenatal medication therapy, to planned early birth of the affected fetus. Recommendations depend on whether the SVT is intermittent or sustained, the gestational age of the fetus, the presence or absence of hydrops, parental wishes, and presence of congenital heart disease (Api & Carvalho, 2008; Kleinman & Nehgme, 2004; Srinivasin & Strasburger, 2008).

Observation is often used when the pregnancy is close to term, the tachycardic episodes are short lived, and there is no evidence of fetal hydrops (Api & Carvalho, 2008). Decision making regarding medical management of SVT should weigh the risks of prematurity against the risks of cardiac failure and poor oxygen delivery *in utero*. Generally, birth is recommended for term fetuses without hydrops. However, if the term fetus has hydrops, the fetus is usually treated *in utero*, and birth usually then occurs after the SVT has converted. If the fetus is preterm, intrauterine conversion therapy is usually initiated along with assessment of fetal lung maturity. In these cases, the risks of preterm birth and its associated complications should be weighed against the risks of a continued cardiac arrhythmia and its associated complications (Api & Carvalho, 2008; Kleinman & Nehgme, 2004; Strasburger, 2005). If the lungs are deemed mature and the conversion of the SVT has been achieved, birth should proceed. However, if the lungs are immature, intrauterine conversion therapy is recommended along with steroid therapy. After the lungs are mature and conversion is achieved, birth should be considered (Sharland, 2001; Strasburger, 2000; Tanel & Rhodes, 2001).

In nonhydropic fetuses, digoxin therapy may be the first-line medication choice. Initially, digoxin is administered to the mother intravenously because oral administration can result in erratic absorption rates as a result of delayed gastric emptying during pregnancy (Api & Strasburger, 2008; Strasburger, 2000; Strasburger et al., 2007). After adequate digitalization with intravenous (IV) digoxin has been accomplished and the fetus has converted to normal sinus rhythm, the mother can be switched to the oral form for maintenance, which is continued until birth (Kleinman & Nehgme, 2004). It is important to note that the dosage of digoxin may need to be as much as 100% higher (twice the normal dose) than is required in the adult, non pregnant woman (Api & Strasburger, 2008;

Larmay & Strasburger, 2004; Strasburger et al., 2007). It is recommended that frequent maternal digoxin levels be drawn; the therapeutic range is 0.8–2.0 ng/mL (Api & Strasburger, 2008; Kleinman & Nehgme, 2004; Larmay & Strasburger, 2004).

The hydropic fetus with SVT remains a therapeutic challenge. Digoxin alone may be ineffective because the transfer of digoxin from the mother to the fetus is poor; adequate fetal blood levels may not be achieved even with near toxic maternal blood levels (Api & Strasburger, 2008; Jaeggi & Nii, 2005; Maeno et al., 2009; Srinivasin & Strasburger, 2008). In these cases, switching to or adding additional medications, such as adenosine, amiodarone, sotalol, and flecainide, may be necessary (Api & Carvalho, 2008; Maeno et al., 2009; Srinivasin & Strasburger, 2008; Strasburger et al., 2007). There is no consensus as to the best line of approach to treatment (Srinivasin & Strasburger, 2008; Suri, Keepanaseril, Aggarwal, & Vijayvergiya, 2009). Rasiah et al. (2011) routinely use flecainide as the first-line drug. Kleinman and Nehgme (2004) recommend a protocol whereby propranolol is added as the second-line medication and flecainide is third line. Oudijk et al. (2002) do not recommend use of verapamil because it may increase fetal mortality.

Sotalol is another medication used for fetal SVT. It is a Class III cardiac medication that has beta-blocker effects normally seen in Class II agents, as well as the potassium channel blocker effect of the Class III cardiac medications. In addition, it has almost complete placental transfer (Api & Strasburger, 2008). If sotalol is used, it is important to discontinue propranolol and flecainide for 72 hours to allow clearance of these medications from the system; digoxin may be continued (Kleinman & Nehgme, 2004). If SVT continues after these medications, amiodarone can be considered. However, sotalol must be discontinued for 96 hours and the dosage of digoxin halved prior to beginning amiodarone therapy (Kleinman & Nehgme, 2004).

There have also been cases in which medications have been injected directly into the fetus, using the intramuscular, intraperitoneal, and umbilical vein routes. In these studies, there have been reports of increased conversion rates back to normal sinus rhythm (Api & Carvalho, 2008; Rasiah et al., 2011; Srinivasin & Strasburger, 2008; Strasburger et al., 2007). Use of fetal routes may require repetitive invasive procedures, potentially exposing both the woman and her fetus to subsequent problems, such as infection and hemorrhage. Strasburger (2000) advocates direct intramuscular injection of the fetus rather than using the umbilical cord for this purpose if a more direct fetal route is deemed necessary.

Bradyarrhythmias: Sinus Bradycardia and Atrioventricular Blocks

Bradycardia is defined as a baseline FHR below 110 bpm (Macones et al., 2008). Intermittent periods of bradycardia are considered benign when accompanied by moderate variability (Menihan & Kopel, 2008). Although transient FHRs less than 110 bpm may be normal, sustained bradycardia requires further assessment and evaluation. The eventual prognosis is dependent on the cause of the bradycardia, the ventricular rate, and the presence or absence of structural cardiac abnormalities (Wren, 2006).

Sinus Bradycardia

Sinus bradycardia is a FHR less than110 bpm sustained for more than 10 minutes (Figure 11-6); the fetal ECG displays normal P waves occurring in routine relationship preceding each QRS complex (see Figure 11-6). Sinus bradycardia is evaluated in relation to the entire clinical picture and may reflect an abnormal fetal or maternal condition, such as maternal or fetal compromise (Menihan & Kopel, 2008); increased vagal tone (Simpson, 2008; Strasburger, 2000); maternal hypothermia (Simpson, 2008); medications such as beta-blocking agents (Strasburger, 2000); fetal hypothyroidism (Kleinman & Nehgme, 2004); placental insufficiency (Kleinman & Nehgme, 2004); intrauterine growth restriction (Strasburger, 2000); or prolonged QT syndrome (Jaeggi & Friedberg, 2008; Larmay & Strasburger, 2004; Strasburger, 2000).

Figure 11-6 Fetal Tracing: Sinus Bradycardia (Fetal Scalp Electrode and Tocodynamometer)

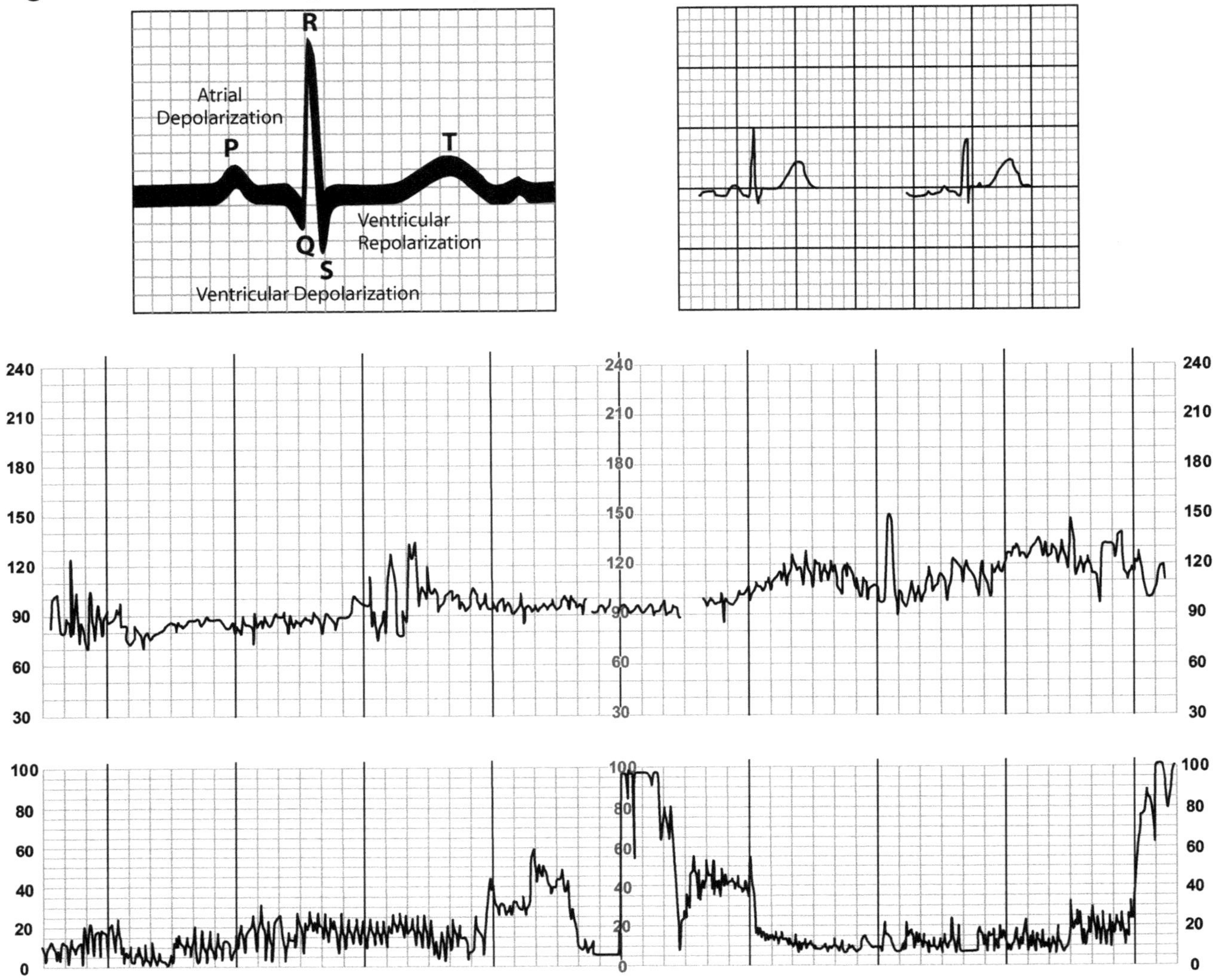

Interventions

Management of sinus bradycardia includes identification of any underlying etiology and determination of fetal well-being. Management of an identified underlying pathology will depend on the specific problem and whether or not fetal well-being can be confirmed.

If moderate variability is present and no underlying pathology is identified, continued observation is warranted and intervention may not be necessary; however, the primary provider should be notified of the FHR findings. In cases where the bradycardia is thought to be a result of fetal hypoxia, urgent delivery is warranted (Jaeggi & Friedburg, 2008).

Atrioventricular Blocks

AV blocks are categorized according to the severity of the block. The three degrees of AV block are first, second, and third (complete). In all blocks, impulse conduction through the AV node is abnormal.

All impulses are conducted through the AV node in first-degree block, but a delay in impulse conduction produces prolonged P-R intervals (Jaeggi & Nii, 2005; Kleinman & Nehgme, 2004; Sonesson, 2010). First-degree blocks are difficult to recognize in the fetus because the FHR is within normal range and therefore will not be observable on the EFM tracing. They may be due to structural anomalies, although diagnosis of such an anomaly may be difficult (Kleinman & Nehgme, 2004; Strasburger, 2005).

Second-degree AV block represents intermittent failure of conduction of some of the atrial impulses through the AV node and may be manifested as occasional loss of conduction through the AV node or as several consecutive dropped beats (Jaeggi & Friedburg, 2008; Kleinman & Nehgme, 2004; Sonesson, 2010). This may occur in association with a rapid atrial rate caused by SVT, atrial flutter or atrial fibrillation, or in association with conduction system disease. When associated with conduction system disease, second-degree block may progress to third-degree, or complete, heart block (Jaeggi & Friedburg, 2008; Kleinman & Nehgme, 2004).

Maternal collagen vascular disease and cardiac structural defects are two causes of second-degree block (Jaeggi & Friedburg, 2008; Kleinman & Nehgme, 2004; Strasburger, 2000). The relationship between maternal collagen disease and AV block centers on the anti-SSA/Ro or anti-SSB/La antibodies developed by the mother. These antibodies cross the placenta, binding to fetal cardiac tissue, including the AV node and the atrial and ventricular myocardium (Kleinman et al., 2004). An inflammatory reaction occurs, leading to fibrosis, calcification, and eventual interruption of the fetal conduction pathway, producing the AV block (Kleinman et al., 2004; Larmay & Strasburger, 2004; Strasburger, 2000; Strasburger et al., 2007). These cardiac manifestations are usually detected between 20 and 24 weeks' gestation (Jaeggi et al., 2010). One recent study by Jaeggi et al. (2010) found that only fetuses of anti-Ro mothers with high titers, regardless of the levels of anti-La, had a potential for developing complete heart block. They also found that high anti-La titers appeared to be a marker for more benign cardiac disease, though there may be other noncardiac manifestations. Further research in this area is recommended by the authors (Jaeggi et al., 2010). Third-degree, or complete, AV block may also be seen in the fetus (Figure 11-7). Third-degree heart block represents the complete absence of conduction of the impulse from the SA node through the AV node. There is a complete dissociation between the atrial and ventricular contractions, creating P waves that have no relationship to the QRS complexes (see Figure 11-7). As a result, there is a higher atrial rate (within the normal range as atrial contraction is stimulated by the SA node) and a much slower ventricular rate (Jaeggi & Friedburg, 2008; Jaeggi & Nii, 2005; Kleinman & Nehgme, 2004; Sonesson, 2010; Strasburger, 2005; Wren, 2006). This ventricular rate is initiated by an ectopic focus below the level of the block (Wren, 2006).

Third-degree blocks are caused by cardiac structural defects, such as transposition of the great arteries, fetal cytomegalovirus or other infections, antiphospholipid antibody syndrome, or the presence of maternal anti-SSA/Ro or anti-SSB/La antibodies, which are present with maternal lupus (Bianchi et al., 2010; Kleinman & Nehgme, 2004; Kleinman et al., 2004; Strasburger, 2000). These antibodies cross the placenta and destroy the fetal cardiac conductive tissues, specifically the AV node (Kleinman et al., 2004; Larmay & Strasburger, 2004; Tanel & Rhodes, 2001; Wren, 2006). Maternal rheumatoid arthritis and other collagen diseases have also been associated with fetal third-degree heart block (Kleinman & Nehgme, 2004; Larmay & Strasburger, 2004).

In up to approximately 50% of fetuses with third-degree heart block, congenital heart disease is also present (Jaeggi & Friedburg, 2008; Jaeggi & Nii, 2005; Strasburger, 2000). Third-degree AV block also may be associated with regurgitation of the mitral or tricuspid valves, damage to the His-Purkinje tissues, inflammation of the AV node and bundle of His, or damage to the fetal myocardium, all leading to congestive cardiomyopathy (Strasburger, 2000; Tulzer, 2000).

Treatment

Treatment of second- and third-degree AV block is essentially the same. If the woman has high anti-SSA/Ro or anti-SSB/La titers, use of steroids that cross the placenta (dexamethasone or betamethasone) may improve fetal cardiac function or prevent further manifestations of

Figure 11-7 Fetal Tracing: Third-Degree Atrioventricular Block (Ultrasound and Tocodynamometer)

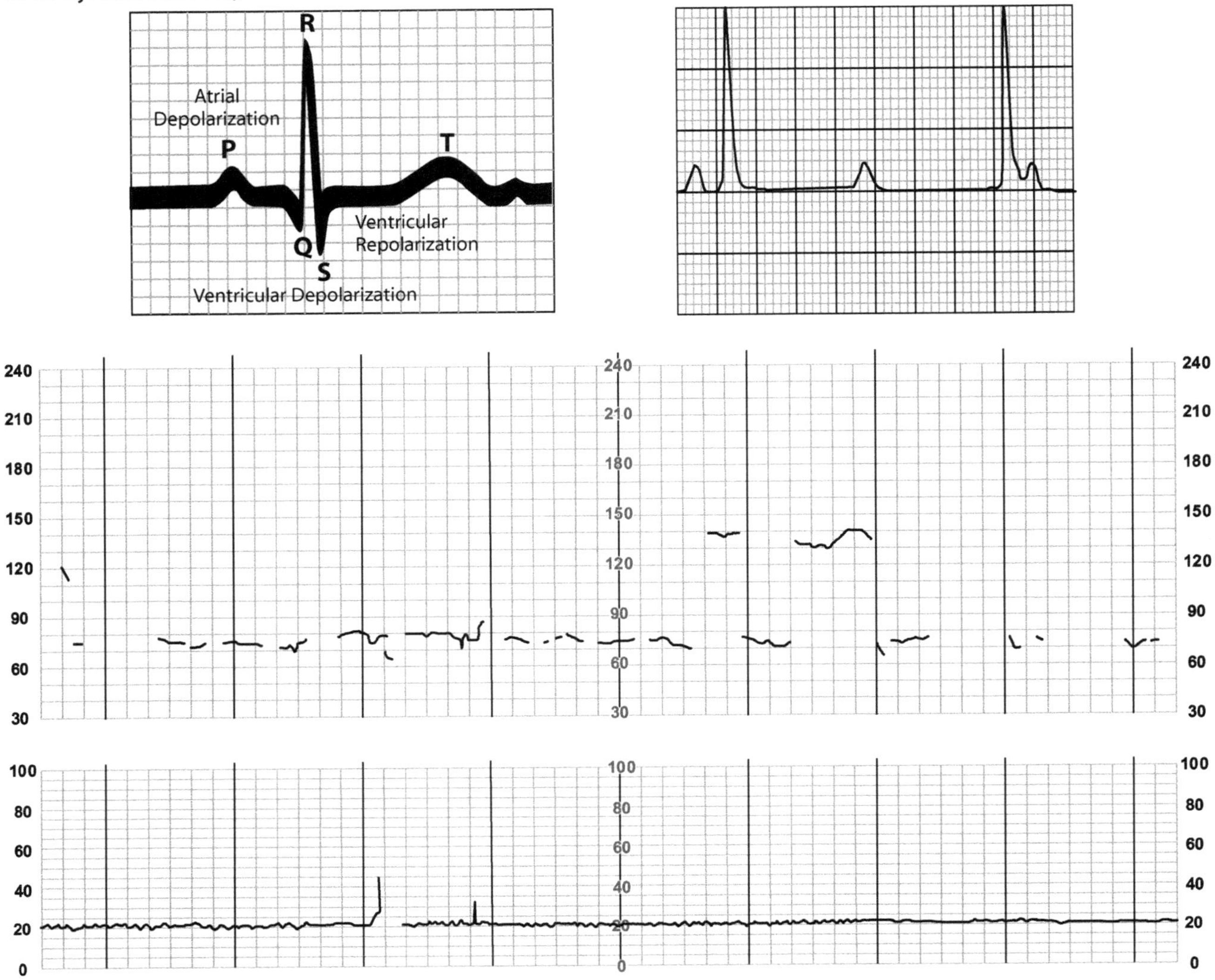

the disease process, such as cardiomyopathy (Jaeggi & Friedburg, 2008; Jaeggi et al., 2004; Strasburger et al., 2007). Steroids are withheld if there is a specific contraindication for their use (Jaeggi & Nii, 2005; Kleinman & Nehgme, 2004). Steroid-induced oligohydramnios has been reported and, as a result, close monitoring of amniotic fluid levels is recommended (Hutter, Silverman, & Jaeggi, 2010; Jaeggi & Friedburg, 2008). If oligohydramnios occurs, the dosage of the steroid should then be titrated downward. Other therapies are directed toward increasing the FHR with a beta-sympathomimetic such as terbutaline or salbutamol (Bianchi et al., 2010; Jaeggi et al., 2004; Jaeggi & Friedburg, 2008). There has been some reported success using dexamethasone and adding a beta-stimulant if the FHR remains below 55 bpm (Hutter et al., 2010; Jaeggi & Friedburg, 2008). Other therapies, such as maternal administration of immunoglobulin or early pacing of the fetus *in utero*, are not recommended because no successful outcomes have been achieved to date (Hutter et al., 2010; Kleinman et al., 2004).

Hydropic fetuses are more difficult to manage. Overall the prognosis is not favorable, and current treatment modalities have not improved outcomes for these fetuses (Fesslova et al., 2009; Kleinman & Nehgme, 2004; Rasiah et al., 2011). In a case report by Matsubara et al. (2008), hydrops was diagnosed in a fetus experiencing complete heart block, with a ventricular rate below 55 bpm. After ritodrine administration for 12 days, the hydrops resolved, though amniotic fluid volume and fetal growth were adversely affected. As a result, the infant was delivered and treatment continued postnatally, including medication and pacemaker insertion. Factors such as a baseline FHR above 55 bpm, absence of structural defects, and absence of hydrops improve the prognosis (Jaeggi & Nii, 2005; Strasburger, 2005).

After birth, fetal epicardial or endocardial leads can be placed temporarily to pace the heart (Feslova et al., 2009; Larmay & Strasburger, 2004). Following temporary pacing, permanent pacemaker implantation should be investigated. Permanent pacemaker implantation is usually required in neonates with structural cardiac disease and in approximately 50% of women with isolated AV block. The recommended criteria for pacemaker application in neonates with isolated block include (1) symptomatic fetus or neonate, (2) resting heart rate less than 50–55 bpm, and (3) presence of wide complex escape rhythms (Larmay & Strasburger, 2004; Strasburger et al., 2007).

LESS COMMON FETAL ARRHYTHMIAS

Other types of fetal arrhythmias are occasionally seen. Rhythm disturbances are classified based on their origin and are referred to as atrial, supraventricular, atrioventricular, or ventricular arrhythmias. An irregular pattern or "skipped beats" may be observed with ultrasonography or a fetoscope. The underlying causes, fetal responses, and sequelae vary according to the specific type of arrhythmia. The fetal rhythm disturbances that clinicians are most likely to see (SVT and AV blocks, also known as junctional rhythms) have been discussed. This section covers other atrial and ventricular fetal arrhythmias sometimes seen in clinical practice.

Atrial Arrhythmias

Premature atrial contractions (PACs), atrial flutter, and atrial fibrillation originate from an atrial pacemaker other than the SA node and demonstrate changes in electrical activity on the fetal ECG.

Premature Atrial Contractions

Premature atrial contractions (PACs; Figure 11-8) may be associated with redundancy or an aneurysm of the flap covering the foramen ovale; maternal caffeine, nicotine, or alcohol use; or maternal hyperthyroidism (Larmay & Strasburger, 2004; Sklansky, 2009; Strasburger, 2000; Strasburger et al., 2007). Most often seen in the third trimester, PACs are characterized by an early atrial contraction (Api & Carvalho, 2008). They exhibit a premature P wave and may be followed by a normal QRS complex (see Figure 11-8). PACs can be either conducted or nonconducted. They are said to be conducted if the impulse is carried down the conduction system, producing a subsequent ventricular contraction. Nonconducted PACs occur with the discharge of an ectopic atrial focus that is too premature to move through the AV node. Because it partially penetrates the AV junction, the premature depolarization is followed by a pause (called a compensatory pause) until the AV node recovers sufficiently to conduct the next sinus node-initiated impulse (Strasburger, 2000) (see Figure 11-8).

PACs also can occur in patterns described by the frequency of PAC occurrence. *Bigeminy* occurs when premature atrial contractions alternate with normal sinus beats. The pattern will be one normal beat (normal P-QRS relationship) followed by one premature beat or PAC (Kleinman & Nehgme, 2004). *Trigeminy* occurs when there is a premature atrial contraction every third beat. The pattern will be two normal beats (normal P-QRS relationship) and one premature beat or PAC. In either case, the fetal tracing will show vertical spikes with upward and downward strokes. The upward stroke represents the PAC, and the downward stroke represents the compensatory pause. The baseline FHR will be seen intermittently between these upward and downward strokes. Treatment, if needed, is geared toward the avoidance of caffeine products and beta-sympathomimetics (Larmay & Strasburger, 2004; Strasburger et al., 2007). Most resolve spontaneously (Api & Carvalho, 2008; Srinivasin & Strasburger, 2008).

Figure 11-8 Fetal Tracing: Premature Atrial Contractions (Fetal Scalp Electrode and Tocodynamometer)

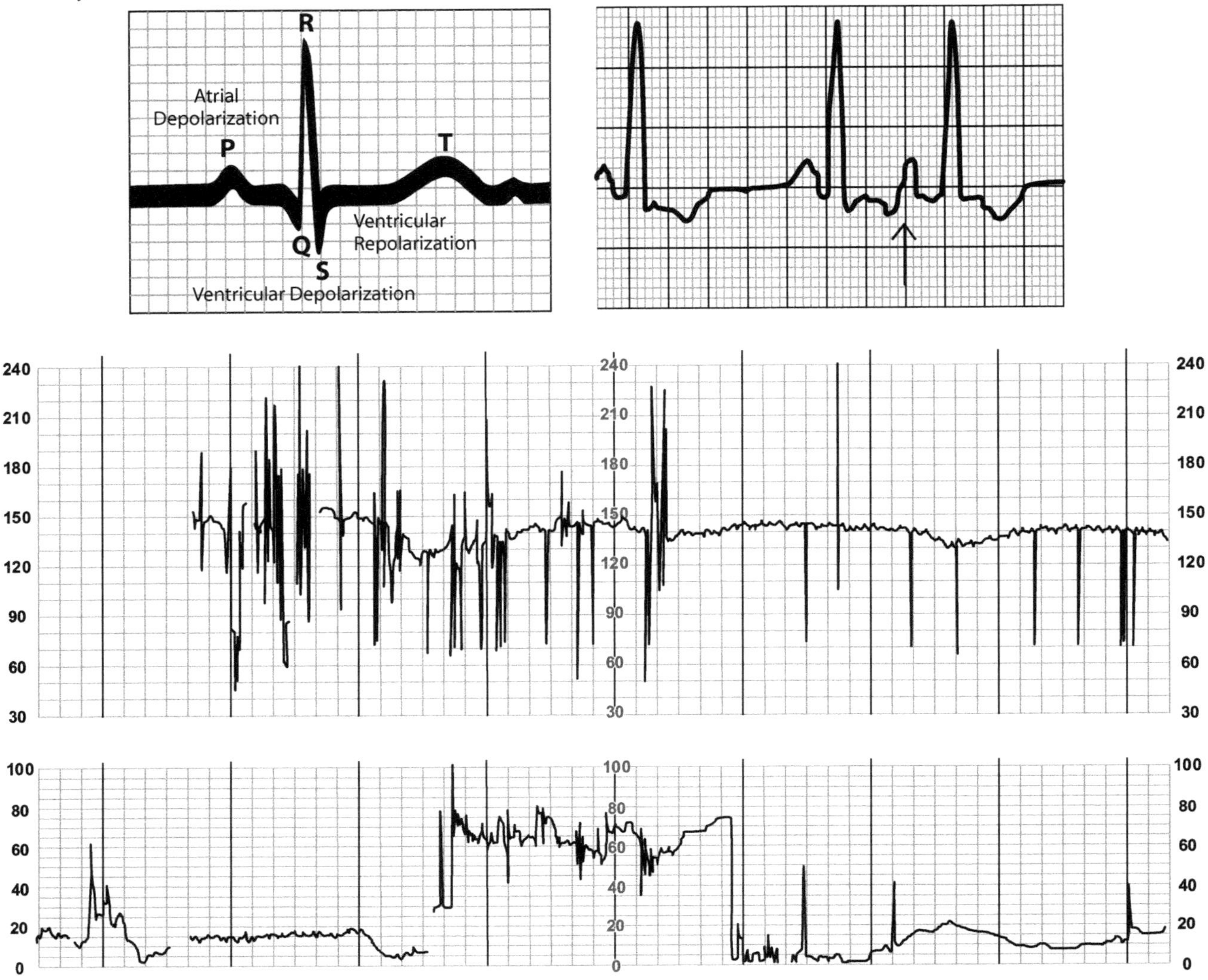

Atrial Flutter

There is a strong association between atrial flutter and SVT because atrial flutter is also due to the reentry of impulses around a circular pathway (Api & Carvalho, 2008; Strasburger, 2005). However, instead of involving the AV node as seen with SVT, the reentrant pathway in atrial flutter is found within the atrial wall. The ECG reading will usually display regularly recurring saw toothed atrial activity instead of the normal P wave. Atrial rates can approach 300–500 bpm in the fetus and 300–360 bpm in the neonate (Kleinman & Nehgme, 2004; Strasburger et al., 2007; Srinivasin & Strasburger, 2008). Because of the significantly increased atrial rate, the AV node slows or blocks some of these impulses, resulting in varying ventricular rates between 100 and 300 bpm (Kleinman et al., 2004; Larmay & Strasburger, 2004; Sklansky, 2009). In addition, the fetal tracing may show half counting of the FHR, as with SVT (Figure 11-9). This arrhythmia may be due to atrial dilatation, as occurs with some atrial structural defects, including deformity of the tricuspid valve; mitral regurgitation; atrial septal defects; hypoplastic left heart; chromosomal abnormalities; cardiomyopathy; or reentrant SVT (Kleinman et al., 2004; Larmay & Strasburger, 2004; Strasburger et al., 2007).

Figure 11-9 Fetal Tracing: Atrial Flutter (Ultrasound and Tocodynamometer)

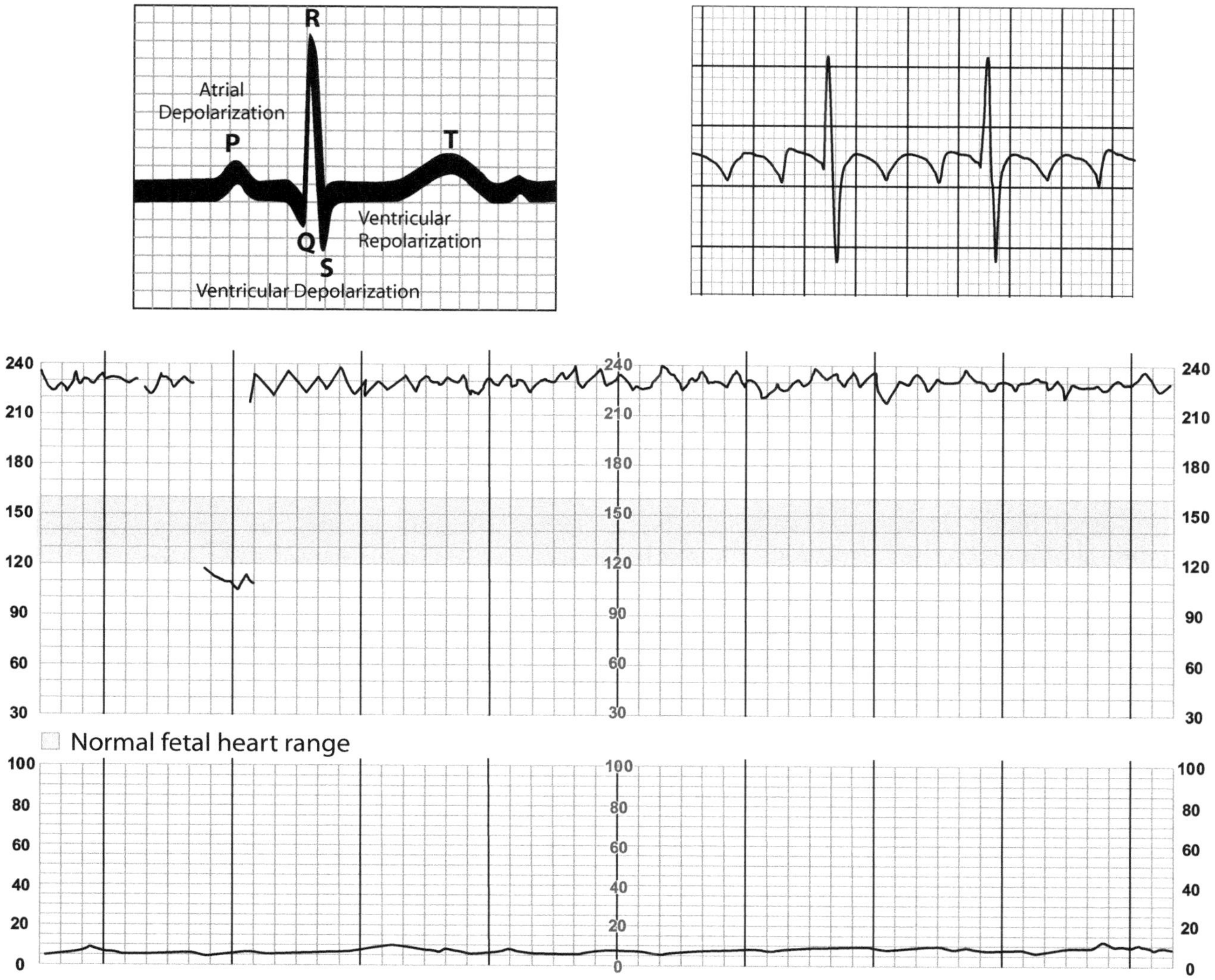

Atrial Fibrillation

Atrial fibrillation occurs even less frequently than atrial flutter (Kleinman & Nehgme, 2004; Strasburger, 2000). Atrial fibrillation may be associated with fetomaternal hemorrhage, Wolff-Parkinson-White (WPW) syndrome, or cardiac structural abnormalities, with the latter contributing most often to the high mortality rate. As with atrial flutter, many of these impulses are blocked at the AV node, resulting in ventricular rates that vary from 60–200 bpm. The ECG will often show low-amplitude irregular atrial activity with QRS complexes of various sizes.

Treatment of Atrial Flutter and Fibrillation

With atrial arrhythmias, as with SVT, the administration of digoxin or flecainide is used initially in the antepartum period to control ventricular response of the fetal heart (Api & Strasburger, 2008; Kleinman & Nehgme, 2004). After an adequate ventricular response is accomplished with digoxin, it is maintained (Kleinman & Nehgme, 2004). If digoxin is not effective in converting the arrhythmia, Class I medications such as procainamide slow the flutter rate, favoring AV node conduction (Joglar & Page, 2001; Kleinman & Nehgme, 2004; Tanel & Rhodes, 2001). Class III medications such as sotalol or amiodarone can also be used to convert atrial flutter (Api & Carvalho, 2008; Kleinman & Nehgme, 2004; Larmay & Strasburger, 2004; Strasburger, 2005). Although amiodarone has a long half-life, it has been associated with fetal cretinism and, as a result, is often not recommended (Schmolling et al., 2000; Vautier-Rit et al., 2000; Vlagsma, Hallensleben, & Meijboom, 2001). Some studies have suggested that sotalol should be the first-line agent for fetuses with atrial flutter (Api & Carvalho, 2008). Verapamil is not recommended because it relies on an immature myocardium to allow for passage of calcium to the fetal heart (Joglar & Page, 2001; Kleinman et al., 2004).

Treatment for atrial fibrillation is similar to that for atrial flutter. However, because of the difficulty in converting this pattern to a normal sinus rhythm using digoxin alone, other more potent cardiac medications, as noted previously, may be needed in place of digoxin.

Premature Ventricular Contractions

Not as common as PACs, premature ventricular contractions (PVCs) are caused by stimulation of an ectopic ventricular focus, producing ventricular contractions that are independent of those originating in the atrium. There may be a compensatory pause after the PVC, during which time the ventricles will not respond to stimuli originating from the SA node. On the ECG, the PVC will be displayed as a bizarre, wide QRS complex without a P wave. The T wave can be in a direction opposite that of the QRS complex (Figure 11-10). The fetal monitor tracing will show a vertical spike with each PVC. Similar to PACs, PVCs can occur as *bigeminy* (occurring every second beat), *trigeminy* (occurring every third beat), or at random intervals. The fetal heart baseline may be obscured if the PVCs are occurring frequently (see Figure 11-10).

Fetal PVCs are rare (Srinivasin & Strasburger, 2008). They can be caused by cardiac anomalies; fetal hydrops; cardiomyopathies; myocarditis; digitalis toxicity; and maternal use of caffeine, nicotine, alcohol, or cocaine. In rare instances, hyperkalemia caused by maternal hyperemesis may also produce fetal PVCs (Kleinman & Nehgme, 2004; Larmay & Strasburger, 2004; Strasburger et al., 2007). As with PACs, most are benign and resolve spontaneously.

CONSEQUENCES OF FETAL ARRHYTHMIAS

Fetal arrhythmias affect fetuses along a continuum from no apparent effect to the development of dilated cardiomyopathy, fetal hydrops, and progression to fetal death. The prognosis depends on a variety of factors, including the associated pathology, the type of arrhythmia, the FHR (because this determines cardiac output), how quickly the arrhythmia is diagnosed, and fetal response to treatment. Presence or absence of fetal hydrops is often the determining factor when considering treatment options.

"Cardiomyopathy" is a broad term that can be subdivided into specific categories, including dilated cardiomyopathy, which is characterized by ventricular dilation and impaired contractility (Fujioka & Kitaura, 2001; Sivasankaran, Sharland, & Simpson, 2005). Dilated cardiomyopathy can be due to infectious agents, such as rubella, coxsackie B, cytomegalovirus, parvovirus, herpes, and toxoplasmosis, or may be associated with heart block, SVT, or PVCs (Api & Carvalho, 2008; Jaeggi & Nii, 2005; Strasburger, 2000; Srinivasin & Strasburger, 2008). Therapies include specific antibiotics and antiviral, fetal administration of IVIG and/or administration of corticosteroids (Pedra et al., 2002).

Cardiomyopathy also may result from complications of pregnancy such as twin-twin transfusion. In this syndrome, there are vascular anastomoses between the placentas, producing an unbalanced transfusion of blood from the donor twin to the recipient (Harkness & Crombleholme, 2005; Huber & Hecher, 2004; Jain & Fisk, 2004). One twin becomes hypervolemic while the other twin becomes hypovolemic. The hypervolemic twin manifests with fluid overload, polyuria, polyhydramnios, hypertension, myocardial hypertrophy, and hemorrhagic infarctions in the kidneys. The hypovolemic twin manifests with growth restriction, decreased renal perfusion, oliguria, oligohydramnios, and

Figure 11-10 Fetal Tracing: Premature Ventricular Contractions (Fetal Scalp Electrode and Tocodynamometer)

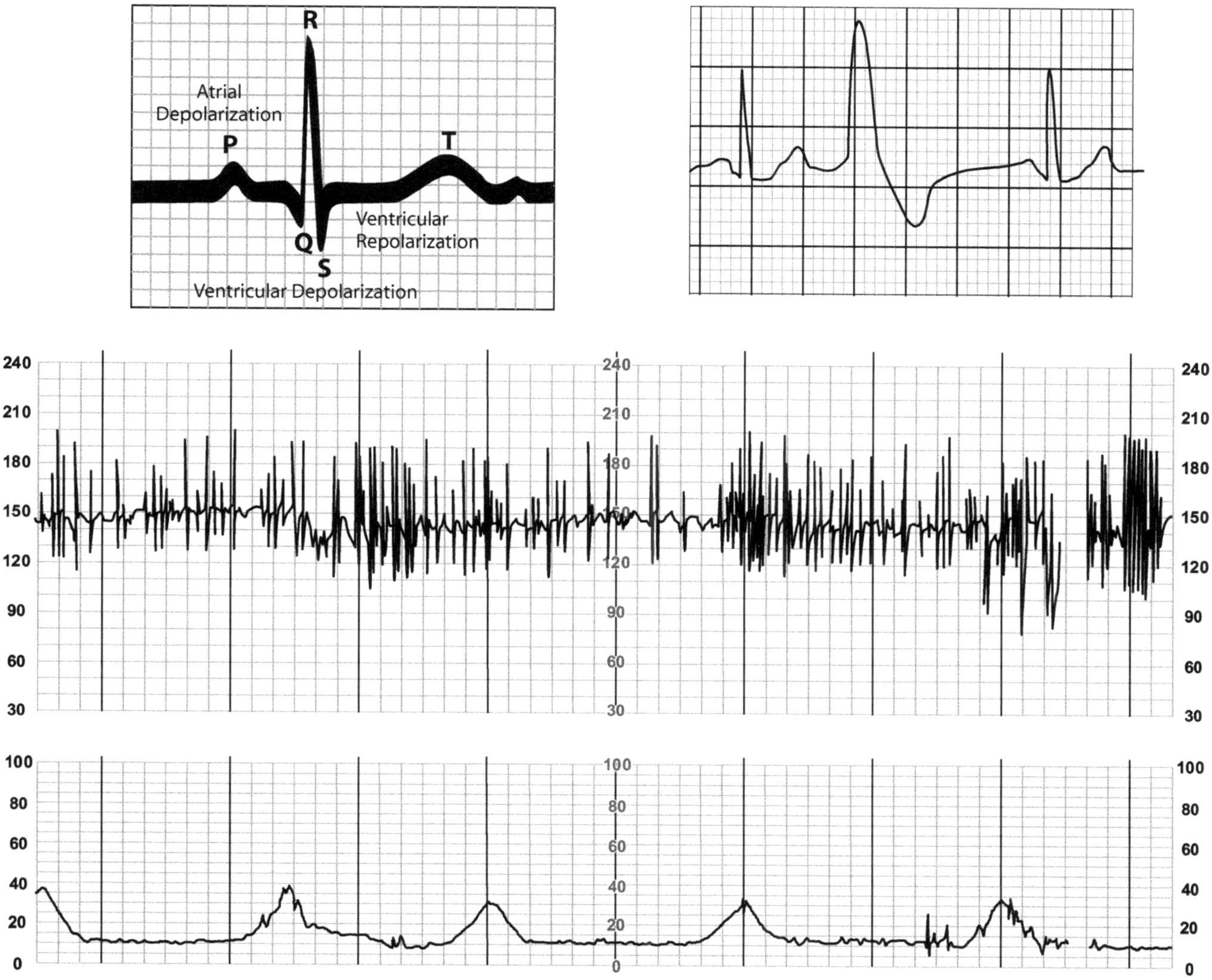

renal hypoperfusion (Harkness & Crombleholme, 2005; Huber & Hecher, 2004; Jain & Fisk, 2004). Both twins may develop cardiomyopathy and/or congestive heart failure and die *in utero* if untreated (Harkness & Crombleholme, 2005; Jain & Fisk, 2004; Pedra et al., 2002).

Fetal hydrops is defined as edema in two or more fetal compartments (anasarca) such as the abdomen, scalp, skin, liver, and spleen. Pericardial and/or pleural effusion may also occur; it is the manifestation of fetal congestive heart failure (Api & Carvalho, 2008; Kleinman & Nehgme, 2004; Strasburger, 2000; Srinivasin & Strasburger, 2008). It is hypothesized that the development of fetal hydrops is related to alterations in the pressures within the heart. Normally, the pressures in the right atrium are greater than those found in the left atrium, one of the factors responsible for maintaining a patent foramen ovale. With some arrhythmias—specifically SVT, atrial flutter, and AV blocks—the pressure in the left atrium is increased. This produces an increased back pressure, resulting in increased pressure in the right atrium, and eventually in the venous system. Increased venous pressures cause interstitial fluid accumulation, producing edema and effusion. To complicate the situation, hepatic synthesis of albumin may be compromised as a result of the decreased hepatic circulation, further contributing to edema formation (Kleinman & Nehgme, 2004; Srinivasin & Strasburger, 2008). As a result of increased venous pressure, there is a secondary increase in aldosterone, renin, norepinephrine, and angiotensin I; this produces vasoconstriction, further worsening the edema (Hamdan & Cassady, 2006).

Fetal death is related to the severity of the edema and associated conditions such as cardiac anomalies. Most cases report a 60–90% mortality, although there have been improvements in these figures in some recent reports (Hamdan & Cassady, 2006; Rasiah et al., 2011). With SVT, fetal mortality can range between 8% and 30%, with the presence of hydrops adversely affecting the outcome (Rasiah et al., 2011). These numbers do not tell the entire story, however. To save the fetus' life, birth may be the only option. In these cases, the difficulties associated with premature birth must be overcome. In general, the earlier the hydrops occurs in gestation, the poorer the prognosis (Hamdan & Cassady, 2006).

TREATMENT ISSUES

Treatment of fetal arrhythmias is a complex process that depends on the type of pattern, gestational age of the fetus, status of the mother, and the presence of indicators of fetal decompensation (Strasburger, 2000). It requires a multidisciplinary team approach, an accurate diagnosis, and an individualized treatment plan for both the woman and her fetus.

Studies have indicated that most referrals for fetal heart irregularities are due to irregularities or "skipped beats." Many have resolved spontaneously prior to diagnosis. In those that have not resolved, a definitive diagnosis should be obtained (Kleinman & Nehgme, 2004; Rasiah et al., 2011; Srinivasin & Strasburger, 2008). After the diagnosis and the risk-benefit analysis to both mother and fetus are determined, medical treatment can be initiated.

Regardless of the situation, parents should be offered pretreatment counseling. Discussion of treatment options requires openness and cultural sensitivity on the part of the medical and nursing team. Options may range from conservative management, to *in utero* treatment, to pregnancy termination, or to planned preterm birth. Table 11-2 describes a selection of treatment recommendations. For example, in cases of SVT or atrial flutter, there is much support for a conservative management scheme in which cases of intermittent fetal tachycardia without evidence of fetal hemodynamic compromise are observed closely, possibly avoiding the need for potentially dangerous pharmacotherapy (Api & Carvalho, 2008; Jaeggi & Nii, 2005; Larmay & Strasburger, 2004; Strasburger, 2000).

If needed, medications that have the longest record of safety should be considered as the first-line agents for treating arrhythmic patterns (Joglar & Page, 2001). The risks inherent in antiarrhythmic therapy depend largely on the electrophysiologic mechanisms of the rhythm disturbance and the pattern observed. Use of antiarrhythmic agents also requires knowledge of pharmacology, underlying electrophysiologic mechanisms, and the electrophysiologic and hemodynamic effect of the agents. Treatment for tachyarrhythmias can be difficult and is often associated with significant morbidity and mortality. None of the antiarrhythmic agents is without significant risk to the fetus, the woman, or both, and all have a variety of side effects, including the possibility of producing an arrhythmia in the mother (Kleinman & Nehgme, 2004; Rasiah et al., 2011). The half-life of these medications also must be considered when they are changed or a combined regimen of antiarrhythmic agents is used. Fetal excretion is primarily placental or renal. If the medication metabolites are excreted in the urine, reingestion must be considered (Kleinman & Nehgme, 2004).

Individual responses of the woman and her fetus to each agent should be observed during treatment. The decision to treat fetal arrhythmias should be based on an understanding of the natural history and precise mechanism of the rhythm disturbances as well as the pharmacology of the specific antiarrhythmic agent. It cannot be predicated simply on the basis of presence of arrhythmia or on the frequency of episodes of fetal tachycardia (Kleinman & Nehgme, 2004).

Antiarrhythmic therapy should be initiated on an inpatient basis with close observation of both mother and fetus, including external fetal heart monitoring for 12–24 hours (Kleinman & Nehgme, 2004; Larmay & Strasburger, 2004; Strasburger, 2000). Trending FHR patterns may provide additional information regarding changing patterns over the course of time, medication dosages and effectiveness, resolution of hydrops (if present), and other interventions utilized

TABLE 11-2 Medication Therapy

MEDICATION	INDICATED USE	RECOMMENDED MATERNAL DOSAGE (TRANSPLACENTAL ADMINISTRATION)*	SIDE EFFECTS	EFFECTIVENESS
*If information available for direct fetal administration, this is indicated in Recommended Maternal Dosage column (in bold)				
Adenosine (Class IV, FDA Class C)	Supraventricular arrhythmias	**IV: 100–200 mcg/kg of EFW via rapid IV bolus into umbilical vein; fetal therapy via maternal IV not recommended** PO: Not available	Bronchospasm (with asthmatic women); dyspnea; transient arrhythmias (bradycardia) after cardioversion; known to ↑ AV block	Assists in identifying SVT (reentrant in nature); does not prevent recurrent SVT (Jaeggi & Nii, 2005; Kleinman et al., 2004).
Amiodarone (Class III, FDA Class D)	Supraventricular arrhythmias; ventricular arrhythmias	IV: 5 mg/kg over 20 min; 500–1000 mg over 24 hr, then oral administration PO: Loading dose: 1200–1600 mg divided in two doses for 7–14 days; then 400–800 mg every day for 1–3 wk Maintenance: 200–800 mg/day (Kleinman & Nehgme, 2004; Strasburger, 2000) 1200 mg/day for 4–6 days with maintenance oral dose of 600–900 mg/day (Api & Carvalho, 2008). **Direct fetal dose: 2.5–5 mg/kg estimated fetal weight, into umbilical vein, given over 10 minutes to avoid severe bradycardia and cardiac arrest (Api & Carvalho, 2008)**	Can ↑ digoxin level; maternal–fetal hypo- or hyperthyroidism; corneal microdeposits; prematurity; low birth weight, congenital malformations; photosensitivity; life-threatening pulmonary alveolitis (not found to be dose related); hepatitis; myopathy; neuropath; nausea; rash; alopecia; tremors; insomnia; nightmares; fetal cretinism; hypotension	Considered "last resort" drug; not recommended for use unless adequate doses of other antiarrhythmic drugs are unsuccessful or not tolerated; adverse reactions require discontinuation in about 20% of women; can be found in breast milk for several weeks after administration (Kleinman et al., 2004). Poor transplacental transfer though serum levels constantly increase due to long half-life causing gradual increase in fetal compartment (Api & Carvalho, 2008).

(continued)

TABLE 11-2 (Continued)

MEDICATION	INDICATED USE	RECOMMENDED MATERNAL DOSAGE (TRANSPLACENTAL ADMINISTRATION)*	SIDE EFFECTS	EFFECTIVENESS
*If information available for direct fetal administration, this is indicated in Recommended Maternal Dosage column (in bold)				
Digoxin (Glycoside, FDA Class C)	Supraventricular arrhythmias; atrial fibrillation (AF) rate control	IV: 1000–1500 mcg/24 hr (loading only) Maintenance: 0.250–1.0 mg/day PO, two to three divided doses (Api & Carvalho, 2008; Kleinman & Nehgme, 2004; Kleinman et al., 2004). **Direct fetal dose: 70 μg in 3–4 divided doses IM over 24 hours (Weiner & Thompson, 1988)**	Toxicity = arrhythmias; nausea and vomiting; anorexia; diarrhea; malaise; fatigue; confusion; facial pain; insomnia; depression; vertigo and colored vision may occur at low serum levels, especially if hypokalemia or hypomagnesemia is present; interacts with other antiarrhythmic agents such as quinidine, verapamil, amiodarone, and propafenone; can also interact with erythromycin; give lower dosage if woman is in renal failure	Contraindicated in ventricular arrhythmias/WPW syndrome; may not be as effective in hydropic fetuses due to poor absorption; requires frequent ECG monitoring to assess toxicity (Kleinman & Nehgme, 2004). Target maternal plasma levels: 2.0–2.5 ng/ml (Api & Carvalho, 2008).
Disopyramide (Class I-A, FDA Class C)	Supraventricular arrhythmias; ventricular tachyarrhythmias	PO: Loading dose: 300 mg Maintenance: 100–200 mg q6h	Hypotension; negative inotropic effect; torsades de pointes; induction of uterine contractions; vagolytic effects; zero interaction with digoxin; interacts with Class III cardiac agents	Rarely used in children; very limited experience in fetuses; other alternatives are available; may stimulate uterine. contractions (Briggs, Freeman, & Yaffe, 2011; Kleinman et al., 2004; Vautier-Rit et al., 2000).
Flecainide (Class I-C, FDA Class C)	Supraventricular arrhythmias; ventricular tachyarrhythmias	IV: Not available in United States PO: 100–400 mg/day in divided doses twice a day (Api & Carvalho, 2008; Briggs et al., 2011; Kleinman et al., 2004)	Narrow therapeutic range; lightheadedness, visual disturbances, nausea; may cause arrhythmias, interacts with many antiarrhythmics	Probably safe with structurally normal hearts (Briggs et al., 2011; Kleinman et al., 2004). Target maternal plasma levels: 200–1000 ng/ml (Api & Carvalho, 2008).
Phenytoin (Class I-B, FDA Class D)	Ventricular arrhythmias; arrhythmias due to digoxin toxicity (Briggs et al., 2011)	IV: Not available in United States PO: 100–400 mg twice a day	Hypotension; vertigo; lethargy; dysarthria; mental retardation; gingivitis; macrocytic anemia; lupus; pulmonary infiltrates; growth restriction; fetal hydantoin syndrome	Prolonged QT interval syndrome; better alternative therapies are available; caution advised with breastfeeding (Joglar & Page, 2001).

(continued)

MEDICATION	INDICATED USE	RECOMMENDED MATERNAL DOSAGE (TRANSPLACENTAL ADMINISTRATION)*	SIDE EFFECTS	EFFECTIVENESS
*If information available for direct fetal administration, this is indicated in Recommended Maternal Dosage column (in bold)				
Procainamide (Class I-A, FDA Class C)	Supraventricular arrhythmias; ventricular tachyarrhythmias	IV: 100 mg bolus over 2 min, up to 25 mg/min to 1 g over first hour Maintenance: 2–6 mg/min PO: 1 g; then up to 500 mg q3h (Kleinman et al., 2004; Strasburger et al., 2007) IV: 600 mg over 20 min PO: 3000–6000 mg/day divided q6h (Strasburger, 2000)	Hypotension with IV; limit oral use to 3–6 months (in women with lupus), gastrointestinal symptoms; agranulocytosis; interacts with Class III cardiac drugs, causing torsades de pointes; fetal levels may exceed maternal	Long record of safety; oral dose frequency requirement may result in noncompliance (Briggs et al, 2011); rarely effective; frequency of dosing limits and side effects limit compliance (Kleinman et al., 2004).
Propafenone (Class I-C, FDA Class C)	Supraventricular arrhythmias; ventricular arrhythmias	IV: Not available in United States PO: 150–300 mg three times a day	Increases digoxin level; prolongs QRS complex; negative inotropic effects; proarrhythmias; gastrointestinal side effects common; avoid in women with coronary artery disease or ventricular dysfunction	Effective in treating arrhythmias associated with WPW syndrome, ventricular premature complexes, and nonsustained ventricular tachycardia (Joglar & Page, 2001); used to treat refractory ventricular tachycardia (Briggs et al., 2011).
Propranolol (Class II, FDA Class C/D)	Supraventricular arrhythmias; ventricular tachyarrhythmias	IV: 1–6 mg slowly PO: 40–160 mg q6h (Kleinman et al., 2004) 80–320 mg/24 hr, divided q6–8h (Strasburger, 2000)	Bronchospasm; central nervous system depression; heart block/↓ inotropic effect; may blunt hypoglycemia in women with diabetes; may affect glucose tolerance in women with non-insulin-dependent diabetes; maternal hypotension; contraindicated in sick sinus syndrome and Raynaud's disease; may cause neonatal respiratory depression, apnea, hypoglycemia, or bradycardia	Has been successful in suppressing ectopy in fetuses with reentrant SVT (especially if recurrent) (Briggs et al., 2011; Kleinman & Nehgme, 2004); may depress respirations or cause hypoglycemia in neonate; possibly associated with low birth weight (Kleinman & Nehgme, 2004).

(continued)

TABLE 11-2 (Continued)

MEDICATION	INDICATED USE	RECOMMENDED MATERNAL DOSAGE (TRANSPLACENTAL ADMINISTRATION)*	SIDE EFFECTS	EFFECTIVENESS
*If information available for direct fetal administration, this is indicated in Recommended Maternal Dosage column (in bold)				
Quinidine (Class I-A, FDA Class C)	Supraventricular arrhythmias; ventricular arrhythmias	PO: 200–300 mg q6h; 300–600 mg q8–12h if sustained dosage used	Hypotension; gastrointestinal effects; torsades de pointes; ↑ digoxin levels; monitor QRS/QTc intervals; maternal/neonatal thrombocytopenia; idiosyncratic reactions (angioedema/vascular collapse) may occur more commonly; eighth nerve toxicity (Briggs et al., 2011; Joglar & Page, 2001)	Does ↑ mortality; can result in increase in existing atrial arrhythmias/ ventricular tachycardia resulting in sudden death (Joglar & Page, 2001).
Sotalol (Class III, FDA Class B/D)	Supraventricular arrhythmias; ventricular tachyarrhythmias; atrial tachycardias	IV: Not available in United States PO: 80–320 mg twice a day (Kleinman & Nehgme, 2004) 40–180 mg twice a day (Strasburger, 2000) 80–160 mg twice a day (Api & Carvalho, 2008)	Monitor QT interval with ECG and electrolyte levels is recommended (Api & Carvalho, 2008). Torsades de pointes with hypokalemia; negative inotropic effect; sinus bradycardia; AV block; arrhythmias more common in renal failure, in females (Kleinman & Nehgme, 2004). Fetal death, neurologic sequelae (Briggs et al., 2011).	More successful experience with atrial flutter than with SVT (Kleinman & Nehgme, 2004). Placental transfer almost complete (maternal plasma levels = fetal levels (Api & Carvalho, 2008; Oudijk et al., 2003).
Verapamil (Class IV, FDA Class C)	Supraventricular arrhythmias	IV: 5–10 mg over 30–60 sec PO: 80–160 mg three times a day	Calcium channel blocker; negative inotropic agent; ↑ serum digoxin levels; ↓ SA and AV node function; maternal hypotension; contraindicated in sick sinus syndrome with magnesium sulfate therapy, second- or third-degree heart block, shock, congestive heart failure, and with concomitant beta-blocker therapy; fetal bradycardia; heart block; may cause ventricular fibrillation if given to woman in ventricular tachycardia; fatigue, headache, dizziness, skin rash, peripheral edema	IV use for treatment of SVT with cardiac failure is contraindicated in neonates; exercise caution, if used at all, in fetuses (Kleinman & Nehgme, 2004).

(Strasburger, 2005). Continuous maternal ECG monitoring also is indicated, and some clinicians recommend daily 12-lead ECGs (Kleinman & Nehgme, 2004; Strasburger, 2000).

Antiarrhythmic agents are classified according to their predominant effects on cardiac activity. The classes of antiarrhythmic agents are Class IA, IB, IC, II, III, and IV (Table 11-3). For example, Class I agents block the voltage-sensitive sodium channels in the same manner as anesthetics. Class I agents generally cause a decrease in excitability and conduction velocity within the heart and are subdivided into three groups according to their effect on the duration of the action potential. Class II agents, the beta-blocking agents, attenuate adrenergic activity and indirectly block fast sodium channels. Class III agents block potassium channels, prolonging repolarization. Class IV agents block the calcium channels, slowing conduction through the SA and AV nodes (Quintana & Sinert, 2006). Table 11-2 lists the antiarrhythmic medications that may be used to treat fetal arrhythmias.

Women previously taking medications with proarrhythmic effects—that is, medications that can change a normal sinus rhythm pattern to arrhythmic patterns, such as beta-adrenergic sympathomimetics—should discontinue such medications, if possible. Regardless of the pattern, all neonates will need care using a multidisciplinary team approach involving obstetric, pediatric and adult cardiology, and neonatology personnel until a definitive diagnosis can be established.

PROGNOSIS

The prognosis of a fetus with an arrhythmia depends on a variety of issues, including the associated pathology, the type of pattern, the presence or absence of hydrops, the FHR, and the adequacy of prescribed treatment, including medications. Identifying these variables will help guide the multidisciplinary team to an individualized care plan for both the woman and her fetus. Neonates with arrhythmias should be evaluated by means of a 12-lead ECG to assess ventricular function, especially preexcitation as seen in WPW syndrome, or for junctional reciprocating tachycardia. Should ectopy be found, an echocardiogram is indicated to rule out

TABLE 11-3 Classification of Antidysrhythmic Medications

CLASSIFICATION	MECHANISM OF ACTION	COMMENT
IA	Beta-adrenoreceptor blocker	Blocks cells that are discharging at abnormally high rates (slows phase 0 depolarization)
IB	Na^+ channel blocker	Blocks cells that are depolarizing or firing rapidly shortening repolarization (shortens phase 3 repolarization)
IC	Na^+ channel blocker	Markedly slows conduction in all cardiac tissue (markedly slows phase 0 depolarization)
II	Beta-adrenoreceptor blocker	Depresses automaticity, prolongs AV conduction, and decreases heart rate and contractility; used to treat supraventricular arrhythmias caused by increased sympathetic nervous system activity; also used for atrial flutter, atrial fibrillation, and AV node reentrant tachycardia (suppresses phase 4 depolarization)
III	K^+ channel blocker	Blocks potassium channels diminishing outward potassium current during repolarization (prolongs phase 3 repolarization)
IV	Ca^{2+} channel blocker	Blocks open or inactivated calcium channels, slowing phase 4 spontaneous depolarization and slowing conduction in tissues dependent on calcium current, that is, AV node (shortens action potential)

Joglar & Page (2001); Quintana & Sinert (2006).

cardiac structural defects. Neonates with controlled SVT are usually given prophylactic treatment for 6–12 months (Larmay & Strasburger, 2004). Neonates with atrial flutter alone and no evidence of WPW syndrome usually require short-term prophylaxis of less than 3–6 months if not cardioverted soon after birth (Strasburger, 2000). The prognosis for full-term neonates is excellent; prematurity complicated with hydrops contributes to neonatal morbidity and mortality (Strasburger, 2000).

A fetus with documented complete AV block should be delivered at a tertiary care center where emergency cardiac pacing can be achieved quickly if needed (Strasburger, 2000). For a fetus with isolated complete AV block complicated by hydrops fetalis, a heart rate below 50 bpm, and a mother with a negative maternal anti-SSA antibody status, the prognosis is very poor (Jaeggi et al., 2004). The same is true for fetuses with complete AV block that is associated with structural cardiac disease (Sharland, 2001) or cardiomyopathy (Jaeggi et al., 2004).

SUMMARY

Fetal arrhythmias are encountered fairly regularly in the clinical care of pregnant women. When a rhythm abnormality is identified by either electronic monitoring or auscultation, the clinician should communicate the presence of an irregular rhythm to appropriate personnel and document the information appropriately. Multidisciplinary involvement is typically needed after an arrhythmia is recognized. Clinicians caring for these women should possess knowledge of maternal–fetal physiology, fetal cardiac anatomy and physiology, pathophysiology of the arrhythmic patterns, assessment technology, treatment modalities, and prognoses appropriate to her or his education, training, and clinical responsibility. This information will allow the clinician to assess the tracing and participate in the multidisciplinary team that develops a comprehensive individualized care plan and to guide or assist with the interventions necessary to obtain the best outcome possible for the fetus/neonate and the family.

REFERENCES

American Heart Association (2012). *Cardiovascular conditions: What is an arrhythmia?* Retrieved from http://www.heart.org/idc/groups/heart-public/@wcm/@hcm/documents/downloadable/ucm_300290.pdf

Api, O., & Carvalho, J. S. (2008). Fetal dysrhythmias. *Best Practice and Research Clinical Obstetrics and Gynaecology, 22*(1), 31–48.

Bianchi, D., Crombleholme, T., D'Alton, M., & Malone, F. (2010). *Fetology: Diagnosis and management of the fetal patient* (2nd ed.). Philadelphia, PA: McGraw-Hill.

Blackburn, S. (2012). *Maternal, fetal, and neonatal physiology: A clinical perspective* (4th ed.). St. Louis, MO: Saunders.

Briggs, G. G., Freeman, R. K., & Yaffe, S. J. (2011). *Drugs in pregnancy and lactation: A reference guide to fetal and neonatal risk* (9th ed.). Philadelphia, PA: Lippincott Williams & Wilkins.

Cabaniss, M. L., & Ross, M. G. (2010). *Fetal monitoring interpretation* (2nd ed.). Philadelphia, PA: Lippincott Williams & Wilkins.

Carvalho, J. S., Prefumo, F., Ciardelli, V., Sairam, S., Bhide, A., & Shinebourne, E. A. (2007). Evaluation of fetal arrhythmias from simultaneous pulsed wave Doppler in pulmonary artery and vein. *Heart, 93*(11), 1448–1453.

Comani, S., Liberati, M., Mantini, D., Gabriele, E., Brisinda, D., Di Luzio, S., . . . Romani, G. L. (2004). Characterization of fetal arrhythmias by means of fetal magnetocardiography in three cases of difficult ultrasonographic imaging. *Pacing and Clinical Electrophysiology, 27*(12), 1647–1655.

Fesslova, V., Vignati, G., Brucato, A., De Sanctis, M., Butera, G., Pisoni, M. P., . . . Meroni, P. L. (2009). The impact of treatment of the fetus by maternal therapy on the fetal and postnatal outcomes for fetuses diagnosed with isolated complete atrioventricular block. *Cardiology in the Young, 19*(3), 282–290. doi:10.1017/S1047951109004053

Fujioka, S., & Kitaura, Y. (2001). Coxsackie B virus infection in idiopathic dilated cardiomyopathy: Clinical and pharmacological implications. *BioDrugs, 15*(12), 791–799.

Hamdan, A. H., & Cassady, G. (2006). *Pediatric hydropsfetalis.* Retrieved from http://www.emedicine.com/ped/topic1042.htm

Harkness, U. F., & Crombleholme, T. M. (2005). Twin–twin transfusion syndrome: Where do we go from here? *Seminars in Perinatology, 29*(5), 296–304.

Huber, A., & Hecher, K. (2004). How can we diagnose and manage twin-twin transfusion syndrome? *Best Practice and Research Clinical Obstetrics & Gynaecology, 18*(4), 543–556.

Hutter, D., Silverman, E. D., & Jaeggi, E. T. (2010). The benefits of transplacental treatment of isolated congenital complete heart block associated with maternal anti-Ro/SSA antibodies: A review. *Scandinavian Journal of Immunology, 72*(3), 235–241. doi:10.1111/j.1365-3083.2010.02440.x

Jaeggi, E. T., & Friedberg, M. K. (2008). Diagnosis and management of fetal bradyarrhythmias. *Pacing and Clinical Electrophysiology, 31*(1, Suppl. 1), S50–S53. doi:10.1111/j.1540-8159.2008.00957.x

Jaeggi, E., Laskin, C., Hamilton, R., Kingdom, J., & Silverman, E. (2010). The importance of the level of maternal anti-Ro/SSA antibodies as a prognostic marker of the development of cardiac neonatal lupus erythematosus a propspective study of 186 antibody-exposed fetuses and infants. *Journal of the American College of Cardiology, 55*(24), 2778–2784. doi:10.1016/j.jacc.2010.02.042

Jaeggi, E. T., & Nii, M. (2005). Fetal brady- and tachyarrhythmias: New and accepted diagnostic and treatment methods. *Seminars in Fetal and Neonatal Medicine, 10*(6), 504–514.

Jain, V., & Fisk, N. M. (2004). The twin-twin transfusion syndrome. *Clinical Obstetrics and Gynecology, 47*(1), 181–202.

Joglar, J. A., & Page, R. L. (2001). Antiarrhythmic drugs in pregnancy. *Current Opinion in Cardiology, 16*(1), 40–45.

Kleinman, C. S., & Nehgme, R. A. (2004). Cardiac arrhythmias in the human fetus. *Pediatric Cardiology, 25*(3), 234–251.

Kumar, S., & O'Brien, A. (2004). Recent developments in fetal medicine. *British Medical Journal, 328*(7446), 1002–1006.

Larmay, H. J., & Strasburger, J. F. (2004). Differential diagnosis and management of the fetus and newborn with an irregular or abnormal heart rate. *Pediatric Clinics of North America, 51*(4),1033–1050.

Macones, G. A., Hankins, G. D. V., Spong, C. Y., Hauth, J., & Moore, T.. (2008). The 2008 National Institute of Child Health and Human Development workshop report on electronic fetal monitoring: Update on definitions, interpretation, and research guidelines. *Obstetrics and Gynecology, 112*(3), 661–666, doi:10.1097/AOG.0b013e3181841395; *Journal of Obstetric, Gynecologic and Neonatal Nurses, 37*(5), 510–515. doi:10.1111/j.1552-6909.2008.00284.x

Maeno, Y., Hirose, A., Kanbe, T., & Hori, D. (2009). Fetal arrhythmia: Prenatal diagnosis and perinatal management. *Journal of Obstetrics and Gynaecology Research, 35*(4),623–629.doi:10.1111/j.1447-0756.2009.01080.x

Matsubara, S., Morimatsu, Y., Shiraishi, H., Kuwata, T., Ohkuchi, A., Izumi, A., . . . Suzuki, M. (2008). Fetus with heart failure due to congenital atrioventricular block treated by maternally administered ritodrine. *Archives of Gynecology and Obstetrics, 278*(1), 85–88.

Menihan, C. A., & Kopel, E. (2008). *Electronic fetal monitoring: Concepts and applications* (2nd ed.). Philadelphia, PA: Lippincott Williams & Wilkins.

Moore, K. L., Persaud, T. V. N., & Torchia, M. G. (2013). *The developing human: Clinically oriented embryology* (9th ed.). Philadelphia, PA: Saunders.

Oudijk, M. A., Ruskamp, J. M., Ambachtsheer, B. E., Ververs, T. F., Stoutenbeek, P., Visser, G. H., & Meijboom, E. J. (2002). Drug treatment of fetal tachycardias. *Paediatric Drugs, 4*(1), 49–63.

Oudijk, M. A., Ruskamp, J. M., Ververs, F. F., Ambachtsheer, E. B., Stoutenbeek, P., Visser, G. H., & Meijboom, E. J. (2003). Treatment of fetal tachycardia with sotalol: Transplacental pharmacokinetics and pharmacodynamics. *Journal of the American College of Cardiology, 42*(4), 765–770.

Pedra, S. R., Smallhorn, J. F., Ryan, G., Chitayat, D., Taylor, G. P., Khan, R., . . . Hornberger, L. K. (2002). Fetal cardiomyopathies: Pathogenic mechanisms, hemodynamic findings and clinical outcomes. *Circulation, 106*, 585–591.

Pickoff, A. S. (2011). Developmental electrophysiology in the fetus and neonate. In R. A Polin, W. W. Fox, & S. H. Abman (Eds.), *Fetal and neonatal physiology* (4th ed., pp. 733–756). Philadelphia, PA: Elsevier.

Quintana, E. C., & Sinert, R. (2006). *Antidysrhythmic toxicity.* Retrieved from: http://www.emedicine.com/emerg/topic45.htm

Rasiah, S. V., Ewer, A. K., Miller, P., & Kilby, M. D. (2011). Prenatal diagnosis, management and outcome of fetal dysrhythmia: A teriary fetal medicine centre experience over an eight-year period. *Fetal Diagnosis and Therapy, 30*(2), 122–127. doi: 10.1159/000325464

Schmolling, J., Renke, K., Richter, O., Pfeiffer, K., Schlebusch, H., & Holler, T. (2000). Digoxin, flecainide, and amiodarone transfer across the placenta and the effects of an elevated umbilical venous pressure on the transfer rate. *Therapeutic Drug Monitor, 22*(5), 582–588.

Seferović, P. M., Ristić, A. D., Maksimović, R., Simeunović, D. S., Ristic, G. G., Radovanovic, G., . . . Matucci-Cerinic, M. (2006). Cardiac arrhythmias and conduction disturbances in autoimmune rheumatic diseases. *Rheumatology, 45*(Suppl. 4), iv39–iv42.

Sharland, G. (2001). Fetal cardiology. *Seminars in Neonatology, 6*(1), 3–15.

Simpson, K. R. (2008). Fetal assessment during labor. In K. R. Simpson & P. A. Creehan (Eds.), *Perinatal nursing* (3rd ed., pp. 399–442). Philadelphia, PA: Lippincott Williams and Wilkins.

Sivasankaran, S., Sharland, G. K., & Simpson, J. M. (2005). Dilated cardiomyopathy presenting during fetal life. *Cardiology in the Young, 15*(4), 409–416.

Sklansky, M. (2009). Fetal cardiac malformations and arrhythmias: Detection, diagnosis, management and prognosis. In R. K. Creasy, R. Resnik, J. D. Iams, C. J. Lockwwod, & T. R. Moore (Eds.), *Creasy & Resnik's maternal–fetal medicine: Principles and practice* (6th ed., pp.305–346). Philadelphia, PA: Saunders.

Snarr, B. S., Wessels, A., & McQuinn, T. C. (2011). Cardiovascular development. In R. A Polin, W. W. Fox, & S. H. Abman (Eds.), *Fetal and neonatal physiology* (4th ed., pp.696–703). Philadelphia, PA: Elsevier.

Sonesson, S. E. (2010). Diagnosing foetal atrioventricular heart blocks. *Scandinavian Journal of Immunology,* 72(3), 205–212. doi:10.1111/j.1365-3083.2010.02434.x

Srinivasin, S., & Strasburger, J. (2008). Overview of fetal arrhythmias. *Current Opinion in Pediatrics, 20*(5), 522–531. doi:10.1097/MOP.0b013e32830f93ec

Strasburger, J. F. (2000). Fetal arrhythmias. *Progress in Pediatric Cardiology, 11*(1), 1–17.

Strasburger, J. F. (2005). Prenatal diagnosis of fetal arrhythmias. *Clinics in Perinatology, 32*(4), 891–912, vii.

Strasburger, J. F., Cheulkar, B., & Wichman, H. J. (2007). Perinatal arrhythmias: Diagnosis and management. *Clinics in Perinatology, 34*(4), 627–652, vii–viii.

Suri, V., Keepanaseril, A., Aggarwal, N., & Vijayvergiya, R. (2009). Prenatal management with digoxin and sotalol combination for fetal supraventricular tachycardia: Case report and review of literature. *Indian Journal of Medical Science, 65*(9), 411–414. doi:10.4103/0019-5359.56117

Tanel, R. E., & Rhodes, L. A. (2001). Fetal and neonatal arrhythmias. *Clinics in Perinatology, 28*(1), 187–207, vii.

Trines, J., & Hornberger, L. K. (2004). Evolution of heart disease in utero. *Pediatric Cardiology,* 25(3), 287–298.

Tulzer, G. (2000). Fetal cardiology. *Current Opinion in Pediatrics, 12*(5), 492–496.

Vautier-Rit, S., Dufour, P., Vaksmann, G., Subtil, D., Vaast, P., Valat, A. S., . . . Puech, F. (2000). Fetal arrhythmias: Diagnosis, prognosis, treatment, apropos of 33 cases. *Gynecologic and Obstetric Fertility, 28*(10), 729–737.

Vlagsma, R., Hallensleben, E., & Meijboom, E. J. (2001). Supraventricular tachycardia and premature atrial contractions in fetus. *Nederlands Tijdschrift Voor Geneeskunde, 145*(7), 295–299.

Weiner, C. P., & Thompson, M. I. (1988). Direct treatment of fetal super ventricular tachycardia after failed transplacental therapy. *American Journal of Obstetrics and Gynecology, 158(3,* Pt. 1), 570–573.

Wren, C. (2006). Cardiac arrhythmias in the fetus and newborn. *Seminars in Fetal and Neonatal Medicine, 11*(3), 182–190.

Glossary of Key Terms

Abrupt—Timing from onset to nadir or peak of FHR change is <30 seconds. Refers to characteristics of periodic or episodic FHR changes.

Acceleration—Abrupt transitory increase in the fetal heart rate from the baseline rate; associated with sympathetic nervous stimulation. When using EFM to assess FHR data in the term fetus, an acceleration is a visually apparent abrupt increase in FHR peaking at least 15 beats per minute above the FHR baseline, lasting at least 15 seconds from onset to return to baseline. In the fetus under 32 completed weeks' gestation, an acceleration increases at least 10 beats per minute above baseline and lasts at least 10 seconds from onset to return to baseline.

Acidemia—Abnormal excess hydrogen ion concentration in the blood due to accumulation of acid or consumption of base.

Acidosis—Abnormal excess hydrogen ion concentration in tissues due to accumulation of acid or consumption of base.

Adrenergic response—Activated by, characteristic of, or secreting epinephrine or substances with similar activity. The term is applied to nerve fibers transmitting norepinephrine at a synapse when a nerve impulse passes (i.e., sympathetic fibers).

Aerobic metabolism—Growing, living, or occurring in the presence of oxygen; requiring oxygen for respiration. Specifically, the chemical process of using oxygen to produce energy from carbohydrates (sugars). This process is also called aerobic respiration, oxidative metabolism, and cellular respiration.

Alkalosis—Abnormal deficit of hydrogen ion in the tissues, resulting in an increase in pH value (decreased hydrogen ion concentration) above normal.

Amnioinfusion—Instillation of fluid into the uterus through an intrauterine catheter. Used to increase amniotic fluid volume in situations of oligohydramnios or umbilical cord compression with associated variable decelerations.

Amniotic Fluid Index (AFI)—Amount of amniotic fluid measured by ultrasonography in centimeters. AFI is expressed as the sum of the measurements of the deepest amniotic fluid pocket in all four abdominal quadrants. AFV has replaced the use of AFI.

Amniotic Fluid Volume (AFV)—Amount of amniotic fluid in the single deepest vertical pocket measured by ultrasonography in centimeters. Used to evaluate uteroplacental function and olgiohydramnios. A pocket greater than 2 cm is considered evidence of adequate amniotic fluid; less than 2 cm should prompt further evaluation. AFV is the preferred measure compared with AFI based on clinical trial results, thus ACOG currently recommends using AFV.

Amplitude—Distance between high and low points of the FHR tracing oscillations. Describes the range of variation in fetal heart rate changes from peak to trough.

Anaerobic metabolism—Chemical processes of energy production from carbohydrates that take place in the absence of oxygen.

Antenatal—Before birth; used synonymously with prenatal.

Antepartum—Period of pregnancy occurring before labor or childbirth.

Antiarrhythmic therapy—Medication regimens used to treat fetal arrhythmias.

Arrhythmia—Any deviation from a normal heart rate; a heart rate without rhythm. Describes FHRs that are too fast (>160 bpm), too slow (<110 bpm), sporadic, or irregular. An arrhythmia may be associated with disordered impulse formation, disordered impulse conduction, or a combination of both. The term is sometimes used interchangeably with dysrhythmia.

Artifact—Inaccurate variation or absence of FHR on the fetal monitor tracing due to mechanical or technical limitations or electrical interference of the monitoring system.

Aspartate aminotransferase (AST)—Enzyme that contributes to protein metabolism. This enzyme is present in the liver and is important in the biosynthesis of amino acids as it catalyzes the reversible transfer of an amino group between glutamic and aspartic acid. The former term was SGOT (serum glutamic-oxaloacetic transaminase). When cell damage occurs, especially in the liver (as seen with severe preeclampsia, HELLP syndrome, or trauma), AST is released into the tissues and bloodstream and AST levels are increased.

Atrial fibrillation—Tachycardiac atrial FHR is rarely identified in the fetus. Often accompanied by a variable degree of AV block that will cause the ventricular rate to vary from 60 to 200 bpm.

Atrial flutter—Extremely rapid tachyarrythmia resulting from reentrant electrical conduction. The atrial rate may range from 300–500 bpm in the fetus and

300–360 bpm in the neonate. The AV node slows or blocks transmission of some of the atrial electrical impulses, resulting in a variable ventricular response. The ventricular rate usually ranges from 190 to 240 bpm. The relationship between atrial and ventricular impulses may be fixed (2:1 or 3:1 AV block) and regular, or variable and irregular (e.g., varying degrees of AV block).

Atrioventricular (AV) arrhythmias—Arrythmias resulting from a defect in the AV junction that disrupts or changes conduction of impulses through the AV node. AV arrhythmias consist of second- and third-degree AV block.

Auscultation—Auditory assessment made by listening for sounds within the body, such as fetal heart sounds. Fetal heart sounds are auscultated to determine rate and rhythm. Technically, "true" auscultation of fetal heart sounds is performed with a fetoscope or stethoscope (e.g., Pinard), but this term also includes the use of a hand-held Doppler ultrasound device to assess the FHR through detection of heart motion by ultrasound.

Autocorrelation—Computerized comparison of consecutive points of waveforms generated by an electronic fetal monitor. Comparison is based on ultrasound waves reflected from the moving fetal heart valves. Current EFM terminology and practices assume the use of this technology in generating EFM data.

Automaticity—Inherent ability of cardiac muscle cells to depolarize spontaneously. Exhibited most strongly by the SA node, the AV node, the bundle of His, and the Purkinje fibers, but can be expressed by any cardiac muscle cell.

Baroreceptors—Pressure-sensitive stretch receptors in carotid sinus and aortic arch that detect changes in blood pressure. Stimulation of fetal baroreceptors alters the FHR by stimulating the autonomic nervous system to increase or decrease the FHR via the sympathetic or parasympathetic branch.

Base deficit—Measures the amount of base buffer reserves below normal levels. A large positive base deficit (e.g., >12 mEq/liter) indicates that base buffers have been used to buffer acids, that sufficient base reserves are not present, and that metabolic acidosis is present.

Base excess—Measures the amount of base buffer reserves above normal levels. A large negative base excess [e.g.,< −12 mEq/liter (−13, −14, etc.)] indicates that base buffers have been used to buffer acids, that sufficient base reserves are not present, and that metabolic acidosis is present.

Baseline fetal heart rate—Approximate mean FHR rounded to increments of 5 beats per minute (bpm) during a 10-minute period, excluding accelerations and decelerations and periods of marked FHR variability (more than 25 bpm). There must be at least 2 minutes of identifiable baseline segments (not necessarily contiguous) in any 10-minute period, or the baseline for that period is indeterminate.

Baseline fetal heart rate variability—Fluctuations in the baseline FHR that are irregular in amplitude and frequency. The fluctuations are visually quantitated as the amplitude of the peak-to-trough in bpm. Variability is a characteristic of the baseline: it is determined in a 10-minute period excluding accelerations and decelerations, and quantified as **absent** (visually undetectable), **minimal** (visually detectable but ≤5 bpm), **moderate** (6–25 bpm), or **marked** (>25 bpm).

Beta-adrenergic receptors—Cellular binding sites sensitive to epinephrine and norepinephrine. Myometrial smooth muscle beta-2 receptors are highly sensitive to epinephrine and have a high affinity to bind with terbutaline.

Betamimetic drugs—Medications that mimic stimulation of the sympathetic nervous system. Specifically in myometrial cells they have a relaxant or depressant effect on uterine contractility. (Sometimes referred to as sympathomimetic or betasympathomimetic.)

Biophysical Profile (BPP)—Antenatal assessment of fetal well-being that combines NST results with multiple physiologic parameters observed with real-time ultrasound. The BPP includes the assessment of five parameters: fetal breathing movement, gross body movement, fetal tone, amniotic fluid volume, and fetal heart rate reactivity (NST).

Bishop score—Method for determining cervical readiness for induction of labor by scoring five components: cervical dilation, effacement, consistency, position, and station of the presenting part. Higher scores (≥6) are associated with successful induction of labor.

Bradyarrhythmia—Slow heart rate rhythm usually occurring when FHR is below 90 beats per minute (e.g., sinus bradycardia or heart block).

Bradycardia—Baseline FHR below 110 beats per minute for a period of 10 minutes or more.

Cardiotocography—Monitoring of the fetal heart rate and uterine activity during labor and birth. Also referred to as cardiotokography.

Category I FHR patterns—FHR tracings demonstrating normal baseline rate, moderate variability, and the absence of late or variable decelerations. Accelerations and early decelerations may or may not be present. Tracings with these features are strongly predictive of normal fetal acid-base status at the time of observation.

Catgory II FHR patterns—Tracings that cannot be classified as either category I or category III patterns. These tracings are not predictive of abnormal acid-base status, but there is not enough evidence to classify them in category I or III.

Category III FHR patterns—Tracings exhibiting a sinusoidal pattern or exhibiting absent variability in conjunction with bradycardia or recurrent late or variable decelerations. These tracings are predictive of abnormal fetal acid-base status at the time of observation.

Chain of authority—Definition of the lines of authority and responsibility for clinical problem resolution within an organization. Describes the persons to contact and the order in which to contact them when differences of opinion about clinical management of patients cannot be resolved directly between providers.

Chemoreceptor—Sensory nerve endings or cells stimulated by increased or decreased blood concentrations of a chemical substance. Sensitive to change in oxygen, carbon dioxide, and pH levels in the blood. Chemoreceptors are located in the aortic and carotid bodies and in the medulla.

Compensatory response to hypoxemia—Describes the ability of the fetus to adjust to low blood oxygen levels by drawing on fetal reserves and mobilizing physiologic responses to maintain central oxygenation. The presence of moderate variability implies adequate physiologic compensation and fetal reserves.

Competence validation—Process of documenting the verification of an individual's knowledge and skills according to predetermined criteria.

Computer analysis (CA)—Use of artificial intelligence (AI) to objectively analyze FHR signals according to predetermined algorithms. CA can also alert care providers, interpret patterns, and offer management options.

Conductivity—Capacity of the cardiac cells to conduct a current through the cells.

Conflict management—Process of managing professional disagreements through effective interpersonal communication and/or within the mechanisms of institutional policies, procedures, and protocols. May involve implementing the chain of command or authority.

Contraction Stress Test (CST)—Assessment of the FHR response to uterine activity typically conducted in the antenatal period. A CST may be assessed when there are at least three contractions of at least 40 seconds' duration in 10 minutes. Contractions may be spontaneous, induced by oxytocin administration, or induced with endogenous oxytocin via nipple or breast stimulation. The presence of late decelerations in response to these contractions (a positive CST) may be an indicator of fetal compromise.

Deceleration—Transitory decrease in the FHR from the baseline rate.

Digyzotic—Pertaining to or derived from two separate zygotes (fertilized ova), as in twin gestation occurring from two fertilized ova. Results in fraternal twins.

Doppler—Instrument that emits ultrasound waves and receives a return signal. In the context of FHR monitoring, a Doppler usually refers to a hand-held ultrasound device used to detect the FHR. It converts the sound waves reflected from the motion of the heart valves into a fetal heart rate.

Doppler velocimetry—Use of specialized ultrasonography to measure the blood flow velocity in the uterine artery, umbilical arteries, and fetal middle cerebral artery. Also referred to as Doppler flow.

Early deceleration—Early decelerations are visually apparent gradual decreases in the FHR. The onset, nadir, and recovery of early decelerations generally occur coincident with the onset, peak, and recovery of uterine contractions. Early decelerations are typically symmetrical in shape.

Electronic fetal monitoring—Auditory and visual assessment of the FHR and uterine activity with data generated by fetal monitor technology. The data generated includes an auditory FHR signal, a digital or graphic display of FHR and UA data, and a permanent record on paper or computerized storage.

Episodic changes—Accelerations or decelerations of the FHR that are not associated with uterine contractions.

Excitability—Readiness of the cardiac cells to respond to a stimulus or irritation.

External fetal monitoring—Collection and assessment of FHR and UA data using an ultrasound transducer to monitor the fetal heart rate and a tocodynamometer to monitor uterine contractions.

Extrinsic influences—Factors outside the fetus that may affect fetal oxygenation and FHR characteristics (e.g., maternal, placental, or umbilical cord factors).

False-negative—When an assessment incorrectly identifies a compromised fetus as healthy.

False-positive—When an assessment incorrectly identifies a healthy fetus as compromised.

Favorable physiologic response—FHR response predictive of a fetus that is able to respond appropriately to the environment and maintain fetal reserves.

Fetal attitude—Relationship of the fetal parts to each other, especially referring to the position of the fetal head in relation to the fetal body when the vertex is presenting. The vertex may be flexed, deflexed, or extended.

Fetal lie—Relationship of the fetal body to the maternal body. Fetal lie may be longitudinal (fetal body is parallel to maternal spine), transverse (fetal body is perpendicular to maternal spine), or oblique (fetal body is at an angle between longitudinal and transverse lie).

Fetal presentation—Lowest part of the fetus that comes out of the uterus first. Most often the presentation is vertex (occiput first), but it can also be breech (buttocks or feet first), shoulder (shoulder first), face or brow (face or brow first), or compound (hand with head or foot with buttocks).

Fetal reserve—Ability to maintain tissue oxygenation and essential physiologic function in response to decreased availability of oxygen or other physiologic stressors. This term is also used to refer to the excess amount of oxygen available to the fetus beyond that normally required for metabolism.

Fetal scalp blood sampling—Collection of small sample of blood from the fetal scalp via a capillary tube that is analyzed for pH level by a blood gas machine. An invasive method of assessing pH level of the fetus. Requires ruptured membranes and lancing the fetal scalp.

Fetal scalp stimulation—Indirect method of assessing acid-base status of the fetus by rubbing the fetal head to elicit anacceleration. Can be performed with or without ruptured membranes. Scalp stimulation is performed during a period of baseline FHR. It is not a resuscitative measure, and should not be performed during decelerations.

Fetal surveillance—Assessment of fetal well-being via indirect methods such as auscultation, electronic fetal monitoring, and antepartum testing.

Fetoscope—Stethoscope adapted for auscultation of the FHR (also known as DeLee fetoscope).

First-generation monitor—Electronic fetal monitor that uses a refractory window and peak-to-peak comparison of fetal heart waveforms generated by an external ultrasound transducer. FHR was calculated by averaging peaks. Current EFM terminology and practices assume the use of autocorrelation techniques that are not available in first-generation monitors.

Funic souffle (bruit)—Soft "blowing" sound heard on auscultation over the umbilical cord. The rate is synchronous with the FHR.

Gradual—Timing from onset to nadir or peak of FHR change is ≥30 seconds. Refers to characteristics of periodic and episodic changes in the FHR.

Heart block—Atrioventricular (AV) conduction defect in which the electrical impulses in the heart are not conducted normally from the atrium to the ventricles via AV nodes. Results in bradycardia.

Hydrops fetalis—Generalized edema in the abdomen, scalp, liver, and spleen of the fetus. Hydrops is a serious and often life-threatening condition resulting from cardiac pump failure. Hydrops may result from immune disorders such as Rh incompatibility or nonimmune causes such as cardiac malformations, cardiac arrhythmias, anemia, or twin-to-twin transfusion syndrome.

Hydrostatic pressure—Pressure exerted by a fluid in a closed system, such as pressure created by amniotic fluid in the uterus. An intrauterine pressure catheter measures hydrostatic pressure in the uterus during and between uterine contractions.

Hyperstimulation—Retired term for excessive uterine activity.

Hypoxemia—Low levels of oxygen in the blood.

Hypoxia—Low levels of oxygen in the tissue; oxygen levels inadequate to meet metabolic needs of the tissue.

Indeterminate—Not definitely or precisely determined or fixed; not leading to a definite end or result. Category II FHR patterns are indeterminate: they are not predictive of abnormal fetal acid-base status, yet there is not adequate evidence at present to classify these as category I or category III. Category II FHR tracings require evaluation and continued surveillance and reevaluation, taking into account the entire associated clinical circumstances.

Intermittent auscultation—Auditory assessment of the FHR at intervals either by fetoscope or hand-held Doppler.

Intermittent decelerations—Occur with fewer than 50% of contractions in a 20-minute period.

Internal fetal monitoring—Invasive assessment of the FHR or uterine contractions or both. A fetal spiral electrode provides auditory and visual fetal heart ECG data. An intrauterine pressure catheter provides visual intrauterine pressure measurements during and between contractions.

Intrapartum—Period of pregnancy that includes labor and birth.

Intrauterine pressure catheter (IUPC)—Catheter used to directly measure intrauterine pressure during and between uterine contractions; may be fluid filled or sensor tipped.

Intrinsic factors—Internal fetal regulatory mechanisms that control the heart rate, including the sympathetic, parasympathetic, and central nervous systems, and baroreceptor, chemoreceptor, and hormonal responses.

Kleihauer-Betke test—Blood analysis to detect the presence and relative amount of fetal hemoglobin in the maternal blood specimen. When a blood specimen is stained on a slide, cells characterized with fetal hemoglobin can be viewed and counted to determine the ratio of fetal blood cells to maternal blood cells. Used to detect and/or estimate the severity of fetal–maternal hemorrhage.

Late deceleration—Late decelerations are visually apparent gradual decreases in the FHR that are associated with uterine contractions. Late decelerations are delayed in timing, meaning the deceleration reaches its nadir (lowest point) after the peak of the contraction. In most cases the onset, nadir, and recovery of the deceleration occur after the respective onset, peak, and resolution of the contraction as well. Late decelerations are typically symmetrical in shape.

Leopold's maneuvers—Systematic method of abdominal palpation to assess fetal position, attitude, and lie.

Long-term variability—Frequency of oscillations (cycles) in the FHR over 1 minute. In current practice, FHR variability is visually assessed as a unit and no distinction is made between short-term and long-term variation in the heart rate.

Medulla oblongata—Lower portion of the brainstem; the relay center for the parasympathetic and sympathetic nervous system.

Meta-analysis—Research strategy used to analyze findings from multiple studies. The process includes defining the hypotheses, standardized terminology, independent and dependent variables, and instruments; defining key words for literature review; defining study inclusion and exclusion criteria; and performing analysis using specialized statistical techniques.

Metabolic acidosis—Decrease in blood pH due to an increase in hydrogen ion concentration, decrease in PO_2, and consumption of buffer bases (expressed as an increased base deficit or base excess). The PCO_2 may be normal.

Metabolic alkalosis—Increase in blood pH due to a decreased hydrogen ion concentration and associated with decreased PCO_2.

Mixed acidosis—Combination of metabolic and respiratory acidosis, reflected as a decrease in pH, decrease in PO_2, increase in PCO_2, and increase in base deficit or excess.

Modified biophysical profile—Antepartum test for fetal well-being consisting of an NST and an amniotic fluid volume.

Monozygotic—Pertaining to or derived from a single zygote (fertilized ovum), as in twin gestation occurring from asingle fertilized ovum. Results in identical twins.

Montevideo units—Total pressure in mmHg for all uterine contractions within a 10-minute timeframe. Calculated by measuring the peak intensity or amplitude (in mmHg) for each contraction occurring in a 10-minute period and adding the numbers together. Contraction amplitude is the difference between the resting tone and the peak of the contraction (in mmHg). It is important to note that these calculations are dependent on the accuracy of IUPC data.

Nadir—Lowest FHR value in a deceleration. With electronic monitoring, it is visually the lowest point in the deceleration curve.

Neurohormonal response—Physiologic response involving both neural and hormonal mechanisms.

Nonhypoxic reflex response—FHR response to an event not associated with decreased PO_2. Fetus quickly responds to change caused by an event (e.g., baroreceptor and vagal response affecting fetal blood pressure because of brief compression of the umbilical cord).

Nonreassuring fetal heart rate pattern—"Nonreassuring fetal status" describes the clinician's interpretation of data regarding fetal status (i.e., the clinician is not reassured by the findings). This term acknowledges the imprecision inherent in the interpretation of the data. Therefore, the diagnosis of nonreassuring fetal status can be consistent with the delivery of a vigorous neonate" (ACOG, 2005). This term is no longer recommended for interpretation of fetal heart monitoring data, but is used in multiple studies to refer to various FHR characteristics that might now be classified as category II or III patterns.

Nonstress test (NST)—Antepartum fetal assessment test used to assess fetal well-being. The FHR is monitored for two accelerations (in a term fetus, FHR increases at least 15 bpm above baseline, lasting for 15 seconds from the time the FHR leaves the baseline to the time it returns to the baseline) in 20 minutes. In a fetus under 32 weeks' gestation,accelerations are increases of at least 10 bpm for 10 seconds duration. The presence of accelerations indicates adequate fetal oxygenation.

Oxytocic—Having the effect of stimulating the uterus to contract.

Parity (P)—Number of pregnancies that have resulted in birth. The TPAL method of describing gravidity (the number of pregnancies, including the present pregnancy) refers to the number of term births (T), preterm births (P), abortions (A), and living children (L) (e.g., gravida 3, para 1102).

Parasympathetic nervous system—Part of autonomic nervous system. Includes the vagus nerve, which decreases the heart rate when stimulated.

Perinatal—Occurring during, or pertaining to, the periods before, during, or after the time of birth up to 28 days after delivery.

Periodic changes—Accelerations or decelerations of the FHR that are associated with uterine contractions.

Phonocardiography—Graphic representation of heart sounds and murmurs, and includes pulse tracings (carotid, apex, and jugular pulse).

Piezoelectric effect—Crystals in the ultrasound transducer generate sound waves that are reflected back from moving structures. A shift in frequency of the waveforms reflected is used to identify the FHR.

Postterm or postdates pregnancy—Pregnancy lasting beyond 42 completed weeks of gestation.

Premature atrial contraction (PAC)—Characterized by the early discharge of an atrial focus, as seen by a premature P wave followed by a narrow, normal-appearing QRS complex. Can be either conducted (i.e., PAC followed by a ventricular contraction, then a compensatory pause followed by normal sinus rhythm) or nonconducted (i.e., PAC followed by compensatory pause). Often followed by an incomplete compensatory pause, produced by the incomplete depolarization of the fetal heart.

Premature rupture of membranes (PROM)—Rupture of membranes that occurs after 37 completed weeks of gestation, without signs and symptoms of labor.

Premature ventricular contraction (PVC)—Premature depolarization in the heart with resultant irregularity in the heart rate and rhythm. PVCs will show no P wave, and the premature QRS is bizarre and wide, with the T wave usually directed opposite to the polarity of the QRS complex. The full compensatory pause may or may not be present.

Preterm PROM (PPROM)—Rupture of membranes that occurs prior to 37 completed weeks of gestation, without signs and symptoms of labor.

Prolonged deceleration—Prolonged decelerations are visually apparent decreases in the FHR that drop at least 15 bpm below baseline and last at least 2 minutes but less than 10 minutes from their onset to the return to baseline.

Pseudosinusoidal pattern—Sinusoidal-appearing, undulating FHR pattern of short duration that is both preceded and followed by an FHR with normal characteristics.

Psychological safety—Psychologically safe environment in which people do not fear negative repercussions such as retaliation, humiliation, or belittlement from speaking up about their ideas or concerns (Edmondson, 1999).

Pulse oximetry—Additional method of assessing the fetal status during labor with internal oxygen saturation monitor. The monitor is placed on the fetal cheek via a vaginal exam. An SpO_2 result of 30% or more is considered reassuring and means the fetus is adequately oxygenated. Also referred to as fetal pulse oximetry or fetal oxygen saturation monitoring. While used in some research settings, this technology is not in use in general clinical practice in the United States.

Reassuring—Descriptive term reflecting the clinician's conclusion that he or she can be reasonably assured of fetal well-being at the present time, based on available assessment data. This term is no longer recommended for use in describing interpretation of EFM data, but is used at times to refer to the clinician's interpretation of antepartum testing results (e.g., an 8/10 or 10/10 biophysical profile score). The term is used in multiple research reports to refer to various FHR characteristics that might now be classified as category I FHR patterns.

Recurrent decelerations—Occurring with at least 50% of the contractions in a 20-minute period.

Refractory window—Inhibitory period in which the electronic ultrasound transducer does not attempt to count the incoming signal. Mechanism in first-generation fetal monitors.

Respiratory acidosis—Decrease in pH due to increased CO_2 and carbonic acid in the blood. Base deficit or excess maybe within normal range. If pulmonary or placental exchange is increased, the amount of CO_2 in the extracellular tissue may decrease.

Respiratory alkalosis—Increase in pH due to decreased hydrogen ion concentration and a decrease in PCO_2 (often associated with hyperventilation).

Rhythm—Regularity or irregularity of the baseline FHR.

Second-generation monitor—Electronic ultrasound fetal monitor that uses multiple comparison points in the waveforms generated by the external ultrasound transducer. Rate calculated by autocorrelation. Current EFM terminology and practice assume the use of this technique in the generation of FHR data.

Short-term variability—Changes in the FHR from one beat to the next. Measures the R-to-R intervals of subsequent fetal cardiac cycles (QRS). Historically, short-term variability and long-term variability were assessed independently of each other and an internal electrode was necessary for assessment of short-term variability. In current clinical practice FHR variability is visually assessed as a unit by peak-to-trough amplitude fluctuations regardless of electronic monitoring method. No distinction is made between short- and long-term FHR variation.

Sinusoidal pattern—Visually apparent undulating smooth sine wavelike pattern in FHR baseline with a cycle frequency of 3–5 per minute, which persists for at least 20 minutes. There is an absence of accelerations and no response to uterine contractions, fetal movement, or stimulation.

Solid sensor-tipped IUPC—Intrauterine pressure catheter that has a microprocessor transducer at the catheter tip that measures the intrauterine pressure directly.

Specificity—Probability that a test will be negative when the infection or specific condition being tested for is not present.

Spiral electrode—Internal device for recording the FHR that is applied directly to the fetal presenting part and receives signals from the electrocardiac impulses of the fetal heart. Used to directly determine FHR based on changes in the R-to-R intervals in successive QRS complexes.

Strain gauge—Pressure transducer that electronically converts uterine pressure changes exerted on a diaphragm into mmHg. Component of closed pressure system using a fluid-filled intrauterine catheter.

Supraventricular arrhythmias—Rhythm disturbances that originate above the ventricles (i.e., in the atria).

Supraventricular tachycardia—Sustained, rapid, regular atrial arrhythmia resulting from reentrant electrical conduction in the atria or the establishment of an irritable ectopic focus taking on the role of pacemaker.

The rate may range from 210 to 320 bpm, but SVT rates are typically between 240 and 260 bpm. May be intermittent or sustained. Supraventricular tachycardia is often characterized by a fixed R-to-R interval with P waves preceding each QRS complex, as identified by ECG.

Sympathetic nervous system—Part of the autonomic nervous system. Stimulation results in FHR increase.

Tachycardia—Baseline FHR above 160 beats per minute for a period of 10 minutes or more.

Tachysystole—Greater than five contractions in 10 minutes, averaged over 30 minutes. Uterine activity is quantified as the number of contractions in 10 minutes over an average of 30 minutes, and tachysystole is further qualified by the presence or absence of associated FHR decelerations.

Tocodynamometer (tocotransducer)—Transducer on an electronic fetal monitor that externally detects abdominal pressure or contour changes resulting from uterine contractions and transmits this information to the monitor to be displayed in graphic form.

Tocolytic—Medication that diminishes or stops uterine activity by altering smooth muscle activity.

Tonus—Intensity of uterine tone or intrauterine pressure between uterine contractions.

Ultrasound transducer—External monitor that detects movement of the fetal heart valves opening and closing through transmission of a sound wave and Doppler shift. Monitor processor converts reflected sound waves into an electronic signal corresponding to the FHR.

Uterine bruit—Sound heard when listening to the blood flow in the maternal uterine vessels (also known as "uterinesoufflé"). Synchronous with maternal pulse.

Variable deceleration—Visually apparent, abrupt (onset to nadir <30 seconds) decrease in the FHR below baseline. The decrease is calculated from onset to the beginning of the nadir of the deceleration. The FHR decreases ≥15 bpm, lasting ≥15 sec and <2 minutes in duration. May occur with or without relationship to uterine contractions. When variable decelerations are associated with uterine contractions, their onset, depth, and duration typically vary with successive uterine contractions.

Ventricular arrhythmias—Rhythm disturbances originating from the ventricles, as a result of premature electrical discharge below the AV junction.

Vibroacoustic stimulation (VAS)—Method of assessing fetal well-being in the antepartum and intrapartum periods using sound from an artificial larynx to elicit an acceleration. May also be referred to as fetal acoustic stimulation or simply acoustic stimulation.

REFERENCES

American College of Obstetricians and Gynecologists. (2005). *Inappropriate use of the terms fetal distress and birthasphyxia* (ACOG Committee Opinion No. 326). Washington, DC: Author.

Edmondson, A. (1999). Psychological safety and learning behavior in work teams. *Administrative Science Quarterly,44*(2), 350–383.

Appendix A

PRACTICE CASE ANSWER SHEET

Case Study Exercise: ________________

1. Baseline FHR:

2. Variability

	a. Absent (undetectable)	________
	b. Minimal (>0 but ≤5 bpm)	________
	c. Moderate (6–25 bpm)	________
	d. Marked (>25 bpm)	________
	e. Unable to determine	________

3. Contractions

	Frequency:	________
	Duration:	________
	Intensity:	________
	Resting tonus:	________

4. Accelerations and decelerations. When present, circle P if periodic or E if episodic.

Accelerations	P	E
Early decelerations	P	
Variable decelerations	P	E
Late decelerations	P	
Prolonged decelerations	P	E
None present		

5. Interpretation

	Category I	________
	Category II	________
	Category III	________

6. List possible underlying physiologic mechanisms or rationales for observed patterns.

7. List in order of priority the physiologic goal(s) for observed patterns.

8. List actions and interventions indicated based on overall interpretation (physiologic based, instrumentation based, and further assessments).

Index

Note: Page numbers followed by *b* indicate boxes; *f* indicates figures; *t* indicates tables.

B

C

Q

R

S

T

Lightning Source UK Ltd.
Milton Keynes UK
UKHW050854010320
359537UK00003B/10